BRIEF
NINTH EDITION

Core
Concepts
in Health

Paul M. Insel

Walton T. Roth
Stanford University

Kirstan Price
Developmental Editor

Boston   Burr Ridge, IL   Dubuque, IA   Madison, WI   New York
San Francisco   St. Louis   Bangkok   Bogotá   Caracas   Kuala Lumpur
Lisbon   London   Madrid   Mexico City   Milan   Montreal   New Delhi
Santiago   Seoul   Singapore   Sydney   Taipei   Toronto

chap
6

102

100

McGraw-Hill Higher Education

A Division of The **McGraw-Hill** *Companies*

2 3 4 5 6 7 8 9 0 BAN/BAN 0 9 8 7 6 5 4 3 2 1

Library of Congress Cataloging-in-Publication Data

Core concepts in health/[editors] Paul M. Insel, Walton T. Roth; Kirstan Price, developmental editor—9th ed.
    p. cm.
    Includes bibliographical references and index.
    ISBN 0-7674-2558-8
    1. Health—Handbooks, manuals, etc.   I. Insel, Paul M.   II. Roth, Walton T.   III. Price, Kirstan
RA776.C83 2001
613—dc21   2001030399

Sponsoring editor, Holly Allen; developmental editors, Kirstan Price, Kathleen Engelberg, Susan Shook Malloy, Star MacKenzie, Elisa Adams; production editor, Melissa Williams; manuscript editor, Joan Pendleton; art director, Jeanne M. Schreiber; design manager, Violeta Diaz; text and cover designer, Ellen Pettengell; art editor, Robin Mouat; illustrators, Joan Carol, Emma Ghiselli, Robin Mouat, Kristin Mount, Susan Seed, John and Judy Waller, Pamela Drury Wattenmaker; photo editor, Brian Pecko; cover photograph © Cliff Riedinger/Natural Selection Stock Photography; proofreader, Julianna Scott Fein; manufacturing manager, Randy Hurst. The text was set in 10.5/12 Berkeley Book by GTS Graphics, Inc. and printed on acid-free 45# Chromatone LG by Banta Book Group.

www.mhhe.com

PHOTO CREDITS

Chapter 1 p. 1, © Rudi Von Briel/PhotoEdit; p. 9, © David Young-Wolff/PhotoEdit; p. 11, © Spencer Grant/PhotoEdit; p. 17, © Bob Collins/The Image Works; p. 18, © Kent Meireis/The Image Works

Chapter 2 p. 21, © Bob Daemmrich/Stock Boston; p. 25, © David Young-Wolff/PhotoEdit; p. 32, © Clive Bryant/PhotoEdit; p. 36, © Jim Cummins/FPG International

Chapter 3 p. 41, © Bob Daemmrich/Stock Boston; p. 43, © Gary A. Conner/PhotoEdit; p. 47, © David Young-Wolff/PhotoEdit; p. 54, © J. Pickerell/The Image Works

Chapter 4 p. 59, © Michael Schwarz/The Image Works; p. 60, © Myrleen Cate/PhotoEdit; p. 67, © David Young-Wolff/PhotoEdit; p. 72, © Laura Dwight/PhotoEdit

Chapter 5 p. 76, © Richard Hutching/PhotoEdit; p. 83, © David Young-Wolff/PhotoEdit; p. 88, © Michelle Bridwell/PhotoEdit; p. 99, © Amy Ramey/PhotoEdit

Chapter 6 p. 104, © Joel Gordon; p. 105, © Dion Ogust/The Image Works; p. 107, © Joel Gordon; p. 109, © Joel Gordon; p. 113, © Joel Gordon; p. 121L, © Andrew Holbrooke/ The Image Works; p. 121R, © A. Ramey/Stock Boston

Chapter 7 p. 130, © Bonnie Kamin; p. 132, © Myrleen Cate/PhotoEdit; p. 143, © Richard Hutchings/PhotoEdit; p. 145, © James Marshall/The Image Works

Chapter 8 p. 154, © Joel Gordon; p. 155, © David Young-Wolff/PhotoEdit; p. 173, © Joel Gordon

Chapter 9 p. 183, © N. Richmond/The Image Works; p. 185, © Joel Gordon; p. 195, © Myrleen Cate/PhotoEdit; p. 199, © Bob Daemmrich/Stock Boston

Chapter 10 p. 216, © Collins/The Image Works; p. 226, © David Davis/Photo Researchers, Inc.; p. 228, © David Madison Photography; p. 232, © David Young-Wolff/PhotoEdit

Chapter 11 p. 236, © Willie L. Hill, Jr./The Image Works; p. 243, © Richard B. Levine; p. 249, © Aaron Haupt/Photo Researchers, Inc.; p. 253, © Fred Gebhart

Chapter 12 p. 258, © Spencer Grant/PhotoEdit; p. 272, © Lawrence Migdale/Stock Boston; p. 280, © Jeff Greenberg/PhotoEdit

Chapter 13 p. 293, © Sonda Dawes/The Image Works; p. 295, © Alán Gallegos/AG Photograph; p. 315, © N. Richmond/The Image Works; p. 317, © Phillip Hayson/Photo Researchers, Inc.

Chapter 14 p. 324, © Woinarowicz/The Image Works; p. 331, © M. Greenlar/The Image Works; p. 335, © Steve Martson/The Image Works

Chapter 15 p. 346, © Bonnie Kamin; p. 350, © David K. Crow/PhotoEdit; p. 354, © Cindy Charles/PhotoEdit/PictureQuest; p. 358, © W. Hill, Jr./The Image Works

Chapter 16 p. 369, © J. Nourouk/PhotoEdit; p. 374, © Bob Daemmrich/Stock Boston; p. 379, © Jonathan Nourok/PhotoEdit; p. 386, © Bob Mahoney/The Image Works

Chapter 17 p. 391, © Tony Prettyman/PhotoEdit; p. 393, © David Young-Wolff/PhotoEdit

Preface

Now in its ninth edition, *Core Concepts in Health* has maintained its leadership in the field of health education for more than 25 years. Since we pioneered the concept of self-responsibility for personal health in 1976, hundreds of thousands of students have used our book to become active, informed participants in their own health care. Each edition of *Core Concepts* has brought improvements and refinements, but the principles underlying the book have remained the same. Our commitment to these principles has never been stronger than it is today, and it is reflected as fully in this Brief Edition as in the Ninth Edition of *Core Concepts* on which this edition is based. We have prepared the Brief Edition to accommodate instructors whose courses—sometimes carrying only one hour of credit—afford too little time for the complete range of topics and the level of detail of the larger edition.

OUR GOALS

Our goals in writing this book can be stated simply:

- To present scientifically based, accurate, up-to-date information in an accessible format.
- To involve students in taking responsibility for their health and well-being.
- To instill a sense of competence and personal power in students.

The first of these goals means making expert knowledge about health and health care available to the individual. *Core Concepts* brings scientifically based, accurate, up-to-date information to students about topics and issues that concern them—exercise, stress, nutrition, weight management, contraception, intimate relationships, HIV infection, drugs, alcohol, and a multitude of others. Current, complete, and straightforward coverage is balanced with "user-friendly" features designed to make the text appealing. Written in an engaging, easy-to-read style and presented in a colorful, open format, *Core Concepts* invites the student to read, learn, and remember. Boxes, tables, artwork, photographs, and many other features highlight areas of special interest throughout the book.

The second of our goals is to involve students in taking responsibility for their health. *Core Concepts* uses innovative pedagogy and unique interactive features to get students thinking about how the material they're reading relates to their own lives. We invite them to examine their emotions about the issues under discussion, to consider their per-

sonal values and beliefs, and to analyze their health-related behaviors. Beyond this, for students who want to change behaviors that detract from a healthy lifestyle, we offer guidelines and tools, ranging from samples of health journals and personal contracts to detailed assessments and behavior change strategies.

Perhaps our third goal in writing *Core Concepts in Health* is the most important: to instill a sense of competence and personal power in the students who read the book. Everyone has the ability to monitor, understand, and affect his or her own health. Although medical and health professionals possess impressive skills and have access to a huge body of knowledge that benefits everyone in our society, people can help to minimize the amount of professional care they actually require in their lifetime by taking care of themselves—taking charge of their health—from an early age. Our hope is that *Core Concepts* will continue to help young people make this exciting discovery—that they have the power to shape their own futures.

ORGANIZATION AND CONTENT OF THE BRIEF NINTH EDITION

The Brief Ninth Edition of *Core Concepts* focuses on the health issues and concerns of greatest importance to students. The general content of this edition remains essentially the same as the Brief Eigth Edition, with coverage of stress, psychological health, intimate relationships and communication, sexuality, substance use and abuse, nutrition, exercise, weight management, cardiovascular disease, cancer, infectious diseases, aging, and environmental health. New to the Brief Ninth Edition is Chapter 15, "Conventional and Complementary Medicine: Skills for the Health Care Consumer," which provides consumer-oriented coverage of both conventional Western medicine and widely used complementary and alternative practices. Topics include the basic premises of conventional medicine; the scientific method and the U.S. drug approvals process; guidelines for choosing a primary care physician; strategies for safe use of over-the-counter and prescription medications; general characteristics of complementary and alternative medicine (CAM); descriptions of such CAM practices as acupuncture, chiropractic, homeopathy, and herbal remedies; consumer guidelines for evaluating CAM practitioners and therapies; and health insurance options.

The ninth edition also includes a greater emphasis on the development of total wellness, with expanded coverage of spiritual wellness and the close connections between mind and body. New and updated topics include paths to spiritual wellness; global religious views on tobacco use; the effects of stress on the brain and the immune system; and the benefits of close connections with others. Chapter 4 has been expanded to include more information on the benefits of intimate relationships and additional strategies for building and maintaining healthy interpersonal relationships. Suggested journal writing activities throughout the book help students to further explore their feelings and values.

For the ninth edition, all chapters were carefully reviewed, revised, and updated. The latest information from scientific and health-related research is incorporated in the text, and newly emerging topics and issues are discussed. The following list gives a sample of some of the current concerns addressed in the ninth edition:

- Healthy People 2010 objectives
- Dietary Guidelines for Americans, 2000 Edition, and Dietary Reference Intakes
- Complementary and alternative medicine
- Causes and prevention of violence
- Ecstasy, GHB, and other "club drugs"
- West Nile virus and other emerging infections
- Emergency contraception and other new methods of contraception
- Mifepristone (RU-486)
- Dietary supplement labeling and safety issues
- Health and safety effects of cell phone use
- Implications of the Human Genome Project
- Women's health issues
- Effective communication
- Genetically modified foods, organic foods, food irradiation, food safety, and other nutrition issues
- Campus safety
- Spiritual wellness
- Carpal tunnel syndrome
- Health risks of cigars, bidis, and spit tobacco

Of course, the health field is dynamic, with new discoveries, advances, trends, and theories reported every week. Ongoing research—on the role of diet in cancer prevention, for example, or on new treatments for HIV infection—continually changes our understanding of the human body and how it works in health and disease. For this reason, no health book can claim to have the final word on every topic. Yet within these limits, *Core Concepts* does present the latest available information and scientific thinking on innumerable topics.

To help students keep up with rapidly advancing knowledge about health issues, the Brief Ninth Edition also includes coverage of a key source of up-to-date information—the Internet. Each chapter includes an annotated list of World Wide Web sites that students can use as a launching point for further exploration of important topics. Chapter 1 also includes guidelines for evaluating health information from the Web.

 Each chapter in the ninth edition is also closely tied to the Web site developed as a companion to the text. Boxes, illustrations, tables, and sections of text marked with the special new World Wide Web icon have corresponding links and activities on the *Core Concepts in Health* Online Learning Center (http://www.mhhe.com/insel9). The Web site and other online supplements are described below in greater detail.

FEATURES OF THE BRIEF NINTH EDITION

As a concise version of the ninth edition of *Core Concepts in Health,* this Brief Edition builds on the features that attracted and held our readers' interest in the previous eight editions. One of the most popular features has always been the **boxes,** which allow us to explore a wide range of current topics in greater detail than is possible in the text itself. More than one-third of the boxes are new to the ninth edition, and many others have been significantly revised or updated. The boxes are divided into six categories, each marked with a unique icon and label.

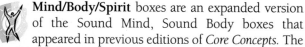 New to the ninth edition, **In the News** boxes focus on current health issues that have recently been highlighted in the media. Topics covered include the Human Genome Project, same-sex marriage and civil unions, cybersex, club drugs, genetically modified foods, cell phones and distracted driving, mifepristone (RU-486), and emerging infectious diseases. Each In the News box is accompanied by the new World Wide Web icon, indicating that the *Core Concepts* Online Learning Center has links to Internet resources students can use to learn more about the topic of the box.

Mind/Body/Spirit boxes are an expanded version of the Sound Mind, Sound Body boxes that appeared in previous editions of *Core Concepts.* The new label reflects their broader focus and greater emphasis on spiritual wellness and the close connections between people's feelings and states of mind and their physical health. Included in Mind/Body/Spirit boxes are topics such as paths to spiritual wellness, religious views of tobacco use, sexual decision making and personal values, expressive writing and chronic conditions, how exercise fosters emotional wellness, and how stress affects the brain and the immune system. These boxes emphasize that all the dimensions of wellness must be developed in order for an individual to achieve optimal health and well-being.

Take Charge boxes distill from each chapter the practical advice students need in order to apply information to their own lives. By referring to these boxes, students can easily find ways to foster friendships, for example; to become more physically active; to enhance support in their relationships; to increase the amount of whole grains in their diets; and to help a friend who has a problem with tobacco, alcohol, or other drugs or has an eating disorder.

Critical Consumer boxes emphasize the key theme of critical thinking by helping students develop and apply critical thinking skills, thereby allowing them to make sound choices related to health and well-being. Critical Consumer boxes provide specific guidelines for evaluating health news and Web sites, using food labels to make dietary choices, selecting exercise footwear, evaluating dietary supplements, and so on.

Dimensions of Diversity boxes are part of our commitment to reflect and respond to the diversity of the student population. These boxes give students the opportunity to identify any special health risks that affect them because of who they are as individuals or as members of a group. They also broaden students' perspectives by exposing them to a wide variety of viewpoints on health-related issues. The different dimensions reflected include gender, ethnicity, socioeconomic status, and age. The principles embodied by these boxes are described in Chapter 1; topics covered in later chapters include special cardiovascular disease risks for women and African Americans, exercise for people with disabilities, drug use in rural areas and links between poverty and poor environmental health.

In addition, some Dimensions of Diversity boxes highlight health issues and practices in other parts of the world, allowing students to see what Americans share with people in other societies and how they differ. Students have the opportunity to learn about attitudes toward death in other countries, the pattern of HIV infection around the world, and other topics of interest.

In Focus boxes highlight current wellness topics of particular interest. Topics include bicycle helmets, shyness, Alzheimer's disease, headaches, diabetes, and carpal tunnel syndrome.

In addition to the box program, many new and refined features are included in the ninth edition of *Core Concepts*. **Vital Statistics** tables and figures highlight important facts and figures in a memorable format that often reveals surprising contrasts and connections. From tables and figures marked with the Vital Statistics label, students can learn about drinking and drug use among college students, world population growth, trends in public opinion about abortion, leading casues of death and disability in the United States, the relationship between victims and offenders in violent crime, and a wealth of other information. For students who grasp a subject best when it is displayed graphically, numerically, or in a table, the Vital Statistics feature provides alternative ways of approaching and understanding the text. In addition, for each Vital Statistics table and figure, the *Core Concepts* Online Learning Center has links to sites where students can find the latest statistics and information.

Core Concepts features a wealth of attractive and helpful **illustrations,** more than 20 of which are new to the ninth edition. The anatomical art, which has been prepared by medical illustrators, is both visually appealing and highly informative. These illustrations help students understand such important information as how blood flows through the heart, how alcohol affects the body, and how to use a condom. New topics illustrated for the ninth edition include diabetes, types of stroke, alcohol consumption by college students, and the vegetarian food pyramid. These lively and abundant illustrations will particularly benefit those students who learn best from visual images

Many of the illustrations in the ninth edition are marked with the new CD icon, indicating that they appear in an enhanced format on *Core Concepts Interactive,* the student CD-ROM that accompanies the text. From self-guided mini-tutorials on the CD-ROM, students can learn more about the stress response, the effects of alcohol and tobacco use, physical processes of aging, immediate and long-term effects of physical activity, the greenhouse effect, and many other topics. The CD-ROM is described in more detail below.

New to the ninth edition, **Communicate!** exercises suggest strategies and activities for improving communication skills in ways that will enhance wellness. Communicate! covers all aspects of communication, from interpersonal communication and communication with oneself to mass communication, from assertive speaking to empathic listening, and from methods of persuasion to critical evaluation of public messages. These exercises appear at appropriate points throughout each chapter.

Also new to the ninth edition are chapter-ending **Tips for Today** sections. These provide a very brief distillation of the major message of each chapter, followed by suggestions for a few simple things that students can try right away. Tips for Today are designed to encourage students and to build their confidence by giving them easy steps they can take immediately to improve their wellness.

Take Action, appearing at the end of every chapter, suggests hands-on exercises and projects that students can undertake to extend and deepen their grasp of the material. Suggested projects include interviews, investigations of campus or community resources, and experimentation with some of the behavior change techniques suggested in the text. Special care has been taken to ensure that the projects are both feasible and worthwhile.

Journal Entry also appears at the end of each chapter. These entries suggest ways for students to use their Health Journal (which we recommend they keep while using *Core Concepts*) to think about topics and issues, explore their own views, and express their thoughts in written form. They are designed to help students deepen their awareness and understanding of their own health-related behaviors. (Journal Entry questions also appear on the *Core Concepts* Online Learning Center in a format that enables students to e-mail their responses to their instructors.)

Making wise choices about health requires students to sort through and evaluate health information. To help students become skilled evaluators, each chapter contains at least one **Critical Thinking Journal Entry.** These entries help students develop their critical thinking skills, including finding relevant information, separating fact from opinion, recognizing faulty reasoning, evaluating information, and assessing the credibility of sources. Critical Thinking Journal Entry questions do not have right or wrong answers; rather, they ask students to analyze, evaluate, or take a stand on a particular issue.

The **Behavior Change Strategies** that conclude many chapters offer specific behavior management/modification plans relating to the chapter's topic. Based on the principles of behavior management that are carefully explained in Chapter 1, these strategies will help students change unhealthy or counterproductive behaviors. Included are strategies for dealing with test anxiety, quitting smoking, planning a personal exercise program, phasing in a healthier diet, and many other practical plans for change.

Designed for quick reference is the **Appendix,** "Nutritional Content of Popular Items from Fast-Food Restaurants." It provides a handy guide to the nutritional content of commonly ordered items at popular fast-food restaurants. Students can use the information to make healthier fast-food choices and to plan their daily food intake. "First Aid at a Glance" from the Red Cross appears inside the back cover of the text, providing information that can save lives. These guides offer students the kind of information they can keep and use for years to come.

An innovative **built-in Study Guide** is included in the back of the book. Printed on perforated pages for easy removal, the study guide provides sample test questions for each chapter to help students prepare for examinations. Also included are 17 Wellness Worksheets, which provide additional opportunities for self-assessment.

LEARNING AIDS

Although all the features of *Core Concepts in Health* are designed to facilitate learning, several specific learning aids have also been incorporated in the text. Learning objectives labeled **Looking Ahead** appear on the opening page of each chapter, identifying major concepts and

helping to guide students in their reading and review of the text. Important terms appear in boldface type in the text and are defined in a **running glossary,** helping students handle a large and complex new vocabulary. A pronunciation guide to all the key terms appears on the student CD-ROM.

Chapter summaries offer students a concise review and a way to make sure they have grasped the most important concepts in the chapter. Also found at the end of every chapter are **Selected Bibliographies** and sections called **For More Information** that contain annotated lists of books, newsletters, hotlines, organizations, and Web sites that students can use to extend and broaden their knowledge or pursue subjects of interest to them. A complete **Index** at the end of the book includes references to glossary terms in boldface type.

TEACHING TOOLS

Available to qualified adopters of the Brief Ninth Edition of *Core Concepts in Health* is a comprehensive package of supplementary materials that enhance teaching and learning. Included in the package are the following items:

- Instructor's Resource Binder
- Transparency Acetates
- Instructor's CD-ROM
- Students on Health Custom Video and McGraw-Hill Health and Wellness Custom Video
- Computerized Test Bank
- *Core Concepts in Health* Online Learning Center
- *Core Concepts Interactive* Student CD-ROM
- Wellness Worksheets
- *Mayfield's Quick View Guide to the Internet for Students of Health, Physical Education, and Exercise Science, Version 2.0*
- Nutrition and Weight Management Journal
- Additional videos, software, and other multimedia
- PageOut, PowerWeb, and other distance learning and online instruction options

The **Instructor's Resource Binder,** contains a variety of helpful teaching materials in an easy-to-use form.

- The **Instructor's Resource Guide,** prepared for the ninth edition by Cathy Kennedy, Colorado State University, includes learning objectives, extended chapter outlines, classroom activities, Internet resources, selected Healthy People 2010 objectives, and health crossword puzzles. The **examination questions** included in the Instructor's Resource Guide have been completely revised and updated for the ninth edition by Kathy McGinnis, San Diego City College. The text bank contains nearly 1600 multiple choice and true-false questions. The answer key lists the page number in the text where each answer is found.

• More than 150 **transparency masters and handouts** are provided as additional lecture resources. The transparency masters include tables, graphs, and key points from the text; illustrations of many body systems are also provided.

• A complete set of **Wellness Worksheets**, a student learning aid described below, is also included in the Instructor's Resource Binder.

Expanded for the ninth edition, the set of 80 **transparency acetates** provide material suitable for lecture and discussion. The acetates do not duplicate the transparency masters in the Instructor's Resource Binder, and many of them are from sources other than the text.

The **Instructor's CD-ROM**, expanded for the ninth edition, contains annotated PowerPoint® lecture outlines, an image set, transparency acetates, and an electronic version of the Instructor's Resource Guide, including the transparency masters and handouts. Also available on the CD-ROM is a new **Integrated Teaching Solutions** tool, which allows the user to create customized chapter lecture outlines keyed to all the supplements available with the text.

Two **customized videos** are available with the ninth edition. The **McGraw-Hill Health and Wellness Custom Video**, new for the ninth edition, includes brief video segments with additional information on health topics such as nutrition, exercise, and heart disease. **Students on Health** was filmed exclusively for *Core Concepts* with students at college campuses across the country. The 8–10-minute segments focus on key wellness concerns and are designed to stimulate critical thinking and class discussion. The accompanying Instructor's Video Guide provides summaries of each segment and discussion questions.

A **computerized test bank** is available to qualified adopters. Diploma, developed by Brownstone Research Group, allows instructors to design tests using the examination questions included with *Core Concepts in Health* and/or incorporating their own questions. It is available in both Windows and Macintosh formats.

Updated and expanded for the ninth edition, the *Core Concepts in Health* Online Learning Center includes a variety of tools for both instructors and students. Password-protected instructor's resources include links to professional resources and downloadable versions of the PowerPoint slides, acetates, image set, Wellness Worksheets, and Instructor's Resource Guide. The Integrated Teaching Solutions tool is also available online. Student resources include a wide variety of elements keyed to each chapter in the text: chapter outlines and learning objectives, interactive study guide questions, glossary flashcards with a pronunciation guide, interactive crossword puzzles, Journal Entry exercises, Internet activities

that guide students in locating and evaluating health-related Web sites, In the News and Vital Statistics Web links, and extensive sets of health and wellness Web links. In addition, the Online Learning Center includes a Behavior Change Workbook and information on career opportunities in health. All of the resources in the Online Learning Center can also be used with PageOut, Web CT, Blackboard, and other options for online courses.

The *Core Concepts Interactive* Student CD-ROM is also expanded and updated for the ninth edition. Packaged with each copy of the text, this interactive CD-ROM provides many helpful learning aids and wellness tools. Resources include interactive quizzes and wellness self-assessments, self-guided tutorials on special topics, a pronunciation guide to key terms, an electronic fitness log, and a guide to using the Internet.

The more than 100 **Wellness Worksheets** available with the ninth edition help students become more involved in their own wellness and better prepared to implement successful behavior change. The worksheets include assessment tools, Internet activities, and knowledge-based reviews of key concepts. They are available shrink-wrapped with the text in an easy-to-use pad.

Other practical items for the student can also be shrink-wrapped with the text:

• The **Nutrition and Weight Management Journal** guides students in assessing their current diet and making appropriate changes.

• Available in a new edition is *Mayfield's Quick View Guide to the Internet for Students of Health, Physical Education, and Exercise Science, Version 2.0*, by Jennifer Campbell Koella and Michael Keene, University of Tennessee, Knoxville. In addition to listing useful Web links, it provides step-by-step instructions on how to access the Internet; how to find, evaluate, and use online information about wellness; and many other topics.

Additional videos, software, and other multimedia are available to qualified adopters. The video library includes tapes on topics such as stress, AIDS, violence, nutrition, alcohol use, and many more. DINE Healthy software provides an easy way for students to evaluate their diets and track the energy expenditure of their activities. HealthQuest software contains interactive assessments, behavior change activities, current articles, video clips, Web links, and many other resources.

McGraw-Hill also offers a wide variety of **digital solutions** to help instructors put courses online. **PageOut** is a simple program that enables instructors to easily develop Web sites for their courses. PageOut can be used to create a course home page, an instructor home page, an interactive syllabus that can be linked to elements in the Online Learning Center, Web links, online discussion areas, an online grade book, and much more. The Online Learning Center can also be customized to work with products like WebCT and Blackboard. **PowerWeb** is a student Internet resource that includes articles from the Annual Editions series, weekly updates with assessments, informative and timely world news, Web links, research and study tools, and interactive exercises. For more information on these and other digital solutions offered by McGraw-Hill, contact your local representative or visit our Web site (http://www.mhhe.com/solutions).

A NOTE OF THANKS

The efforts of innumerable people have gone into producing this ninth edition of *Core Concepts in Health*. The book has benefited immensely from their thoughtful commentaries, expert knowledge and opinions, and many helpful suggestions. We are deeply grateful for their participation in the project.

Academic Contributors

David Antonuccio, Ph.D., Department of Psychiatry and Behavioral Sciences, University of Nevada School of Medicine
Alcohol and Tobacco

Roger Baxter, M.D., Internist and Infectious Disease Specialist, Kaiser Permanente Medical Center, Oakland, California; Associate Clinical Professor, University of California, San Francisco
Immunity and Infection

Andrea T. Borchers, Ph.D., Carl L. Keen, Ph.D., and M. Eric Gershwin, M.D., Division of Rheumatology, Allergy, and Clinical Immunology, University of California at Davis School of Medicine
Conventional and Complementary Medicine: Skills for the Health Care Consumer

Virginia Brooke, Ph.D., University of Texas Medical Branch at Galveston
The Challenge of Aging

Boyce Burge, Ph.D., Institute for Human Nutrition
Cardiovascular Disease and Cancer

Theodore C. Dumas, Ph.D., Stanford University
Stress: The Constant Challenge

Thomas Fahey, Ed.D., California State University, Chico
Exercise for Health and Fitness

Michael R. Hoadley, Ph.D., University of South Dakota
Personal Safety: Protecting Yourself from Unintentional Injuries and Violence

Paul M. Insel, Ph.D., Stanford University
Taking Charge of Your Health

Shepard A. Insel, Ed.D.
Intimate Relationships and Commmunication

Nancy Kemp, M.D.
Contraception and Abortion; Alcohol and Tobacco; Cardiovascular Disease and Cancer; Immunity and Infection

Charles Ksir, Ph.D., University of Wyoming
The Use and Abuse of Psychoactive Drugs

Jessica McAlpine, M.D., Department of Gynecology and Obstetrics, Stanford University Medical Center
Sexuality, Pregnancy, and Childbirth

Joyce D. Nash, Ph.D., Clinical Psychologist in private practice (San Francisco and Palo Alto)
Weight Management

David Quadagno, Ph.D., Florida State University
Sexuality, Pregnancy, and Childbirth

Walton T. Roth, M.D., Stanford University
Psychological Health

James H. Rothenberger, M.P.H., and Lynn C. Faust, M.P.H., University of Minnesota
Environmental Health

David S. Sobel, M.D., M.P.H., Director of Patient Education and Health Promotion, Kaiser Permanente Northern California
Conventional and Complementary Medicine: Skills for the Health Care Consumer

Albert Lee Strickland and Lynne Ann DeSpelder, Cabrillo College
The Challenge of Aging

Mae V. Tinklenberg, R.N., N.P., M.S.
Contraception and Abortion

R. Elaine Turner, Ph.D., R.D., University of Florida
Nutrition Basics

Academic Advisers and Reviewers

Rick Barnes, East Carolina University

Lois Beach, State University of New York at Plattsburgh

M. Betsy Bergen, Kansas State University

Penny J. Brynildson, Bethel College

Sandra Minor Bulmer, Southern Connecticut State University

Patricia A. Cost, Weber State University

Claire B. Elkins, Saddleback Community College

Natalie Erlich, Oklahoma State University

Sally J. Ford, Pima Community College

Marianne Frauenknecht, Western Michigan University

Kathy French, University of Central Arkansas

Daniel S. Gerber, University of Massachusetts at Amherst

Roger B. Imbrogno, Merced College

Richard Madson, Palm Beach Community College

Bobby C. Martin, Hampton University

La Tonya D. Mouzon, Southern Illinois University
at Carbondale

Miguel A. Pérez, California State University Fresno

Kerry J. Redican, Virginia Polytechnical Institute and
State University

Connie Reynolds, Utah Valley State

Jan S. Richter, University of Central Oklahoma

Thea Siria Spatz, University of Arkansas at Little Rock

Ladona Tornabene, University of South Dakota

Beatrice G. Wallace, Southside Virginia Community
College

Helen Welle-Graf, Georgia Southern University

Scott D. Winnail, University of Wyoming

Kristin Jacoby Yusko, University of Maryland
College Park

Finally, we would like to thank the staff at Mayfield
Publishing Company, particularly the members of the *Core*

Concepts book team. First, we are indebted to Kirstan Price
for her dedication and her extraordinary creative energies,
which have helped to make this book such a success.
Thanks also go to Holly Allen, Sponsoring Editor; Kate
Engelberg, Susan Shook Malloy, Star MacKenzie, and Elisa
Adams, Developmental Editors; Jennifer Hardy, Develop-
mental Editing Assistant; Kara Indelli, Editorial Assistant;
Linda Toy, Production Director; Melissa Williams, Senior
Production Editor; Jeanne M. Schreiber, Art Director;
Robin Mouat, Art Editor; Marty Granahan, Permissions
Editor; Brian Pecko, Photo Editor; Randy Hurst, Manufac-
turing Manager; Matt Ballantyne, Production Assistant;
Kristin Davis, Marketing Manager; Jay Bauer, Marketing
Communications Specialist. To all we express our deep
appreciation.

Paul M. Insel
Walton T. Roth

Brief Contents

Contents

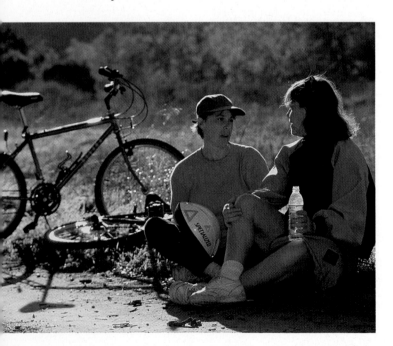

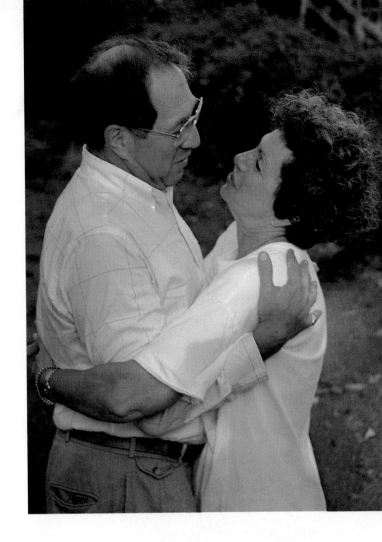

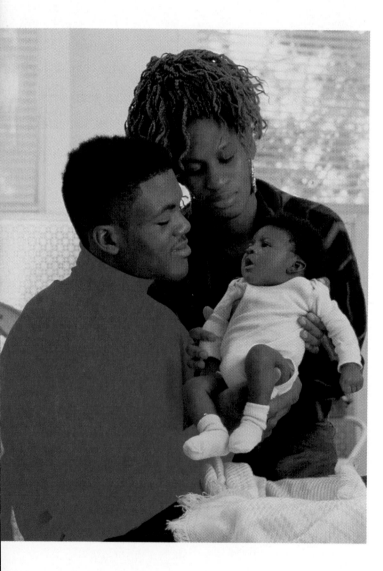

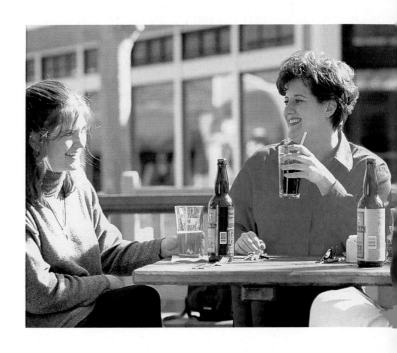

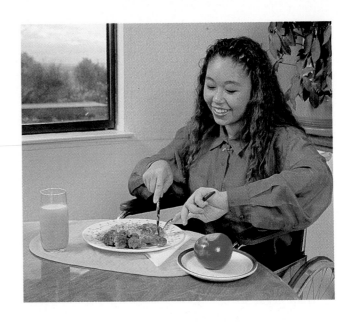

Chapter 9
NUTRITION BASICS   183

NUTRITIONAL REQUIREMENTS: COMPONENTS OF A HEALTHY DIET   183

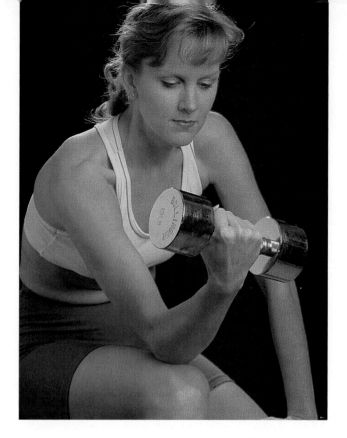

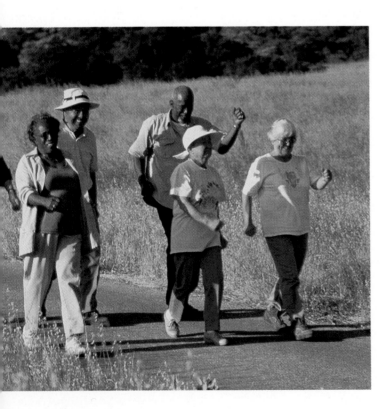

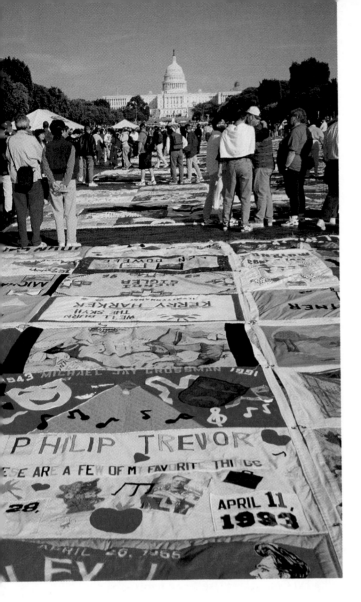

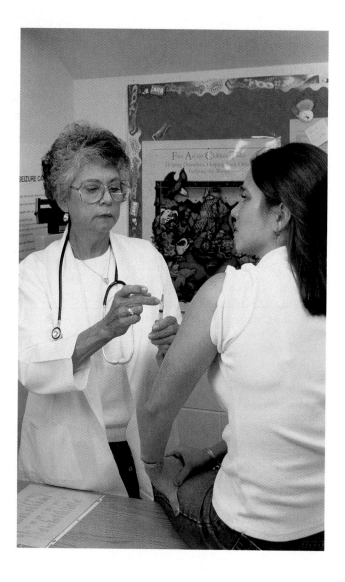

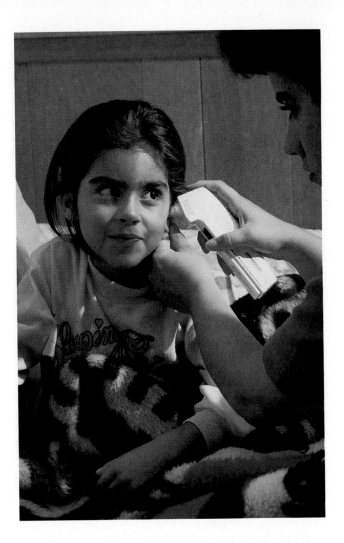

BOXES

In the News

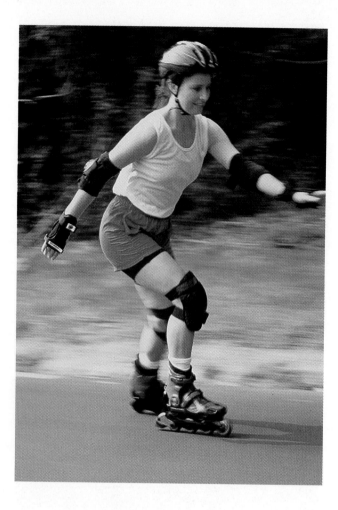

Mind/Body/Spirit

Dimensions of Diversity

Critical Consumer

Take Charge

In Focus

TOPICS OF SPECIAL CONCERN TO WOMEN

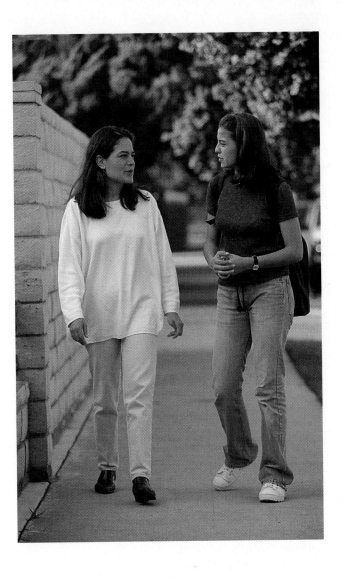

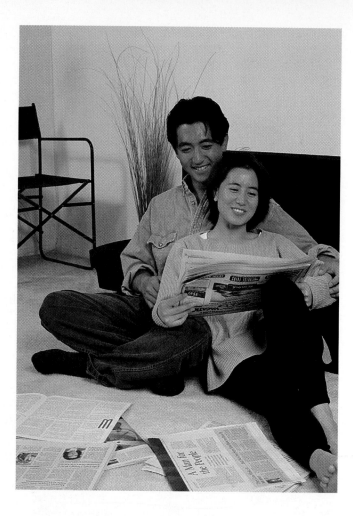

*Note: The health issues and conditions listed here include those that
disproportionately influence or affect women or men, For more information, see the index under gender, women, men, and any of the special
topics listed here.*

Taking Charge of Your Health

1

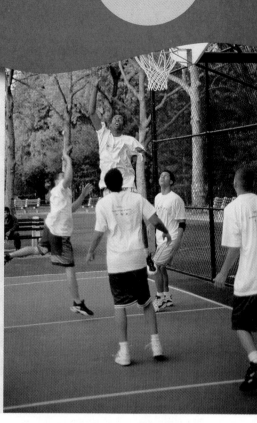

LOOKING AHEAD

After reading this chapter, you should be able to

• Describe the six dimensions of wellness and a wellness lifestyle

• Identify major goals of the national Healthy People initiative

• Explain the importance of personal decision making and behavior change in achieving a wellness lifestyle

• Describe the steps in creating a behavior management plan to change a health-related behavior

• Describe the influence of gender, ethnicity, income, and disability on health

• Discuss the available sources of health information and how to think critically about them

A first-year college student resolves to meet the challenge of making new friends. A long-sedentary senior starts riding her bike to school every day instead of taking the bus. A busy graduate student volunteers to plant trees in a blighted inner-city neighborhood. What do these people have in common? Each is striving for optimal health and well-being. Not satisfied to be merely free of major illness, these individuals want more. They want to live life actively, energetically, and fully, in a state of optimal personal, interpersonal, and environmental well-being. They have taken charge of their health and are on the path to wellness.

WELLNESS: THE NEW HEALTH GOAL

Wellness is an expanded idea of health. Many people think of health as being just the absence of physical disease. But wellness transcends this concept of health—for example, when individuals with serious illnesses or disabilities rise above their physical or mental limitations to live rich, meaningful, vital lives. Some aspects of health

are determined by your genes, your age, and other factors that may be beyond your control. But true wellness is largely determined by the decisions you make about how to live your life. In this book, we will use the terms *health* and *wellness* interchangeably to mean the ability to live life fully—with vitality and meaning.

The Dimensions of Wellness

No matter what your age or health status, you can optimize your health in each of the following six interrelated dimensions. Wellness in any dimension is not a static goal but a dynamic process of change and growth (Figure 1-1).

wellness Optimal health and vitality, encompassing physical, emotional, intellectual, spiritual, interpersonal, social, and environmental well-being.

Terms

1

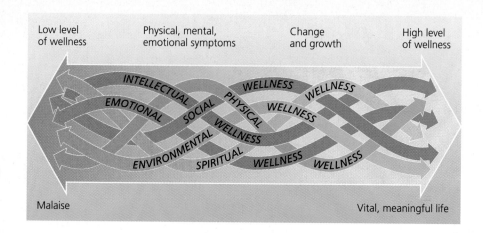

Low level of wellness   Physical, mental, emotional symptoms   Change and growth   High level of wellness

INTELLECTUAL WELLNESS WELLNESS
EMOTIONAL SOCIAL PHYSICAL WELLNESS
WELLNESS
ENVIRONMENTAL SPIRITUAL WELLNESS WELLNESS

Malaise   Vital, meaningful life

Figure 1-1 The wellness continuum. Wellness is composed of six interrelated dimensions, all of which must be developed in order to achieve overall wellness.

Physical Wellness Optimal physical health requires eating well, exercising, avoiding harmful habits, making responsible decisions about sex, learning about and recognizing the symptoms of disease, getting regular medical and dental checkups, and taking steps to prevent injuries at home, on the road, and on the job. The habits you develop and the decisions you make today will largely determine not only how many years you will live, but also the quality of your life during those years.

Emotional Wellness Optimism, trust, self-esteem, self-acceptance, self-confidence, self-control, satisfying relationships, and an ability to share feelings are just some of the qualities and aspects of emotional wellness. Emotional health is a dynamic state that fluctuates with your physical, intellectual, spiritual, interpersonal and social, and environmental health. Maintaining emotional wellness requires monitoring and exploring your thoughts and feelings, identifying obstacles to emotional well-being, and finding solutions to emotional problems, with the help of a therapist if necessary.

Intellectual Wellness The hallmarks of intellectual health include an openness to new ideas, a capacity to question and think critically, and the motivation to master new skills, as well as a sense of humor, creativity, and curiosity. An active mind is essential to overall wellness, for learning about, evaluating, and storing health-related information. Your mind detects problems, finds solutions, and directs behavior. People who enjoy intellectual

wellness never stop learning. They relish new experiences and challenges and actively seek them out.

Spiritual Wellness To enjoy spiritual health is to possess a set of guiding beliefs, principles, or values that give meaning and purpose to your life, especially during difficult times. Spiritual wellness involves the capacity for love, compassion, forgiveness, altruism, joy, and fulfillment. It is an antidote to cynicism, anger, fear, anxiety, self-absorption, and pessimism. Spirituality transcends the individual and can be a common bond among people. Organized religions help many people develop spiritual health. Many others find meaning and purpose in their lives on their own—through nature, art, meditation, political action, or good works.

Interpersonal and Social Wellness Satisfying relationships are basic to both physical and emotional health. We need to have mutually loving, supportive people in our lives. Developing interpersonal wellness means learning good communication skills, developing the capacity for intimacy, and cultivating a support network of caring friends and/or family members. Social wellness requires participating in and contributing to your community, country, and world.

Environmental or Planetary Wellness Increasingly, personal health depends on the health of the planet—from the safety of the food supply to the degree of violence in a society. Other examples of environmental threats to health are ultraviolet radiation in sunlight, air and water pollution, lead in old house paint, and secondhand tobacco smoke in indoor air. Wellness requires learning about and protecting yourself against such hazards—and doing what you can to reduce or eliminate them, either on your own or with others.

The six dimensions of wellness interact continuously, influencing and being influenced by one another. Making a change in one dimension often affects some or all of the others. Maintaining good health is a dynamic process,

Terms

infectious disease A disease that is communicable from one person to another; caused by invading microorganisms such as bacteria and viruses.

chronic disease A disease that develops and continues over a long period of time; usually caused by a variety of factors, including lifestyle factors.

1. The persistent presence of a support network
2. Chronic positive expectations; the tendency to frame events in a constructive light
3. Episodic outbreaks of joyful, happy experiences
4. A sense of spiritual involvement
5. A tendency to adapt to changing conditions
6. Rapid response and recovery of stress response systems to repeated challenges
7. An increased appetite for physical activity
8. A tendency to identify and communicate feelings
9. Repeated episodes of gratitude and generosity
10. A persistent sense of humor

SOURCE: Ten warning signs of good health. 1996. *Mind/Body Health Newsletter* 5(1). Reprinted by permission.

and increasing your level of wellness in one area of life often influences many others.

💿 New Opportunities, New Responsibilities

Wellness is a relatively recent concept. A century ago, people considered themselves lucky just to survive to adulthood. A child born in 1900, for example, could expect to live only about 47 years. Many people died as a result of common **infectious diseases** and poor environmental conditions (unrefrigerated food, poor sanitation, air and water pollution). However, over the past 100 years, the average life span has nearly doubled, thanks largely to the development of vaccines and antibiotics to prevent and fight infectious diseases and to public health campaigns to improve environmental conditions (Figure 1-2).

But a different set of diseases has emerged as our major health threat, and heart disease, cancer, and stroke are now the top three causes of death in the United States (Table 1-1). Treating these and other **chronic diseases** has proved enormously expensive and difficult. It has become clear that the best treatment for these diseases is prevention—people having a greater awareness about health and about taking care of their bodies.

The good news is that people do have some control over whether they develop heart disease, cancer, and other chronic diseases. People make choices every day that either increase or decrease their risks for these diseases—lifestyle choices involving such behaviors as exercise, diet, smoking, and drinking. Health care professionals can provide information, advice, and encouragement—but the rest is up to each of us.

🖥️ National Wellness Goals: The Healthy People Initiative

You may think of health and wellness as personal concerns, goals that you strive for on your own for your own benefit. But the U.S. government also has a vital interest in the health of all Americans. A healthy population is the nation's greatest resource, the source of its vitality, creativ-

ity, and wealth. Poor health, in contrast, drains the nation's resources and raises national health care costs. As the embodiment of our society's values, the federal government also has a humane interest in people's health.

The U.S. government's national Healthy People initiative seeks to prevent unnecessary disease and disability and to achieve a better quality of life for all Americans. Healthy People reports, published first in 1980 and revised every decade, set national health goals based on 10-year agendas. Each report includes both broad goals and specific targets in many different areas of wellness. The latest report, *Healthy People 2010,* proposes two broad national goals:

• *Increase quality and years of healthy life.* The life expectancy of Americans has increased significantly in the past century; however, people can expect poor health to limit their activities and cause distress during the last 15% of their lives (Figure 1-3). Health-related quality of life calls for a full range of functional capacity to enable people to work, play, and maintain satisfying relationships.

• *Eliminate health disparities among Americans.* Many health problems today disproportionately affect certain American populations—for example, ethnic minorities, people of low socioeconomic status or educational attainment, and people with disabilities. *Healthy People 2010* calls for eliminating disparities in health status, health risks, and use of preventive services among all population groups within the next decade.

Giving substance to these broad goals are hundreds of specific objectives—measurable targets for the year 2010—in many different focus areas that relate to wellness, including fitness, nutrition, safety, substance abuse, health care, and chronic and infectious diseases. Examples of health promotion objectives from *Healthy People 2010,* as well as estimates of our progress toward these targets, appear in Table 1-2. *Healthy People 2010* reflects the changing attitude of Americans: an emerging sense of personal responsibility as the key to good health. The primary concerns of *Healthy People 2010* are the principal

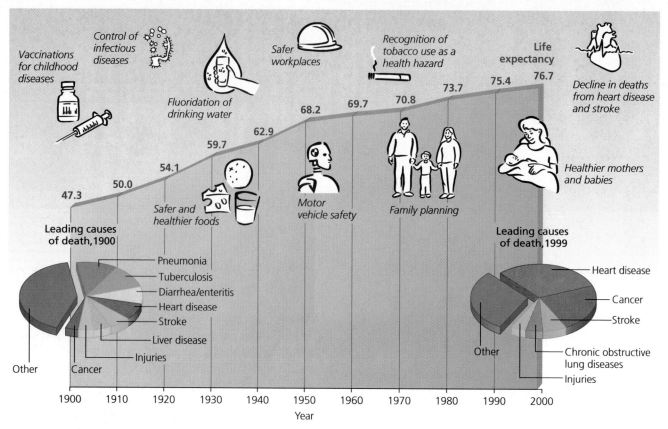

Vaccinations for childhood diseases

Control of infectious diseases

Fluoridation of drinking water

Safer workplaces

Recognition of tobacco use as a health hazard

Life expectancy

Decline in deaths from heart disease and stroke

Safer and healthier foods

Motor vehicle safety

Family planning

Healthier mothers and babies

47.3   50.0   54.1   59.7   62.9   68.2   69.7   70.8   73.7   75.4   76.7

Leading causes of death, 1900

Pneumonia
Tuberculosis
Diarrhea/enteritis
Heart disease
Stroke
Liver disease
Injuries

Other   Cancer

Leading causes of death, 1999

Heart disease
Cancer
Stroke
Chronic obstructive lung diseases
Injuries

Other

1900 1910 1920 1930 1940 1950 1960 1970 1980 1990 2000

Year

VITAL STATISTICS

Figure 1-2 Public health achievements of the twentieth century. During the twentieth century, public health achievements greatly improved the quality of life for Americans, and life expectancy rose from 47 to 77. A dramatic shift in the leading causes of death also occurred, with deaths from infectious diseases declining from more than 33% of all deaths to just 2.2%. Heart disease, cancer, and stroke are now responsible for more than 50% of all deaths among Americans.   SOURCES: National Center for Health Statistics. 2000. *Health, United States, 2000, with Adolescent Health Chartbook.* Hyattsville, Md.: National Center for Health Statistics. Centers for Disease Control and Prevention. 1999. Ten great public health achievements—United States, 1900–1999. *Morbidity and Mortality Weekly Report* 48(50): 1141. National Center for Health Statistics. 2001. United States life tables, 1998. *National Vital Statistics Reports* 48(18): 29–34.

topics covered in this book. In many ways, personal wellness goals are not different from the national aspirations.

Health Issues for Diverse Populations

Americans are a diverse people. Our ancestry is European, African, Asian, Pacific Islander, Latin American, and Native American. We live in cities, suburbs, and rural areas and work at every imaginable occupation. In no other country in the world do so many diverse people live and work together every day. And in no other country is the understanding and tolerance of differences so much a part of the political and cultural ideal. We are at heart a nation of diversity, and, though we often fall short of our goal, we strive for justice and equality among all.

When it comes to health, most differences among people are insignificant; most health issues concern us all

equally. We all need to eat well, exercise, manage stress, and cultivate satisfying personal relationships. We need to know how to protect ourselves from heart disease, cancer, sexually transmitted diseases, and injuries. We need to know how to use the health care system.

But some of our differences, as individuals and as members of groups, do have important implications for health. Some of us, for example, have a genetic predisposition for developing certain health problems, such as high cholesterol. Some of us have grown up eating foods that raise our risk of heart disease or obesity. Some of us live in an environment that increases the chance that we will smoke cigarettes or abuse alcohol. These health-related differences among individuals and groups can be biological—determined genetically—or cultural—acquired as patterns of behavior through daily interactions with our families, communities, and society. Many

Table 1-1   **Leading Causes of Death in the United States**

Rank	Cause of Death	Number of Deaths	Percent of Total Deaths	Female/Male Ratio*	Lifestyle Factors
1	Heart disease	724,859	31.0	51/49	D I S A
2	Cancer	541,532	23.2	48/52	D I S A
3	Stroke	158,448	6.8	61/39	D I S
4	Chronic obstructive lung diseases	112,584	4.8	49/51	S
5	Unintentional injuries	97,835	4.2	36/64	S A
	Motor-vehicle-related	(43,501)	(1.9)	33/67	
	All others	(54,334)	(2.3)	37/63	
6	Pneumonia and influenza	91,871	3.9	55/45	S
7	Diabetes mellitus	64,751	2.8	54/46	D I S
8	Suicide	30,575	1.3	20/80	A
9	Kidney diseases	26,182	1.1	52/48	D
10	Chronic liver disease and cirrhosis	25,192	1.1	35/65	A
	All causes	2,337,256			

Key: D Cause of death in which diet plays a part
I Cause of death in which an inactive lifestyle plays a part
S Cause of death in which smoking plays a part
A Cause of death in which excessive alcohol consumption plays a part

*Ratio of females to males who died of each cause. For example, an equal number of women and men died of heart disease, but only about half as many women as men died of motor-vehicle-related injuries.

SOURCE: National Center for Health Statistics. 2000. Deaths: Final data for 1998. *National Vital Statistics Reports* 48(11).

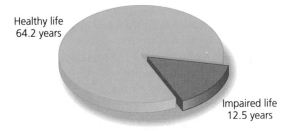

Healthy life 64.2 years

Impaired life 12.5 years

Life expectancy 76.7 years

Figure 1-3   Quantity of life versus quality of life. Years of healthy life as a proportion of life expectancy in the U.S. population. SOURCES: U.S. Department of Health and Human Services. 2000. *Healthy People 2010.* 2nd ed. Washington, D.C.: DHHS. National Center for Health Statistics. 2000. Deaths: Final data for 1998. *National Vital Statistics Reports* 48(11).

health conditions are a function of biology and culture combined. A person can have a genetic predisposition for a disease, for example, but won't actually develop the disease itself unless certain lifestyle factors are present, such as stress or a poor diet.

When we talk about health issues for diverse populations, we face two related dangers. The first is the danger of stereotyping, of talking about people as groups rather than as individuals. It's certainly true that every person is an individual with a unique genetic endowment and unique life experiences. But many of these influences are shared with others of similar genetic and cultural background. Statements about these group similarities can be useful; for example, they can alert people to areas that may be of special concern for them and their families.

The second danger is that of overgeneralizing, of ignoring the extensive biological and cultural diversity that exists among peoples who are grouped together. Groups labeled Latino or Hispanic, for example, include Mexican Americans, Puerto Ricans, people from South and Central America, and other Spanish-speaking peoples. It's important to keep these considerations in mind whenever you read about culturally diverse populations.

Health-related differences among groups can be identified and described in the context of several different dimensions. Those highlighted in *Healthy People 2010* are gender, ethnicity, income and education, disability, geographic location, and sexual orientation.

Gender   Men and women have different life expectancies, different reproductive concerns, and different incidences of many diseases, including heart disease, cancer, stroke, and cirrhosis. Men are more likely to develop heart disease in middle age. They have higher rates of deaths from injuries, suicide, homicide, and HIV/AIDS.

Table 1-2 Selected *Healthy People 2010* Objectives

Objective	Estimate of Current Status (%)	Goal (%)
Increase the proportion of people age 18 and older who engage regularly, preferably daily, in moderate physical activity for at least 30 minutes per day.	15	30
Increase the proportion of people age 2 and older who consume at least three daily servings of vegetables, with at least one-third being dark-green or orange vegetables.	3	50
Increase the prevalence of healthy weight among all people age 20 and older.	42	60
Reduce the proportion of adults 18 and older who use cigarettes.	24	12
Reduce the proportion of college students reporting binge drinking during the past 2 weeks.	39	20
Increase the proportion of sexually active persons who use condoms.	23	50
Increase the proportion of adults who take protective measures to reduce the risk of skin cancer (sunscreens, sun-protective clothing, and so on).	47	75
Increase the use of safety belts by motor vehicle occupants.	69	92
Increase the number of residences with a functioning smoke alarm on every floor.	87	100
Increase the proportion of persons with health insurance.	83	100

SOURCE: U.S. Department of Health and Human Services. 2000. *Healthy People 2010.* 2nd ed. Washington, D.C.: DHHS.

Women are more affected by issues involving contraception and reproductive choices. They are at greater risk for Alzheimer's disease and for major depression. They live longer than men, and they are more likely to be poor.

Ethnicity Some genetic diseases are concentrated in certain gene pools, the result of each ethnic group's relatively distinct history. Sickle-cell disease occurs almost exclusively among people of African ancestry. Tay-Sachs disease afflicts people of Eastern European Jewish heritage. Cystic fibrosis is more common among Northern Europeans. In addition to biological differences, many cultural differences occur along ethnic lines. Ethnic groups may vary in their traditional diets; their patterns of family and interpersonal relationships; their attitudes toward tobacco, alcohol, and other drugs; and their health beliefs and practices.

Income and Education Inequalities in income and education underlie many of the health disparities among Americans. Income and education are closely related, and groups with the highest poverty rates and least education have the worst health status. People with low incomes and less education have higher rates of infant mortality, traumatic injury and violent death, and many diseases, including heart disease, diabetes, tuberculosis, and HIV infection. They are more likely to eat poorly, be overweight, smoke, drink, and use drugs. They are exposed to more stressors and have less access to health care services. Poverty and low educational attainment are far more important predictors of poor health than any ethnic factor.

Disability People with disabilities are those who have activity limitations, need assistance, or perceive themselves as having a disability. About one in five people in the United States has some level of disability, and the rate is rising, especially among younger segments of the population. People with disabilities are more likely to be inactive and overweight. They report more days of depression and fewer days of vitality than people without activity limitations. Many people with disabilities also lack access to health care services.

Geographic Location About one in four Americans currently lives in a rural area—a place with fewer than 2500 residents. People living in rural areas are less likely to be physically active, to use safety belts, or to obtain screening tests for preventive health care. They have less access to timely emergency services and much higher rates of injury-related death than people living in urban areas. They are also more likely to lack health insurance.

Sexual Orientation The 1–5% of Americans who identify themselves as homosexual or bisexual make up a diverse community with varied health concerns. Their emotional wellness and personal safety are affected by

Compared to the U.S. population as a whole, American ethnic minorities have higher rates of death and disability from many causes. These disparities result from a complex mix of genetic variations, environmental factors, and health behaviors, and it is often difficult to separate factors related to ethnicity from those associated with socioeconomic status and educational attainment. Achieving the *Healthy People 2010* goal of eliminating all health disparities will require a national effort to identify and address the underlying causes of these disparities, including poverty, lack of access to quality health care, environmental hazards in homes and neighborhoods, and the need for disease prevention programs tailored to specific community needs.

The federal government collects population and health information on five broad ethnic minority groups in American society: blacks, or African Americans; Hispanics, or Latinos; Asian Americans; American Indians and Alaska Natives; and Native Hawaiian and other Pacific Islander Americans. Each group has some specific health concerns.

Blacks, or African Americans

On the 2000 census, about 12.9% of the population reported that they were either African American or African American *and* one or more other races. (Census 2000 allowed respondents to choose more than one race, so percentages reflect both those who reported only one race and those who reported two or more races). Although African Americans are represented in every socioeconomic group, nearly 30% live below the poverty line. The health status of blacks lags behind that of the total population in several areas, including life expectancy and incidence of chronic and infectious diseases.

The leading causes of death among African Americans are the same as for the general population, but blacks have a higher infant mortality rate and a lower suicide rate. The death rate for HIV infection and homicide among blacks is about six to eight times the rate for whites. African Americans also die from stroke at almost twice the rate of whites. Strokes are related to high blood pressure, which is much more common among blacks than in the general population. Diabetes, another risk factor for cardiovascular disease, is a special concern for black women, especially those who are overweight. African American men face a 60% greater risk of prostate cancer than whites, giving them the highest prostate cancer risk of any group in the world.

Hispanics, or Latinos

About 12.5% of the population reported that they were of Spanish/Hispanic/Latino origin on Census 2000. They are a diverse group, with roots in Mexico, Puerto Rico, Cuba, and South and Central America. Many Latinos are of mixed Spanish and American Indian descent or of mixed Spanish, Indian, and African American descent.

Overall, the leading causes of death for Latinos are the same as those for the general population—heart disease and cancer—but Latinos tend to have lower rates of death from heart disease and cancer than non-Hispanic whites and African Americans. Hispanics have higher rates of death from diabetes, homicide, HIV infection, and infant mortality than non-Hispanic whites, but they have lower rates of death from suicide and lung cancer. Some special concerns are diabetes, gallbladder disease, and obesity, all probably related to American Indian

descent. The birth rate among Latinos is higher than that of the general population, and contraceptive use is relatively low.

Asian Americans

About 4.2% of the population reported that they were Asian American, alone or in combination with one or more other races. They include people who trace their ancestry to countries in the Far East, Southeast Asia, or the Indian subcontinent, including Japan, China, Vietnam, Laos, Cambodia, Korea, the Philippines, India, and Pakistan. Numbering 11.8 million people, they speak more than 30 different languages and represent a similar number of distinct cultures.

Asian Americans have lower death rates overall than does the general population. For example, the death rate for coronary heart disease is 40% lower for Asian American men than for white men. However, health differences exist among these groups. For example, Southeast Asian men have higher rates of lung cancer, smoking, and liver cancer than the rest of the population; Vietnamese American women have higher rates of cervical cancer. Among recent immigrants from Southeast Asia, tuberculosis and hepatitis B are serious health problems. Many Asian Americans lack health insurance, and more than 20% have no regular source of health care.

American Indians and Alaska Natives

American Indians and Alaska Natives, alone or in combination with one or more other races, represent about 1.5% of the population. Most embrace a tribal identity, such as Sioux, Navaho, or Hopi, rather than the identity of American Indian or Alaska Native. American Indians and Alaska Natives have lower rates of death from heart disease, stroke, and cancer than the general population, but they also have high rates of early death. For those under 45, leading causes of death include unintentional injuries, homicide, suicide, and cirrhosis; many of these problems are linked to alcohol abuse. Smoking rates are also high. Diabetes is prevalent, occurring at twice the rate for the general population; in some tribes, more than 20% of all adults are affected, and the Pimas of Arizona have the highest known prevalence of diabetes of any population in the world. American Indians and Alaska Natives have a high teen birth rate and a high infant mortality rate; more than 10% of children and 20% of adults have no regular source of health care.

Native Hawaiian and Other Pacific Islander Americans

Native Hawaiians and other Pacific Islander Americans trace their ancestry to the original peoples of Hawaii, Guam, Samoa, or other Pacific Islands; they represent less than 1% of the total population. Native Hawaiians have a higher overall death rate than whites and higher rates of many diseases, including hypertension, diabetes, lung cancer, stroke, and asthma. The high rate of smoking and high prevalence of overweight and obesity among Native Hawaiians and other Pacific Islander Americans may contribute to these conditions. In addition, many Native Hawaiians and other Pacific Islander Americans lack health insurance and access to regular health care. Among some Pacific Islander populations, the rate of infant mortality is more than double that of the general population.

In June 2000, government and private-sector researchers announced that they had completed a rough draft of the human genome. Their findings pave the way for many potential health benefits but also raise many difficult ethical issues.

Genome Basics

Your genome consists of the complete set of genetic material in your cells—the master blueprint for all cellular structures and activities. The nucleus of each cell contains 23 pairs of chromosomes, which are made up of tightly packed coils of deoxyribonucleic acid (DNA). DNA consists of two long strands wound around each other in a spiral, ladderlike structure referred to as a double helix. The rungs of the ladder are made from pairings of four different nucleotide bases: adenine, thymine, cytosine, and guanine, or A, T, C, and G. When researchers say they have mapped the genome, they mean they have sequenced the entire string of billions of A's, T's, C's, and G's.

A gene is a smaller unit of DNA made up of a specific sequence of hundreds or thousands of nucleotide base pairs. You have two copies of each gene—one inherited from each parent. Each of the estimated 30,000–40,000 genes in your DNA controls the production of a particular protein. Proteins serve both as the structural material for your body and as the regulators of all chemical reactions and metabolic processes. Many diseases are thought to be caused or promoted by an absence or excess of particular proteins. About 3% of the total human genome is made of genes; the function of the other 97%, called "junk" DNA, isn't completely understood.

Further work is needed to transform the draft of the genome into information useful for improving human health. Once the sequence is completed and checked, the next step will be to locate genes and identify the structure and function of the proteins they make. Researchers will also look closely at variations among individuals. Humans differ from one another at the rate of only about one base in every thousand (0.1%). Most of these differences occur in junk DNA and have no effect on health. However, some variations occur at critical spots that cause a gene to make the wrong protein. By sequencing the genomes of many individuals, it should be possible to identify the specific gene variations linked to increased risk for particular diseases.

Vast Promise

Researchers hope to use the deciphered human genome to improve health and quality of life for all people. Some likely developments include the following:

- *Personalized risk assessment:* A study of your genes could replace family history and other indirect clues as a means of determining your risk of particular diseases. Individualized lifestyle and medical screening advice may someday replace blanket public health recommendations.

- *Pharmacogenomics:* Genetic information could help physicians prescribe medications based on individual drug sensitivities and the likelihood that a particular disorder will respond to a particular drug.

- *Gene therapy and other new treatments:* Gene research will help develop new therapies that will directly affect the underlying biological mechanisms—genes and proteins—of serious disorders such as asthma, diabetes, and cancer.

Limitations and Troubling Questions

Despite the many potential benefits of knowledge of the genome, there are limitations to what this information can do for human health. Errors in our genes are responsible for an estimated 3000 to 4000 clearly hereditary conditions, including sickle-cell disease, Huntington's disease, and cystic fibrosis. Altered genes also play a part in heart disease, cancer, stroke, diabetes, and many other common conditions. However, in these more common and complex disorders, genetic alterations serve only to increase an individual's risk. The disease itself results from the interaction of many genes with environmental and behavioral factors. It will be much more difficult to develop tests and therapies for disorders with complex causes.

In addition, access to information about the human genome and the genes of individuals raises many difficult ethical issues. Privacy and discrimination are key concerns. If genetic testing can identify years in advance who will get sick and who will not, employers and health insurance companies could save millions of dollars by not hiring or enrolling people whose genes show them to be at increased risk for disease. This is especially troubling because it is likely that tests for genetic susceptibility to many conditions will be available years, perhaps decades, before any gene-based treatments are developed. Chapter 16 has more information on genetic testing.

Other questions relate to potential uses of tools for altering the genome. Do we have enough information to know how knocking out "bad" genes will affect our species? For example, the gene alteration that causes sickle-cell disease must be present in both copies of the gene for a person to develop the disorder; people with only one copy of the altered gene have an increased resistance to malaria. If the gene for sickle-cell disease were eliminated, would many more people succumb to malaria? What other unknown effects might we cause by tinkering with the genome? In addition, if it becomes easy to change ourselves and our children, will we become less tolerant of people who have such "conditions" as short stature or baldness?

The Role of Behavior and Environmental Factors

Most common disorders result from the complex interaction of many different genes, environmental factors, and lifestyle choices. For example, researchers have identified genes that increase a woman's risk for breast cancer, but these genes explain only a small proportion of cases. Behavior and environment exert a powerful influence on health and the risk of disease. This power can be seen in the 33% increase in the incidence of diabetes that has occurred among Americans since 1990. This huge increase is not due to any sudden change in our genes; it is the result of increasing rates of obesity due to poor dietary choices and lack of physical activity.

It's important not to adopt a position of biological determinism—a belief that your genes inevitably completely control your future health. Genomics research will certainly lead to a better understanding of the underlying causes of disease and to new techniques for diagnosis and treatment. However, your health, both in terms of your lifestyle choices and your use of genetic information, is still in your own hands.

factors relating to personal, family, and social acceptance of their sexual orientation. Gay, lesbian, and bisexual teens are more likely to engage in risky behaviors such as unsafe sex and drug use; they are also more likely to be depressed and to attempt suicide. HIV/AIDS is a major concern for gay men, and gay men and lesbians may have higher rates of substance abuse, depression, and suicide.

These are just some of the differences among people and groups that can influence wellness. Boxes labeled Dimensions of Diversity examine special wellness challenges and solutions of diverse population groups in the United States and around the world.

CHOOSING WELLNESS

Each of us has the option and the responsibility to decide what kind of future we want—one characterized by zestful living or one marked by symptoms and declining energy. The message of this book is that wellness is something everyone can have. Achieving it requires knowledge, self-awareness, motivation, and effort—but the benefits last a lifetime. Optimal health comes mostly from a healthy lifestyle, patterns of behavior that promote and support your health now and as you get older.

Factors That Influence Wellness

Scientific research is continuously revealing new connections between our habits and emotions and the level of health we enjoy. For example, heart disease, the nation's number one killer, is associated with cigarette smoking, high levels of stress, habitually hostile and suspicious attitudes toward people and the world, a diet high in fat and low in fiber, and a sedentary way of life. Other habits are beneficial. Regular exercise, for example, can help prevent heart disease, high blood pressure, diabetes, osteoporosis, and depression and may reduce the risk of colon cancer, stroke, and back injury. As we learn more about how our actions affect our bodies and minds, we can make informed choices for a healthier life.

Of course, behavior isn't the only factor involved in wellness. Our heredity, the environment we live in, and whether we have access to adequate health care are other important influences. These factors, which vary for both individuals and groups, can interact in ways that produce either health or disease. For example, a sedentary lifestyle combined with a genetic predisposition for diabetes can greatly increase a person's risk of developing the disease. If this person also lacks adequate health care, he or she is much more likely to suffer dangerous complications from diabetes and have a lower quality of life.

But in many cases, behavior can tip the balance toward good health, even when heredity or environment is a negative factor. For example, if you have a family history of

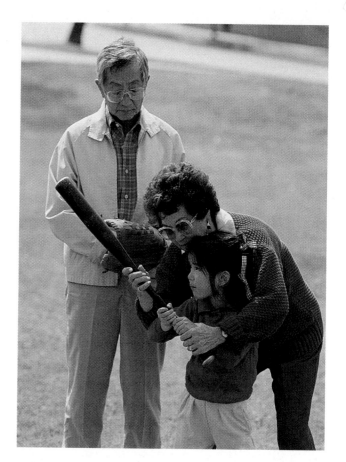

With wellness come health and vitality throughout the life span.

obesity, you can maintain a normal weight by being careful to balance calorie intake against activities that burn calories. If your life is highly stressful, you can lessen the chances of heart disease and stroke by learning ways to manage and cope with stress. If you live in an area with severe air pollution, you can reduce the risk of lung disease by not smoking. You can also take an active role in improving your environment. Behaviors like these enable you to make a difference in how great an impact heredity and environment will have on your health.

A Wellness Profile

What does it mean to be healthy today? A basic list of important behaviors and habits includes the following:

- Having a sense of responsibility for your own health and taking an active rather than a passive stance toward your life
- Learning to manage stress in effective ways
- Maintaining high self-esteem and mentally healthy ways of interacting with other people
- Understanding your sexuality and having satisfying intimate relationships

- Avoiding tobacco and other drugs; using alcohol responsibly, if at all
- Eating well, exercising, and maintaining a healthy weight
- Knowing the facts about cardiovascular disease, cancer, infections, sexually transmitted diseases, and injuries and using your knowledge to protect yourself against them
- Understanding the health care system and using it intelligently
- Knowing when to treat your illnesses yourself and when to seek help
- Understanding the natural processes of aging and dying and accepting the limits of human existence
- Understanding how the environment affects your health and taking appropriate action to improve it

Incorporating these behaviors into your daily life may seem like a tall order, and in a sense it is the work of a lifetime. But the habits you establish now are crucial: They tend to set lifelong patterns. Some behaviors do more than set up patterns—they produce permanent changes in your health. If you become addicted to drugs or alcohol at age 20, for example, you may be able to kick the habit, but you will always face the struggle of a recovering addict. If you contract gonorrhea, you may discover later that your reproductive organs were damaged without your realizing it, making you infertile or sterile. Some things just can't be reversed or corrected.

> **COMMUNICATE!** To get started thinking and talking about health behaviors, ask some of your close family members what they think wellness is. Are they aware of its many dimensions? Do they know, for example, that spending time with friends, having a spiritual practice, and keeping an active mind all contribute to wellness? Do they have some ideas about wellness that haven't occurred to you? What can you learn from them, and what can they learn from you?

Ww. HOW DO YOU REACH WELLNESS?

Your life may not resemble the one described by the wellness profile at all. You probably have a number of healthy habits and some others that place your health at risk. Taking big steps toward wellness may at first seem like too

much work, but as you make progress, it gets easier. At first you'll be rewarded with a greater sense of control over your life, a feeling of empowerment, higher self-esteem, and more joy. These benefits will encourage you to make further improvements. Over time, you'll come to know what wellness feels like—more energy; greater vitality; deeper feelings of curiosity, interest, and enjoyment; and a higher quality of life.

Ww. Getting Serious About Your Health

Before you can start changing a health-related behavior, you have to know that the behavior is problematic and that you *can* change it. To make good decisions, you need information about relevant topics and issues, including what resources are available to help you change.

Examining Your Current Health Habits Have you considered how your current lifestyle is affecting your health today and how it will affect your health in the future? Do you know which of your current habits enhance your health and which detract from it? Begin your journey toward wellness with self-assessment: Think about your own behavior, and talk with friends and family members about what they've noticed about your lifestyle and your health.

Many people start to consider changing a behavior when they get help from others. An observation from a friend, family member, or physician can help you see yourself as others do and may get you thinking about your behavior in a new way. Landmark events can also get you thinking about behavior change. A birthday, the birth of a child, or the death of someone close to you can be powerful motivators for thinking seriously about behaviors that affect wellness. New information can also help you get started. As you read this text, you may find yourself reevaluating some of your health-related behaviors. This could be a great opportunity to make healthful changes that will stay with you for the rest of your life.

Choosing a Target Behavior To maximize your chances of success, don't try to change all your problem behaviors at once—to quit smoking, give up high-fat foods, start jogging, avoid drugs, get more sleep. Working on even one behavior change will make high demands on your energy. Concentrate on one behavior that you want to change, your **target behavior,** and work on it systematically. Start with something simple, like snacking on candy between afternoon classes or always driving to a particular class instead of walking or biking.

Obtaining Information About Your Target Behavior Once you've chosen a target behavior, you need to find out more about it. You need to know its risks and benefits for you—both now and in the future. How is your target behavior affecting your level of wellness today? What diseases or conditions does this behavior place you at risk for? What effect would changing your behavior have on your health? As a starting point, use material from this text and from the resources listed in the For More Information section at the end of each chapter.

Finding Outside Help   Have you identified a particularly challenging target behavior, something like alcohol addiction, excessive overeating, or depression that interferes with your ability to function or places you at a serious health risk? Outside help is often needed for changing behaviors or conditions that may be too deeply rooted or too serious for a self-management approach. If this is the case, don't be stopped by the seriousness of the problem—there are many resources available to help you solve it. On campus, the student health center or campus counseling center may be a source of assistance. Many communities offer a variety of services through adult education, health departments, and private agencies. Consult the yellow pages, your physician, your local health department, or the United Way; the latter often sponsors local referral services.

Building Motivation for Change

Knowledge is a necessary ingredient for behavior change, but it isn't usually enough to make people act. Millions of people smoke or have sedentary lifestyles, for example, even though they know it's bad for their health. To succeed at behavior change, you need strong motivation.

Examining the Pros and Cons of Change   Health behaviors have short-term and long-term benefits and costs associated with them. For example, in the short term, an inactive lifestyle allows for more time to watch TV and hang out with friends but leaves a person less able to participate in recreational activities. In the long term, it increases risk for heart disease, cancer, stroke, and premature death. For successful behavior change, you must believe that the benefits of changing outweigh the costs.

Do a careful analysis of the short-term and long-term benefits and costs of continuing your current (target) behavior and of changing to a new, healthier behavior. Focus on the effects that are most meaningful to you, including those that are tied to your personal identity and values. For example, if you see yourself as an active person who is a good role model for others, then adopting behaviors such as regular physical activity and adequate sleep would support your personal identity. If you value independence and control over your life, then quitting smoking would be consistent with your values and goals. To complete your analysis, ask friends and family members about the effects of your behavior on them. For example, a younger sister may tell you that your smoking habit influenced her decision to take up smoking.

Pay special attention to the short-term benefits of behavior change, as these can be an important motivating

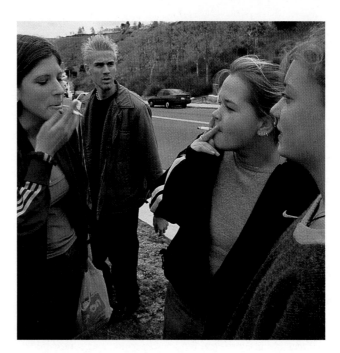

Changing powerful, long-standing habits requires motivation, commitment, and a belief that we are in control of our own behavior. To quit smoking, these young women must overcome a habit that is supported by their addiction to nicotine and by their social environment.

force. Although some people are motivated by long-term goals, such as avoiding a disease that may hit them in 30 years, most are more likely to be moved to action by shorter-term, more personal goals. Feeling better, doing better in school, improving at a sport, reducing stress, and increasing self-esteem are common short-term benefits of health behavior change.

Boosting Self-Efficacy   When you start thinking about changing a health behavior, a big factor in your eventual success is whether you have confidence in yourself and in your ability to change. **Self-efficacy** refers to your belief in your ability to successfully take action and perform a specific task. Strategies for boosting self-efficacy include developing an internal locus of control, using visualization and self-talk, and obtaining encouragement from supportive people.

LOCUS OF CONTROL   Who do you believe is controlling your life? Is it your parents, friends, or school? Is it "fate"? Or is it you? **Locus of control** refers to the figurative "place" a person designates as the source of responsibility for the events in his or her life. People who believe they are in control of their own lives are said to have an internal locus of control. Those who believe that factors beyond their control—heredity, friends and family, the environment, fate, luck, or other outside forces—are more important in determining the events of their lives are said to have an external locus of control.

Making sound choices about your own wellness requires critical thinking. In order to choose and implement healthy behaviors, you must be able to identify accurate information about health in general and your own personal risk factors in particular. You must be able to evaluate health-related products and services such as exercise shoes, fast food, health insurance, and medical treatments. Thinking critically is crucial if you are to take advantage of all the opportunities you have to optimize your health and well-being.

General Strategies

A key first step in sharpening your critical thinking skills is to look carefully at your sources of health information. Critical thinking involves knowing where and how to find relevant information, how to separate fact from opinion, how to recognize faulty reasoning, how to evaluate information, and how to assess the credibility of sources. The following strategies can help you sort through the health information you receive from common sources, including television, newspapers, magazines, books, advertisements, Web sites, and friends and family members.

- *Go to the original source.* Media reports often simplify the results of medical research. Find out for yourself what a study really reported, and determine whether it was based on good science. What type of study was it? Was it published in a recognized medical journal? Was it an animal study or did it involve people? Did the study include a large num-ber of people? What did the authors of the study actually report in their findings?

- *Watch for misleading language.* Reports that feature "breakthroughs" or "dramatic proof" are probably hype. Some studies will find that a behavior "contributes to" or is "associated with" an outcome; this does not imply a proven cause-and-effect relationship. Information may also be distorted by an author's point of view. Carefully read or listen to information in order to understand its implications.

- *Distinguish between research reports and public health advice.* If a study finds a link between a particular vitamin and cancer, that should not necessarily lead you to change your behavior. But if the Surgeon General or the American Cancer Society advises you to eat less fat or quit smoking, you can assume that many studies point in this direction and that this is advice you should follow.

- *Remember that anecdotes are not facts.* Sometimes we do get helpful health information from our friends and family. But just because your cousin Bertha lost 10 pounds on Dr. Amazing's new protein diet doesn't mean it's a safe, effective way for you to lose weight. Before you make a big change in your lifestyle, verify the information with your physician, this text, or other reliable sources.

- *Be skeptical, and use your common sense.* If a report seems too good to be true, it probably is. Be especially wary of information contained in advertisements. The goal of an ad is to sell you something, to create a feeling of need for a product where no real need exists. Evaluate "scientific" claims carefully, and beware of quackery.

For lifestyle management, an internal locus of control is an advantage because it reinforces motivation and commitment. For example, if you believe you can take action to reduce your hereditary risk of breast cancer, you will be motivated to follow guidelines for early detection of the disease. If you find yourself attributing too much influence to outside forces, gather more information about your target behavior. Make a list of all the ways that behavior change will improve your health. If you recognize and accept that you are in charge of your life, you're well on your way to wellness.

VISUALIZATION AND SELF-TALK   One of the best ways to boost your confidence and self-efficacy is to visualize yourself successfully engaging in a new, healthier behavior. Imagine yourself turning down cigarettes, going for a regular after-dinner walk, or choosing healthier snacks. Also visualize yourself enjoying all the short-term and long-term benefits that behavior change will bring. Create a new self-image: What will you and your life be like when you become a nonsmoker, a regular exerciser, or a healthy eater?

You can also use self-talk, the internal dialogue you carry on with yourself, to increase your confidence in your ability to change. Counter any self-defeating patterns of thought with more positive or realistic thoughts:

"Behavior change is difficult, but if I work at it, I will succeed," or "I am a strong, capable person, and I can maintain my commitment to change." Refer to Chapter 3 for more on self-talk.

ROLE MODELS AND OTHER SUPPORTIVE INDIVIDUALS   Social support can also make a big difference in your level of motivation and your chances of success. Perhaps you know people who have reached the goal you are striving for; they could be role models or mentors for you, providing information and support for your efforts. Gain strength from their experiences, and tell yourself, "If they can do it, so can I."

In addition, find a buddy who wants to make the same changes you do and who can take an active role in your behavior change program. For example, an exercise buddy can provide companionship and encouragement for times when you might be tempted to skip that morning jog. Or you and a friend can watch to be sure that you both have only one alcoholic beverage at a party. If necessary, look beyond your current social network at possible new sources of help, such as a support group.

Identifying and Overcoming Key Barriers to Change

Have you tried and failed to change your target behavior in the past? Don't let past failures discourage you; they

• *Make choices that are right for you.* Your roommate swears by swimming; you prefer aerobics. Your sister takes a yoga class to help her manage stress; your brother unwinds by walking in the woods. Friends and family members can be a great source of ideas and inspiration, but each of us needs to find a wellness lifestyle that works for us.

Internet Resources

More than half of all Internet users report having surfed for health information. Evaluating health information from online sources poses special challenges and requires additional critical thinking skills. When reviewing a health-related Web site, ask the following questions:

• *What is the source of the information? Who is the author or sponsor of the Web page?* Web sites maintained by government agencies, professional associations, or established academic or medical institutions are likely to present trustworthy information. Many other groups and individuals post accurate information, but it is important to look at the qualifications of the people who are behind the site. (Check the home page or click on an "about us" or "who we are" link.)

• *How often is the site updated?* Look for sites that are updated frequently. Also check the "last modified" date of any specific Web page on a site.

• *What is the purpose of the page? Does the site promote particular products or procedures? Are there obvious reasons for bias?*

Be wary of information from sites that sell specific products, use testimonials as evidence, appear to have a social or political agenda, or ask for money.

• *What do other sources say about a topic?* Be cautious of claims or information that appears at only one site or comes from a chat room or bulletin board.

• *Does the site conform to any set of guidelines or criteria for quality and accuracy?* Look for sites that identify themselves as conforming to some code or set of principles, such as those set forth by the Health on the Net Foundation or the American Medical Association. These codes include criteria such as use of information from respected sources and disclosure of the site's sponsors.

Additional strategies for locating and assessing health-related information from the Internet can be found on the *Core Concepts in Health* Online Learning Center (http://www.mhhe.com/insel9).

You will find boxes labeled Critical Consumer throughout the text to help you develop and apply your critical thinking skills. In addition, be sure to work through the Critical Thinking Journal Entry activities at the end of each chapter. Developing the ability to think critically and independently about health issues will serve you well throughout your life.

can be a great source of information you can use to boost your chances of future success. Make a list of the problems and challenges you faced in your previous behavior change attempts; to this, add the short-term costs of behavior change that you identified in your analysis of the pros and cons of change. Once you've listed these key barriers to change, develop a practical plan for overcoming each one. For example, if you always smoke when you're with certain friends, practice in advance how you will turn down the next cigarette you are offered.

Self-talk can also help overcome barriers. Make behavior change a priority in your life, and plan to commit the necessary time and effort. Ask yourself: How much time and energy will behavior change *really* require? Isn't the effort worth all the short- and long-term benefits?

Enhancing Your Readiness to Change

The transtheoretical, or "stages of change," model, developed by psychologists James Prochaska and Carlo DiClemente, has been shown to be an effective approach to lifestyle self-management. According to this model, you move through six well-defined stages as you work to change your target behavior. Try to identify your current stage, and then adopt appropriate strategies to move forward in the cycle of change:

• *Precontemplation: No intention of changing behavior.* If you're at this stage, try raising your consciousness of your target behavior and its effects on you and those around you. Ask yourself what has prevented you from changing in the past. Get the facts about your target behavior and the local resources available to help you with change.

• *Contemplation: Intending to take action within 6 months.* Begin keeping a written record of your target behavior and work on your analysis of the pros and cons of change. Try to boost self-efficacy through visualization, self-talk, and the support of other people.

• *Preparation: Planning to take action within a month.* At this stage, your next step is to create a specific plan for change (see the following section of the chapter).

• *Action: Outwardly changing behavior.* This stage requires the greatest commitment of time and energy to keep from reverting to old, unhealthy patterns of behavior. You'll need to use all the plans and strategies that you developed to this point.

• *Maintenance: Successful behavior change 6 or more months earlier.* To guard against slips and relapses during the maintenance stage, continue with the positive strategies you used in earlier stages.

Date __November 5__   Day   M (TU) W TH F SA SU

Time of day	M/S	Food eaten	Cals.	H	Where did you eat?	What else were you doing?	How did someone else influence you?	What made you want to eat what you did?	Emotions and feelings?	Thoughts and concerns?
7:30	M	1 C Crispix cereal 1/2 C skim milk coffee, black 1 C orange juice	110 40 — 120	3	dorm cafeteria	reading newspaper	eating w/ friends, but I ate what I usually eat	I always eat cereal in the morning	a little keyed up & worried	thinking about quiz in class today
10:30	S	1 apple	90	1	library	studying	alone	felt tired & wanted to wake up	tired	worried about next class
12:30	M	1 C chili 1 roll 1 pat butter 1 orange 2 oatmeal cookies 1 soda	290 120 35 60 120 150	2	cafeteria terrace	talking	eating w/ friends; we decided to eat at the cafeteria	wanted to be part of group	excited and happy	interested in hearing everyone's plans for the weekend

M/S = Meal or snack   H = Hunger rating (0–3)

Figure 1-4   Sample health journal entries.

For some behaviors, such as addictions, you may reach the sixth and final stage, *termination.* At this point, you are no longer tempted to lapse back into your old habits; you have a new self-image and total self-efficacy with regard to your target behavior.

Developing Skills for Change: Creating a Personalized Plan

Once you are committed to making a change, it's time to put together a detailed plan of action. Your key to success is a well-thought-out plan that sets goals, anticipates problems, and includes rewards.

1. Monitor Your Behavior and Gather Data   Begin by keeping careful records of the behavior you wish to change (your target behavior) and the circumstances surrounding it. Keep these records in a health journal, a notebook in which you write the details of your behavior along with observations and comments. Note exactly what the activity was, when and where it happened, what you were doing, and what your feelings were at the time (see the sample journal in Figure 1-4). Keep your journal for a week or two to get some solid information about the behavior you want to change.

2. Analyze the Data and Identify Patterns   After you have collected data on the behavior, analyze the data to identify patterns. When are you most hungry? When are

you most likely to overeat? What events seem to trigger your appetite? Perhaps you are especially hungry at mid-morning or when you put off eating dinner until 9:00. Perhaps you overindulge in food and drink when you go to a particular restaurant or when you're with certain friends. Be sure to note the connections between your feelings and such external cues as time of day, location, situation, and the actions of others around you. Do you always think of having a cigarette when you read the newspaper? Do you always bite your fingernails when you're studying?

3. Set Realistic, Specific Goals   Don't set an impossibly difficult overall goal for your program—going from a sedentary lifestyle to running a marathon within 2 months, for example. Working toward more realistic, achievable goals will greatly increase your chances of success. Your goal should also be specific and measurable, something you can easily track. Instead of a vague general goal such as improving eating habits or being more physically active, set a specific target—eating five servings of fruits and vegetables each day or walking or biking for 30 minutes at least 5 days per week.

Whatever your ultimate goal, it's a good idea to break it down into a few small steps. Your plan will seem less overwhelming and more manageable, increasing the chances that you'll stick to it. You'll also build in more opportunities to reward yourself (discussed in step 4), as well as milestones you can use to measure your progress. If you plan to lose 15 pounds, for example, you'll find it easier to take off 5 pounds at a time. If you want to start an exercise program, begin by taking 10- to 15-minute walks a few times per week. Take the easier steps first and work up to the harder steps. With each small success, you'll build your confidence and self-efficacy.

4. Devise a Strategy or Plan of Action   Next, you need to develop specific strategies and techniques that will support your day-to-day efforts at behavior change.

OBTAIN INFORMATION AND SUPPLIES   Identify campus and community resources that can provide practical help—for example, a stop-smoking course or a walking club. Take any necessary preparatory steps, such as signing up for a stress-management workshop or purchasing walking shoes, nicotine replacement patches, or a special calendar to track your progress.

MODIFY YOUR ENVIRONMENT   You can be more effective in changing behavior if you control the environmental cues that provoke it. This might mean not having cigarettes or certain foods or drinks in the house, not going to parties where you're tempted to overindulge, or not spending time with particular people, at least for a while. If your health journal reveals that you always get a candy bar at a certain vending machine, change your route so you don't pass by it. If you always end up taking a coffee break and chatting with friends when you go to the library to study, choose a different place to study, such as your room.

You can change the cues in your environment so they trigger the new behavior you want instead of the old one. Tape a picture of a cyclist speeding down a hill on your TV screen. Leave your exercise shoes in plain view. Put a chart of your progress in a special place at home to make your goals highly visible and inspire you to keep going. When you're trying to change an ingrained habit, small cues can play an important part in keeping you on track.

REWARD YOURSELF   Another very powerful way to affect your target behavior is to set up a reward system that will reinforce your efforts. Most people find it difficult to change long-standing habits for rewards they can't see right away. Giving yourself instant, real rewards for good behavior along the way will help you stick with a plan to change your behavior.

Carefully plan your reward payoffs and what they will be. Make a list of your activities and favorite events to use as rewards. They should be special, inexpensive, and preferably unrelated to food or alcohol. Depending on what you like to do, you might treat yourself to a concert, a ball game, a new CD, a long-distance phone call to a friend, a day off from studying for a long hike in the woods—whatever is rewarding to you.

INVOLVE THE PEOPLE AROUND YOU   Rewards and support can also come from family and friends. Tell them about your plan, and ask for their help. Encourage them to be active, interested participants. Ask them to support you when you set aside time to go running or avoid second helpings at Thanksgiving dinner. To help friends and family members who will be involved in your program respond appropriately, you may want to create a specific list of dos and don'ts.

PLAN AHEAD FOR CHALLENGING SITUATIONS   Take time out now to list situations and people that have the potential to derail your program and to develop possible coping mechanisms. For example, if you think that you'll have trouble exercising during finals week, schedule short bouts of physical activity as stress-reducing study breaks. If a visit to a friend who smokes is likely to tempt you to lapse, plan to bring nicotine patches, chewing gum, and a copy of your behavior change contract to strengthen your resolve.

5. Make a Commitment by Signing a Personal Contract   A serious personal contract—one that commits your word—can result in a higher chance of follow-through than will a casual, offhand promise. Your contract can help prevent procrastination by specifying the important dates and can also serve as a reminder of your personal commitment to change. Your contract should include a statement of your goal and your commitment to reaching it. Include details of your plan: the date you'll begin, the steps you'll use to measure your progress, the concrete strategies you've developed for promoting change, and the date you expect to reach your final goal. Have someone—preferably someone who will be actively helping you with your program—sign your contract as a witness.

A Sample Behavior Change Plan   Let's take the example of Michael, who wants to improve his diet. By monitoring his eating habits in his health journal for several weeks, he gets a good sense of his typical diet—what he eats and where he eats it. Through self-assessment and investigation, he discovers that he currently consumes only about one serving of fruit per week, much less than the recommended two to four servings per day. He also finds out that fruit is a major source of fiber, vitamins, minerals, and other substances important for good health. He sets the target of eating three servings of fruit per day as the overall goal for his behavior change plan. Then, Michael develops a specific plan for change, which he describes in a contract that commits him to reaching his goal (Figure 1-5). Once Michael has signed his contract, he's ready to take action.

You can apply the general behavior change planning framework presented in this chapter to any target behavior. Additional examples of behavior change plans are

I agree to increase my consumption of fruit from one serving per week to three servings per day. I will begin my program on __10/5__ and plan to reach my final goal by __12/7__. I have divided my program into three parts, with three separate goals. For each step in my program, I will give myself the reward listed.

1. I will begin to have a serving of fruit with breakfast on __10/5__.
   (Reward: _baseball game_)
2. I will begin to have a serving of fruit with lunch on __10/26__.
   (Reward: _music CD_)
3. I will begin to substitute fruit juice for soda for one snack each day on __11/16__.
   (Reward: _Concert_)

My plan for increasing fruit consumption includes the following strategies:
1. _Keeping my dorm room refrigerator stocked with easy-to-carry fruit and fruit juice._
2. _Packing fruit in my book backpack every day._
3. _Placing reminders to buy, carry, and eat fruit in my dorm room, backpack, and wallet._
4. _Buying lunch at a place that serves fruit or fruit juice._

I understand that it is important for me to make a strong personal effort to make the change in my behavior. I sign this contract as an indication of my personal commitment to reach my goal.

Michael Cook   9/28

Witness: _Katie Lim_   9/28

Figure 1-5 A sample behavior change contract.

presented in the Behavior Change Strategy sections that appear at the end of many chapters.

Putting Your Plan into Action

The starting date has arrived, and you are ready to put your plan into action. This stage requires commitment, the resolve to stick with the plan no matter what temptations you encounter. Remember all the good reasons you have to make the change—and remember that *you* are the boss. Use all your strategies to make your plan work. Make sure your environment is change-friendly, and obtain as much support and encouragement from others as possible. Keep track of your progress in your health journal, and give yourself regular rewards. And don't forget to give yourself a pat on the back—congratulate yourself, notice how much better you look or feel, and feel good about how far you've come and how you've gained control of your behavior.

Staying with It

As you continue with your program, don't be surprised when you run up against obstacles; they're inevitable. In fact, it's a good idea to expect problems and give yourself time to step back, see how you're doing, and make some changes before going on again. If you find your program is grinding to a halt, try to identify what is blocking your progress, and revise your plan if necessary. Consider whether the people around you are supportive, and evaluate your own levels of motivation and commitment. High levels of stress can also derail a behavior change program. If stress is a problem for you, consider making stress management your highest priority for behavior change (see Chapter 2).

COMMUNICATE! How do others see your future? Ask a couple of close friends how they see you 5, 10, and 20 years from now. Which of their predictions do you like? For instance, do they see you as happy, healthy, successful? Which predictions do you hope won't come true? What can you do now to control these outcomes?

BEING HEALTHY FOR LIFE

Your first few behavior change projects may never go beyond the planning stage. Those that do may not all succeed. But as you taste success by beginning to see

Changing behavior takes motivation. But how do you get motivated? The following strategies may help:

- Write down the potential benefits of the change. If you want to lose weight, your list might include increased ease of movement, energy, and self-confidence.

- Now write down the costs of not changing.

- Frequently visualize yourself achieving your goal and enjoying its benefits. If you want to manage time more effectively, picture yourself as a confident, organized person who systematically tackles important tasks and sets aside time each day for relaxation, exercise, and friends.

- Discount obstacles to change. Counter thoughts such as "I'll never have time to shop for and prepare healthy foods" with thoughts such as "Lots of other people have done it and so can I."

- Bombard yourself with propaganda. Subscribe to a self-improvement magazine. Take a class dealing with the change you want to make. Read books and watch talk shows on the subject. Post motivational phrases or pictures on your refrigerator or over your desk. Listen to motiva-tional tapes in the car. Talk to people who have already made the change you want to make.

- Build up your confidence. Remind yourself of other goals you've achieved. At the end of each day, mentally review your good decisions and actions. See yourself as a capable person, one who is in charge of his or her health.

- Create choices. You will be more likely to exercise every day if you have two or three types of exercise to choose from, and more likely to quit smoking if you've identified more than one way to distract yourself when you crave a cigarette. Get ideas from people who have been successful, and adapt some of their strategies to suit you.

- If you slip, keep trying. Research suggests that four out of five people will experience some degree of backsliding when they try to change a behavior. Only one in four succeeds the first time around. If you retain your commitment to change even when you lapse, you are still farther along the path to change than before you made the commitment. Try again. And again, if necessary.

progress and changes, you'll start to experience new and surprising positive feelings about yourself. You'll probably find that you're less likely to buckle under stress. You may begin opening doors to a new world of enjoyable physical and social events. You may accomplish things you never thought possible—winning a race, climbing a mountain, quitting smoking, having a lean, muscular body. Being healthy takes extra effort, but the paybacks in energy and vitality are priceless.

Once you've started, don't stop. Remember that maintaining good health is an ongoing process. Tackle one area at a time, but make a careful inventory of your health strengths and weaknesses and lay out a long-range plan. Take on the easier problems first, and then use what you have learned to attack more difficult areas. Look over your shoulder to make sure you don't fall into old habits. Keep informed about the latest health news and trends; research is constantly providing new information that directly affects daily choices and habits.

You can't completely control every aspect of your health. At least three other factors—heredity, health care, and environment—play important roles in your well-being. But you can make a difference—you can help create an environment around you that supports wellness for everyone. You can help support nonsmoking areas in public places. You can speak up in favor of more nutritious foods and better physical fitness facilities. You can include nonalcoholic drinks at your parties. You can vote for measures that improve access to health care for all people and support

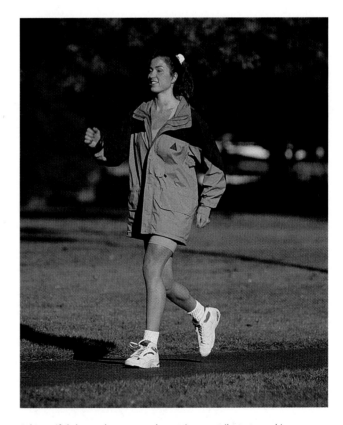

A beautiful day and a spectacular setting contribute to making exercise a satisfying and pleasurable experience. Choosing the right activity and doing it the right way are important elements in a successful health behavior change program.

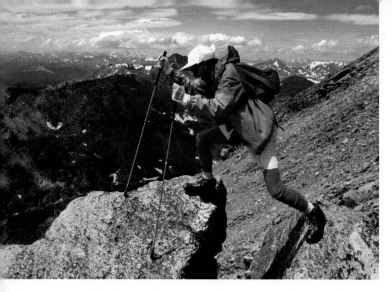

This retiree spends leisure time hiking and climbing mountains. If you want to enjoy vigor and health in *your* middle and old age, begin now to make the choices that will give you lifelong vitality.

politicians who sponsor them. You can also work on larger environmental challenges: air and water pollution, traffic congestion, overcrowding and overpopulation, and many others.

In your lifetime, you can choose to take an active role in the movement toward increased awareness, greater individual responsibility and control, healthier lifestyles, and a healthier planet. Your choices and actions will have a tremendous impact on your present and future wellness. The door is open, and the time is now—you simply have to begin.

Tips for Today

You are in charge of your health! Many of the decisions you make every day have an impact on the quality of your life, both now and in the future. By making positive choices, large and small, you help ensure a lifetime of wellness.

Right now you can

- Go for a 15-minute walk.

- Have an orange, a nectarine, or a plum for a snack.

- Call a friend and arrange a time to catch up with each other.

- Start thinking about whether you have a health behavior you'd like to change. If you do, consider the elements of a behavior change strategy. For example,

  - Begin a mental list of the pros and cons of the behavior.

  - Think of one or two rewards that will be meaningful to you as you reach interim goals.

- Think of someone who will support you in your attempts to make a behavior change—either someone who might want to make the same change you're contemplating or someone you can trust to provide you with encouragement. Talk to that person about your plan, get his or her feedback, and ask for his or her support.

SUMMARY

- Wellness is the ability to live life fully, with vitality and meaning. Wellness is dynamic and multidimensional; it incorporates physical, emotional, intellectual, spiritual, interpersonal and social, and environmental dimensions.

- As chronic diseases have become the leading cause of death in the United States, people have recognized that they have greater control over, and greater responsibility for, their health than ever before.

- The Healthy People initiative seeks to achieve a better quality of life for all Americans. The broad goals of the *Healthy People 2010* report are to increase quality and years of healthy life and to eliminate health disparities among Americans.

- Health-related differences among people that have implications for wellness can be described in the context of gender, ethnicity, income and education, disability, geographic location, and sexual orientation.

- Although heredity, environment, and health care all play roles in wellness and disease, a healthy lifestyle can mitigate their effects.

- To make lifestyle changes, you need information about yourself, your health habits, and resources available to help you change.

- You can increase your motivation for behavior change by examining the benefits and costs of change, boosting self-efficacy, and identifying and overcoming key barriers to change.

- The stages of change model describes six stages that people move through as they try to change their behavior: precontemplation, contemplation, preparation, action, maintenance, and termination.

- A specific plan for change can be developed by (1) monitoring behavior by keeping a journal; (2) analyzing the recorded data; (3) setting specific goals; (4) devising strategies for modifying the environment, rewarding yourself, and involving others; and (5) making a personal contract.

- Although we cannot control every aspect of our health, we can make a difference in helping create an environment that supports wellness for everyone.

1. Ask some older members of your family (parents and grandparents) what they recall about patterns of health and disease when they were young. Do they remember any large outbreaks of infectious disease? Did any of their friends or relatives die while very young or die of a disease that can now be treated? How have health concerns changed during their lifetime?

2. Choose a person you consider a role model, and interview him or her. What do you admire about this person? What can you borrow from his or her experiences and strategies for success?

1. Purchase a small notebook to use as your health journal throughout this course. At the end of each chapter, we include suggestions for journal entries—opportunities to think about topics and issues, explore and formulate your own views, and express your thoughts in written form. These exercises are intended to help you deepen your understanding of health topics and your own behaviors in relation to them. For your first journal entry, make a list of the positive behaviors that enhance your health (such as jogging and getting enough sleep). Consider what additions you can make to the list or how you can strengthen or reinforce these behaviors. (Don't forget to congratulate yourself for these positive aspects of your life.) Next, list the behaviors that detract from wellness (such as smoking and eating a lot of candy). Consider which of these behaviors you might be able to change. Use these lists as the basis for self-evaluation as you proceed through this book.

2. Think about what troubled you most during the past week. In your health journal, write down the names of three or four people who might be able to help you with whatever troubled you. If the problem persists, consider starting at the top of your list and talking to this person about it.

3. Think of the last time you did something you knew to be unhealthy primarily because those around you were doing it. How could you have restructured the situation or changed the environmental cues so that you could have avoided the behavior? In your health journal, describe several possible actions that will help you avoid the behavior the next time you're in a similar situation.

4. Make a list in your health journal of rewards that are meaningful to you. Add to the list as you think of new things to use. Refer to this list of rewards when you're developing plans for behavior change.

5. *Critical Thinking* In this book, several Journal Entry items are designed to help you sharpen your critical thinking skills. For your first Critical Thinking journal entry, write a short essay describing your sources of health information. Do you rely on newspaper or magazine articles? On television? On a particular Web site? On friends and family? What criteria do you use to evaluate this information, to assess its credibility, and to make decisions about your health?

Books

Columbia University's Health Education Program. 1998. *The "Go Ask Alice" Book of Answers.* New York: Henry Holt. *Presents answers to a variety of student-oriented health questions from the popular "Go Ask Alice" Web site.*

Prochaska, J. O., J. C. Norcross, and C. C. DiClemente. 1994. *Changing for Good: The Revolutionary Program That Explains the Six Stages of Change and Teaches You How to Free Yourself from Bad Habits.* New York: Morrow. *Outlines the authors' model of behavior change and offers suggestions and advice for each stage of change.*

Ridley, M. 2000. *Genome: The Autobiography of a Species in 23 Chapters.* New York: HarperCollins. *Describes the findings from the Human Genome Project and their implications for individuals and society as a whole.*

Swartzberg, J. E., and S. Margen. 2001. *The Complete Home Wellness Handbook.* New York: Rebus. *Provides information and strategies for promoting health and well-being throughout the life span.*

Newsletters

Consumer Reports on Health (800-234-2188; http://www.ConsumerReports.org)

Harvard Health Letter (800-829-9045; http://www.health.harvard.edu/newsletters)

Harvard Men's Health Watch (800-829-3341)

Harvard Women's Health Watch (800-829-5921)

HealthNews (800-848-9155)

Mayo Clinic Health Letter (800-333-9037)

University of California at Berkeley Wellness Letter (904-445-6414; http://www.wellnessletter.com)

WWW. Organizations, Hotlines, and Web Sites

The Internet addresses (also called uniform resource locators, or URLs) listed here were accurate at the time of publication. Up-to-date links to these and many other wellness-oriented Web sites are provided on the links pages of the *Core Concepts in Health* Online Learning Center (http://www.mhhe.com/insel9).

Centers for Disease Control and Prevention. Through phone, fax, and the Internet, the CDC provides a wide variety of health information.

> 404-332-4555 (CDC Infoline); 888-CDC-FAXX (CDC FAX)
> http://www.cdc.gov

Many other government Web sites provide access to health-related materials:

> Agency for Healthcare Research and Quality: http://www.ahrq.gov/consumer
> National Institutes of Health: http://www.nih.gov
> National Library of Medicine, MedlinePlus:
> http://www.nlm.nih.gov/medlineplus
> U.S. Consumer Gateway—Health:
> http://www.consumer.gov/health.htm

Go Ask Alice. Sponsored by the Columbia University Health Service, this site provides answers to student questions about stress, sexuality, fitness, and many other wellness topics.

> http://www.goaskalice.columbia.edu

Healthfinder. A gateway to online publications, Web sites, support and self-help groups, and agencies and organizations that produce reliable health information.

> http://www.healthfinder.gov

Healthy People 2010. Provides information on Healthy People objectives and priority areas.

> 202-205-8583; 301-468-5960
> http://web.health.gov/healthypeople

National Health Information Center (NHIC). Puts consumers in touch with the organizations that are best able to provide answers to health-related questions.

> 800-336-4797
> http://www.health.gov/nhic

National Women's Health Information Center. Provides information and answers to frequently asked questions.

> 800-994-WOMAN
> http://www.4woman.org

NOAH: New York Online Access to Health. Provides consumer health information in both English and Spanish.

> http://www.noah-health.org

The following are just a few of the many sites that provide consumer-oriented information on a variety of health issues:

InteliHealth: http://www.intelihealth.com
Mayo Health Oasis: http://www.mayohealth.org
Medscape Healthwatch: http://healthwatch.medscape.com
OnHealth: http://www.onhealth.com
WebMD: http://webmd.com

The following sites provide daily health news updates:

CNN/Health: http://www.cnn.com/HEALTH
HealthScout: http://www.healthscout.com
Yahoo Health News: http://dailynews.yahoo.com/h/hl
Your Health Daily: http://www.yourhealthdaily.com

SELECTED BIBLIOGRAPHY

American Cancer Society. 2001. *Cancer Facts and Figures—2001.* Atlanta: American Cancer Society.

American Heart Association. 2001. *2001 Heart and Stroke Statistical Update.* Dallas: American Heart Association.

Baker, C. 1999. *Your Genes, Your Choices: Exploring the Issues Raised by Genetic Research.* Washington, D.C.: American Association for the Advancement of Science.

Centers for Disease Control and Prevention. 1999. Achievements in public health, 1900–1999: Tobacco use, United States. *Morbidity and Mortality Weekly Report* 48(43): 986–993.

Centers for Disease Control and Prevention. 1999. Ten great public health achievements—United States, 1900–1999. *Morbidity and Mortality Weekly Report* 48(50): 1141.

Centers for Disease Control and Prevention. 2000. State- and sex-specific prevalence of selected characteristics—Behavioral Risk Factor Surveillance System. *MMWR Surveillance Summaries* 49(SS-6).

Centers for Disease Control and Prevention, Division of Nutrition and Physical Activity. 1999. *Promoting Physical Activity: A Guide for Community Action.* Champaign, Ill.: Human Kinetics.

Collins, F. S., and V. A. McKusick. 2001. Implications of the Human Genome Project for medical science. *Journal of the American Medical Association* 285(5): 540–544.

Cubbin, C., F. B. LeClere, and G. S. Smith. 2000. Socioeconomic status and the occurrence of fatal and nonfatal injury in the United States. *American Journal of Public Health* 90(1): 70–77.

Holtzman, N. A., and T. M. Marteau. 2000. Will genetics revolutionize medicine? *New England Journal of Medicine* 343(2): 141–144.

Martin, G., and J. Pear. 1999. *Behaviour Modification: What It Is and How to Do It,* 6th ed. Upper Saddle River, N.J.: Prentice-Hall.

Nathan, D. G., P. B. Fontanarosa, and J. D. Wilson. 2001. Opportunities for medical research in the 21st century. *Journal of the American Medical Association* 285(5): 533–534.

National Center for Health Statistics. 2000. Deaths: Final data for 1998. *National Vital Statistics Reports* 48(11).

National Center for Health Statistics. 2000. *Health, United States, 2000, with Adolescent Health Chartbook.* Hyattsville, Md.: National Center for Health Statistics.

Pink slip in your genes. 2001. *Scientific American,* January.

Schank, M. J. 1999. Self-health appraisal: Learning the difficulties of lifestyle change. *Journal of Nursing Education* 38(1): 10–12.

Schlicht, J., J. Godin, and D. C. Camaione. 1999. How to help your clients stick with an exercise program: Build self-efficacy to promote exercise adherence. *ACSM's Health and Fitness Journal* 3(6): 27–31.

Stages of change: Getting to where you want to be. 2000. *Harvard Heart Letter,* April.

U.S. Bureau of the Census. 1999. *Poverty 1998* (http://www.census.gov/hhes/poverty/poverty98/pv98est1.html; retrieved August 1, 2000).

U.S. Bureau of the Census. 2001. *Census 2000 Brief: Overview of Race and Hispanic Origin.* Washington, D.C.: U.S. Bureau of the Census.

U.S. Department of Health and Human Services. 1999. *Eliminating Racial and Ethnic Disparities in Health* (http://raceandhealth.hhs.gov/sidebars/sbinitOver.htm; retrieved July 31, 2000).

U.S. Department of Health and Human Services. 2000. *Healthy People 2010.* 2nd ed. Washington, D.C.: DHHS.

U.S. Department of Health and Human Services, Office of Minority Health. 1998. *Asian Americans and Pacific Islanders: Executive Overview* (http://www.omhrc.gov/overview2.htm; retrieved July 31, 2000).

Zimmerman, G. L., C. G. Olsen, and M. F. Bosworth. 2000. A "stages of change" approach to helping patients change behavior. *American Family Physician* 61(5): 1409–1416.

Stress: The Constant Challenge

LOOKING AHEAD

After reading this chapter, you should be able to

- Explain what stress is and how people react to it—physically, emotionally, and behaviorally

- Describe the relationship between stress and disease

- List common sources of stress

- Describe techniques for preventing and managing stress

- Put together a step-by-step plan for successfully managing the stress in your life

Everybody talks about stress. People say they're "overstressed" or "stressed out." They may blame stress for headaches or ulcers, and they may try to combat stress with aerobics classes—or drugs. But what is stress? And why is it important to manage it wisely?

Most people associate stress with negative events: the death of a close relative or friend, financial problems, or other unpleasant life changes that create nervous tension. But stress isn't merely nervous tension. And it isn't something to be avoided at all costs. Consider this list of common stressful situations or events: interviewing for a job, running in a race, being accepted to college, going out on a date, watching a basketball game, and getting a promotion.

Obviously, stress doesn't arise just from unpleasant situations. Stress can also be associated with physical challenges and the achievement of personal goals. Physical and psychological stress-producing factors can be either pleasant or unpleasant. What is crucial is how you respond, whether in positive, life-enhancing ways or in negative, counterproductive ways.

As a college student, you may be in one of the most stressful periods of your life. You may be on your own for the first time, or you may be juggling the demands of college with the responsibilities of a job, a family, or both. Financial pressures may be intense. Housing and transportation may be sources of additional hassles. You're also meeting new people, engaging in new activities, learning new information and skills, and setting a new course for your life. Good and bad, all these changes and challenges are likely to have a powerful effect on you, both physically and psychologically. Respond ineffectively to stress, and eventually it will take a toll on your sense of wellness. Learn effective responses, however, and you will enhance your health and gain a feeling of control over your life.

WHAT IS STRESS?

Just what is stress, if such vastly different situations can cause it? In common usage, "stress" refers to two different things: situations that trigger physical and emotional reactions *and* the reactions themselves. In this text, we'll use the more precise term **stressor** for situations that trigger physical and emotional reactions and the term **stress response** for those reactions. A date and a final exam, then, are stressors; sweaty palms and a pounding heart are symptoms of the stress response. We'll use the term stress to describe the general physical and emotional state that accompanies the stress response. A person on a date or taking a final exam experiences stress.

Physical Responses to Stressors

Imagine you are waiting to cross a street, perhaps daydreaming about a movie you saw last week. The light turns green and you step off the curb. Almost before you see it, you feel a car speeding toward you. With just a fraction of a second to spare, you leap safely out of harm's way. In that split second of danger and in the moments following it, you have experienced a predictable series of physical reactions. Your body has gone from a relaxed state to one prepared for physical action to cope with a threat to your life. Two major control systems in your body are responsible for your physical response to stressors: the nervous system and the endocrine system.

Actions of the Nervous System   The nervous system consists primarily of the brain, spinal cord, and nerves. Part of the nervous system is under voluntary control: commanding your arm to reach for a chocolate, for instance. The part that is not under conscious supervision, such as what controls the digestion of the chocolate, is known as the **autonomic nervous system.** In addition to digestion, it controls heart rate, breathing, blood pressure, and hundreds of other functions you normally take for granted.

The autonomic nervous system consists of two divisions. The **parasympathetic division** is in control when you are relaxed; it aids in digesting food, storing energy, and promoting growth. In contrast, the **sympathetic division** is activated during arousal or when there is an emergency, such as severe pain, anger, or fear. Sympathetic nerves act on many targets—on nearly every organ, sweat gland, blood vessel, and muscle, in fact—to enable your body to handle an emergency. In general, it commands your body to stop storing energy and instead to mobilize all energy resources to respond to the crisis.

Actions of the Endocrine System   One important target of the sympathetic nervous system is the **endocrine system.** This system of glands, tissues, and cells helps control body functions by releasing **hormones** and other chemical messengers into the bloodstream. Chemicals released into the blood are relatively free to travel throughout the body; however, stress hormones act only on those organs that have specialized stress hormone receptors.

How do both systems work together in an emergency? Let's go back to your close call with that car. As you first sense the car speeding toward you, your sympathetic nervous system prompts the **hypothalamus,** a control center in the brain, to release a chemical messenger to the

Terms

stressor Any physical or psychological event or condition that produces stress.

stress response The physiological changes associated with stress.

stress The collective physiological and emotional responses to any stimulus that disturbs an individual's homeostasis.

autonomic nervous system The branch of the peripheral nervous system that, largely without conscious thought, controls basic body processes; consists of the sympathetic and parasympathetic divisions.

parasympathetic division A division of the autonomic system that moderates the excitatory effect of the sympathetic division, slowing metabolism and restoring energy supplies.

sympathetic division A division of the autonomic nervous system that reacts to danger or other challenges by almost instantly accelerating body processes.

endocrine system The system of glands, tissues, and cells that secrete hormones into the bloodstream to influence metabolism and other body processes.

hormone A chemical messenger produced in the body and transported by the bloodstream to target cells or organs for specific regulation of their activities.

hypothalamus A part of the brain that activates, controls, and integrates the autonomic mechanisms, endocrine activities, and many body functions.

pituitary gland The "master gland," closely linked with the hypothalamus, that controls other endocrine glands and secretes hormones that regulate growth, maturation, and reproduction.

adrenocorticotropic hormone (ACTH) A hormone, formed in the pituitary gland, that stimulates the outer layer of the adrenal gland to secrete its hormones.

adrenal glands Two glands, one lying atop each kidney, their outer layer (cortex) producing steroid hormones such as cortisol, and their inner core (medulla) producing the hormones epinephrine and norepinephrine.

cortisol A steroid hormone secreted by the cortex (outer layer) of the adrenal gland; also called *hydrocortisone.*

epinephrine A hormone secreted by the medulla (inner core) of the adrenal gland; also called *adrenaline,* the "fear hormone."

norepinephrine A hormone secreted by the medulla (inner core) of the adrenal gland; also called *noradrenaline,* the "anger hormone."

endorphins Brain secretions that have pain-inhibiting effects.

fight-or-flight reaction A defense reaction that prepares an individual for conflict or escape by triggering hormonal, cardiovascular, metabolic, and other changes.

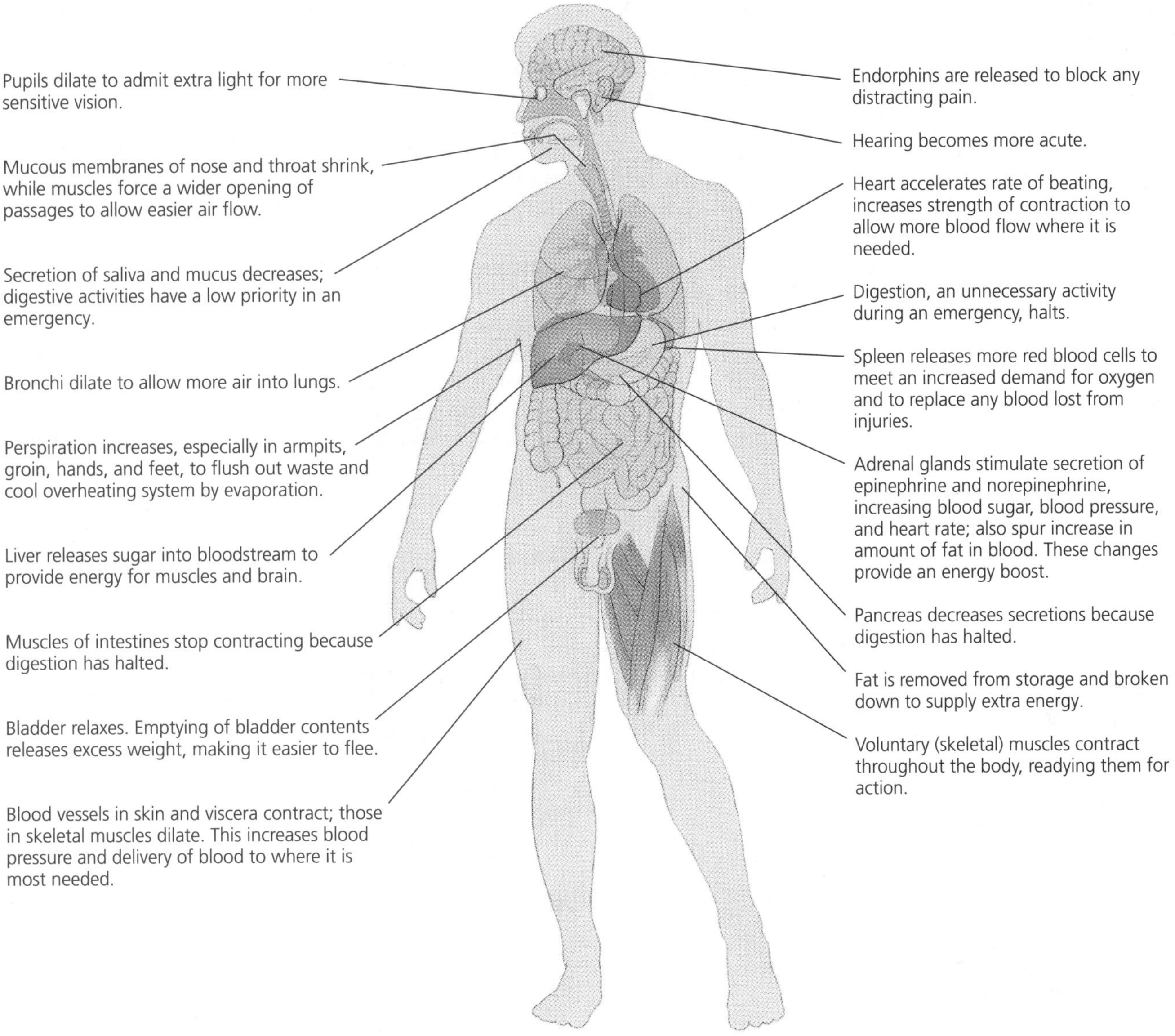

Pupils dilate to admit extra light for more sensitive vision.

Mucous membranes of nose and throat shrink, while muscles force a wider opening of passages to allow easier air flow.

Secretion of saliva and mucus decreases; digestive activities have a low priority in an emergency.

Bronchi dilate to allow more air into lungs.

Perspiration increases, especially in armpits, groin, hands, and feet, to flush out waste and cool overheating system by evaporation.

Liver releases sugar into bloodstream to provide energy for muscles and brain.

Muscles of intestines stop contracting because digestion has halted.

Bladder relaxes. Emptying of bladder contents releases excess weight, making it easier to flee.

Blood vessels in skin and viscera contract; those in skeletal muscles dilate. This increases blood pressure and delivery of blood to where it is most needed.

Endorphins are released to block any distracting pain.

Hearing becomes more acute.

Heart accelerates rate of beating, increases strength of contraction to allow more blood flow where it is needed.

Digestion, an unnecessary activity during an emergency, halts.

Spleen releases more red blood cells to meet an increased demand for oxygen and to replace any blood lost from injuries.

Adrenal glands stimulate secretion of epinephrine and norepinephrine, increasing blood sugar, blood pressure, and heart rate; also spur increase in amount of fat in blood. These changes provide an energy boost.

Pancreas decreases secretions because digestion has halted.

Fat is removed from storage and broken down to supply extra energy.

Voluntary (skeletal) muscles contract throughout the body, readying them for action.

Figure 2-1 The fight-or-flight reaction. In response to a stressor, the autonomic nervous system and the endocrine system cause physical changes that prepare the body to deal with an emergency.

nearby **pituitary gland.** In turn, the pituitary gland releases **adrenocorticotropic hormone (ACTH)** into the bloodstream. When ACTH reaches the **adrenal glands,** located just above the kidneys, it stimulates them to release **cortisol** and other key hormones into the bloodstream. Simultaneously, sympathetic nerves instruct your adrenal glands to release the hormones **epinephrine,** or adrenaline, and **norepinephrine,** which in turn trigger a series of profound changes as they circulate throughout your body (Figure 2-1). Your hearing and vision become more acute. Bronchi dilate to allow more air into your lungs. Your heart rate accelerates and blood pressure increases to ensure that your blood—and the oxygen, nutrients, and hormones it carries—will be rapidly distributed where needed. Your liver releases extra sugar into your bloodstream to provide an energy boost for your muscles and brain. **Endorphins** are released to relieve pain in case of injury. Blood cell production increases.

Taken together, these almost-instantaneous physical changes are called the **fight-or-flight reaction.** They give you the heightened reflexes and strength you need to dodge the car or deal with other stressors. Although these physical changes may vary in intensity, the same basic set of physical reactions occurs in response to any type of stressor, positive or negative.

The Return to Homeostasis Once a stressful situation ends, the parasympathetic division of your autonomic nervous system takes command and halts the reaction. It initiates the adjustments necessary to restore homeostasis, a state in which blood pressure, heart rate, hormone levels, and other vital functions are maintained within a narrow range of normal. Your parasympathetic nervous system calms your body down, slowing a rapid heartbeat, drying sweaty palms, and returning breathing to normal. Gradually, your body resumes its normal "housekeeping" functions, such as digestion and temperature regulation. Damage that may have been sustained during the fight-or-flight reaction is repaired. The day after you narrowly dodge the car, you wake up feeling fine. In this way, your body can grow, repair itself, and acquire reserves of energy. When the next crisis comes, you'll be ready to respond—instantly—again.

The Fight-or-Flight Reaction in Modern Life The fight-or-flight reaction is a part of our biological heritage, a survival mechanism that has served humankind well. It enables our bodies to quickly prepare to escape from an injury or to engage in a physical battle. In modern life, however, the fight-or-flight reaction is often absurdly inappropriate. Many of the stressors we face in everyday life do not require a physical response—for example, an exam, a mess left by a roommate, or a red traffic light. The fight-or-flight reaction prepares the body for physical action regardless of whether such action is a necessary or appropriate response to a particular stressor.

Emotional and Behavioral Responses to Stressors

The physical response to a stressor may vary in intensity from person to person and situation to situation, but we all experience a similar set of physical changes—the fight-or-flight reaction. Emotionally and behaviorally, however, there is a great deal of variation in how people view potential stressors and how people respond to them.

Effective and Ineffective Responses Our emotional and behavioral responses to stressors are as critical to our overall experience of stress as are our physical responses. Common emotional responses to stressors include anxiety, depression, and fear. Although emotional responses are determined in part by inborn personality, we often can moderate or learn to control them. Coping techniques are discussed in detail later in the chapter.

Our behavioral responses—controlled by the **somatic nervous system,** which manages our conscious actions — are under our control. Effective behavioral responses can promote wellness and enable us to function at our best. Ineffective behavioral responses to stressors can impair wellness and can become stressors themselves. Depending on the stressor involved, effective behavioral responses may include talking, laughing, exercising, meditating, learning time-management skills, or finding a more compatible roommate. Inappropriate behavioral responses include overeating and using tobacco, alcohol, or other drugs. Emotional and behavioral responses to stressors depend on a complex set of factors that includes personality, cultural background, gender, and past experiences.

Personality and Stress Some people seem to be nervous, irritable, and easily upset by minor annoyances; others are calm and composed even in difficult situations. Scientists remain unsure just why this is or how the brain's complex emotional mechanisms work. But personality, the sum of behavioral and emotional tendencies, clearly affects how people perceive and react to stressors. To investigate the links among personality, stress, and overall wellness, researchers have looked at different constellations of characteristics, or "personality types."

TYPE A AND B PERSONALITIES Cardiologists Meyer Friedman and Ray Rosenman describe people with "Type A personalities" as ultracompetitive, controlling, impatient, aggressive, and hostile. Type A people tend to react more explosively to stressors, and they are upset by events that others would consider only mild annoyances. On the other hand, Type B individuals are relaxed, contemplative, and much less hurried. They tend to be less frustrated by the flow of daily events and more tolerant of the behavior of others. Studies indicate that certain characteristics of the Type A pattern—anger, cynicism, and hostility—increase the risk of heart disease. Type A people may also have a higher perceived stress level and more problems coping with stress.

THE HARDY PERSONALITY Researchers have also looked at personality traits that seem to enable people to deal more successfully with stress. Psychologist Suzanne Kobasa examined "hardiness," a particular form of optimism. She found that people with a hardy personality view potential stressors as challenges and opportunities for growth and learning, rather than as burdens. Hardy people tend to perceive fewer situations as stressful, and their reaction to stressors tends to be less intense. They are committed to their activities, have a sense of inner purpose, and feel at least partly in control of events in their lives.

Is there anything people can do to change their personality and become more stress-resistant? It is unlikely that

Terms

homeostasis A state of stability and consistency in an individual's physiological functioning.

somatic nervous system The branch of the peripheral nervous system that governs motor functions and sensory information; largely under our conscious control.

general adaptation syndrome (GAS) A pattern of stress responses consisting of three stages: alarm, resistance, and exhaustion.

eustress Stress resulting from a pleasant stressor.

distress Stress resulting from an unpleasant stressor.

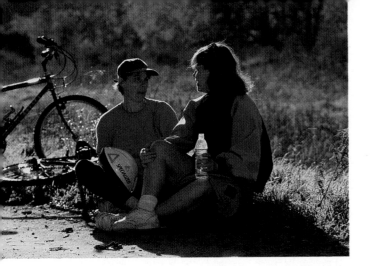

A person's emotional and behavioral responses to stressors depend on many different factors, including personality, gender, and cultural background. Research suggests that women are more likely than men to respond to stressors by seeking social support.

more likely to respond behaviorally with a pattern of "tend-and-befriend"—nurturing friends and family and seeking social support and social contacts. Rather than becoming aggressive or withdrawing from difficult situations, women are more likely to act to create and enhance their social networks in ways that reduce stress.

Past Experiences   Your past experiences significantly influence your response to stressors. For example, if you were unprepared for the first speech you gave in your speech class and performed poorly, you will probably experience greater anxiety in response to future assignments. If you had performed better, your confidence and sense of control would increase, and you would probably experience less stress with future speeches. Effective behavioral responses, such as careful preparation and visualizing yourself giving a successful speech, can help overcome the effects of negative past experiences.

COMMUNICATE!   It is all too easy to mistake the source of stress. Recall a situation in which you lost your temper at a friend or family member. Were you under stress from a different source at the time? Try to practice coming up with a better way to handle such an encounter next time. For example, "I know you want to talk about who's responsible for getting the car fixed, but I'm really under pressure to finish this assignment right now. Can we talk later?"

you can change your basic personality. However, you can change your typical behaviors and patterns of thinking and develop positive techniques for coping with stressors. Strategies for successful stress management are described later in the chapter.

Cultural Background   We all know that cultural stereotypes are exaggerations and that a variety of personalities exist within every ethnic group. However, people of various cultures do differ in their values, lifestyles, and what they consider to be acceptable behavior. It's not surprising that perceiving and dealing with stress are also influenced by the family and the culture in which you are brought up. Suppose you go out on a date with someone who doesn't say much. You might worry that the person is behaving this way because he or she doesn't like you, and you may experience stress as a result. If you are quiet by nature and because of your cultural background, you'll probably feel things are going just fine.

Gender   Like cultural background, our gender role—the activities, abilities, and behaviors our culture expects of us based on whether we're male or female—also affects our experience of stress. Some behavioral responses to stressors, such as crying or openly expressing anger, may be deemed more appropriate for one gender than the other. Strict adherence to gender roles can thus place limits on how a person responds to stress and can itself become a source of stress. Adherence to traditional gender roles can also affect the perception of a potential stressor. For example, if a man derives most of his sense of self-worth from his work, retirement may be a more stressful life change for him than for a woman whose self-image is based on several different roles.

Although both men and women experience the fight-or-flight physiological response to stress, women are

STRESS AND DISEASE

The role of stress in health and disease is complex, and much remains to be learned. However, mounting evidence suggests that stress—interacting with a person's genetic predisposition, personality, social environment, and health-related behaviors—can increase vulnerability to numerous ailments. A variety of related theories have been proposed to explain the relationship between stress and disease.

The General Adaptation Syndrome

Biologist Hans Selye, working in the 1930s and 1940s, was one of the first scientists to develop a comprehensive theory of stress and disease. Selye coined the term **general adaptation syndrome (GAS)** to describe what he believed was a universal and predictable response pattern to all stressors. He recognized that stressors could be pleasant, such as attending a party, or unpleasant, such as getting a flat tire or a bad grade. He called stress triggered by a pleasant stressor **eustress** and stress triggered by an unpleasant stressor **distress.** The sequence of physical responses associated with GAS is the same for both eustress and distress and occurs in three stages: alarm, resistance, and exhaustion (Figure 2-2).

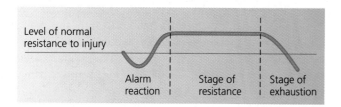

Figure 2-2 The general adaptation syndrome. Selye observed a predictable sequence of responses to stress. During the alarm phase, a lower resistance to injury is evident. With continued stress, resistance to injury is actually enhanced. With prolonged exposure to repeated stressors, exhaustion sets in, with a return of low resistance levels seen during acute stress.

Alarm This stage includes the complex sequence of events brought on by the activation of the sympathetic nervous system and the endocrine system—the fight-or-flight reaction. During this stage, the body is more susceptible to disease or injury because it is geared up to deal with a crisis. A person in this phase may experience headaches, indigestion, and anxiety.

Resistance With continued stress, Selye theorized that the body developed a new level of homeostasis in which it was more resistant to disease and injury than it normally would be. During the resistance stage, a person can cope with normal life and added stress.

Exhaustion As you might imagine, both the mobilization of forces during the alarm reaction and the maintenance of homeostasis during the resistance stage require a considerable amount of energy. If a stressor persists or if several stressors occur in succession, general exhaustion results. This is not the sort of exhaustion people complain of after a long, busy day. It's a life-threatening type of physiological exhaustion characterized by such symptoms as distorted perceptions and disorganized thinking.

Allostatic Load

While Selye's model of GAS is still viewed as a key contribution to modern stress theory, some aspects of it are now discounted. For example, increased susceptibility to disease after repeated or prolonged stress is now thought to be due to the effects of the stress response itself rather than to a depletion of resources (Selye's exhaustion state). In particular, long-term overexposure to stress hormones such as cortisol has been linked with health problems. Researchers have termed the long-term wear and tear of the stress response the *allostatic load*. An individual's allostatic load is dependent on many factors, including ge-

netics, life experiences, and emotional and behavioral responses to stressors. A high allostatic load may be due to frequent stressors, poor adaptation to common stressors, an inability to shut down the stress response, or imbalances in the stress response of different body systems. Researchers have linked high allostatic load with heart disease, hypertension, obesity, and reduced brain and immune system functioning. In other words, when your allostatic load exceeds your ability to cope, you are more likely to get sick.

Psychoneuroimmunology

One of the most fruitful areas of current research into the relationship between stress and disease is **psychoneuroimmunology (PNI).** PNI is the study of the interactions among the nervous system, the endocrine system, and the immune system. The underlying premise of PNI is that stress, through the actions of the nervous and endocrine systems, impairs the immune system and thereby affects health.

Researchers have discovered a complex network of nerve and chemical connections between the nervous and endocrine systems and the immune system. We have already seen that the hormones and other chemical messengers released during the stress response produce profound physical changes to prepare the body to deal with a stressor. These compounds also affect the immune system. For example, increased levels of cortisol are linked to a decreased number of immune system cells, or lymphocytes. Epinephrine and norepinephrine appear to promote the release of lymphocytes but at the same time reduce their efficiency.

The nervous, endocrine, and immune systems share other connections. Scientists have identified hormone-like substances called neuropeptides that appear to translate emotions into physiological events. Neuropeptides are produced and received by both brain and immune cells, so that the brain and the immune system share a biochemical "language," which is also the language of emotions. The biochemical changes that accompany particular emotions can strongly influence the functioning of the immune system; some emotions may suppress lymphocyte function, while others promote it.

Links Between Stress and Specific Conditions

People who have unresolved chronic stress in their lives or who handle stressors poorly are at risk for a wide range of health problems. In the short term, the problem might just be a cold, a stiff neck, or a stomachache. Over the long term, the problems can be more severe—cardiovascular disease, high blood pressure, or impairment of the immune system.

Cardiovascular Disease During the stress response, heart rate increases and blood vessels constrict, causing

Like a computer that registers information in response to typing on a keyboard, your brain is able to respond to and store information about changes in your environment. Unlike a computer, your brain has the attribute of plasticity—it physically changes its structure and function in response to experience. Also unlike a computer, your brain is altered by psychological stress. Moderate stress enhances the ability to acquire information and remember daily events, while high levels of acute stress can impair learning. For example, people can often remember minute details following a fender bender but can't recall the events surrounding a major car crash. Thus, it is good to be a little bit nervous before an exam—but not highly anxious.

The effects of stress on brain form and function are apparent in a structure called the hippocampus, which is involved in learning and memory. High levels of chronic stress cause brain cells (neurons) in the hippocampus to shrink in size or die, thus impairing learning and memory. Exciting new research in neuroscience has revealed that the hippocampus actually grows new neurons during adulthood. However, stress acts to reduce new cell birth in the hippocampus, reducing the replacement of lost neurons. Together, these effects of stress result in fewer neurons and fewer connections between neurons in the hippocampus, thus decreasing the capacity for information processing. People who are depressed or who suffer from post-traumatic stress disorder have higher levels of stress hormones in their bloodstream and smaller hippocampi than others. Even in the absence of a serious disorder, it is thought that the accumulation of stress effects across the life span can contribute to brain aging. Thus, the way you cope with stress can affect the way your brain works both immediately and over the long term.

blood pressure to rise. Chronic high blood pressure is a major cause of *atherosclerosis,* a disease in which the lining of the blood vessels becomes damaged and caked with fatty deposits. These deposits can block arteries, causing heart attacks and strokes. Recent research suggests that certain types of emotional responses increase a person's risk of cardiovascular disease. So-called hot reactors, people who exhibit extreme increases in heart rate and blood pressure in response to emotional stressors, may face an increased risk of cardiovascular problems.

Altered Functioning of the Immune System   Sometimes you seem to get sick when you can least afford it—during exam week, when you're going on vacation, or when you have a big job interview. As research in PNI suggests, this is more than mere coincidence. Some of the health problems linked to stress-related changes in immune function include vulnerability to colds and other infections, asthma and allergy attacks, increased risk of cancer, and flare-ups of chronic diseases such as genital herpes.

Other Health Problems   Many other health problems may be caused or worsened by uncontrolled stress:

- Digestive problems such as stomachaches, diarrhea, constipation, irritable bowel syndrome, and ulcers
- Tension headaches and migraines
- Insomnia and fatigue
- Injuries, including on-the-job injuries caused by repetitive strain
- Menstrual irregularities, impotence, and pregnancy complications
- Psychological problems, including depression, anxiety, eating disorders, and post-traumatic stress disorder (PTSD), which afflicts people who have suffered or witnessed severe trauma

COMMON SOURCES OF STRESS

We are surrounded by stressors—at home, at school, on the job, and within ourselves. Being able to recognize potential sources of stress is an important step in successfully managing the stress in our lives.

Major Life Changes

Any major change in your life that requires adjustment and accommodation can be a source of stress. Early adulthood and the college years are typically associated with many significant changes, such as moving out of the family home, establishing new relationships, setting educational and career goals, and developing a sense of identity and purpose. Even changes typically thought of as positive—graduation, job promotion, marriage—can be stressful.

Clusters of major life changes may be linked to the development of health problems in some people. Research indicates that some life changes, particularly those that are perceived negatively, can affect health. However, personality and coping skills are important moderating influences. People with a strong support network and a stress-resistant personality are less likely to become ill in response to major life changes than people with fewer internal and external resources.

Daily Hassles

Have you done any of the following in the past week?

- Misplaced your keys, wallet, or an assignment

Headaches come in various types but are often grouped into three major categories: tension headaches, migraines, and cluster headaches. Other types of headaches have underlying organic causes, such as sinus congestion or infection.

Tension Headaches

Approximately 90% of all headaches are tension headaches, characterized by a dull, steady pain, usually on both sides of the head. It may feel as though a band of pressure is tightening around the head, and the pain may extend to the neck and shoulders. Acute tension headaches may last from hours to days, while chronic tension headaches may occur almost every day for months or even years. Psychological stress, poor posture, and immobility are the leading causes of tension headaches. There is no cure, but the pain can be relieved with over-the-counter painkillers and with therapies such as massage, relaxation, hot or cold showers, and rest.

If your headaches are frequent, keep a diary with details about the events surrounding each one. Are your headaches associated with late nights, academic deadlines, or long periods spent sitting at a computer? If you can identify the stressors that are consistently associated with your headaches, you can begin to gain more control over the situation. If you suffer persistent tension headaches, you should consult your physician.

Migraines

Migraines typically progress through a series of stages lasting from several minutes to several days. They may produce a variety of symptoms, including throbbing pain that starts on one side of the head and may spread; heightened sensitivity to light; visual disturbances such as flashing lights; nausea; and fatigue. About 70% of migraine sufferers are women, and migraine headaches may have a genetic component. Research suggests that people who get migraines may have abnormally excitable nerve cells in their brains. When triggered, these nerve cells send a wave of electrical activity throughout the brain, which in turn causes migraine symptoms. Potential triggers include menstruation, stress, fatigue, atmospheric changes, specific sounds or odors, and certain foods. The frequency of attacks varies from a few in a lifetime to several per week.

Keeping a headache journal can help a migraine sufferer identify headache triggers—the first step to avoiding them. In addition, many new treatments can help reduce the frequency, severity, and duration of migraines.

Cluster Headaches

Cluster headaches are extremely severe headaches that cause intense pain in and around one eye. They usually occur in clusters of one to three headaches each day over a period of weeks or months, alternating with periods of remission in which no headaches occur. About 90% of people with cluster headaches are male. There is no known cause or cure for cluster headaches, but a number of treatments are available. During cluster periods, refrain from smoking cigarettes and drinking alcohol because these activities can trigger attacks.

- Had an argument with a troublesome neighbor, coworker, or customer
- Waited in a long line
- Been stuck in traffic or had another problem with transportation
- Worried about money
- Been upset about the weather

While major life changes are undoubtedly stressful, they seldom occur regularly. Psychologist Richard Lazarus has proposed that minor problems—life's daily hassles—can be an even greater source of stress because they occur much more often. People who perceive hassles negatively are likely to experience a moderate stress response every time they are faced with one. Over time, this can take a significant toll on health. Researchers have found that for some people, daily hassles contribute to a general decrease in overall wellness.

College Stressors

College is a time of major life changes and abundant minor hassles. You will be learning new information and skills and making major decisions about your future. You may be away from home for the first time, or you may be adding extra responsibilities to a life already filled with job and family.

Academic Stressors   Exams, grades, and choosing a major are among the many academic stressors faced by college students. In addition to an increased workload compared to that in high school, many students are unpleasantly surprised by a more rigorous evaluation of their work in college. Higher-quality efforts are expected of college students, so earning good grades takes more effort and dedication. Careful planning and preparation can help make academic stressors more predictable and manageable.

Students close to graduation may find themselves faced with the need to plan for life after college—a potentially daunting task. Remember that you'll have many opportunities to change career paths in the future, and the training and life experience gained from one path can often be transferred to other endeavors.

Interpersonal Stressors   The college years often involve such potential stressors as establishing new rela-

The college experience has the potential, and the intention, of making you a more mature individual with the capacity to function successfully in the real world. Any experience with so much influence over your immediate state of mind and long-term behavior is bound to be stressful. The fact that college is stressful is not a new discovery. UCLA's Higher Education Research Institute has been surveying first-year college students since 1966. The 1999 survey revealed that, more than ever, college students feel overwhelmed with responsibility and under immense pressure to excel. These feelings stem from increased demands in college (more college students report that they will work full-time while in college), a highly competitive job market, and, on average, a decreased preparedness on the part of incoming students compared to past years (high school grade inflation is greater than ever). Interestingly, many stressors associated with the college experience have little to do with scholastics directly. These stressors include things like relationship difficulties, adjusting to a stranger as a roommate, leaving home, financial worries, and lack of privacy.

Twice as many female as male students report they frequently feel overwhelmed. This could be due to a real difference in stress perception between genders or to a gender-related difference in the likelihood of honestly reporting stress levels. However, more women than men are concerned that they will not have enough money to finish their schooling. Female students also report that they spend more time studying, doing volunteer work, and tending to housework or child-care responsibilities; male students report more time exercising, playing sports, watching television, and playing computer and video games. These survey results suggest that women spend more time than men on goal-oriented activities, which may contribute to the gender difference in perceived stress.

Irrespective of gender, college *is* stressful. For you to fully realize your college expectations, you will need to evaluate your stress levels, identify the common stressors that you experience, and learn successful coping techniques.

SOURCE: UCLA Higher Education Research Institute. 2001. *An Overview of the 2000 Freshman Norms* (http://www.gseis.ucla.edu/heri/00_exec_summary.htm; retrieved January 22, 2001). UCLA Higher Education Research Institute. 2000. *An Overview of the 1999 Freshman Norms* (http://www.gseis.ucla.edu/heri/test/executive.htm; retrieved February 1, 2000).

tionships and balancing multiple roles—student, employee, friend, spouse, parent, and so on. You'll have the opportunity to meet new people and make new friends at the start of every term and in every new class and activity. Social engagements may be exhilarating for some and painful for others. Viewed as an exciting challenge or an odious necessity, interacting with others involves attention, on-the-spot decision making, and energy expenditure—and is stressful. Be yourself, go with the flow, and try not to be overly concerned with being liked by everyone you meet.

Time-Related Pressures   Do you accept too many responsibilities or manage your time poorly? Time pressures are a problem for most students, but they may be particularly acute for those who also have job and family responsibilities. Most people do have enough time to fulfill all of their responsibilities, but they don't manage their time or their priorities effectively. For these people, it's important to make a plan and *stick to it*. Effective time-management-strategies are described in the next section.

Financial Concerns   As young adults leave home and become independent, financial responsibilities such as paying tuition, taking out loans, and managing living expenses are likely to arise. Most students live off savings from full-time summer jobs and part-time jobs during the school year, and many take out loans in order to pay tu-

ition. Some students work full-time and support a family while taking college courses. Regardless of your situation, try to avoid extravagant spending and excessive worry about finances. Instead, use your resources to pursue academic achievements that will help enhance your future financial picture.

Job-Related Stressors

In recent surveys, Americans rate their jobs as one of the key sources of stress in their lives. Tight schedules and overtime contribute to time-related pressures, and worries about job performance, salary, and job security are a source of stress for some people. Interactions with bosses, coworkers, and customers can also contribute to stress. High levels of job stress are also common for people who are left out of important decisions relating to their jobs. When workers are given the opportunity to shape how their jobs are performed, job satisfaction goes up and stress levels go down.

If job-related (or college-related) stress is severe or chronic, the result can be **burnout**, a state of physical, mental, and emotional exhaustion. Burnout occurs most

burnout A state of physical, mental, and emotional exhaustion.

Terms

Stress is universal, but some groups within the United States face unique stressors and have higher-than-average rates of stress-related physical and emotional problems. These include women, ethnic minorities, the economically disadvantaged, and people with disabilities. Many of the unique stressors that affect special populations stem from prejudice—biased, negative attitudes toward a group of people.

Discrimination occurs when people act according to their prejudices; it can be blatant or subtle. Blatant examples of discrimination are not common, but they are major stressors, akin to significant life changes. Examples include a swastika painted on a Jewish studies house, the defacement of a sculpture honoring the achievements of gay men, and sexual harassment during a fraternity party. More subtle acts may occur much more frequently. For example, an African American student in a mostly white college town feels that shopkeepers are keeping an eye on him, a student using a wheelchair has difficulty with narrow aisles and high counters at local stores, and a female business executive finds that restaurants always assume the lunch check should go to her male clients. Some of these social stressors are unique to certain groups, and it may be difficult for other people to understand how serious such stressors can be.

Women and minorities also often face additional job-related stressors because of stereotypes and discrimination. They make less money than white males in comparable jobs and with comparable levels of education. Women are more likely to face sexual harassment on the job. As employment opportunities have expanded for women, they also often find themselves balancing multiple roles—employee, parent, spouse, caregiver to aging parents, and so on. Women who work outside the home still do most of the housework, and time-related stress can be severe. All these types of stressors can contribute to higher levels of stress-related health problems.

often in highly motivated and driven individuals who come to feel that their work is not recognized or that they are not accomplishing their goals. People in the helping professions—teachers, social workers, caregivers, police officers, and so on—are also prone to burnout. For some people who suffer from burnout, a vacation or leave of absence may be appropriate. For others, a reduced work schedule, better communication with superiors, or a change in job goals may be necessary.

Social Stressors

Although social support is a key buffer against stress, your interactions with others can also be a source of stress themselves. As mentioned earlier, the college years are a time of great change in interpersonal relationships. The community and society in which you live can also be major sources of stress. Social stressors include prejudice and discrimination. You may feel stress as you try to relate to people of other ethnic or socioeconomic groups. As a member of a particular ethnic group, you may feel pressure to assimilate into mainstream society. If English is not your first language, you face the added burden of conducting many daily activities in a language with which you may not be completely comfortable.

Other stressors are found in the environment and in ourselves. Environmental stressors—external conditions or events that cause stress—include loud noises, unpleasant smells, and natural disasters. Internal stressors can occur as we put pressure on ourselves to reach personal goals and evaluate our progress and performance. Physical and emotional states such as illness and exhaustion are other examples of internal stressors.

TECHNIQUES FOR MANAGING STRESS

What can you do about all this stress? A great deal. And the effort is well worth the time: People who manage stress effectively not only are healthier but also have more time to enjoy life and accomplish their goals.

Social Support and Communication

People need people. Sharing fears, frustrations, and joys not only makes life richer but also seems to contribute to the well-being of body and mind. Allow yourself time to nourish and maintain a network of people at home, at work, at school, or in your community that you can count on for emotional support, feedback, and nurturance. Communication skills, discussed in detail in Chapter 4, can be critical in forming and maintaining intimate relationships.

Exercise

Exercise helps maintain a healthy body and mind. One study found that just a brisk 10-minute walk leaves people feeling more relaxed and energetic for up to 2 hours. Researchers have also found that people who exercise regularly react with milder physical stress responses before, during, and after exposure to stressors. People who took three brisk 45-minute walks a week for 3 months reported that they perceived fewer daily hassles. Their sense of wellness also increased.

It's not hard to incorporate light to moderate exercise into your day. Walk to class or bike to the store instead of driving. Use the stairs instead of the elevator. Take a walk with a friend instead of getting a cup of coffee. Go bowling, play tennis, or roller-skate instead of seeing a movie.

Meaningful connections with others can play a key role in stress management and overall wellness. A sense of isolation can lead to chronic stress, which in turn can increase one's susceptibility to temporary illnesses like colds and to chronic illnesses like heart disease. Although the mechanism isn't clear, social isolation can be as significant to mortality rates as factors like smoking, high blood pressure, and obesity.

There is no single best pattern of social support that works for everyone. However, research suggests that having a variety of types of relationships may be important for wellness. To help determine whether your social network measures up, circle true or false for the following statements.

T   F   1. If I needed an emergency loan of $100, there is someone I could get it from.

T   F   2. There is someone who takes pride in my accomplishments.

T   F   3. I often meet or talk with family or friends.

T   F   4. Most people I know think highly of me.

T   F   5. If I needed an early morning ride to the airport, there's no one I would feel comfortable asking to take me.

T   F   6. I feel there is no one with whom I can share my most private worries and fears.

T   F   7. Most of my friends are more successful making changes in their lives than I am.

T   F   8. I would have a hard time finding someone to go with me on a day trip to the beach or country.

To calculate your score, add the number of true answers to questions 1–4 and the number of false answers to questions 5–8. If your score is 4 or more, you should have enough support to protect your health. If your score is 3 or less, you may need to reach out. There are a variety of things you can do to strengthen your social ties:

- *Foster friendships.* Keep in regular contact with your friends. Offer respect, trust, and acceptance, and provide help and support in times of need.

- *Keep your family ties strong.* Stay in touch with the family members you feel close to. Participate in family activities and celebrations.

- *Get involved with a group.* Do volunteer work, take a class, attend a lecture series, join a religious group. Choose activities that are meaningful to you and that include direct involvement with other people.

- *Build your communication skills.* The more you share your feelings with others, the closer the bonds between you will become. When others are speaking, be a considerate and attentive listener.

Individual relationships change over the course of your life, but it's never too late to build friendships or become more involved in your community. Your investment of time and energy in your social network will pay off—in a brighter outlook now, and in better health and well-being for the future.

SOURCE: Friends can be good medicine. 1998. *Mind/Body Newsletter* 7(1): 3–6. QUIZ SOURCE: Japenga, A. 1995. A family of friends. *Health,* November/December, 94. Adapted with permission. Copyright © 1995 Health.

Make a habit of taking a brisk after-dinner stroll. Plan hikes and easy bike outings for the weekends.

Nutrition

A healthy diet will give you an energy bank to draw on whenever you experience stress. Eating wisely also will enhance your feelings of self-control and self-esteem. Learning the principles of sound nutrition is easy, and sensible eating habits rapidly become second nature when practiced regularly. One special nutrition tip for stress management: Avoid or limit caffeine. (For more on sound nutrition, see Chapter 9.)

Sleep

Lack of sleep can be both a cause and an effect of excess stress. Without sufficient sleep, our mental and physical processes steadily deteriorate. We get headaches, feel irritable, are unable to concentrate, forget things, and may be more susceptible to illness. Fatigue and sleep deprivation are major factors in many fatal car, truck, and train crashes. Extreme sleep deprivation can lead to hallucinations and other psychotic symptoms. Adequate sleep, on the other hand, improves mood, fosters feelings of competence and self-worth, and supports optimal mental and emotional functioning. If you are sleep-deprived, sleeping extra hours may significantly improve your daytime alertness and mental abilities.

Nearly everyone, at some time in life, has trouble falling asleep or staying asleep—a condition known as insomnia. Strategies for overcoming insomnia include going to bed at the same time every night and getting up at the same time every morning; avoiding tobacco, caffeine in the later part of the day, and alcohol before bedtime; exercising every day, but not too close to bedtime; using your bed only for sleeping, not for eating, reading, or watching TV; and relaxing and having a light snack before you go to bed.

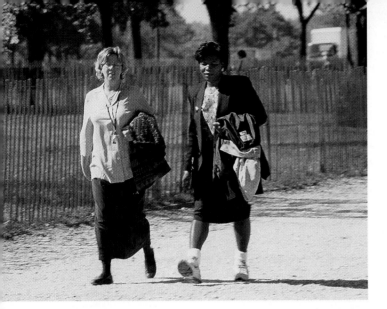

Exercise is a particularly effective antidote to stress. A lunchtime walk gives these coworkers a chance to both exercise and foster friendships.

Time Management

A surprising number of the stressors in most people's lives relate to time. Many people never seem to have enough time, and they always seem to feel overwhelmed by the pace of their lives. Others have too much time on their hands and are often bored. Learning to manage your time successfully is crucial to coping with the stressors you face every day. Three common factors that negatively impact time management for college students are perfectionism, overcommitment, and procrastination. If these or other time-related stressors are a problem for you, try some or all of the following strategies for managing your time more productively and creatively:

• *Set priorities.* Divide your tasks into three groups: essential, important, and trivial. Focus on the first two. Ignore the third.

• *Schedule tasks for peak efficiency.* You've undoubtedly noticed you're most productive at certain times of the day (or night). Schedule as many of your tasks for those hours as you can, and stick to your schedule.

• *Set realistic goals, and write them down.* Attainable goals spur you on. Impossible goals, by definition, cause frustration and failure. Fully commit yourself to achieving your goals by putting them in writing.

• *Budget enough time.* For each project you undertake, calculate how long it will take to complete. Then tack on another 10–15%, or even 25%, as a buffer against interruptions or unanticipated problems.

• *Break down long-term goals into short-term ones.* Instead of waiting for or relying on large blocks of time, use short amounts of time to start a project or keep it moving.

• *Visualize the achievement of your goals.* By mentally rehearsing your performance of a task, you will be able to reach your goal more smoothly.

• *Keep track of the tasks you put off.* Analyze the reasons why you procrastinate. If the task is difficult or unpleasant, look for ways to make it easier or more fun. If you hate cleaning up your room, break the work into 10-minute tasks. If you find the readings for one of your classes particularly difficult, choose an especially nice setting for your reading, and then reward yourself each time you complete a section or chapter.

• *Consider doing your least favorite tasks first.* Once you have the most unpleasant ones out of the way, you can work on the projects you enjoy more.

• *Consolidate tasks when possible.* For example, try walking to the store so that you run your errands and exercise in the same block of time.

• *Identify quick transitional tasks.* Keep a list of 5-minute tasks you can do while waiting or between other tasks, such as watering your plants, doing the dishes, or checking a homework assignment.

• *Delegate responsibility.* Asking for help when you have too much to do is no cop-out; it's good time management. Just don't delegate to others the jobs you know you should do yourself, such as researching a paper.

• *Say no when necessary.* If the demands made on you don't seem reasonable, say no—tactfully, but without guilt or apology.

• *Give yourself a break.* Allow time for play—free, unstructured time when you ignore the clock. Don't consider this a waste of time. Play renews you and enables you to work more efficiently.

• *Stop thinking or talking about what you're going to do, and just do it!* Sometimes the best solution for procrastination is to stop waiting for the right moment and just get started. You will probably find that things are not as bad as you feared, and your momentum will keep you going.

COMMUNICATE! Learning to say no—whether to extra work or extra play—is an important part of effective time management. If you don't have enough time for something that your friends are pressuring you to do, you may need to use assertive communication to maintain control of your own time. Begin by knowing your priorities and believing in your right to decide what you will do. Remain calm in the face of pressure and don't feel guilty about saying no. For example, "I'd like to go to the club with you, but I have to get started on my English paper. I have only this week to work on it, and it's important to me. I'm sorry you don't have anyone else to go with right now—I could go on Friday if you're available then."

Cognitive Techniques

Some stressors arise in our own minds. Ideas, beliefs, perceptions, and patterns of thinking can add to our stress level. Each of the techniques described below can help you change unhealthy thought patterns to ones that will help you cope with stress. As with any skill, mastering these techniques takes practice and patience.

Think and Act Constructively Worrying, someone once said, is like shoveling smoke. Think back to the worries you had last week. How many of them were needless? Think about things you *can* control. Try to stand aside from the problem, consider the positive steps you can take to solve it, and then carry them out.

Take Control A situation often feels more stressful if you feel you're not in control of it. Time may seem to be slipping away before a big exam, for example. Unexpected obstacles may appear in your path, throwing you off course. When you feel your environment is controlling you instead of the other way around, take charge! Concentrate on what is possible to control, and set realistic goals. Be confident of your ability to succeed.

Problem-Solve When you find yourself stewing over a problem, take a moment to sit down with a piece of paper and go through a formal process of problem solving. Within a few minutes you can generate a plan:

1. Define the problem in one or two sentences.
2. Identify the causes of the problem.
3. Consider alternative solutions; don't just stop with the most obvious one.
4. Weigh positive and negative consequences for each alternative.
5. Make a decision—choose a solution.
6. Make a list of what you will need to do to carry out your decision.
7. Begin to act on your list; if you're unable to do that, temporarily turn to other things.
8. Evaluate the outcome and revise your approach if necessary.

Modify Your Expectations Expectations are exhausting and restricting. The fewer expectations you have, the more you can live spontaneously and joyfully. The more you expect from others, the more often you will feel let down. And trying to meet the expectations others have of you is often futile.

Maintain Positivity If you catch your mind beating up on you—"Late for class again! You can't even cope with college! How do you expect to ever hold down a professional job?"—change your inner dialogue. Talk to yourself as you would to a child you love: "You're a smart, capable person. You've solved other problems; you'll handle this one. Tomorrow you'll simply schedule things so you get to class with a few minutes to spare." (Chapter 3 has more information on self-talk.)

Cultivate Your Sense of Humor When it comes to stress, laughter may be the best medicine. Even a fleeting smile produces changes in your autonomic nervous system that can lift your spirits. And a few minutes of belly laughing can be as invigorating as brisk exercise. Hearty laughter elevates your heart rate, aids digestion, eases pain, and triggers the release of endorphins and other pleasurable and stimulating chemicals in the brain. After a good laugh, your muscles go slack; your pulse and blood pressure dip below normal. You are relaxed. Cultivate the ability to laugh at yourself, and you'll have a handy and instantly effective stress reliever. Try some of the following strategies:

• Keep a humor journal. Write down funny things that you and others say, including unintentional slips of the tongue. Collect funny and clever sayings and cartoons that make you smile.

• Collect some funny props—clown noses, "arrow" headbands, Groucho glasses—that you can put on the next time you feel stressed or anxious. Or simply try making funny faces in front of a mirror.

• Watch funny films and television programs. In a study of college students, those who watched an episode of *Seinfeld* prior to giving an impromptu speech were less anxious and had a lower heart rate than those who didn't watch the program.

Go with the Flow Remember that the branch that bends in the storm doesn't break. Try to flow with your life, accepting the things you can't change. Be forgiving of faults, your own and those of others. Instead of anticipating happiness at some indefinite point in the future, realize that pleasure is integral to being alive. You can create it every day of your life. View challenges as an opportunity to learn and grow. Be flexible.

Relaxation Techniques

First identified and described by Herbert Benson of the Harvard Medical School, the **relaxation response** is a physiological state characterized by a feeling of warmth and quiet mental alertness. This is the opposite of the fight-or-flight reaction. When the relaxation response is triggered by a relaxation technique, heart rate, breathing,

relaxation response A physiological state characterized by a feeling of warmth and quiet mental alertness.

Terms

The Basic Technique

1. Pick a word, phrase, or object to focus on. If you like, you can choose a word or phrase that has a deep meaning for you, but any word or phrase will work. Some meditators prefer to focus on their breathing.

2. Take a comfortable position in a quiet environment, and close your eyes if you're not focusing on an object.

3. Relax your muscles.

4. Breathe slowly and naturally. If you're using a focus word or phrase, silently repeat it each time you exhale. If you're using an object, focus on it as you breathe.

5. Keep a passive attitude. Disregard thoughts that drift in.

6. Continue for 10–20 minutes, once or twice a day.

7. After you've finished, sit quietly for a few minutes with your eyes first closed and then open. Then stand up.

Suggestions

- Allow relaxation to occur at its own pace; don't try to force it. Don't be surprised if you can't tune your mind out for more than a few seconds at a time.

- If you want to time your session, peek at a watch or clock occasionally, but don't set a jarring alarm.

- The technique works best on an empty stomach, before a meal or about 2 hours after eating. Avoid times of day when you're tired—unless you want to fall asleep.

- Although you'll feel refreshed even after the first session, it may take a month or more to get noticeable results. Be patient.

and metabolism slow down. Blood pressure and oxygen consumption decrease. At the same time, blood flow to the brain and skin increases, and brain waves shift from an alert beta rhythm to a relaxed alpha rhythm. Practiced regularly, relaxation techniques can counteract the debilitating effects of stress. If one technique doesn't seem to work well enough for you after you've given it a good try, try another one.

Progressive Relaxation   Unlike most of the others, this simple method requires no imagination, willpower, or self-suggestion. You simply tense, and then relax, the muscles in your body, group by group. The technique, also known as deep muscle relaxation, helps you become aware of the muscle tension that occurs when you're under stress. When you consciously relax those muscles, other systems of the body get the message and ease up on the stress response.

Start, for example, with your right fist. Inhale as you tense it. Exhale as you relax it. Repeat. Next, contract and relax your right upper arm. Repeat. Do the same with your left arm. Then, beginning at your forehead and ending at your feet, contract and relax your other muscle groups. Repeat each contraction at least once, breathing in as you tense, breathing out as you relax. To speed up the process, tense and relax more muscles at one time—both arms simultaneously, for instance. With practice, you'll be able to relax very quickly and effectively by clenching and releasing only your fists.

Visualization   Also known as using imagery, **visualization** lets you daydream without guilt. Next time you feel stressed, close your eyes. Imagine yourself floating on a cloud, sitting on a mountaintop, or lying in a meadow. What do you see and hear? Is it cold out? Or damp? What do you smell? What do you taste? Involve all your senses. Your body will respond as if your imagery were real. An alternative: Close your eyes and imagine a deep purple light filling your body. Now change the color into a soothing gold. As the color lightens, so should your distress.

Visualization can also be used to rehearse for an upcoming event and enhance performance. By experiencing an event ahead of time in your mind, you can practice coping with any difficulties that may arise. Think positively, and you can "psych yourself up" for a successful experience.

Meditation   The need to periodically stop our incessant mental chatter is so great that, from ancient times, hundreds of forms of **meditation** have developed in cultures all over the world. Meditation is a way of telling the mind to be quiet for a while. Because meditation has been at the core of many Eastern religions and philosophies, it has acquired an "Eastern" mystique that has caused some people to shy away from it. Yet meditation requires no special knowledge or background. Whatever philosophical, religious, or emotional reasons may be given for meditation, its power derives from its ability to elicit the relaxation response. Regular practice of meditation will subtly carry over into your daily life, encouraging physical and emotional balance no matter what confronts you.

Deep Breathing   Your breathing pattern is closely tied to your stress level. Deep, slow breathing is associated with relaxation. Rapid, shallow, often irregular breathing occurs during the stress response. With practice, you can

Diaphragmatic Breathing

1. Lie on your back with your body relaxed.

2. Place one hand on your chest and one on your abdomen. (You will use your hands to monitor the depth and location of your breathing.)

3. Inhale slowly and deeply through your nose into your abdomen. Your abdomen should push up as far as is comfortable. Your chest should expand only a little and only in conjunction with the movement of your abdomen.

4. Exhale gently through your mouth.

5. Continue for about 5–10 minutes per session. Focus on the sound and feel of your breathing.

Breathing In Relaxation, Breathing Out Tension

1. Assume a comfortable position, lying on your back or sitting in a chair.

2. Inhale slowly and deeply into your abdomen. Imagine the inhaled, warm air flowing to all parts of your body. Say to yourself, "Breathe in relaxation."

3. Exhale from your abdomen. Imagine tension flowing out of your body. Say to yourself, "Breathe out tension."

4. Pause before you inhale.

5. Continue for 5–10 minutes or until no tension remains.

Chest Expansion

1. Sit in a comfortable chair, or stand.

2. Inhale slowly and deeply into your abdomen as you raise your arms out to the sides. Pull your shoulders and arms back and lift your chin slightly so that your chest opens up.

3. Exhale gradually as you lower your arms and chin, and return to the starting position.

4. Repeat 5–10 times or until your breathing is deep and regular and your body feels relaxed and energized.

Quick Tension Release

1. Inhale into your abdomen slowly and deeply as you count slowly to four.

2. Exhale slowly as you again count slowly to four. As you exhale, concentrate on relaxing your face, neck, shoulders, and chest.

3. Repeat several times. With each exhalation, feel more tension leaving your body.

SOURCES: Stop stress with a deep breath. 1996. *Health,* October, 53. Breathing for health and relaxation. 1995. *Mental Medicine Update* 4(2): 3–6. When you're stressed, catch your breath. 1995. *Mayo Clinic Health Letter,* December 5.

learn to slow and quiet your breathing pattern, thereby also quieting your mind and relaxing your body. Breathing techniques can be used for on-the-spot tension relief, as well as for long-term stress reduction.

The primary goal of many breathing exercises is to change your breathing pattern from chest breathing to diaphragmatic ("belly") breathing. During the day, most adults breathe by expanding their chest and raising their shoulders rather than by expanding their abdomen. This pattern of chest breathing is associated with stress, a sedentary lifestyle, restrictive clothing, and cultural preferences for a large chest and a small waist. Diaphragmatic breathing, which involves free expansion of the diaphragm and lower abdomen, is the pattern of breathing characteristic of children and sleeping adults. (The diaphragm is a sheet of muscle and connective tissue that divides the chest and abdominal cavities.) Diaphragmatic breathing is slower and deeper than chest breathing.

Other Relaxation Techniques

- *Hatha yoga* involves a series of physical postures, called *asanas,* that stretch and relax different parts of the body; the emphasis is on breathing, stretching, body awareness, and balance. Proper technique is necessary to obtain maximum benefits from yoga, so qualified instruction is recommended.

- *T'ai chi ch'uan,* a martial art that developed in China, consists of a series of slow, fluid, elegant movements that promote relaxation and concentration as well as the development of body awareness, balance, muscular strength, and flexibility. As with yoga, it's best to begin with some qualified instruction.

- *Listening to music* can influence pulse, blood pressure, and the electrical activity of muscles; music therapy can be effective in reducing depression and anxiety and in pain management. Set aside a time to listen to music that makes you feel relaxed; formal music therapy can also focus on stress management.

visualization A technique for promoting relaxation or improving performance that involves creating or re-creating vivid mental pictures of a place or an experience; also called *imagery.*

meditation A technique for quieting the mind by focusing on a particular word, object (such as a candle flame), or process (such as breathing).

Terms

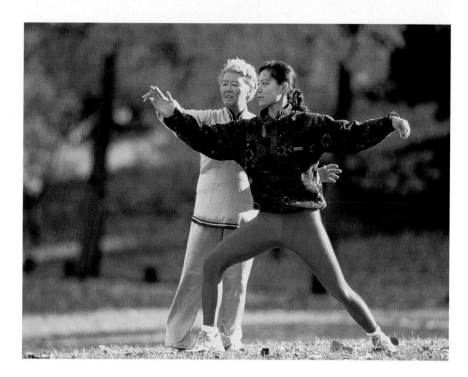

T'ai chi ch'uan is among the many techniques for inducing the relaxation response. In addition to helping this woman manage stress, regular practice of t'ai chi will also improve her balance and increase her muscular strength and flexibility.

Other relaxation techniques include biofeedback, massage, hypnosis, and autogenic training. To learn more about these and other techniques for inducing the relaxation response, refer to For More Information at the end of the chapter.

Counterproductive Coping Strategies

College is a time when you'll learn to adapt to new and challenging situations and gain skills that will last a lifetime. It is also a time when many people develop habits, in response to stress, that are counterproductive and unhealthy and that may also last well beyond graduation.

- *Tobacco:* The nicotine in cigarettes and other tobacco products can make you feel relaxed and even increase your ability to concentrate, but it is highly addictive. Smoking causes cancer, heart disease, impotence, and many other health problems and is the leading preventable cause of death in the United States.

- *Alcohol:* Having a few drinks might make you feel temporarily at ease, and drinking until you're intoxicated may help you forget your current stressors. However, using alcohol to deal with stress places you at risk for all the short-term and long-term problems associated with alcohol abuse. It also does nothing to address the actual causes of stress in your life.

- *Other drugs:* Altering your body chemistry in order to cope with stress is a strategy that has many pitfalls and does not directly address your stressors.

For example, caffeine raises cortisol levels and blood pressure and disrupts sleep. Marijuana can elicit panic attacks with repeated use, and some research suggests that it enhances the stress response.

- *Binge eating:* The feelings of satiation and sedation that follow eating produce a relaxed state that reduces stress. However, regular use of eating as a means of coping with stress may lead to binge eating, a risky behavior associated with weight gain and serious eating disorders.

Refer to later chapters for more information on these unhealthy coping strategies: tobacco and alcohol (Chapter 8), drug use (Chapter 7), nutrition (Chapter 9), and eating disorders (Chapter 11).

CREATING A PERSONAL PLAN FOR MANAGING STRESS

No single strategy or program for managing stress will work for everyone, but you can use the principles of behavior management described in Chapter 1 to tailor a plan specifically to your needs.

Identifying Stressors

Before you can learn to manage the stressors in your life, you have to identify them. A strategy many experts recommend is keeping a stress journal for a week or two. Keep a log of your daily activities, and assign a rating to your stress level for every hour. Each time you feel or express a stress response, record the time and the circumstances in your journal. Note what you were doing at the time, what you were thinking or feeling, and the outcome of your response.

After keeping your journal for a few weeks, you should be able to identify your key stressors and spot patterns in how you respond to them. Take note of the people, places, events, and patterns of thought and behavior that cause you the most stress. You may notice, for example, that mornings are usually the most stressful part of your day. Or you may discover that when you're angry at your roommate, you're apt to respond with behaviors that only make matters worse. Once you've outlined the general pattern of stress in your life, you may want to focus on a particularly problematic stressor or on an inappropriate behavioral response you've identified. Keep a stress log for another week or two that focuses just on the early morning hours, for example, or just on your arguments with your roommate. The more information you gather, the easier it will be to develop effective strategies for coping with the stressors in your life.

Designing Your Plan

Now that you've identified the key stressors in your life, it's time to choose the techniques that will work best for you and create an action plan for change. Finding a buddy to work with you can make the process more fun and increase your chances of success. Some experts recommend drawing up a formal contract with yourself.

Whether or not you complete a contract, it's important to design rewards into your plan. You might treat yourself to a special breakfast in a favorite restaurant on the weekend (as long as you eat a nutritious breakfast every weekday morning). If you practice your relaxation technique faithfully, you might reward yourself with a long bath or an hour of pleasure reading at the end of the day. It's also important to evaluate your plan regularly and redesign it as your needs change. Under times of increased stress, for example, you might want to focus on good eating, exercise, and relaxation habits. Over time, your new stress-management skills will become almost automatic. You'll feel better, accomplish more, and reduce your risk of disease.

Getting Help

If the techniques discussed so far don't provide you with enough relief from the stress in your life, you might want to read more about specific areas you wish to work on, consult a peer counselor, join a support group, or participate in a few psychotherapy sessions. Excellent self-help guides can be found in bookstores or the library.

Your student health center or student affairs office can tell you whether your campus has a peer counseling program. They can also probably help you locate an appropriate support group. Short-term psychotherapy is another useful option.

SUMMARY

- When confronted with a stressor, the body undergoes a set of physical changes known as the fight-or-flight reaction. The sympathetic nervous system and endocrine system act on many targets in the body to prepare it for action—even if the situation does not require physical action.

- Emotional and behavioral responses to stressors vary among individuals. Ineffective responses increase stress but can be moderated or changed.

- Factors that influence emotional and behavioral responses to stressors include personality, cultural background, gender, and past experiences.

- The general adaptation syndrome (GAS) has three stages: alarm, resistance, and exhaustion.

- A high allostatic load characterized by prolonged or repeated exposure to stress hormones can increase a person's risk of health problems.

- Psychoneuroimmunology (PNI) looks at how the physiological changes of the stress response affect the immune system and the risk of illness.

- Health problems linked to stress include cardiovascular disease, colds and other infections, asthma and allergies, cancer, flare-ups of chronic diseases, and psychological problems.

Are you a person who doesn't perform as well as you should on tests? Do you find that anxiety interferes with your ability to study effectively before the test and to think clearly in the test situation? If so, you may be experiencing test anxiety—an ineffective response to a stressful situation that can be replaced with more effective responses. If test anxiety is a problem for you, try some of the following strategies:

- Before the test, find out everything you can about it—its format, the material to be covered, the grading criteria. Ask the instructor for practice materials. Study in advance; don't just cram the night before. Avoid all-nighters.

- Devise a study plan. This might include forming a study group with one or more classmates or outlining what you will study, when, where, and for how long. Generate your own questions and answer them.

- Once in the test situation, sit away from possible distractions, listen carefully to instructions, and ask for clarification if you don't understand a direction.

- During the test, answer the easiest questions first. If you don't know an answer and there is no penalty for incorrect

answers, guess. If there are several questions you have difficulty answering, review the ones you have already handled. Figure out approximately how much time you have to cover each question.

- For math problems, try to estimate the answer before doing the precise calculations.

- For true-false questions, look for qualifiers such as *always* and *never*. Such questions are likely to be false.

- For essay questions, look for key words in the question that indicate what the instructor is looking for in the answer. Develop a brief outline of your answer, sketching out what you will cover. Stick to your outline, and keep track of the time you're spending on your answer. Don't let yourself get caught with unanswered questions when time is up.

- Remain calm and focused throughout the test. Don't let negative thoughts rattle you. Avoid worrying about past performance, how others are doing, or the negative consequences of a poor test grade. If you start to become nervous, take some deep breaths and relax your muscles completely for a minute or so.

- A cluster of major life events can lead to increased stress and an increased risk of health problems. Minor daily hassles increase stress if they are perceived negatively.

- Sources of stress associated with college may be academic, interpersonal, time-related, or financial pressures. Job-related stress is common, particularly for employees who have little control over decisions relating to their jobs.

- New and changing relationships, prejudice, and discrimination are examples of social stressors.

- Social support, exercise, nutrition, sleep, and time management are effective at reducing stress.

- Cognitive techniques for managing stress involve developing new and healthy patterns of thinking,

such as practicing problem solving, monitoring self-talk, and cultivating a sense of humor.

- The relaxation response is the opposite of the fight-or-flight reaction. Techniques that trigger it include progressive relaxation, imagery, meditation, and deep breathing. Counterproductive coping strategies include smoking, drinking, and binge eating.

- A successful individualized plan for coping with stress begins with the use of a stress journal or log to identify and study stressors and inappropriate behavioral responses. Completing a contract and recruiting a buddy can help your plan succeed.

TAKE ACTION

1. Choose a friend or family member who seems to deal particularly well with stress. Interview that person about his or her methods of managing stress. What strategies does he or she use? What can you learn from that person that can be applied to your own life?

2. Investigate the services available in your community—such as peer counseling, support groups, and

time-management classes—to help people deal with stress. If possible, visit or gather information on one or more of them. Write a description and evaluation of their services, including your personal reactions.

3. Reread the stress-management techniques described in this chapter, and choose one to try for a week. If possible, select a behavior or strategy, such as regular

exercise or systematic time management, that you've never tried before. After a trial period, evaluate the effectiveness of the strategy you chose. Did your stress level decrease during the week? Were you better able to deal with daily hassles and any more severe stressors that you encountered?

1. Watch for the physical changes of the stress response when you're in stressful situations. In your health journal, keep a stress log in which you note how many times in a day you experience the stress response to some degree. Also include a brief description of the circumstances surrounding your stress response. Is your life more or less stressful than you expected?

2. Make a list of the daily hassles you commonly encounter, such as being awakened early by loud neighbors, standing in a long line for lunch, or repeatedly misplacing your keys. Divide your list into two groups: avoidable and unavoidable. For each stressor that is potentially avoidable, describe a strategy for eliminating it from your life. For stressors that are unavoidable, make a list of effective coping mechanisms.

3. Critical Thinking Some techniques for stress management, including meditation and hypnosis, are considered strange or unscientific by some people. Find out more about one such technique through library or Internet research. What evidence can you find to support or oppose the idea that the technique can help people manage stress? Based on your research, write a brief essay in your health journal stating your opinion. As you consider the evidence, be sure to look closely at your sources of information.

FOR MORE INFORMATION

Books and Articles

Benson, H. 2000. *The Relaxation Response.* New York: Avon, Wholecare. *An expanded and updated edition of the 1975 classic on relaxation techniques and their physical benefits.*

Dement, W. C. 1999. *The Promise of Sleep.* New York: Delacorte. *An exploration of sleep and its effects on wellness by a prominent sleep researcher.*

Girdano, D. A., D. Dusek, and G. S. Everly. 2001. *Controlling Stress and Tension,* 6th ed. New York: Allyn & Bacon. *An easy-to-understand guide to identifying and combating stressors.*

Justice, B. 2000. *Who Gets Sick: How Beliefs, Moods, and Thoughts Affect Health.* Los Angeles: Jeremy Tarcher. *Explores what is known today about the role of thought and emotion in health and illness.*

Sapolsky, R. M. 1998. *Why Zebras Don't Get Ulcers: An Updated Guide to Stress-Related Diseases and Coping.* New York: W. H. Freeman. *An entertaining look at the effects of stress on the body and the relationship between stress and disease.*

WW Organizations and Web Sites

American Music Therapy Association. Provides information about music therapy and about how to find a certified therapist.
301-589-3300
http://www.musictherapy.org

American Psychological Association. Provides information on stress management and psychological disorders.
202-336-5500; 800-964-2000 (referrals)
http://www.apa.org; http://helping.apa.org

Association for Applied Psychophysiology and Biofeedback. Provides information about biofeedback and referrals to certified biofeedback practitioners.

800-477-8892
http://www.aapb.org

Center for Anxiety and Stress Treatment. A commercial site that also includes an anxiety symptom checklist and a list of stress-busting tips for work stress.
http://www.stressrelease.com

The Humor Project. A clearinghouse for information and practical ideas related to humor.
518-587-8770
http://www.humorproject.com

National Institute for Occupational Safety and Health (NIOSH). Provides information and links on job stress.
http://www.cdc.gov/niosh/stresshp.html

National Institute of Mental Health (NIMH). Publishes informative brochures about stress and stress management as well as other aspects of mental health.
800-421-4211; 301-443-4513
http://www.nimh.nih.gov

National Sleep Foundation. Provides information about sleep and how to overcome sleep problems such as insomnia and jet lag; brochures are available from the Web site or via fax.
202-347-3471; 202-347-3472 (fax)
877-BE-AWAKE (daytime sleepiness screening)
http://www.sleepfoundation.org

Student Counseling Virtual Pamphlet Collection. Links to online pamphlets from student counseling centers at colleges and universities across the country; topics include stress, sleep, and time management.
http://counseling.uchicago.edu/vpc

See also the listings for Chapters 1 and 3.

Bowman, M. A., et al. 2000. Changes in functional status related to health maintenance visits to family physicians. *Journal of Family Practice* 49(5): 428–433.

Bremner, J. D. 1999. Does stress damage the brain? *Biological Psychiatry* 45(7): 797–805.

Bremner, J. D., et al. 2000. Hippocampal volume reduction in major depression. *American Journal of Psychiatry* 157(1): 115–118.

Brown, E. S., A. J. Rush, and B. S. McEwen. 1999. Hippocampal remodeling and damage by corticosteroids: Implications for mood disorders. *Neuropsychopharmacology* 21(4): 474–484.

Cerbone, F. G., and C. L. Larison. 2000. A bibliographic essay: The relationship between stress and substance use. *Substance Use and Misuse* 35(5): 757–786.

Daun, J. M., R. W. Ball, and J. G. Cannon. 2000. Glucocorticoid sensitivity of interleukin-1 agonist and antagonist secretion: The effects of age and gender. *American Journal of Physiological Regulation and Integrative and Comparative Physiology* 278(4): R855–862.

de Quervain, D. J., et al. 2000. Acute cortisone administration impairs retrieval of long-term declarative memory in humans. *Nature Neuroscience* 3(4): 313–314.

Gang, A., et al. 2001. Psychological stress perturbs epidermal permeability barrier homeostasis: Implications for the pathogenesis of stress-associated skin disorders. *Archives of Dermatology* 137(1): 53–59.

Jacobs, B. L., H. van Praag, and F. H. Gage. 2000. Adult brain neurogenesis and psychiatry: A novel theory of depression. *Molecular Psychiatry* 5(3): 262–269.

Kimata, H. 2001. Effect of humor on allergen-induced wheal reactions. *Journal of the American Medical Association* 285(6): 738.

Lacey, K., et al. 2000. A prospective study of neuroendocrine and immune alterations associated with the stress of an oral academic examination among graduate students. *Psychoneuroendocrinology* 25(4): 339–356.

Maes, M., et al. 1999. The effects of psychological stress on leukocyte subset distribution in humans: Evidence of immune activation. *Neuropsychobiology* 39(1): 1–9.

McEwen, B. S. 1998. Protective and damaging effects of stress mediators. *New England Journal of Medicine* 338(3): 171–179.

Nordstrom, C. K., et al. 2001. Work-related stress and early atherosclerosis. *Epidemiology* 12(2): 180–185.

Sapolsky, R. M., L. M. Romero, and A. U. Munck. 2000. How do glucocorticoids influence stress responses? Integrating permissive, suppressive, stimulatory, and preparative actions. *Endocrine Reviews* 21(1): 55–89.

Scheufele, P. M. 2000. Effects of progressive relaxation and classical music on measurements of attention, relaxation, and stress responses. *Journal of Behavioral Medicine* 23(2): 207–228.

Shepard, J. D., et al. 2000. Additive pressure effects of caffeine and stress in male medical students at risk for hypertension. *American Journal of Hypertension* 13(5 Pt. 1): 475–481.

Siegman, A. W., et al. 2000. Antagonistic behavior, dominance, hostility, and coronary heart disease. *Psychosomatic Medicine* 62(2): 248–257.

Skirka, N. 2000. The relationship of hardiness, sense of coherence, sports participation, and gender to perceived stress and psychological symptoms among college students. *Journal of Sports Medicine and Physical Fitness* 40(1): 63–70.

Taylor, S. E., et al. 2000. Biobehavioral responses to stress in females. Tend-and-befriend, not fight-or-flight. *Psychological Review* 107(3): 411–429.

Van Cauter, E., R. Leproult, and L. Plat. 2000. Age-related changes in slow wave sleep and REM sleep and relationship with growth hormone and cortisol levels in healthy men. *Journal of the American Medical Association* 284(7): 861–868.

Weber, B., et al. 2000. Increased diurnal plasma concentrations of cortisone in depressed patients. *Journal of Clinical Endocrinology and Metabolism* 85(3): 1133–1136.

Wolff, G. E., et al. 2000. Differences in daily stress, mood, coping, and eating behavior in binge eating and nonbinge eating college women. *Addictive Behaviors* 25(2): 205–216.

Psychological Health

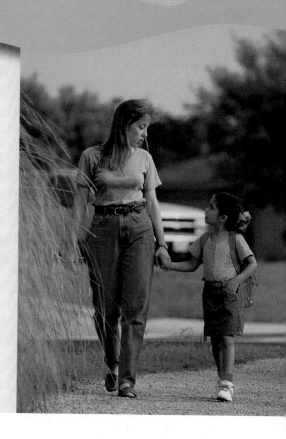

3

LOOKING AHEAD

After reading this chapter, you should be able to

- Describe what it means to be psychologically healthy

- Explain how to develop and maintain a positive self-concept and healthy self-esteem

- Discuss the importance to psychological health of an optimistic outlook, good communication skills, and constructive approaches to dealing with loneliness and anger

- Describe common psychological disorders and list the warning signs of suicide

- Explain the types of help available for psychological problems

What exactly is psychological health? Many people over the centuries have expressed opinions about the nature of psychological (or mental) health. Some even claim that there is no such thing, that psychological health is just a myth. We disagree. We think there is such a thing as psychological health just as there is physical health—and the two are closely interrelated. Just as your body can work well or poorly, giving you pleasure or pain, your mind can also work well or poorly, resulting in happiness or unhappiness. Psychological health is a crucial component of overall wellness. (We are using "mental health" and "psychological health" interchangeably; the latter is the more current term, but it hasn't replaced "mental health" yet.)

If you feel pain and unhappiness rather than pleasure and happiness or if you sense that you could be functioning at a higher level, there may be ways you can help yourself—either on your own or with professional help. This chapter will explain how.

WHAT PSYCHOLOGICAL HEALTH IS NOT

Psychological health is not the same as psychological **normality.** Being mentally normal simply means being close to average. You can define normal body temperature because a few degrees above or below this temperature always means physical sickness. But your ideas and attitudes can vary tremendously without your feeling emotional distress. And psychological diversity is valuable; living in a society of people with varied ideas and lifestyles makes life interesting and challenging.

Conforming to social demands is not necessarily a mark of psychological health. If you don't question what's

---

normality The psychological characteristics attributed to the majority of people in a population at a given time.

Terms

going on around you, you're not fulfilling your potential as a thinking, questioning human being. Never seeking help for personal problems does not mean you are psychologically healthy, any more than seeking help proves you are mentally ill. Unhappy people may not want to seek professional help because they don't want to reveal their problems to others, may fear what their friends might think, or may not know whom to ask for help. People who are severely disturbed psychologically or emotionally may not even realize they need help, or they may become so suspicious of other people that they can only be treated without their consent.

We cannot say people are "mentally ill" or "mentally healthy" on the basis of symptoms alone. Life constantly presents problems. Time and life inevitably alter the environment as well as our minds and bodies, and changes present problems. The symptom of anxiety, for example, can help us face a problem and solve it before it gets too big. Someone who shows no anxiety may be refusing to recognize problems or do anything about them. A person who is anxious for good reason is likely to be judged more psychologically healthy in the long run than someone who is inappropriately calm. Finally, we cannot judge psychological health from the way people look. All too often, a person who seems to be OK and even happy suddenly takes his or her own life.

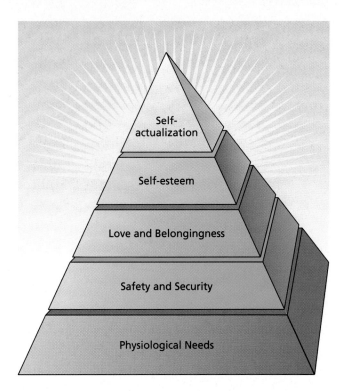

Figure 3-1   Maslow's hierarchy of needs.   SOURCE: Maslow, A. 1970. *Motivation and Personality,* 2nd ed. New York: Harper & Row.

DEFINING PSYCHOLOGICAL HEALTH

It is even harder to say what psychological health *is* than what it is *not.* Psychological health can be defined either negatively as the absence of sickness or positively as the presence of wellness. A positive definition is a more ambitious outlook, one that encourages you to fulfill your own potential. During the 1960s, Abraham Maslow eloquently described an ideal of mental health in his book *Toward a Psychology of Being.* He stated that there is a *hierarchy of needs,* listed here in order of decreasing urgency: physiological needs, safety, being loved, maintaining self-esteem, and self-actualization (Figure 3-1). When urgent needs like the need for food, water, shelter, sleep, and safety are satisfied, less urgent needs take priority. According to Maslow, people who live at their fullest have achieved **self-actualization.** They have fulfilled a good measure of their human potential and share certain qualities.

Realism

Self-actualized people are able to deal with the world as it is and not demand that it be otherwise. If you are realistic, you know the difference between what is and what you want. You also know what you can change and what you cannot. Unrealistic people often spend a great deal of time and energy trying to force the world and other peo-

ple into their ideal picture. Realistic people accept evidence that contradicts what they want to believe, and if it is important evidence, they modify their beliefs.

Acceptance

Psychologically healthy people can largely accept themselves and others. Self-acceptance means having a positive **self-concept,** or self-image, or appropriately high **self-esteem.** They have a positive but realistic mental image of themselves and positive feelings about who they are, what they are capable of, and what roles they play. People who feel good about themselves are likely to live up to their positive self-image and enjoy successes that in turn reinforce these good feelings. A good self-concept is based on a realistic view of personal worth—it does not mean being egocentric or "stuck on yourself."

Autonomy

Psychologically healthy people are able to direct themselves, acting independently of their social environment. **Autonomy** is more than freedom from physical control by something outside the self. Many people, for example, shrink from expressing their feelings because they fear disapproval and rejection. They respond only to what they feel as outside pressure. Behavior such as this is **other-directed.** In contrast, **inner-directed** people find guidance from within, from their own values and feelings.

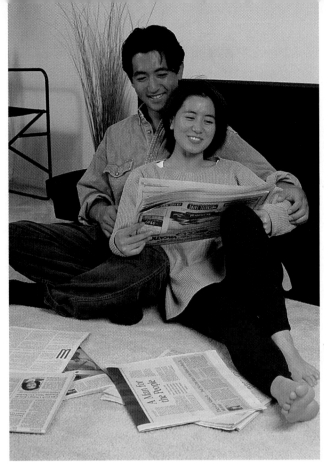

Self-actualized people respond in a genuine, spontaneous way to what happens around them. They are capable of maintaining close interpersonal relationships.

They are not afraid to be themselves. Psychologically free people act because they choose to, not because they are driven or pressured.

Autonomy can give healthy people certain childlike qualities. Very small children have a quality of being "real." They respond in a genuine, spontaneous way to whatever happens. Being genuine means not having to plan words or actions to get approval or make an impression. It means being aware of feelings and being willing to express them—being unself-consciously oneself. This quality is sometimes called **authenticity**; such people are *authentic*, the "real thing."

A Capacity for Intimacy

Healthy people are capable of physical and emotional intimacy. They can expose their feelings and thoughts to other people. They are open to the pleasure of intimate physical contact and to the risks and satisfactions of being close to others in a caring, sensitive way.

Creativity

Psychologically healthy people are creative and have a continuing fresh appreciation for what goes on around

them. They are not necessarily great poets, artists, or musicians, but they do live their everyday lives in creative ways: "A first-rate soup is more creative than a second-rate painting." Creative people seem to see more and to be open to new experiences; they don't fear the unknown. And they don't need to minimize uncertainty or avoid it; they actually find it attractive.

How did Maslow's group achieve their exemplary psychological health, and (more important) how can *we* attain it? Maslow himself did not answer that question, but we have a few suggestions. Undoubtedly it helps to have been treated with respect, love, and understanding as a child, to have experienced stability and to have achieved a sense of mastery. As adults, since we cannot redo the past, we must concentrate on meeting current psychological challenges in ways that will lead to mental wellness.

WW. MEETING LIFE'S CHALLENGES

Life is full of challenges—large and small. Everyone, regardless of heredity and family influences, must learn to cope successfully with new situations and new people.

Growing Up Psychologically

Along the path from birth to old age, we are confronted with a series of challenges. How we respond influences the development of our personality and identity.

Developing an Adult Identity   A primary task beginning in adolescence is the development of an adult identity: a unified sense of self, characterized by attitudes, beliefs, and ways of acting that are genuinely one's own. People with adult identities know who they are, what they are capable of, what roles they play, and their place among their peers. They have a sense of their own uniqueness but also appreciate what they have in common with others. They view themselves realistically and can assess their strengths and weaknesses without relying on the opinions of others. Achieving an identity also

self-actualization The highest level of growth in Maslow's hierarchy.

self-concept The ideas, feelings, and perceptions one has about oneself; also called *self-image*.

self-esteem Satisfaction and confidence in oneself; the valuing of oneself as a person.

autonomy Independence; the sense of being self-directed.

other-directed Guided in behavior by the values and expectations of others.

inner-directed Guided in behavior by an inner set of rules and values.

authenticity Genuineness.

Terms

means that one can form intimate relationships with others while maintaining a strong sense of self.

Our identities evolve as we interact with the world and make choices about what we'd like to do and whom we'd like to model ourselves after. Developing an adult identity is particularly challenging in a heterogeneous, secular, and relatively affluent society like ours, in which many roles are possible, many choices are tolerated, and ample time is allowed for experimenting.

Early identities are often modeled after parents—or the opposite of parents, in rebellion from what they represent. Later, peers, rock stars, sports heroes, and religious figures are added to the list of possible models. Early identities are rarely permanent, but at some point, most of us adopt a more stable, individual identity that ties together the experiences of childhood and the expectations and aspirations of adulthood.

How far have you gotten in developing your adult identity? Write down a list of characteristics you think a friend who knows you well would use to describe you. Rank them from the most to the least important. Your list might include elements such as gender, socioeconomic status, ethnic and/or religious identification, choice of major, interests and talents, attitudes toward drugs and alcohol, style of dress, the kinds of people with whom you typically associate, your expected role in society, and aspects of your personality. Which elements of your identity do you feel are permanent and which do you think may change over time? Are there any characteristics missing from your list that you'd like to add?

Developing Intimacy   Learning to live intimately with others and finding a productive role for yourself in society are other tasks of adulthood—to be able to love and work. People with established identities can form intimate relationships and sexual unions characterized by sharing, open communication, long-term commitment, and love. Those who lack a firm sense of self may have difficulty establishing relationships because they feel overwhelmed by closeness and the needs of another person.

COMMUNICATE!   Self-disclosure is essential to interpersonal relationships, but too much self-disclosure too soon can scare people off. You also want to make a good impression! When you're just getting to know someone, make sure you monitor and control how much you reveal about yourself, especially information that could be construed as negative. Pay attention to feedback from others—do they continue to be interested, or do they show signs of wanting to disengage from the conversation, such as looking around the room or moving away from you? Once you know people better and have begun to develop bonds of friendship, it is appropriate to disclose more personal and intimate information about yourself.

Developing Values and Purpose in Your Life   Values are criteria for judging what is good and bad; they underlie our moral decisions and behavior. As adults we need to assess how far we have evolved morally and what values we actually have adopted, either explicitly or implicitly. Without an awareness of our personal values, our lives may be hurriedly driven forward by immediate desires and the passing demands of others. But are we doing things according to our principles? What are we striving for with our actions? Living according to values means considering your options carefully before making a choice, choosing between options without succumbing to outside pressures that oppose your values, and making a choice and acting on it rather than doing nothing. Your actions and how you justify them proclaim to others what you stand for.

Achieving Healthy Self-Esteem

Having a healthy level of self-esteem means regarding your self, which includes all aspects of your identity, as good, competent, and worthy of love.

Developing a Positive Self-Concept   Ideally, a positive self-concept begins in childhood, based on experiences within the family and outside it. Children need to develop a sense of being loved and being able to give love and to accomplish their goals. If they feel rejected or neglected by their parents, they may fail to develop feelings of self-worth and may grow to have a negative self-concept.

Other components of self-concept are integration and stability. An integrated self-concept is one that you have made for yourself—not someone else's image of you or a mask that doesn't quite fit. Stability depends on the integration of the self and its freedom from contradictions. People who have gotten mixed messages about themselves from parents and friends may have contradictory self-images, which defy integration and make them vulnerable to shifting levels of self-esteem. At times they regard themselves as entirely good, capable, and lovable— an ideal self—and at other times they see themselves as entirely bad, incompetent, and unworthy of love. At neither extreme do such people see themselves or others realistically, and their relationships with other people are filled with misunderstandings and ultimately with conflict.

Meeting Challenges to Self-Esteem   As an adult, you sometimes run into situations that challenge your self-concept: People you care about may tell you they don't love you or feel loved by you, or your attempts to accomplish a goal may end in failure. You can react to such challenges in several ways. The best approach is to acknowledge that something has gone wrong and try again, adjusting your goals to your abilities without radically revising your self-concept. Less productive re-

Spiritual wellness means different things to different people. For many, it involves developing a set of guiding beliefs, principles, or values that give meaning and purpose to life. It helps people achieve a sense of wholeness within themselves and in their relationships with others. Spiritual wellness influences people on an individual level, as well as on a community level, where it can bond people together through compassion, love, forgiveness, and self-sacrifice. For some, spirituality includes a belief in a higher power. Regardless of how it is defined, the development of spiritual wellness is critical for overall health and well-being. Its development is closely tied to the other components of wellness, particularly psychological health.

There are many paths to spiritual wellness. One of the most common in our society is organized religion. Some people object to the notion that organized religion can contribute to psychological health and overall wellness, asserting that it reinforces people's tendency to deny real difficulties and to accept what can and should be changed. Freud criticized religion as wishful thinking; Marx called it an opiate to make the poor accept social injustice. However, many elements of religious belief and practice can promote psychological health.

Organized religion usually involves its members in a community where social and material support is available. Religious organizations offer a social network to those who might otherwise be isolated. The major religions provide paths for transforming the self in ways that can lead to greater happiness and serenity and reduce feelings of anxiety and hopelessness. In Christianity, salvation follows turning away from the selfish ego to God's sovereignty and grace, where a joy is found that frees the believer from anxious self-concern and despair. Islam is the word for a kind of self-surrender leading to peace with God. Buddhism teaches how to detach oneself from selfish desire, leading to compassion for the suffering of others and freedom from fear-engendering illusions. Judaism emphasizes the social and ethical redemption the Jewish community can experience if it follows the laws of God. Religions teach specific techniques for achieving these transformations of the self: prayer, both in groups and in private; meditation; the performance of rituals and ceremonies symbolizing religious truths; and good works and service to others. Christianity's faith and works are perhaps analogous to the cognitive and behavioral components of a program of behavior change.

Spiritual wellness does not require participation in organized religion. Many people find meaning and purpose in other ways. By spending time in nature or working on environmental issues, people can experience continuity with the natural world. Spiritual wellness can come through helping others in one's community or by promoting human rights, peace and harmony among people, and opportunities for human development on a global level. Other people develop spiritual wellness through art or through their personal relationships.

Particularly in the second half of life, people seem to have an urge to view their activities and consciousness from a transcendent perspective. Perhaps it is the approach of death that makes older people tend to take less interest in material possessions and to devote more time to interpersonal and altruistic pursuits. At every age, however, people seem to feel better if they have beliefs about the ultimate purpose of life and their own place in the universe.

sponses are denying that anything went wrong and blaming someone else. The worst reaction is to develop a lasting negative self-concept in which you feel bad, unloved, and ineffective—in other words, to become demoralized.

One method for fighting demoralization is to recognize and test your negative thoughts and assumptions about yourself and others. The first step is to note exactly when an unpleasant emotion—feeling worthless, wanting to give up, feeling depressed—occurs or gets worse, to identify the events or daydreams that trigger that emotion, and to observe whatever thoughts come into your head just before or during the emotional experience. It is helpful to keep a daily journal about such events.

At first, it may be hard to figure out a rational response until hours or days after the event that upset you. But once you get used to noticing the way your mind works, you may be able to catch yourself thinking negatively and change the thought process before it goes too far. This approach is not the same as positive thinking—substituting a positive thought for a negative one. Instead, you simply try to make your thoughts as logical and accurate as possible.

Being Less Defensive

Sometimes our wishes come into conflict with people around us or with our conscience, and we become frustrated and anxious. If we cannot resolve the conflict by changing the external situation, we try to resolve the conflict internally by rearranging our thoughts and feelings. These psychological **defense mechanisms** allow us to protect ourselves against unacceptable thoughts or comfort ourselves when under pressure. Common defense mechanisms include repression, denial, rationalization, daydreaming, and humor. The drawback of many of these coping mechanisms is that although they succeed temporarily, they don't help find solutions to the underlying problem or conflict.

Recognizing your favorite defense mechanisms can be difficult, because they've probably become habits, occur-

defense mechanism A mental mechanism for coping with conflict or anxiety.	Terms

Do your patterns of thinking make events seem worse than they truly are? Do negative beliefs about yourself become self-fulfilling prophecies? Substituting realistic self-talk for negative self-talk can help you build and maintain self-esteem and cope better with the challenges in your life. Here are some examples of common types of **cognitive distortions**, along with suggestions for more accurate and rational responses.

Cognitive Distortion	Negative Self-Talk	Realistic Self-Talk
Focusing on negatives	School is so discouraging—nothing but one hassle after another.	School is pretty challenging and has its difficulties, but there certainly are rewards. It's really a mixture of good and bad.
Expecting the worst	Why would my boss want to meet with me this afternoon if not to fire me?	I wonder why my boss wants to meet with me. I guess I'll just have to wait and see.
Overgeneralizing	(After getting a poor grade on a paper) Just as I thought—I'm incompetent at everything.	I'll start working on the next paper earlier. That way, if I run into problems, I'll have time to consult with the TA.
Minimizing	I won the speech contest, but none of the other speakers was very good. I wouldn't have done as well against stiffer competition.	It may not have been the best speech I'll ever give, but it was good enough to win the contest. I'm really improving as a speaker.
Blaming others	I wouldn't have eaten so much last night if my friends hadn't insisted on going to that restaurant.	I overdid it last night. Next time I'll make different choices.
Expecting perfection	I should have scored 100% on this test. I can't believe I missed that one problem through a careless mistake.	Too bad I missed one problem through carelessness, but overall I did very well on this test. Next time I'll be more careful.
Believing you're the cause of everything	Sarah seems so depressed today. I wish I hadn't had that argument with her yesterday; it must have really upset her.	I wish I had handled the argument better, and in the future I'll try to. But I don't know if Sarah's behavior is related to what I said or even if she's depressed. In any case, I'm not responsible for how Sarah feels or acts; only she can take responsibility for that.
Thinking in black and white	I've got to score 10 points in the game today. Otherwise, I don't belong on the team.	I'm a good player or else I wouldn't be on the team. I'll play my best—that's all I can do.
Magnifying events	They went to a movie without me. I thought we were friends, but I guess I was wrong.	I'm disappointed they didn't ask me to the movie, but it doesn't mean our friendship is over. It's not that big a deal.

SOURCE: Adapted from Schafer, W. 1995. *Stress Management for Wellness,* 3rd ed. Copyright © 1996 by Holt, Rinehart, and Winston. Reprinted by permission of the publisher.

ring unconsciously. But we each have some inkling about how our mind operates. Try to look at yourself as an objective, outside observer would and analyze your thoughts and behavior in a psychologically stressful situation from the past. Having insight into what strategies you typically use can lead to new, less defensive and more effective ways of coping in the future.

Being Optimistic

Many psychologists believe that pessimism is not just a symptom of everyday depression but an important root cause as well. Pessimists not only expect repeated failure and rejection but also perversely accept it as deserved. Pessimists do not see themselves as capable of success, and they irrationally dismiss any evidence of their own accomplishments. This negative point of view is learned, typically at a young age from parents and other authority figures. But as an optimist would tell you, that means it also has the potential of being unlearned.

Pessimists must first recognize and then dispute false, negative predictions they generate about themselves. Learning to be optimistic is easier and more lasting than, for example, learning to eat less. Unlike refusing foods you love, disputing your own negative thoughts is fun—because doing so makes you feel better immediately.

Maintaining Honest Communication

Another important area of psychological functioning is communicating honestly with others. It can be very frustrating for us and for people around us if we cannot express what we want and feel. Others can hardly respond to our needs if they don't know what those needs are. We must recognize what we want to communicate and then express it clearly. Some people know what they want others to do but don't state it clearly because they fear denial of the request, which they interpret as personal rejection. Such people might benefit from **assertiveness** training: learning to insist on their rights and to bargain for what they want. Assertiveness includes being able to say no or yes depending on the situation.

Dealing with Loneliness

The right balance between being alone and being with others is often hard to achieve. Unhappiness with being alone may come from interpreting it as a sign of rejection—that others are not interested in spending time with you. Before you conclude that, be sure that you give others a real chance to get to know you. Examine your patterns of thinking: You may harbor unrealistic expectations about other people—for example, that everyone you meet must like you and, if they don't, you must be terribly flawed.

If you decide that you're not spending enough time with people, take action to change the situation. College life provides many opportunities to meet people. In addition to classes and dorms, there are organizations of all kinds—hiking clubs, religious groups, and so on—that offer a chance to meet others who share your interests.

Dealing with Anger

Popular wisdom has said that you should express your anger rather than suppress it. However, recent studies have questioned this idea by showing that people who are overtly hostile seem to be at higher risk for heart attacks. Furthermore, angry words or actions won't contribute to psychological wellness if they damage important personal or professional relationships or produce feelings of guilt or loss of control. Perhaps the best way to resolve this contradiction is to look at the expression of anger in each situation and distinguish between a gratuitous expression of anger and a reasonable level of self-assertiveness.

Managing Your Own Anger If you feel explosive anger coming on, consider the following two strategies to head it off. First, try to *reframe* what you're thinking at that moment. You'll be less angry at another person if there is a possibility that his or her behavior was not intentionally directed against you. Did the man who cut into your lane on the freeway do it deliberately to spite you, or did he simply fail to see you? Look for possible mitigating factors

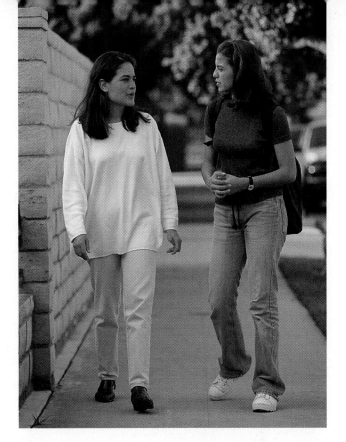

Communication is an important element in any interpersonal relationship. As these women express their thoughts and feelings to each other and listen attentively in response, they enhance their relationship, which in turn supports their psychological well-being.

that would make you less likely to blame him: Maybe he's late for a job interview. If you're angry because you've just been criticized, avoid mentally replaying scenes from the past where you received similar unjust criticisms. Think about what is happening now, and try to act differently than in the past—less defensively and more analytically. Why am I taking it personally? Why am I acting like a jerk just because she did?

Second, until you're able to change your thinking, try do *distract* yourself. Use the old trick of counting to 10 before you respond, or start concentrating on your breathing. If needed, take a longer cooling-off period by leaving the situation until your anger has subsided. This does not mean that you should permanently avoid the issues and people who make you angry. When you've had a chance to think more clearly about the matter, return to it.

cognitive distortion A pattern of thinking that makes events seem worse than they are.

assertiveness Expression that is forceful but not hostile.

Terms

Table 3-1	Lifetime Prevalence of Selected Psychological Disorders Among Americans		
Disorder		**Men (%)**	**Women (%)**
Anxiety disorders			
Simple phobia		6.7	15.7
Social phobia		11.1	15.5
Panic disorder		2.0	5.0
Generalized anxiety disorder		3.6	6.6
Obsessive-compulsive disorder		1.7	2.8
Post-traumatic stress disorder		5.0	10.4
Mood disorders			
Major depressive episode		12.7	21.3
Manic episode		1.6	1.7
Schizophrenia and related disorders		1.0	0.5

SOURCES: U.S. Department of Health and Human Services. 1999. *Mental Health: A Report of the Surgeon General.* Rockville, Md.: DHHS. Weissman, M. M. 1998. Cross-national epidemiology of obsessive-compulsive disorder. *CNS Spectrums* 3(5 Suppl 1): 6–9. Kessler, R.C., et al. 1995. Posttraumatic stress disorder in the National Comorbidity Survey. *Archives of General Psychiatry* 52(12): 1048–1060. Kessler, R. C., et al. 1994. Lifetime and 12-month prevalence of DSM-III-R psychiatric disorders in the United States. *Archives of General Psychiatry* 51(1): 8–19.

Dealing with Anger in Other People   If someone you're with becomes very angry, respond "asymmetrically" by reacting not with anger but with calm. Try to validate the other person by acknowledging that they had a reason to be angry. This does not mean apologizing, if you don't think you're to blame, or accepting verbal abuse, which is always inappropriate. Focus on solving the problem by allowing the individual to explain why he or she is so angry and what can be done to alleviate the situation. Finally, if the person cannot be calmed, it may be best to disengage, at least temporarily. After a time-out, a rational problem-solving approach may be possible.

COMMUNICATE!   You have probably experienced someone else's anger, and perhaps you reacted by becoming angry yourself. But deflecting anger over a minor matter may be more helpful than responding to it directly. The next time someone is angry, see whether you can remain calm long enough to hear the real message behind the person's anger. Is there a way you can respond to what is said, instead of to the way it was said? For instance, instead of "Quit yelling at me!" you might say, "I realize you're upset because I erased your messages. Is there anything I can do to help you find out who called?"

PSYCHOLOGICAL DISORDERS

All of us have felt anxious at times, and in dealing with the anxiety we may have avoided doing something that we wanted to do or should have done. Most of us have had periods of feeling down when we became pessimistic, less energetic, and less able to enjoy life. Many of us have been bothered at times by irrational thoughts or odd feelings. Such feelings and thoughts can be normal responses to the ordinary challenges of life, but when emotions or irrational thoughts start to interfere with daily activities and rob us of our peace of mind, they can be considered symptoms of a psychological disorder (Table 3-1).

Anxiety Disorders

Fear is a basic and useful emotion. It provides motivation for self-protection and for learning to cope with new or potentially dangerous environmental or social situations. Only when fear is out of proportion to real danger can it be considered a problem. **Anxiety** is another word for fear, especially a feeling of fear that is not in response to any definite threat. Only when anxiety is experienced almost daily or in life situations that recur and cannot be avoided can anxiety be called a disorder.

Simple Phobia   The most common and most understandable anxiety disorder, **simple**, or **specific, phobia** is a fear of something definite like lightning or a particular animal or location. Examples of commonly feared animals are snakes, spiders, and dogs; frightening locations are often high places or enclosed spaces. Sometimes, but not always, these fears originate in bad experiences.

Social Phobia   People with **social phobia** fear humiliation or embarrassment while being observed by others. Fear of speaking in public is perhaps the most common phobia of this kind. Extremely shy people can have social fears that extend to almost all social situations.

Panic Disorder   People with **panic disorder** experience sudden unexpected surges in anxiety, accompanied by symptoms such as rapid and strong heartbeat, shortness of breath, loss of physical equilibrium, and a feeling of losing mental control. Such attacks usually begin in one's early twenties and can lead to a fear of being in crowds or closed places or of driving or flying. Sufferers fear that a panic attack will occur in a situation from which escape is difficult (such as while in an elevator), where the attack could be incapacitating and result in a dangerous or embarrassing loss of control (such as while driving a car or shopping), or where no medical help would be available if needed (as when a person is alone away from home). Fears such as these lead to avoidance of situations that might cause trouble. The fears and avoidance may spread

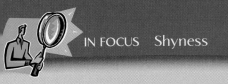

Shyness is a form of social anxiety, a fear of what others will think of one's behavior or appearance. Physical signs include a rapid heartbeat, a nervous stomach, sweating, cold and clammy hands, blushing, dry mouth, and trembling muscles. Shy people are often excessively self-critical, and they engage in very negative self-talk. The accompanying feelings of self-consciousness, embarrassment, and unworthiness can be overwhelming.

To avoid situations that make them anxious, shy people may refrain from making eye contact or speaking up in public. They may shun social gatherings. They may avoid college courses or job promotions that demand more interpersonal interaction or public speaking. The consequences of severe shyness can include social isolation, loneliness, and lost personal and professional opportunities. Very shy people also have higher than average rates of other anxiety and mood disorders and of substance abuse.

Shyness is very common, with 40–50% of Americans describing themselves as shy. However, only 5–10% of adults are so shy that their condition interferes seriously with work, school, daily life, or interpersonal relationships. Shyness is often hidden, and most shy people manage to appear reasonably outgoing, even though they suffer the physical and emotional symptoms of their anxiety. Many shy people do better in structured rather than spontaneous settings.

What causes people to be shy? Research indicates that for some, the trait may be partly inherited. But for shyness, as for many health concerns, biology is not destiny. Many shy children outgrow their shyness, just as others acquire it later in life. Clearly, other factors are involved. The type of attachment between a child and his or her caregiver is important, as are parenting styles. Shyness is more common in cultures where children's failures are attributed to their own actions but successes are attributed to other people or events. People's experiences during critical developmental transitions, such as starting school and entering adolescence, have also been linked to shy-

ness. For adults, the precipitating factor may be an event such as divorce or the loss of a job.

Recent surveys indicate that shyness rates may be rising in the United States. With the advent of technologies such as ATM machines, video games, voice mail, faxes, and e-mail, the opportunities for face-to-face interaction are diminishing. Electronic media can be a wonderful way for shy people to communicate, but it can also allow them to hide from all social interaction. In fact, one study found that greater use of the Internet was associated with a decline in participants' communication with family members, a reduction in the size of their social circles, and an increase in levels of depression and loneliness. It remains to be seen whether the first generation to have cradle-to-grave access to home computers, faxes, and the Internet will experience higher rates of shyness.

Shyness is often undiagnosed, but help is available. Shyness classes, assertiveness training groups, and public speaking clinics are available (see the Behavior Change Strategy at the end of the chapter). For the seriously shy, effective treatments include cognitive-behavioral therapy and antidepressant drugs.

If you're shy, try to remember that shyness is widespread and that there are worse fates. Some degree of shyness has an up side. Shy people tend to be gentle, supportive, kind, and sensitive; they are often exceptional listeners. People who think carefully before they speak or act are less likely to hurt the feelings of others. Shyness may also facilitate cooperation. For any group or society to functon well, a variety of roles is required, and there is a place for quieter, more reflective individuals.

SOURCES: Carducci, B. J. 1999. *Shyness: A Bold New Approach.* New York: Perennial. Kraut, R., et al. 1998. Internet paradox: A social technology that reduces social involvement and psychological well-being? *American Psychologist* 53(9): 1017–1031. Lamberg, L. 1998. Social phobia—not just another name for shyness. *Journal of the American Medical Association* 280(8): 685–686.

---

to a large variety of situations until a person is virtually housebound, a condition called **agoraphobia.**

Generalized Anxiety Disorder

A basic reaction to future threats is to worry about them. **Generalized anxiety disorder (GAD)** is a diagnosis given to people whose worries have taken on a life of their own, pushing out other thoughts and refusing banishment by any effort of will. The topics of the worrying are ordinary concerns: Will I be able to pass the exam next Friday? Where will I get money to get my car fixed? Is my boyfriend really interested in me? But the end result is a persistent feeling of nervousness, often accompanied by depression, which impairs one's ability to enjoy life and to get things done.

Obsessive-Compulsive Disorder

The diagnosis of **obsessive-compulsive disorder (OCD)** is given to people

Terms

anxiety A feeling of fear that is not directed toward any definite threat.

simple (specific) phobia A persistent and excessive fear of a specific object, activity, or situation.

social phobia An excessive fear of performing in public; speaking in public is the most common example.

panic disorder A syndrome of severe anxiety attacks accompanied by physical symptoms.

agoraphobia An anxiety disorder characterized by fear of being alone away from help and avoidance of many different places and situations; in extreme cases, a fear of leaving home. From the Greek for "fear of the public market."

generalized anxiety disorder (GAD) An anxiety disorder characterized by excessive, uncontrollable worry about all kinds of things and anxiety in many situations.

obsessive-compulsive disorder (OCD) An anxiety disorder characterized by uncontrollable, recurring thoughts and the performing of senseless rituals.

with obsessions or compulsions or both. **Obsessions** are recurrent, unwanted thoughts or impulses. Unlike the worries of GAD, they are not ordinary concerns, but improbable fears such as of suddenly committing an antisocial act or of having been contaminated by germs. **Compulsions** are repetitive, difficult-to-resist actions usually associated with obsessions. A common compulsion is hand washing, associated with an obsessive fear of contamination by dirt. Other compulsions are counting and repeatedly checking if something has been done—for example, if a door has been locked or a stove turned off. People with OCD feel anxious, out of control, and embarrassed, and their rituals can occupy much of their time.

Post-Traumatic Stress Disorder People who suffer from **post-traumatic stress disorder (PTSD)** are reacting to severely traumatic events (events that produce a sense of terror and helplessness) such as physical violence to oneself or loved ones. Trauma occurs in personal assaults (rape or military combat), natural disasters (floods, earthquakes), and tragedies like fires and airplane or car crashes. Symptoms include reexperiencing the trauma in dreams and in intrusive memories, trying to avoid anything associated with the trauma, and numbing of feelings. Sleep disturbances and other symptoms of anxiety and depression also commonly occur. Such symptoms can last months or even years.

Therapies for anxiety disorders range from medication to psychological interventions concentrating on a person's thoughts and behavior.

ᵂᵂ. Mood Disorders

We all experience ups and downs in our mood in response to daily events. These temporary mood changes typically don't affect our overall emotional state or level of wellness. A person with a mood disorder, however, experiences emotional disturbances that are intense and persistent enough to affect normal functioning.

Depression The most common mood disorder, **depression** has forms and degrees. It usually involves demoralization and can include the following:

- A feeling of sadness and hopelessness
- Loss of pleasure in doing usual activities
- Poor appetite and weight loss
- Insomnia or disturbed sleep
- Restlessness or, alternatively, fatigue
- Thoughts of worthlessness and guilt
- Trouble concentrating or making decisions
- Thoughts of death or suicide

Not all these features are present in every depressive episode. Sometimes instead of poor appetite and insomnia, the opposite occurs—eating too much and sleeping too long. Amazingly, people can have most of the symptoms of depression without feeling sad or hopeless or in a depressed mood, although they usually do experience a loss of interest or pleasure in things. In some cases, depression is a clear-cut reaction to specific events, such as the loss of a loved one, failing in school, being fired, or the breakup of a relationship, while in other cases no trigger event is obvious.

RECOGNIZING THE WARNING SIGNS OF SUICIDE One of the principal dangers of severe depression is suicide. Although a suicide attempt can occur unpredictably and unaccompanied by depression, the chances are greater if symptoms are numerous and severe. Additional warning signs of suicide include the following:

- Expressing the wish to be dead or revealing contemplated methods
- Increasing social withdrawal and isolation
- A sudden, inexplicable lightening of mood (which can mean the person has finally decided to commit suicide)

Certain risk factors increase the likelihood of suicide:

- A history of previous attempts
- A suicide by a family member or friend
- Readily available means, such as guns or pills
- A history of substance abuse or eating disorders
- Serious medical problems

The groups in the United States with the highest suicide rates are males age 20–34, Native American males, and white males over age 65. Women attempt three times as many suicides as men, yet men succeed at more than three times the rate of women.

Terms

obsession A recurrent, irrational, unwanted thought or impulse.

compulsion An irrational, repetitive, forced action, usually associated with an obsession.

post-traumatic stress disorder (PTSD) An anxiety disorder characterized by reliving traumatic events through dreams, flashbacks, and hallucinations.

depression A mood disorder characterized by loss of interest, sadness, hopelessness, loss of appetite, disturbed sleep, and other physical symptoms.

electroconvulsive therapy (ECT) The use of electric shock to induce brief, generalized seizures; used in the treatment of selected psychological disorders.

seasonal affective disorder (SAD) A mood disorder characterized by seasonal depression, usually occurring in winter, when there is less daylight.

mania A mood disorder characterized by excessive elation, irritability, talkativeness, inflated self-esteem, and expansiveness.

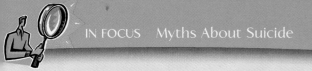

Myth   People who really intend to kill themselves do not let anyone know about it.
Fact   Most people who eventually commit suicide *have* talked about doing it.

Myth   People who made a suicide attempt but survived did not really intend to die.
Fact   This may be true for some, but people who seriously want to end their life may fail because they misjudge what it takes. Even a pharmacist may misjudge the lethal dose of a drug.

Myth   People who succeed in suicide really wanted to die.
Fact   We cannot be sure of that either. Some people are only trying to make a dramatic gesture or plea for help but miscalculate.

Myth   People who really want to kill themselves will do it regardless of any attempts to prevent them.
Fact   Few people are single-minded about suicide even at the moment of attempting it. People who are quite determined to take their life today may change their mind completely tomorrow.

Myth   Suicide is proof of mental illness.
Fact   Many suicides are committed by people who do not meet ordinary criteria for mental illness, although people with depression, schizophrenia, and other psychological disorders have a much higher than average suicide rate.

Myth   People inherit suicidal tendencies.
Fact   Certain kinds of depression that lead to suicide do have a genetic component. But many examples of suicide running in a family can be explained by factors such as psychologically identifying with a family member who committed suicide, often a parent.

Myth   All suicides are irrational.
Fact   By some standards all suicides may seem "irrational." But many people find it at least understandable that someone might want to commit suicide, for example, when approaching the end of a terminal illness or when facing a long prison term.

HELPING YOURSELF OR A FRIEND   If you are severely depressed or know someone who is, expert help from a mental health professional is essential. Don't try to do it all yourself. If you suspect one of your friends is suicidally depressed, try to get him or her to see a professional.

Don't be afraid to discuss the possibility of suicide with people you fear are suicidal. You won't give them an idea they haven't already thought of. And asking direct questions is the best way to determine whether someone seriously intends to commit suicide. Encourage your friend to talk and to take positive steps to improve his or her situation. If you feel there is an immediate danger of suicide, ensure that the person is not left alone, especially when he or she is emotionally upset and more likely to act impulsively. If you must leave your friend alone, have your friend promise not to do anything to harm himself or herself without first calling you. Get qualified help as soon as possible.

If your friend refuses help, you might try to contact your friend's relatives and tell them that you are worried. If the depressed person is a college student, you may need to let someone in your health service or college administration know your concerns. Finally, most communities have emergency help available, often in the form of a hotline telephone counseling service run by a suicide prevention agency (check the yellow pages).

TREATING DEPRESSION   Although treatments are highly effective, only about 35% of people who suffer from depression currently seek treatment. Treatment for depression depends on its severity and on whether the depressed person is suicidal. The best initial treatment for moderate to severe depression is probably a combination of drug therapy and some kind of psychotherapy. "Uppers" such as amphetamines are not good antidepressants; much better are newer prescription antidepressants, although they may take several weeks to begin working. Therefore, when suicidal impulses are strong, hospitalization for a week or so may be necessary. **Electroconvulsive therapy (ECT)** is effective for severe depression when other approaches have failed.

One type of depression is treated in a unique way—by having sufferers sit with eyes open in front of a bright light source for an hour or so early every morning. These patients have **seasonal affective disorder (SAD)**, in which depression worsens during winter months as the number of hours of daylight diminishes and then improves with the lengthening of daylight in the spring and summer. Seasonal depression is more common among people who live at higher latitudes, where there are fewer hours of light in winter. Light therapy may work by extending the perceived length of the day and thus convincing the brain that it is summertime even during the winter months.

Mania and Bipolar Disorder   People who experience **mania**, a less common feature of mood disorders, are restless, have a lot of energy, need little sleep, and often talk nonstop. They may devote themselves to fantastic projects and spend more money than they can afford. Many manic people swing between manic and depressive

Mainstream therapies for depression include medications such as Prozac that are accepted as safe and effective by government regulatory agencies, certain psychotherapies, and light therapy in the case of seasonal affective disorder. Yet, in surveys, 20% of people in the United States who suffer from depression report using unconventional therapies such as acupuncture, body movement therapy, homeopathy, qigong, faith healing, or herbs or other "natural" substances. With the exception of one herb, St. John's wort (*Hypericum perforatum*), these therapies have not been shown to be effective in double-blind placebo-controlled trials. Such trials are the only scientific way to show that a treatment has healing power beyond that of a **placebo.**

St. John's wort, a flowering plant that grows as a weed in the United States, has been reputed to have curative properties since the time of Hippocrates in ancient Greece. Modern pharmacological studies confirm that its active ingredients produce a number of biochemical and physiological changes in animals, although it's still unclear exactly how these changes might affect depression. Data from a number of studies demonstrate that St. John's wort can benefit some people with mild to moderate depression. St. John's wort may cause fewer adverse effects than conventional antidepressants, although the user may experience gastrointestinal disturbances, increased sensitivity to sunlight, dizziness, dry mouth, or other side effects; it should not be taken by pregnant women. In addition, St. John's wort may interact with, and reduce the effectiveness of, certain medications, including oral contraceptives and certain medications for treating heart disease, depression, HIV infection, and seizures.

One reason for the popularity of an herb for depression is that it doesn't require a prescription or any kind of contact with a physician or therapist; for those who are not members of a generous health care plan, an herbal remedy may also be less expensive than a prescription antidepressant. On the other hand, people suffering from depression *should* seek professional advice and not try to get along entirely with self-diagnosis and self-help. St. John's wort doesn't work for everyone, and it is not effective for severe depression. Also, because herbal products are classified as dietary supplements, they are not scrutinized by the regulatory agencies that oversee prescription drugs. Thus, customers have no guarantee that the product contains the herbs and dosages listed on the label.

Finally, although St. John's wort is more effective than a placebo for some people, it may not be as effective as newer prescription antidepressants. Research is currently underway to learn more about St. John's wort—its active ingredients, method of action, level of effectiveness, and possible side effects or drug interactions. Until more is known, caution may be the best approach.

SOURCES: Shelton, R. C. et al. 2001. Effectiveness of St. John's wort in major depression. *Journal of the American Medical Association* 285(15): 1978–1986. National Institute of Mental Health. 2000. *Questions and Answers About St. John's Wort* (http://www.nimh.nih.gov/publicat/stjohnqa. cfm; retrieved August 31, 2000); Ernst, E., J. I. Rand, and C. Stevinson. 1998. Complementary therapies for depression.An overview. *Archives of General Psychiatry* 55: 1026–1032; Wong, A. H., M. Smith, and H. S. Boon. 1998. Herbal remedies in psychiatric practice. *Archives of General Psychiatry* 55: 1033–1044.

states, a syndrome called **bipolar disorder** because of the two opposite poles of mood. Tranquilizers are used to treat individual manic episodes, while drugs like lithium carbonate taken daily can prevent future mood swings.

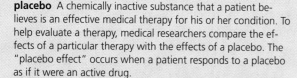

Terms

placebo A chemically inactive substance that a patient believes is an effective medical therapy for his or her condition. To help evaluate a therapy, medical researchers compare the effects of a particular therapy with the effects of a placebo. The "placebo effect" occurs when a patient responds to a placebo as if it were an active drug.

bipolar disorder A mental illness characterized by alternating periods of depression and mania.

schizophrenia A psychological disorder that involves a disturbance in thinking and in perceiving reality.

attention-deficit/hyperactivity disorder (ADHD) A disorder characterized by persistent, pervasive problems with inattention and/or hyperactivity to a degree that is not considered appropriate for a child's developmental stage and that causes significant difficulties in school, work, or relationships.

Schizophrenia

Schizophrenia can be severe and debilitating or quite mild and hardly noticeable. Although people are capable of diagnosing their own depression, they usually don't diagnose their own schizophrenia, because they often can't see that anything is wrong. This disorder is not rare; in fact, 1 in every 100 people has a schizophrenic episode sometime in his or her lifetime, most commonly starting in adolescence. Some general characteristics of schizophrenia include the following:

- *Disorganized thoughts.* Thoughts may be expressed in a vague or confusing way.

- *Inappropriate emotions.* Emotions may be absent or strong but inappropriate.

- *Delusions.* People with delusions—firmly held false beliefs—may think that their minds are controlled by outside forces, that people can read their minds, that they are great personages like Jesus Christ or the president of the United States, or that they are being persecuted by a group like the CIA.

- *Auditory hallucinations.* Schizophrenic people may hear voices when no one is present.

Attention-deficit/hyperactivity disorder (ADHD) is among the most controversial of all psychiatric diagnoses. The American Psychiatric Association (APA) describes ADHD as persistent, pervasive problems with inattention and/or hyperactivity to a degree that is not considered appropriate for a child's developmental stage and that causes significant difficulties in school, at home, and in peer relationships. Symptoms develop before a child is 7 years old and last at least 6 months; some symptoms may persist into adulthood, but the disorder always begins in childhood. The debate over ADHD arises because it is difficult to draw the line between normal degrees of inattention, hyperactivity, and impulsiveness and levels that are pathological and may benefit from treatment.

Some mental health professionals feel that the diagnosis of ADHD is applied too broadly and that large numbers of children who do not meet the criteria for ADHD are unnecessarily exposed to the potentially harmful side effects of psychostimulants used in treatment. Concerned parents and physicians point to the large increase in the use of Ritalin (methylphenidate), the most widely used drug for ADHD, in the past decade and the fact that U.S. children are much more likely than European children to be diagnosed with ADHD and treated with drugs. They feel that ADHD may sometimes be a conveniently simple diagnosis in cases where a child's difficulties are actually due to much more complex family, educational, or social problems. These concerns led to the filing, in 2000, of several class action lawsuits against the APA and the maker of Ritalin.

However, many mental health professionals feel that a strong case can be made for diagnosing some children with ADHD and treating them with medication. Treatment with psychostimu-

lants reduces the core symptoms of ADHD and allows affected individuals to better focus their attention and control impulsive and aggressive behavior. Once treated, affected students do better at school both academically and socially. Without treatment, children with ADHD may be labeled absentminded, rude, and dumb; they may develop low self-esteem and more serious psychological and behavior problems as adolescents and adults.

How many U.S. children have been diagnosed with ADHD and treated with medication? A widespread survey involving all public school children in Maryland found that about 3% of the students were receiving medication for ADHD. Boys were three to four times more likely than girls to be taking medication, and white grade-school students were about twice as likely to be receiving medication as African American, Latino, and Asian American students. What's unclear from these survey findings is how many of the children who are taking medication do not meet the criteria for ADHD and how many children who actually have ADHD remain undiagnosed and untreated. Major government and professional organizations are trying to raise awareness among teachers, parents, and health professionals about how best to identify children with ADHD. Despite these efforts, it is likely that the diagnosis and treatment of ADHD will remain controversial.

SOURCES: Safer, D. J., and M. Malever. 2000. Stimulant treatment in Maryland public schools. *Pediatrics* 106(3): 533–539. Angold, A., et al. 2000. Stimulant treatment for children: A community perspective. *Journal of the American Academy of Child and Adolescent Psychiatry* 39(8): 975–984. Hausman, K. 2000. Parents accuse APA, Novartis of conspiracy over Ritalin sales. *Psychiatric News* 35(15): 1 ff. Frances, A., and M. B. First. 1998. *Your Mental Health.* New York: Scribner.

- *Deteriorating social and work functioning.* Social withdrawal and poor performance at school or work may be so gradual that they are hardly noticed at first.

A schizophrenic person needs help from a mental health professional. Suicide is a risk in schizophrenia, and expert treatment can reduce that risk and minimize the social consequences of the illness by shortening the period when symptoms are active. The key element in treatment is regular medication.

GETTING HELP

Knowing when self-help or professional help is required for mental health problems is usually not as difficult as knowing how to start or where to go.

Self-Help

If you have a personal problem to solve, a smart way to begin is by finding out what you can do on your own. Some problems are specifically addressed in this book. Behavioral and cognitive approaches all involve becoming

more aware of self-defeating actions and ideas and combating them in some way: being more assertive; communicating honestly; raising your self-esteem by counteracting thoughts, people, and actions that undermine it; and confronting, rather than avoiding, the things you fear. Get more information by seeing what books are available in the psychology or self-help sections of libraries and bookstores. But be selective. Watch out for self-help books making fantastic claims that deviate from mainstream approaches.

Some people find it helpful to express their feelings in a journal. Grappling with a painful experience in this way provides an emotional release and can help you develop more constructive ways of dealing with similar situations in the future. Research indicates that using a journal this way can improve physical as well as emotional wellness.

For some people, religious belief and practice may promote psychological health. Religious organizations provide a social network and a supportive community, and religious practices, such as prayer and meditation, offer a path for personal change and transformation.

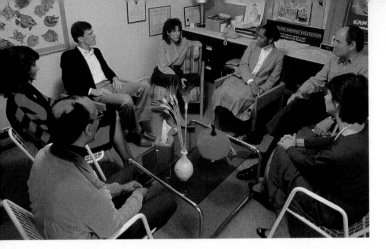

Group therapy is just one of many different approaches to psychological counseling. If you have concerns you would like to discuss with a mental health professional, shop around to find the approach that works for you.

Peer Counseling and Support Groups

Sharing your concerns with others is another helpful way of dealing with psychological health challenges. Just being able to share what's troubling you with an accepting, empathetic person can bring relief. Comparing notes with people who have problems similar to yours can give you new ideas about coping. Many colleges offer peer counseling through a health center or through the psychology or education department. Peer counselors may steer you toward an appropriate campus or community resource or simply offer a sympathetic ear.

Many self-help groups work on the principle of bringing together people with similar problems to share their experiences and support each other. Support groups are typically organized around a specific problem, such as eating disorders or substance abuse.

⩔w. Professional Help

Sometimes self-help or talking to nonprofessionals is not enough. More objective, more expert, or more discreet help is needed. Many people have trouble accepting the need for professional help, and often those who most need help are the most unwilling to get it. You may someday find yourself having to overcome your own reluctance, or that of a friend, about seeking help.

Determining the Need for Professional Help In some cases, professional help is optional. Some people are interested in improving their psychological health in a general way by going into individual or group therapy to learn more about themselves and how to interact with others. Interpersonal friction among family members or between partners often falls in the middle between necessary and optional. Successful help with such problems can mean the difference between a painful divorce and a satisfying relationship.

It's sometimes difficult to determine whether someone needs professional help, but it is important to be aware of behaviors that may indicate a serious problem:

- If depression, anxiety, or other emotional problems begin to interfere seriously with school or work performance or in getting along with others
- If suicide is attempted or is seriously considered (refer to the warning signs earlier in the chapter)
- If symptoms such as hallucinations, delusions, incoherent speech, or loss of memory occur
- If alcohol or drugs are used to the extent that they impair normal functioning during much of the week, if finding or taking drugs occupies much of the week, or if reducing their dosage leads to psychological or physiological withdrawal symptoms

Choosing a Mental Health Professional Mental health workers belong to several different professions and have different roles. Psychiatrists are medical doctors. They are experts in deciding whether a medical disease lies behind psychological symptoms, and they are usually involved in treatment if medication or hospitalization is required. Clinical psychologists typically hold a Ph.D. degree; they are often experts in behavioral and cognitive therapies. Other mental health workers include social workers, licensed counselors, and clergy with special training in pastoral counseling.

Tips for Today

Life inevitably brings change and challenge—they are a part of growth and development. Most of life's psychological challenges can be met with self-help and everyday skills—introspection and insight, honest communication, support from family and friends. Sometimes a psychological problem poses a greater challenge than we can handle on our own; for these situations, professional help is available.

Right now you can

- Consider the areas in your life where you can be creative (one of the qualities associated with self-actualization), whether in music, art, Web page design, party planning, or whatever you truly enjoy. With the knowledge that allowing your creative side to flourish is a valuable use of your time, plan a way to spend an hour or more on this activity this week.

- Sit down and write 100 positive adjectives that describe you (friendly, loyal, athletic, smart, musical, sensitive, and so on). If you can't think of 100 right now, write as many as you can and keep thinking about it over the next day or two until you reach 100.

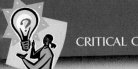

College students are usually in a good position to find convenient, affordable mental health care. Larger schools typically have both health services that employ psychiatrists and psychologists and counseling centers staffed by professionals and peer counselors. Resources in the community may include a school of medicine, a hospital, and a variety of professionals who work independently. It's a good idea to get recommendations from physicians, clergy, friends who have been in therapy, or community agencies rather than pick a name at random.

Financial considerations are also important. Find out how much different services will cost and what your health insurance will cover. If you're not adequately covered by a health plan, don't let that stop you from getting help; investigate low-cost alternatives on campus and in your community. The cost of treatment is linked to how many therapy sessions will be needed, which in turn depends on the type of therapy and the nature of the problem. Psychological therapies focusing on specific problems may require eight or ten sessions at weekly intervals. Therapies aiming for psychological awareness and personality change can last months or years.

Deciding whether a therapist is right for you will require meeting the therapist in person. Before or during your first meeting, find out about the therapist's background and training:

- Does she or he have a degree from an appropriate professional school and a state license to practice?

- Has she or he had experience treating people with problems similar to yours?

- How much will therapy cost?

You have a right to know the answers to these questions and should not hesitate to ask them. After your initial meeting, evaluate your impressions:

- Does the therapist seem like a warm, intelligent person who would be able to help you and interested in doing so?

- Are you comfortable with the personality, values, and beliefs of the therapist?

- Is he or she willing to talk about the techniques in use? Do these techniques make sense to you?

If you answer yes to these questions, this therapist may be satisfactory for you. If you feel uncomfortable—and you're not in need of emergency care—it's worthwhile to set up one-time consultations with one or two others before you make up your mind. Take the time to find someone who feels right for you.

Later in your treatment, evaluate your progress:

- Are you being helped by the treatment?

- If you are displeased, is it because you aren't making progress or because therapy is raising difficult, painful issues you don't want to deal with?

- Can you express dissatisfaction to your therapist? Such feedback can improve your treatment.

If you're convinced your therapy isn't working or is harmful, thank your therapist for her or his efforts, and find another.

- Take a serious look at how you've been feeling the past few weeks. If you have any feelings that are especially difficult to deal with, begin to think about how you can get help with them. Consider consulting the self-help section at the bookstore, talking to a trustworthy friend or peer counselor, or making an appointment with a staff person at the campus counseling center.

SUMMARY

- Psychological health encompasses more than a single particular state of normality. Psychological diversity is valuable among groups of people.

- Defining psychological health as the presence of wellness means that to be healthy you must strive to fulfill your potential. Self-actualized people have high self-esteem and are realistic, inner-directed, authentic, capable of emotional intimacy, and creative.

- Crucial parts of psychological wellness include developing an adult identity, establishing intimate relationships, and developing values and purpose in life, and achieving healthy self-esteem.

- A pessimistic outlook can damage psychological well-being; it can be overcome by developing more realistic self-talk.

- Honest communication requires recognizing what needs to be said and saying it clearly.

- People may be lonely if they haven't developed ways to be happy on their own or if they interpret being alone as a sign of rejection. Lonely people can take action to expand their social contacts.

- Dealing successfully with anger involves distinguishing between a reasonable level of assertiveness and gratuitous expressions of anger, heading off rage, and responding to the anger of others.

- People with psychological disorders have symptoms severe enough to interfere with daily living.

- Anxiety is a fear that is not directed toward any definite threat. Anxiety disorders include simple phobias, social phobias, panic disorder, generalized anxiety disorder, obsessive-compulsive disorder, and post-traumatic stress disorder.

- Depression is a common mood disorder; loss of interest or pleasure in things seems to be its most

Shyness is often the result of both high anxiety levels and lack of key social skills. To help overcome shyness, you need to learn to manage your fear of social situations and to develop social skills such as appropriate eye contact, initiating topics in conversations, and maintaining the flow of conversations. Try some of the following strategies for reducing your anxiety in social situations:

- Refocus your attention away from the physical stress reaction you're experiencing and toward the social task at hand. Your nervousness is probably much less visible than you think.

- Allow a warm-up period for new situations. Realize that you will feel more nervous at first, and take steps to relax and become more comfortable. Refer to the suggestions for deep breathing and other relaxation techniques in Chapter 2.

- If possible, take breaks during anxiety-producing situations. For example, if you're at a party, take a moment to visit the restroom or step outside. Alternate between speaking with good friends and striking up conversations with new acquaintances.

- Practice realistic self-talk. Replace your self-critical thoughts with more supportive ones: "No one else is perfect, and I don't have to be either." "It would have been good if I had thought of a funny story to tell, but I had a very nice talk with my new acquaintance."

Starting and maintaining conversations can be difficult for shy people, who may feel overwhelmed by their physical stress reaction. If small talk is a problem for you, try the following:

- Introduce yourself early in the conversation. If you tend to forget names, repeat your new acquaintance's name to help fix it in your mind ("Nice to meet you, Amelia.").

- Ask questions, and look for shared topics of interest. Simple, open-ended questions like "How's your presentation coming along?" or "How do you know our host?" encourage others to carry the conversation for a while and help bring forth a variety of subjects.

- Take turns talking, and elaborate on your answers. Simple "yes" and "no" answers don't move the conversation along. Try to relate something in your life—a course you're taking or a hobby you have—to something in the other person's life. Match self-disclosure with self-disclosure.

- Have something to say. Expand your mind and become knowledgeable about current events and local or campus news. If you have specialized knowledge about a topic, practice discussing it in ways that both beginners and experts can understand and appreciate.

- If you get stuck for something to say, try giving a compliment ("Great presentation!" or "I love your earrings.") or performing a social grace (pass the chips or get someone a drink).

- Be an active listener. Reward the other person with your full attention and with regular responses. Make frequent eye contact and maintain a relaxed but alert posture.

At first, your new behaviors will likely make you anxious. Don't give up—things *will* get easier. Create lots of opportunities to practice your new behaviors. Eventually, you'll be able to sustain social interactions with comfort and enjoyment. If you find that social anxiety is a major problem for you and self-help techniques don't seem to work, consider looking into a shyness clinic or treatment program on your campus.

SOURCES: Carducci, B. J. 1999. *Shyness: A Bold New Approach*. New York: Perennial. University of Texas at Dallas, Student Counseling Center. 2000. *Overcoming Social Anxiety* (http://www.utdallas.edu/student/slife/counseling/anxiety.html; retrieved August 31, 2000).

universal symptom. Severe depression carries a high risk of suicide, and suicidally depressed people need professional help. Symptoms of mania include exalted moods with unrealistically high self-esteem, little need for sleep, and rapid speech. Mood swings between mania and depression characterize bipolar disorder.

- Schizophrenia is characterized by disorganized thoughts, inappropriate emotions, delusions, auditory hallucinations, and deteriorating social and work performance.

- Help is available in a variety of forms, including self-help, peer counseling, support groups, and therapy with a mental health professional.

TAKE ACTION

1. Investigate the mental health services on your campus and in your community. What services are available? Think about which ones you would feel comfortable using, for either yourself or someone else, should the need ever arise.
2. Many colleges and communities have peer counseling programs, hotline services (for both general problems and specific issues such as rape, suicide, and drug abuse), and other kinds of emergency counseling services. Some programs are staffed by trained volunteers. Investigate such programs in your school (through the health clinic or student services) or community and consider volunteering for one. The training and experience can help you understand both yourself and others.

3. Being assertive rather than passive or aggressive is a valuable skill that everyone can learn. To improve your ability to assert yourself appropriately, sign up for a workshop or class in assertiveness training on your campus or in your community.

1. Do you remember incidents or moments from childhood that stand out as wonderful or horrible? Write a short essay about two such incidents, including what your feelings were and what you think you learned from them. Then describe what you would do now in the same situations and why.

2. *Critical Thinking* In the past, some political candidates have dropped out of a race or been defeated after it was revealed that they had undergone psychiatric treatment or some other form of therapy. Do you think a person who has been treated for a mental illness should be excluded from holding a public office or from any other profession? Why or why not? Does your position depend on the type of illness or the treatment the individual received? In your health journal, write a brief essay explaining your position.

3. Think about a person you respect. Describe him or her in writing, listing the qualities you admire. Do you have any of those qualities? What does your list say about the kind of person you want to be?

FOR MORE INFORMATION

Books

Casey, N. 2001. *Unholy Ghost: Writers on Depression.* New York: William Morrow. *An eloquent collection of essays about depression.*

Frances, A., and M. B. First. 1999. *Your Mental Health: A Layman's Guide to the Psychiatrist's Bible.* New York: Scribner. *A resource-packed reference with information on dozens of mental disorders; based on the APA's DSM-IV.*

Schwartz, S. 2000. *Abnormal Psychology: A Discovery Approach.* Mountain View, Calif.: Mayfield. *Provides a comprehensive introduction to psychological disorders.*

Seligman, M. E. P. 1998. *Learned Optimism.* New York: Pocket Books. *A discussion of the effects of pessimism, optimism, and learned helplessness, with suggestions for change.*

Wolpert, L. 2000. *Malignant Sadness: The Anatomy of Depression.* New York: Free Press. *A look at the nature of depression, with information for people with the disorder and their families.*

WW. Organizations, Hotlines, and Web Sites

American Psychiatric Association (APA). Provides public information by pamphlet or online about a variety of topics, including depression, anxiety, eating disorders, and psychiatric medications.
202-682-6000; 888-357-7924
http://www.psych.org

American Psychological Association Consumer HelpCenter. Provides information about common challenges to psychological health and about how to obtain professional help.
800-964-2000
http://helping.apa.org

Anxiety Disorders Association of America (ADAA). Provides information and resources related to anxiety disorders, including listings of support groups.
301-231-9350
http://www.adaa.org

Internet Mental Health. An encyclopedia of mental health information, including medical diagnostic criteria.
http://www.mentalhealth.com

Mental Health Net. A comprehensive guide to mental health online, including background information and links for many topics.
http://www.cmhc.com

NAMI (National Alliance for the Mentally Ill). Provides information and support for people who are affected by mental illness.
800-950-NAMI (Help Line)
http://www.nami.org

National Depressive and Manic-Depressive Association (NDMDA). Provides educational materials and information about support groups and other resources.
800-82-NDMDA
http://www.ndmda.org

National Institute of Mental Health (NIMH). Provides helpful information about anxiety, depression, eating disorders, and other challenges to psychological health.
800-421-4211 (NIMH information line); 301-443-4513
http://www.nimh.nih.gov

National Mental Health Association. Provides consumer information on a variety of issues, including how to find help.
800-969-NMHA
http://www.nmha.org

National Mental Health Services Knowledge and Exchange Network (KEN). A one-stop source for information and resources relating to mental health.
800-789-CMHS
http://www.mentalhealth.org

Psych Central: Dr. John Grohol's Mental Health Page. A guide to psychology, support, and mental health issues, resources, and people on the Internet.
http://psychcentral.com

Student Counseling Virtual Pamphlet Collection. Provides links to more than 400 pamphlets produced by different student counseling centers; topics range from depression and anxiety to time management and assertiveness.

http://counseling.uchicago.edu/vpc

The following sites include interactive online assessments for various psychological problems:

Depression-screening.org: http://www.depression-screening.org
Freedom from Fear: http://www.freedomfromfear.com
New York University Department of Psychiatry: http://www.med.nyu.edu/Psych/public.html

SELECTED BIBLIOGRAPHY

American Psychiatric Association. 2000. *Diagnostic and Statistical Manual of Mental Disorders,* Fourth Edition, Text Revision *(DSM-IV-TR).* Washington, D.C.: American Psychiatric Association Press.

Baare, W. F., et al. 2001. Volumes of brain structures in twins discordant for schizophrenia. *Archives of General Psychiatry* 58(1): 33–40.

Chang, E. C., and W. B. Bridewell. 1998. Irrational beliefs, optimism, pessimism, and psychological distress: A preliminary examination of differential effects in a college population. *Journal of Clinical Psychology* 54(2): 137–142.

Dodgson, P. G., and J. V. Wood. 1998. Self-esteem and the cognitive accessibility of strengths and weaknesses after failure. *Journal of Personality and Social Psychology* 75(1): 178–197.

Generalized anxiety disorder. 2000. *Journal of the American Medical Association Patient Page* 283(23): 3156.

Hinsie, L. E. 1999. The treatment of schizophrenia: A survey of the literature. *Psychiatric Quarterly* 70(1): 5–26.

Kender, K. S., and C. A. Prescott. 1999. A population-based twin study of lifetime major depression in men and women. *Archives of General Psychiatry* 56(1): 39–44.

Lam, R. W., et al. 2000. Effects of light therapy on suicidal ideation in patients with winter depression. *Journal of Clinical Psychiatry* 61(1): 30–32.

Maruta, T., et al. 2000. Optimists vs. pessimists: Survival rate among medical patients over a 30-year period. *Mayo Clinic Proceedings* 75(2): 140–143.

National Institutes of Health, National Center for Complementary and Alternative Medicine. 2000. *Factsheet: St. John's Wort* (http://nccam.nih.gov/nccam/fcp/factsheets/stjohnswort/stjohnswort.htm; retrieved May 9, 2000).

Nolen-Hoeksema, S., C. Grayson, and J. Larson. 1999. Explaining the gender difference in depressive symptoms. *Journal of Personality and Social Psychology* 77(5): 1061–1072.

Panic disorder. 2000. *Journal of the American Medical Association Patient Page* 283(19): 2612.

Perkonnigg, A., et al. 2000. Traumatic events and posttraumatic stress disorder in the community: Prevalence, risk factors, and comorbidity. *Acta Psychiatrica Scandinavica* 101: 46–59.

Pini, S., et al. 2001. Insight into illness in schizophrenia, schizoaffective disorder, and mood disorders with psychotic features. *American Journal of Psychiatry* 158(1): 122–125.

Raikkonen, K., et al. 1999. Effects of optimism, pessimism, and trait anxiety on ambulatory blood pressure and mood during everyday life. *Journal of Personal and Social Psychology* 76(1): 104–113.

Reynolds, C. F., et al. 1999. Nortriptyline and interpersonal psychotherapy as maintenance therapies for recurrent major depression. *Journal of the American Medical Association* 281: 39–45.

Rothwell, J. D. 2000. *In the Company of Others: An Introduction to Communication.* Mountain View, Calif.: Mayfield.

Schwartz, S. 2000. *Abnormal Psychology: A Discovery Approach.* Mountain View, Calif.: Mayfield.

Sheldon, K. M., and L. Houser-Marko. 2001. Self-concordance, goal attainment, and the pursuit of happiness: Can there be an upward spiral? *Journal of Personality and Social Psychology* 80(1): 152–165.

Snow, V., S. Lascher, and C. Mottur-Pilson. 2000. Pharmacological treatment of acute major depression and dysthymia. *Annals of Internal Medicine* 132(9): 738–742.

Spicer, R. S., and T. R. Miller. 2000. Suicide acts in 8 states: incidence and case fatality rates by demographics and method. *American Journal of Public Health* 90(12): 1885–1891.

Stein, M. B., K. L. Jang, and W. J. Livesley. 1999. Heritability of anxiety sensitivity: A twin study. *American Journal of Psychiatry* 156(2): 246–251.

Treating depression with electroconvulsive therapy. 2001. *Journal of the American Medical Association* 285(10): 1390.

U.S. Department of Health and Human Services. 1999. *Mental Health: A Report of the Surgeon General.* Rockville, Md.: DHHS.

Vaillant, G. E. 1997. *Adaptation to Life.* Boston: Little, Brown.

Van Ameringen, M., C. Mancini, and J. M. Oakman. 1998. The relationship of behavioral inhibition and shyness to anxiety disorder. *Journal of Nervous and Mental Disease* 186(7): 425–431.

Weissman, M. M. 1998. Cross-national epidemiology of obsessive-compulsive disorder. *CNS Spectrums* 3(5 Suppl 1): 6–9.

Williams, J. W., et al. 2000. A systematic review of newer pharmacotherapies for depression in adults: Evidence report summary. *Annals of Internal Medicine* 132(9): 743–756.

Intimate Relationships and Communication

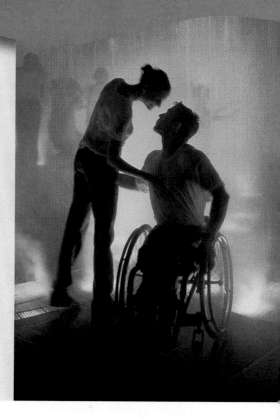

LOOKING AHEAD

After reading this chapter, you should be able to

- Explain the qualities that help people develop intimate relationships
- Describe different types of love relationships and the stages they often go through
- Describe common challenges of forming and maintaining intimate relationships
- Discuss relationship options available to adults today
- List some characteristics of successful families and some potential problems families face
- Explain some of the joys and challenges of being a parent

H uman beings need social relationships; we cannot thrive as solitary creatures. Nor could the human species survive if adults didn't cherish and support each other, if we didn't form strong mutual attachments with our infants, and if we didn't create families in which to raise children. Simply put, people need people.

Although people are held together in relationships by a variety of factors, the foundation of many relationships is love. Love in its many forms—romantic, passionate, platonic, parental—is the wellspring from which much of life's meaning and delight flows. In our culture, it binds us together as partners, parents, children, and friends. People devote tremendous energy to seeking mates, nurturing intimate relationships, keeping up friendships—all for the pleasure of loving and being loved.

Many human needs are satisfied in intimate relationships: the need for approval and affirmation, for companionship, for meaningful ties and a sense of belonging, for sexual satisfaction. Many of society's needs are fulfilled by relationships, too. Overall, healthy intimate relationships are an important contributor to the well-being of both individuals and society.

Ww. DEVELOPING INTIMATE RELATIONSHIPS

People who develop successful intimate relationships believe in themselves and in the people around them. They are willing to give of themselves—to share their ideas, feelings, time, needs—and to accept what others want to give them.

Self-Concept and Self-Esteem

The principal thing that we all bring to our relationships is our *selves*. To have successful relationships, we must first accept and feel good about ourselves. A positive self-concept and a healthy level of self-esteem help us love and respect others. How and where do we acquire a positive sense of self?

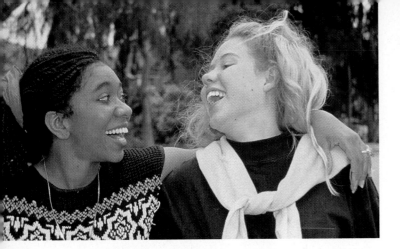

Close relationships without a sexual component are more common than those with sexual activity. Friendship satisfies our need for affection, affirmation, sharing, and companionship.

As discussed in Chapter 3, the roots of our identity and sense of self can be found in childhood, in the relationships we had with our parents and other family members. As adults, we probably have a sense that we're basically lovable, worthwhile people and that we can trust others if, as babies and children, we felt loved, valued, and respected; if adults responded to our needs in a reasonably appropriate way; and if they gave us the freedom to explore and develop a sense of being separate individuals.

Our personal identity isn't fixed or frozen. According to psychologist Erik Erikson, it continues to develop as we encounter and resolve various crises at each stage of life. The fundamental tasks of early childhood are the development of trust during infancy and of autonomy during toddlerhood. From these experiences and interactions we construct our first ideas about who we are.

Another thing we learn in early childhood is **gender role**—the activities, abilities, and characteristics our culture deems appropriate for us based on whether we're male or female. In our society, men have traditionally been expected to work and provide for their families; to be aggressive, competitive, and power-oriented; and to use thinking and logic to solve problems. Women have been expected to take care of home and children; to be cooperative, supportive, and nurturing; and to approach life emotionally and intuitively. Although more egalitarian

gender roles are emerging in our society, the stereotypes we learn in childhood tend to be deeply ingrained.

Our ways of relating to others may also be rooted in childhood. Some researchers have suggested that our adult styles of loving may be based on the style of **attachment** we established in infancy with our mother, father, or other primary caregiver. According to this view, people who are secure in their intimate relationships probably had a secure, trusting, mutually satisfying attachment to their mother, father, or other parenting figure. As adults, they find it relatively easy to get close to others. They don't worry about being abandoned or having someone get too close to them. They feel that other people like them and are generally well intentioned.

Even if people's earliest experiences and relationships were less than ideal, however, they can still establish satisfying relationships in adulthood. People can be resilient and flexible. They have the capacity to change their ideas, beliefs, and behavior patterns. They can learn ways to raise their self-esteem; they can become more trusting, accepting, and appreciative of others; and they can acquire the communication and conflict-resolution skills for maintaining successful relationships. Although it helps to have a good start in life, it may be even more important to begin again, right from where you are.

Friendship

The first relationships we form outside the family are friendships. With members of either the same or the other sex, friendships give people the opportunity to share themselves and discover others. The friendships we form in childhood are important in our development; through them we learn about tolerance, sharing, and trust. Friendships usually include the following characteristics:

- *Companionship.* Friends are relaxed and happy in each other's company. They have common values and interests and spend time together.

- *Respect.* Good friends respect each other's feelings and opinions and work to resolve their differences without demeaning or insulting each other. They also show their respect by being honest with one another.

- *Acceptance.* Friends feel free to be themselves and express their feelings spontaneously without fear of ridicule or criticism.

- *Help.* Sharing time, energy, and even material goods is important to friendship. Friends know they can rely on each other in times of need.

- *Trust.* Friends are secure in the knowledge that they will not intentionally hurt each other.

- *Loyalty.* Friends can count on each other. They stand up for each other in both word and deed.

- *Reciprocity.* There is give-and-take between friends;

- Find people with interests similar to your own. Join a club, participate in sports, do volunteer work, or join a discussion group to meet people with common interests.

- Be a good listener. Take a genuine interest in people. Solicit their opinions, and take time to listen to their problems and ideas.

- Take risks. If you meet someone interesting, ask him or her to join you for a meal or an event you would both enjoy.

- Be trustworthy. Honor all confidences, and don't talk about your friend behind his or her back.

- Tell your friend about yourself. Self-disclosure—letting your friend know about your real concerns and joys—signals trust.

- Be supportive and kind. Be there when your friend is going through a rough time.

- Develop your capacity for intimacy. Intimate relationships are genuine, spontaneous, and caring.

- Don't expect perfection. Like any relationship, your friendship may go through difficult times. Talk through conflicts as they arise.

they share joys and burdens more or less equally over time.

Friendships are usually more stable and longer lasting than intimate partnerships. Friends are often more accepting and less critical than lovers, probably because their expectations are different. Like love relationships, friendships bind society together, providing people with emotional support and buffering them from stress.

> **COMMUNICATE!**   Intimate relationships are crucial for your overall well-being. You can help keep friendships strong by offering your friends support when they share feelings such as anger, disappointment, and frustration. The next time a friend shares a problem with you, listen closely and empathize with her or his feelings. Offer supportive statements and, if appropriate, your help. For example, "I understand your frustration; you've been working very hard on that project. Is there anything I can do to help?"

Love, Sex, and Intimacy

Love is one of the most basic and profound human emotions. It is a powerful force in all our intimate relationships. Love encompasses opposites: affection and anger, excitement and boredom, stability and change, bonds and freedom. Love does not give us perfect happiness, but it does give our lives meaning.

For most people, love, sex, and commitment are closely linked ideals in intimate relationships. Love reflects the positive factors that draw people together and sustain them in a relationship. It includes trust, caring, respect, loyalty, interest in the other, and concern for the other's well-being. Sex brings excitement and passion to the relationship. It intensifies the relationship and adds fascination and pleasure. Commitment, the determination to continue, reflects the stable factors that help maintain the relationship. Responsibility, reliability, and faithfulness are

characteristics of commitment. Although love, sex, and commitment are related, they are not necessarily connected. One can exist without the others. Despite the various "faces" of love, sex, and commitment, most of us long for a special relationship that contains them all.

Other elements can be identified as features of love, such as euphoria, preoccupation with the loved one, idealization of the loved one, and so on, but these tend to be temporary. These characteristics may include **infatuation,** which will fade or deepen into something more substantial. As relationships progress, the central aspects of love and commitment take on more importance.

Another way of looking at love has been proposed by psychologist Robert Sternberg. He sees love as being composed of intimacy, passion, and commitment (Figure 4-1). Intimacy refers to the feelings of warmth and closeness we have with someone we love. Passion refers to romance, attraction, and sexuality. Commitment refers to both the short-term decision that you love someone and the long-term commitment to be in the relationship. According to Sternberg, these three elements can be enlarged, diminished, or combined in different ways, giving different kinds of love.

Men and women tend to have different views of the relationship between love (or intimacy) and sex (or passion). Women generally view sex from the point of view of a relationship, whereas men can more readily separate sex from love, according to many studies.

The Pleasure and Pain of Love   The experience of intense love has confused and tormented lovers throughout history. They live in a tumultuous state of excitement, subject to wildly fluctuating feelings of joy and despair. They lose their appetite, can't sleep, and can think of nothing but the loved one. Is this happiness? Misery? Or both?

The contradictory nature of passionate love can be understood by recognizing that human emotions have two components: physiological arousal and an emotional explanation for the arousal. Love is just one of

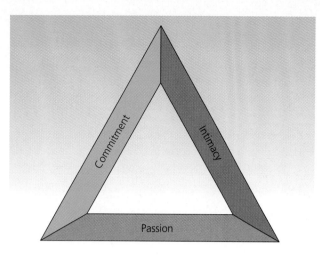

Figure 4-1 The love triangle. SOURCE: Stemberg, R., and M. Barnes. 1988. *The Psychology of Love.* New Haven: Yale University Press, p. 37.

many emotions accompanied by physiological arousal; numerous unpleasant ones can also generate arousal, such as fear, rejection, frustration, and challenge. Although experiences like attraction and sexual desire are pleasant, extreme excitement is similar to fear and is unpleasant. For this reason, passionate love may be too intense to enjoy. Over time, the physical intensity and excitement tend to diminish. When this happens, pleasure may actually increase.

The Transformation of Love   At first, love is likely to be characterized by high levels of passion and rapidly increasing intimacy. After a while, passion decreases as we become habituated to it and to the person. Sometimes intimacy continues to grow at a deeper, less conscious level; at other times, the couple may drift apart. Commitment isn't necessarily diminished by time. It grows more slowly and is maintained as long as we judge the relationship to be successful. If the relationship begins to fade, the level of commitment usually decreases.

The disappearance of romance or passionate love is often experienced as a crisis in a relationship. If a more lasting love fails to emerge, the relationship will likely break up, and each person will search for another who will once again ignite his or her passion. Love does not necessarily have to be intensely passionate. When intensity diminishes, partners often discover a more enduring love. They can now move from absorption in each other to a relationship that includes external goals and projects, friends, and family. In this kind of intimate, more secure love, satisfaction comes not just from the relationship itself but also from achieving other creative goals, such as work or child rearing. The key to successful relationships is in transforming passion into an intimate love, based on closeness, caring, and the promise of a shared future.

Challenges in Relationships

Even in the best of circumstances, there are times when a loving relationship will be tested. Common relationship challenges relate to self-disclosure, commitment, expectations, competitiveness, and jealousy.

Honesty and Openness   Getting close to another person by sharing thoughts and feelings is emotionally risky, but it is necessary for a relationship to deepen. Take your time, and self-disclose at a slow but steady rate—one that doesn't make you feel too vulnerable or your partner too uncomfortable. Over time, you and your partner will learn more about each other and feel more comfortable sharing.

Unequal or Premature Commitment   Sometimes one person in an intimate partnership becomes more serious about the relationship than the other partner. Sometimes a couple makes a premature commitment, and then one of the partners has second thoughts and wants to break off the relationship. Sometimes both partners begin to realize that something is wrong, but each is afraid to tell the other. Most such problems can be dealt with only by honest and sensitive communication.

Unrealistic Expectations   Each partner brings hopes and expectations to a relationship, some of which may be unrealistic. Common expectations that can hurt a relationship include expecting your partner to change; assuming that your partner has all the same opinions, priorities, interests, and goals as you; and believing that a relationship will fulfill all of your personal, financial, intellectual, and social needs.

Competitiveness   If one partner always feels the strong need to compete and win, such as in discussions and arguments, it can detract from the sense of connectedness, interdependence, equality, and mutuality between partners. If competitiveness is a problem for you, ask yourself if your need to win is more important than your partner's feelings or the future of your relationship.

Balancing Time Spent Together and Apart   You may enjoy time together with your partner but you may also want to spend time alone or with other friends. It's important to talk with your partner about what time apart means and to share your feelings about what you expect from the relationship in terms of time together. Differences in expectations about time spent together can mirror differences in ideas about emotional closeness. It's important to remember that every individual is unique and has different needs for distance and closeness in a relationship. In addition, traditional gender roles tend to teach women to be caretakers of relationships and men to be independent and self-reliant.

- *Be aware of the importance of support.* Time and energy spent on support will help both you and your partner deal with stress and create a positive atmosphere that will help when differences or conflicts do occur.

- *Learn to ask for help from your partner.* Try different ways of asking for help and support from your partner and make note of which approaches work best for your relationship.

- *Help your partner the way she or he would like to be helped.* Some people prefer empathy and emotional support, while others like more practical help with problems.

- *Avoid negativity, especially when being asked for help.* Asking for help puts a person in a vulnerable position. If your partner asks for your aid, be gracious and supportive; don't use phrases like "I told you so" or "You should have just . . ." or your partner may learn not to ask for your help at all.

- *Make positive attributions.* If you're unsure about the reasons for your partner's behavior, give her or him the benefit of the doubt. For example, if your partner arrives for a date 30 minutes late and in a bad mood, assume it's because she or he had a bad day rather than attributing it to a character flaw or relationship problem. Offer appropriate support.

- *Help yourself.* Develop coping strategies for times your partner won't be available. These might include things you can do for yourself, such as going for a walk, or other people you can turn to for support.

- *Keep relationship problems separate.* Avoid bringing up relationship problems when you are offering or asking for help.

SOURCE: Plante, T., and K. Sullivan. 2000. *Getting Together and Staying Together: The Stanford Course on Intimate Relationships.* Bloomington, Ind.: 1st Books Library.

Jealousy Some people think that jealousy is a reflection of love, but jealousy actually more accurately reflects insecurity or possessiveness. In its irrational and extreme forms, jealousy can destroy a relationship by its insistent demands and attempts at control. Jealousy is a factor in precipitating violence in dating relationships among both high school and college students, and abusive spouses often use jealousy to justify their violence. (Problems with control and violence in relationships are discusssed in Chapter 00.) People with a healthy level of self-esteem are less likely to feel jealous. When jealousy occurs in a relationship, it's important for the partners to communicate clearly with each other about their feelings.

Successful Relationships

A true intimate relationship is characterized by a conscious sense of connectedness to another person. It emerges after a period of deep sharing, and it reflects a warm, caring, and trusting concern between partners. Successful relationships result in a heightened sense of self-worth for both partners. To build a successful relationship, you need to be able to communicate your needs and wants clearly, listen to your partner, negotiate, and compromise. These skills are described in the next section of the chapter.

Ending a Relationship

Even when a couple starts out with the best of intentions, an intimate relationship may not last. Ending an intimate relationship is usually difficult and painful. If you are involved in a breakup, following these guidelines may help make the ending easier:

- Give the relationship a fair chance before breaking up.

- Be fair and honest, tactful and compassionate.

- If you are the rejected person, give yourself time to resolve your anger and pain.

- Recognize the value in the experience.

Use the recovery period following a breakup for self-renewal. Redirect more of your attention to yourself, and reconnect with people and areas of your life that may have been neglected as a result of the relationship. Time will help heal the pain of the loss of the relationship.

COMMUNICATION

The key to developing and maintaining any type of intimate relationship is good communication.

Nonverbal Communication

As much as 65% of face-to-face communication is nonverbal. Even when we're silent, we're communicating. We send messages when we look at someone or look away, lean forward or sit back, smile or frown. Especially important forms of nonverbal communication are touch, eye contact, and proximity. If someone we're talking to touches our hand or arm, looks into our eyes, and leans toward us when we talk, we get the message that the person is interested in us and cares about what we're saying. If a person keeps looking around the room while we're talking or takes a step backward, we get the impression the person is uninterested or wants to end the conversation.

The ability to interpret nonverbal messages correctly is important to the success of relationships. It's also

Getting Started

- When you want to have a serious discussion with your partner, find a time when you will not be interrupted and a private place.

- Face your partner and maintain eye contact. Use nonverbal feedback to show that you are interested and involved in the communication process.

Being an Effective Speaker

- State your concern or issue as clearly as you can.

- Use "I" statements—statements about how *you* feel—rather than statements beginning with "You," which tell another person how you think he or she feels. When you use "I" statements, you are taking responsibility for your feelings. "You" statements are often blaming or accusatory and will probably get a defensive or resentful response.

- Focus on a specific behavior rather than on the whole person. Be specific about the behavior you like or don't like. Avoid generalizations beginning with "You always" or "You never." Such statements make people feel defensive.

- Make constructive requests. Opening your request with "I would like" keeps the focus on your needs rather than your partner's supposed deficiencies.

- Avoid blaming, accusing, and belittling. Even if you are right, you have little to gain by putting your partner down. When people feel criticized or attacked, they are less able to think rationally or solve problems constructively.

- Ask for action ahead of time. Tell your partner what you would like to have happen in the future; don't wait for him or her to blow it and then express anger or disappointment.

Being an Effective Listener

- Provide appropriate nonverbal feedback (nodding, smiling, making eye contact, and so on).

- Don't interrupt.

- Develop the skill of reflective listening. Don't judge, evaluate, analyze, or offer solutions (unless asked to do so). Your partner may just need to have you there in order to sort out feelings. By jumping in right away to "fix" the problem, you may actually be cutting off communication.

- Don't give unsolicited advice. Giving advice implies that you know more about what a person needs to do than he or she does; therefore, it often evokes anger or resentment.

- Clarify your understanding of what your partner is saying by restating it in your own words and asking if your understanding is correct.

- Be sure you are really listening, not off somewhere in your mind rehearsing your reply. Try to tune in to your partner's feelings as well as the words.

- Let your partner know that you value what he or she is saying and want to understand. Respect for the other person is the cornerstone of effective communication.

---

important, when sending messages, to make sure our body language agrees with our words. When our verbal and nonverbal messages don't correspond, we send a mixed message.

Communication Skills

Three keys to good communication in relationships are self-disclosure, listening, and feedback.

- *Self-disclosure* involves revealing personal information that we ordinarily wouldn't reveal because of the risk involved. It usually increases feelings of closeness and moves the relationship to a deeper level of intimacy. Friends often disclose the most to each other, sharing feelings, experiences, hopes, and disappointments; married couples sometimes share less because they think they already know everything about each other.

- *Listening,* the second component of good communication, is a rare skill. Good listening skills require that we spend more time and energy trying to fully understand another person's "story" and less time judging, evaluating, blaming, advising, analyzing, or trying to control. Empathy, warmth, respect, and genuineness are qualities of skillful listeners. Attentive listening encourages friends or partners to share more and, in turn, to be attentive listeners.

- *Feedback,* a constructive response to another's self-disclosure, is the third key to good communication. Giving positive feedback means acknowledging that the friend's or partner's feelings are valid—no matter how upsetting or troubling—and offering self-disclosure in response. If, for example, your partner discloses unhappiness about your relationship, it is more constructive to say that you're concerned or saddened by that and want to hear more about it than to get angry, to blame, to try to inflict pain, or to withdraw. Self-disclosure and feedback can open the door to change, whereas other responses block communication and change.

Gender and Communication

Many authorities believe that, because of the way they've been raised, men and women generally approach conversation and communication differently. According to this view, men tend to use conversation in a competitive way, perhaps hoping to establish dominance in relationships. When male conversations are over, men often find themselves in a one-up or a one-down position. Women tend to use conversation in a more *affiliative* way, perhaps hoping to establish friendships. They negotiate various degrees of closeness, seeking to give and receive support. Men tend to talk more—though without disclosing more—and listen less. Women tend to use good listening skills like eye contact, frequent nodding, focused attention, and asking relevant questions.

Although these are generalized patterns, they can translate into problems in specific conversations. Even when a man and a woman are talking about the same subject, their unconscious goals may be very different. The woman may be looking for understanding and closeness, while the man may be trying to demonstrate his competence by giving advice and solving problems. Both styles are valid; the problem comes when differences in styles result in poor communication and misunderstanding.

Sometimes communication is not the problem in a relationship—the partners understand each other all too well. The problem is that they're unable or unwilling to change or compromise. Although good communication can't salvage a bad relationship, it does enable couples to see their differences and make more informed decisions.

Conflict and Conflict Resolution

Conflict is natural in intimate relationships. No matter how close two people become, they still remain separate individuals with their own needs, desires, past experiences, and ways of seeing the world. In fact, the closer the relationship, the more opportunities for conflict there will be. Conflict itself isn't dangerous to a relationship; it may simply indicate that the relationship is growing. But if it isn't handled in a constructive way, it will damage—and ultimately destroy—the relationship.

Conflict is often accompanied by anger—a natural emotion, but one that can be difficult to handle. If we express anger, we run the risk of creating distrust, fear, and distance; if we act it out without thinking things through, we can cause the conflict to escalate; if we suppress it, it turns into resentment and hostility. The best way to handle anger in a relationship is to recognize it as a symptom of something that requires attention and needs to be changed. When angry, partners should back off until they calm down and then come back to the issue later and try to resolve it rationally. Negotiation will help dissipate the anger so the conflict can be resolved.

Although the sources of conflict for couples change over time, they primarily revolve around the basic tasks of living together: dividing the housework, handling money, spending time together, and so on. Sexual interaction is also a source of disagreement for many couples.

Although there are numerous theories on and approaches to conflict resolution, some basic strategies are generally useful in successfully negotiating with a partner:

1. *Clarify the issue.* Take responsibility for thinking through your feelings and discovering what's really bothering you. Agree that one partner will speak first and have the chance to speak fully while the other listens. Then reverse the roles. Try to understand the other partner's position fully by repeating what you've heard and asking questions to clarify. Agree to talk only about the topic at hand and not get distracted by other issues. Sum up what your partner has said.

2. *Find out what each person wants.* Ask your partner to express his or her desires. Don't assume you know what your partner wants and speak for him or her.

3. *Identify various alternatives for getting each person what he or she wants.* Practice brainstorming to generate a variety of options.

4. *Decide how to negotiate.* Work out some agreements or plans for change; for example, one partner will do one task and the other will do another task, or one partner will do a task in exchange for something he or she wants. Find a solution that satisfies both partners.

5. *Solidify the agreements.* Go over the plan verbally and write it down, if necessary, to ensure that you both understand and agree to it.

6. *Review and renegotiate.* Decide on a time frame for trying out the new plan, and set a time to discuss how it's working. Make adjustments as needed.

To resolve conflicts, partners have to feel safe in voicing disagreements. They have to trust that the discussion won't get out of control, that they won't be abandoned by the other, and that the partner won't take advantage of their vulnerability. Partners should follow some basic ground rules when they argue, such as avoiding ultimatums, resisting the urge to give the silent treatment. If you and your partner find that you argue again and again over the same issue, it may be better to stop trying to resolve that problem and instead come to accept the differences between you.

COMMUNICATE! A key strategy for effective communication is to use "I" statements that describe how you feel rather than "you" statements to describe how you think another person is acting or feeling. Try thinking of three "you" statements that you would like to make to someone you know, and then translate each one into an "I" statement. For example, "You never do anything to clean up the apartment" could be changed to "I get irritated when I realize that I've been doing most of the housework around the apartment. I'd like to talk about setting up a schedule for sharing the chores." Once you become familiar with "I" statements, try substituting them for "you" statements.

More and more, people are looking to the Internet to find friends and partners. Communications with others in cyberspace can enable people to be themselves in a relaxed atmosphere, to try out other personas, and to confide in others in a private way. The Internet is a good tool for locating people who share your hobbies and interests. If your goal is to communicate with someone about a common interest, e-mail, newsgroups, listservs, and chat rooms are all good options.

People looking for intimate partners are also using the Internet. By getting to know someone online, you can make that "first impression" in the comfort of your living room. In online relationships, people will respond to you based on who you are rather than on your appearance. And with more than 100 million users of the World Wide Web in the United States alone, you have many more people to interact with than on your campus or in your neighborhood.

There are drawbacks to meeting partners online, however. People can misrepresent themselves, pretending to be very different—older or younger or even of a different sex—than they really are. Investing time and emotional resources in an unrealistic romance can be painful. There have also been a few instances in which online romances have become dangerous or even deadly (see Chapter 16 for information on cyberstalking). If you decide to meet someone in person whom you have pre-

viously met only online, here are some strategies that can help keep you safe:

- To increase your chances of meeting people interested in you as a person, avoid sexually oriented Internet sites.

- Until you know much more about a cyberfriend, don't give out personal information, including your real full name, school, or place of employment.

- Schedule a phone conversation or a series of phone conversations before deciding whether or not to meet an online friend in person.

- Don't agree to meet someone face-to-face unless you feel completely comfortable about it. Always meet initially in a public place—a museum, a coffee shop, a restaurant. Bring along a friend to further increase your safety.

Finally, take care that your pursuit of online relationships does not interfere with your other interpersonal relationships and social activities. As described in Chapter 3, researchers have found that extensive use of the Internet is associated with greater loneliness, less communication with family members, and fewer social contacts. To maximize your emotional and interpersonal wellness, use the Internet to widen your circle of friends, not shrink it.

PAIRING AND SINGLEHOOD

Although most people eventually marry, everyone spends some time as a single person, and nearly everyone makes some attempt to find a partner. Intimate relationships are as important for singles as for couples.

Choosing a Partner

Most men and women select partners for long-term relationships through a fairly predictable process, although they may not be consciously aware of it. Most people pair with someone who lives in the same geographic area and who is similar in ethnic and socioeconomic background, educational level, lifestyle, physical attractiveness, and other traits. In simple terms, people select partners like themselves.

First attraction is based on easily observable characteristics: looks, dress, social status, and reciprocated interest. Once the euphoria of romantic love winds down, personality traits and behaviors become more significant factors in how the partners view each other. Through sharing and self-disclosure, they gradually gain a deeper knowledge of each other. The emphasis shifts to basic values, such as religious beliefs, political affiliation, sexual attitudes, and future aspirations regarding career, family, and children. If they are compatible, many people gradually discover deeper, more enduring forms of love.

Perhaps the most important question for potential mates is, How much do we have in common? Although differences add interest to a relationship, similarities increase the chances of a relationship's success. If there are major differences, partners should first ask, How accepting of differences are we? Then, How well do we communicate? Acceptance and communication skills go a long way toward making a relationship work, no matter how different the partners. Areas in which differences can affect the relationship include values, religion, ethnicity, attitudes toward sexuality and gender roles, socioeconomic status, familiarity with the other's culture, and interactions with the extended family.

Dating

Most Americans find romantic partners through some form of dating. They narrow the field through a process of getting to know each other. In the traditional male-female dating pattern, the man takes the lead, initiating the date, while the woman waits to be called. In this pattern, casual dating might evolve into steady or exclusive dating, then engagement, and finally marriage.

For many young people today, traditional dating has given way to a more casual form of getting together in groups. Greater equality between the sexes is at the root of this change. Rather than strictly as couples, people go out in groups, and each person pays his or her way. A man and woman may begin to spend more time together, but often in the group context. If sexual involvement develops, it is more likely to be based on friendship, respect, and common interests than on expectations related to gender roles. In this model, mate selection may progress from getting together to living together to marriage.

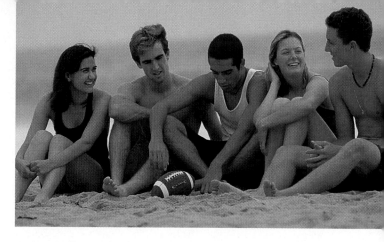

For many college students today, group activities have replaced dating as a way to meet and get to know potential partners.

> **COMMUNICATE!** College offers many opportunities to expand your social network. If you're shy about meeting new people, work out in advance what you will say. The next time you want to strike up a conversation with a new acquaintance, try starting out by introducing yourself. Mention the physical context of the conversation, such as the location, weather, or ongoing event. Ask questions that will engage the other person, such as "Is this the first art history class you've taken?" or "Have you been to a lot of basketball games this season?"

Living Together

According to the U.S. Bureau of the Census, over 4 million heterosexual couples and an estimated 1.5 million gay and lesbian couples are currently living together. Living together, or **cohabitation,** is one of the most rapid and dramatic social changes that has ever occurred in our society. It seems to be gaining acceptance as part of the normal mate selection process. By age 30, about half of all men and women will have cohabited and some employers and communities extend benefits to unmarried domestic partners. The only thing separating those who cohabit from those who don't is religion. Several factors are involved in this change, including greater acceptance of premarital sex, increased availability of contraceptives, the tendency for people to wait longer before getting married, and a larger pool of single and divorced individuals.

Living together provides many of the benefits of marriage: companionship; a setting for an enjoyable and meaningful relationship; the opportunity to develop greater intimacy through learning, compromising, and sharing; a satisfying sex life; and a way to save on living costs. Living together also has certain advantages over marriage. It can give the partners a greater sense of autonomy. Not bound by the social rules and expectations that are part of the institution of marriage, partners may find it easier to keep their identity and more of their independence. Cohabitation doesn't incur the same legal obligations as marriage. If things don't work out, the legal partners may find it easier to leave a relationship that hasn't been legally sanctioned.

But living together has some liabilities, too. In most cases, the legal protections of marriage are absent, such as health insurance benefits and property and inheritance rights. These considerations can be particularly serious if the couple has children, from either former relationships or the current partnership. Since social acceptance of cohabitation is not universal, couples may feel family pressure to marry or otherwise change their living arrangements, especially if they have young children.

Although many people choose cohabitation as a kind of trial marriage, unmarried partnerships tend to be less stable than marriages. There is little evidence that cohabitation before marriage leads to happier or longer-lasting marriages; in fact, some studies have found slightly less marital satisfaction among couples who had previously cohabited.

Gay and Lesbian Partnerships

Regardless of **sexual orientation,** most people look for love in a close, satisfying, committed relationship. Gay and lesbian, or **homosexual,** couples have many similarities with **heterosexual** couples. According to one study, most gay men and lesbians have experienced at least one long-term relationship with a single partner. Like heterosexual relationships, gay and lesbian partnerships provide intimacy, passion, and security.

One difference between heterosexual and homosexual couples is that gay and lesbian couples tend to adopt "best friend" roles in their relationship rather than traditional gender roles. Domestic tasks are shared or split, and both

> **cohabitation** Living together in a sexual relationship without being married.
>
> **sexual orientation** A consistent pattern of emotional and sexual attraction based on biological sex; it exists along a continuum that ranges from exclusive heterosexuality (attraction to people of the other sex) through bisexuality (attraction to people of both sexes) to exclusive homosexuality (attraction to people of one's own sex).
>
> **homosexual** Emotional and sexual attraction to people of one's own sex.
>
> **heterosexual** Emotional and sexual attraction to people of the other sex.

Terms

On July 1, 2000, Vermont became the first state to offer the option of "civil union" to people for whom legal marriage is not an option. This was the date a law went into effect as a result of a Vermont Supreme Court ruling that same-sex couples were entitled to the same benefits and protections given to married couples, including rights relating to medical decisions and health care; parenting, child custody, and child support; inheritance; state income taxes; and other issues.

A civil union is a legal status parallel to civil marriage (the Vermont legislature decided not to use the word *marriage* for these unions), and for the purposes of Vermont law, civil union spouses are treated as legally married. Same-sex couples from other states may travel to Vermont to enter civil unions, but their status back in their home states is unclear. In fact, more than 30 states have enacted "defense of marriage acts" (DOMAs), which attempt to deny the validity of same-sex unions by defining marriage as a union between a man and a woman. There is also a federal DOMA, signed by President Clinton in 1996, which denies to same-sex couples the 1,049 federal benefits of marriage, including federal tax status, Social Security, survivor and pension benefits, and immigration rights. (Currently, the Netherlands is the only country to offer *marriage* and its associated legal benefits to same-sex partners; it began recognizing such unions in April 2001.)

What cases are made for and against civil union and same-sex marriage? Opponents put forth numerous arguments, including that the purpose of marriage is to procreate, that the Bible forbids same-sex unions, that homosexuals are seeking special rights, and that the majority of the population opposes such unions. The primary argument, however, is that same-sex marriage undermines the sanctity and validity of marriage as it is traditionally understood and thus undermines society. Rules and restrictions on who can marry preserve the value of the institution of marriage, according to this view. The underlying assumption of this position is that homosexual behavior is a choice and that people can change their orientation, though the process is difficult.

Proponents of civil union and same-sex marriage believe that homosexuality is outside the control of the individual and results from genetic and environmental factors that create an unchangeable orientation by adolescence or adulthood. The issue of same-sex union is then seen as one of basic civil rights, in which a group is being denied rights on the basis of something as unalterable as skin color. To the argument that marriage has a traditional meaning in our society, proponents respond that, on the contrary, marriage is an evolving institution that changes as society changes. Prior to 1967, marriage between whites and African Americans was prohibited in the United States; before the Civil War, African Americans were not allowed to marry at all. A generation ago, proponents go on, women's rights were restricted, gender roles were rigid, and divorce was rare. Today, most committed couples live together before getting married, many women have children outside of marriage, many families are headed by a single parent, and two-career couples who choose not to have children at all are increasingly common. These and other trends, according to this view, are leading people to broaden their definition of marriage and to see same-sex marriage as just another variation.

Both opponents and proponents point out that marriage is healthy for both men and women and is the main social institution promoting family values; both sides see this assertion as supportive of their position. What remains to be seen is how society in general is going to view same-sex marriage in the future—as a furthering of American values or as an attack on them.

partners usually support themselves financially. Another difference is that gay and lesbian couples often have to deal with societal hostility or ambivalence toward their relationships—in contrast to the social approval given to heterosexual couples. Consequently, community may be more important as a source of identity and social support than it is for heterosexuals.

Singlehood

Despite the prevalence and popularity of marriage, a significant proportion of adults in our society are unmarried—more than 90 million individuals. They are a diverse group, encompassing young people who have not married yet but plan to in the future, people who are living together (gay or heterosexual), divorced and widowed people, and those who would like to marry but haven't found a mate (Figure 4-2).

Several factors contribute to the growing number of single people. One is the changing view of singlehood, which is increasingly being viewed as a legitimate alternative to marriage. Education and career are delaying the age at which young people are marrying. More young people are living with their parents as they complete their education, seek jobs, or strive for financial independence. Many other single people live together without being married. Gay people who would marry their partners if they were legally permitted to do so are counted among the single population. High divorce rates mean more singles, and people who have experienced divorce in their families may have more negative attitudes about marriage and more positive attitudes about singlehood.

Being single doesn't mean not having close relationships, however. Single people may date, enjoy active and fulfilling social lives, and have a variety of sexual experiences and relationships. Other advantages of being single include more opportunities for personal and career development without concern for family obligations and more freedom and control in making life choices. Disadvantages include loneliness and a lack of companionship, as well as economic hardships (mainly for single women). Single men and women both experience some discrimination and often are pressured to get married.

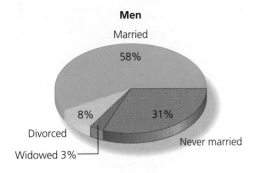

Men

Married
58%

8%

Divorced

Widowed 3%

31%

Never married

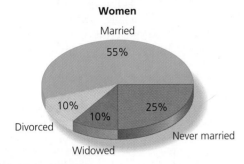

Women

Married
55%

10%

Divorced

10%

Widowed

25%

Never married

VITAL STATISTICS

Figure 4-2   Marital status of the U.S. population age 15 years and older.   SOURCE: U.S. Bureau of the Census. 1999. *Marital Status of the Population 15 Years Old and Over, by Sex and Race: 1950 to Present* (http://www.census.gov/population/socdemo/ms-la/tabms-1.txt; retrieved January 24, 2001).

Nearly everyone has at least one episode of being single in adult life. How enjoyable and valuable this single time is depends on several factors, including how deliberately the person has chosen it; how satisfied the person is with social relationships, standard of living, and job; how comfortable the person feels when alone; and how resourceful and energetic the person is about creating an interesting and fulfilling life.

MARRIAGE

About 95% of all Americans marry at some time in their lives. Marriage continues to remain popular because it satisfies several basic needs. There are many important social, moral, economic, and political aspects of marriage, all of which have changed over the years. In the past, people married mainly for practical reasons, such as raising children or forming an economic unit. Today, people marry more for personal, emotional reasons. This shift places a greater burden on marriage to fulfill certain expectations that are sometimes unreasonably high. People may assume that all their emotional needs will be met by their partner; they may think that fascination and passion will always remain at high levels; they may simply expect to "live happily ever after." When people enter marriage with such preconceptions, it may be harder for them to appreciate the benefits that marriage really offers.

Benefits of Marriage

The primary functions and benefits of marriage are those of any intimate relationship: affection, personal affirmation, companionship, sexual fulfillment, emotional growth. Marriage also provides a setting in which to raise children, although an increasing number of couples choose to remain childless, and people can also choose to raise children without being married. Marriage is also important for providing for the future. By committing themselves to the relationship, people establish themselves with lifelong companions as well as some insurance for their later years.

Issues in Marriage

Although we might like to believe otherwise, love is not enough to make a successful marriage. Couples have to be strong and successful in their relationship before getting married, because relationship problems will be magnified rather than solved by marriage. The following relationship characteristics appear to be the best predictors of a happy marriage:

- The partners have realistic expectations about their relationship.
- Each feels good about the personality of the other.
- They communicate well.
- They have effective ways of resolving conflicts.
- They agree on religious/ethical values.
- They have an egalitarian role relationship.
- They have a good balance of individual versus joint interests and leisure activities.

Once married, couples must face many adjustment tasks. In addition to providing each other with emotional support, they have to negotiate and establish marital roles, establish domestic and career priorities, manage their finances, make sexual adjustments, manage boundaries and relationships with their extended family, and participate in the larger community. Marital roles and responsibilities have undergone profound changes in recent years. Although women still take most of the responsibility for home and children even when they work and although men still suffer more job-related stress and health problems than women do, the trend is toward an equalization of responsibilities.

The Role of Commitment

Coping with all these challenges requires that couples be committed to remaining in the relationship through its inevitable ups and downs. They will need to be tolerant of each other's imperfections and keep their perspective and sense of humor. Commitment is based on conscious choice rather than on feelings, which, by their very nature, are transitory. Commitment is a promise of a shared future, a promise to be together, come what may. Committed

Research studies consistently underscore the importance of strengthening your family and social ties to help maintain emotional and physical wellness. Living alone, or simply feeling alone, can have a negative effect on both your state of mind and your physical health. Married people, on average, live longer than unmarried people—whether single, divorced, or widowed—and they score higher on measures of mental health. Findings suggest that there is something intrinsically beneficial about long-term committed relationships.

People with strong social ties are less likely to become ill and tend to recover more quickly if they do. The benefits of intimate relationships have been demonstrated for a range of conditions: People with strong social support are less likely to catch colds. They recover better from heart attacks and live longer with heart disease. Among men with prostate cancer, those who are married live significantly longer than those who are single, divorced, or widowed; women with breast cancer live longer if they participate in a support group.

What is it about social relationships that supports wellness? Friends and partners may encourage and reinforce healthy habits, such as exercising, eating right, and seeing a physician when needed. In times of illness, a loving partner can provide both practical help and emotional support. Feeling loved, esteemed, and valued brings comfort at a time of vulnerability, reduces anxiety, and mitigates the damaging effects of stress.

Although good relationships may help the sick get better, bad relationships may have the opposite effect. The impact of relationship quality on the course of illness may be partly explained by effects on the immune system: A study of married couples whose fighting went beyond normal conflict and into criticism and name-calling found them to have weaker immune responses than couples whose arguments were more civil. (The immune effects were particularly strong among the wives, leading some researchers to postulate that women may be more aware of and affected by relationship problems.)

Marriage, of course, isn't the only support system available. Whether married or single, if you have supportive people in your life, you are likely to enjoy better physical and emotional health than if you feel isolated and alone. So when you start planning lifestyle changes to improve your health and well-being, don't forget to nurture your relationships with family and friends. Relationships are powerful medicine.

partners put effort and energy into the relationship, no matter how they feel. They take time to attend to their partner, give compliments, and face conflict when necessary. To many people, commitment is a more important goal than living together or marriage.

Separation and Divorce

People marrying today have a 50–55% chance of divorcing. The high rate of divorce in the United States reflects our extremely high expectations for emotional fulfillment and satisfaction in marriage. It also indicates that we no longer believe in the permanence of marriage.

The process of divorce usually begins with an emotional separation. Often one partner is unhappy and looks beyond the relationship for other forms of validation. Dissatisfaction increases until the unhappy partner decides he or she can no longer stay. Physical separation follows, although it may take some time for the relationship to be over emotionally.

Except for the death of a spouse or family member, divorce is the greatest stress-producing event in life. Both men and women experience turmoil, depression, and lowered self-esteem during and after divorce. People experience separation distress and loneliness for about a year and then begin a recovery period of 1–3 years. During this time they gradually construct a postdivorce identity, along with a new pattern of life. Most people are surprised by how long it takes to recover from divorce. Children are especially vulnerable to the trauma of divorce, and sometimes counseling is appropriate to help them adjust to the changes in their lives.

FAMILY LIFE

American families are very different today than they were even a few decades ago. Currently, about half of all families are based on a first marriage; almost one-third are headed by a single parent; the remainder are remarriages or involve some other arrangement. Despite the tremendous variation apparent in American families, certain patterns can still be discerned.

For many young adults, the family life cycle begins with marriage. This first stage, when newlyweds are learning how to live together, ends abruptly when they have a baby. New parents have a new set of responsibilities, and their roles change profoundly and irreversibly: no more spontaneous outings to see a movie or leisurely Sunday mornings sipping coffee and browsing through the newspaper. The third member of the family, the new infant, demands around-the-clock attention.

Deciding to Become a Parent

Many factors have to be taken into account when you are considering parenthood. Following are some questions you should ask yourself and some issues you should consider when making this decision. Some issues are relevant to both men and women; others apply only to women.

- *Your physical health and your age.* Are you in reasonably good health? If not, can you improve your health by changing your lifestyle, perhaps by modifying your diet or giving up cigarettes, alcohol, or drugs? Are you overweight? Do you have physical conditions, such as diabetes or high blood pressure, that will require extra care and medical attention during pregnancy?

- *Your financial circumstances.* Can you afford a child? Will your health insurance cover the costs of pregnancy, delivery, and medical attention for mother and baby before and after the birth. Supplies for the baby are expensive, too. Depending on a variety of factors, the annual cost of raising a child averages about $8,900.

- *Your relationship with your partner.* Are you in a stable relationship, and do both of you want a child? Are your views compatible on such issues as child-rearing goals, the distribution of responsibility for the child, and work and housework obligations?

- *Your educational, career, and child care plans.* Have you completed as much of your education as you want right now? Have you established yourself in a career, if that is something you want to do? Have you investigated parental leave and company-sponsored child care?

- *Your emotional readiness for parenthood.* Do you have the emotional discipline and stamina to nurture an infant? Are you prepared to have a helpless baby completely dependent on you all day and all night? Are you willing to change your lifestyle to provide the best conditions for a baby's development?

- *Your social support system.* Do you have a network of family and friends who will help you with the baby? Are there community resources you can call on for additional assistance? A family's social support system is one of the most important factors affecting its ability to adjust to a baby and cope with new responsibilities.

- *Your personal qualities, attitudes toward children, and aptitude for parenting.* Do you like infants, young children, and adolescents? Do you think time with children is time well spent? Do you have safe ways of handling anger, frustration, and impatience?

Becoming a Parent

Few new parents have any preparation for the job of parenting, yet they have to assume that role literally overnight. They have to learn quickly how to hold a baby, how to change it, how to feed it, how to interpret its cries. No wonder the birth of the first child is one of the most stressful transitions for any couple.

Even couples with an egalitarian relationship before their first child is born find that their marital roles become more traditional with the arrival of the new baby. The father becomes the principal provider and protector, and the mother becomes the primary nurturer. Most research indicates that mothers have to make greater changes in their lives than fathers do. Although men today spend more time caring for their infants than ever before, women still take the ultimate responsibility for seeing that the baby is fed, clean, and comfortable. In addition, women are usually the ones who make job changes; they may quit working or reduce their hours in order to stay home with the baby for several months or more, or they may try to juggle the multiple roles of mother, homemaker, and employee and feel guilty that they never have enough time to do justice to any of these roles.

Parenting and the Family Life Cycle

Sometimes being a parent is a source of unparalleled pleasure and pride—the first smile, the first word, the first home run. But at other times, parenting can seem like an overwhelming responsibility. How can you be sure you're not making some mistake that will stunt your child's physical, psychological, or emotional growth?

There is really no "right" way to raise children to ensure that they become healthy and happy. Of course, parents must provide for basic physical needs, such as food, shelter, clothing, and medical care. They must also help children develop a positive self-concept. But how do parents know how to best accomplish this? Unfortunately, there is no set of hard-and-fast rules to guide parents in all situations.

Exactly what a parent does on any given occasion depends on a variety of factors, including values, beliefs, experience, and both the parent's and the child's personalities. Parents should try to remember that raising a child is an ongoing process. No single action is likely to either form or deform a child's personality forever. The important thing is to keep seeking ways to promote satisfaction for all family members—including the parents! It is also important for parents to develop and maintain confidence in their parenting skills, their common sense—and, above all, their love for their children.

At each stage of the family life cycle, the relationship between parents and children changes. And with those changes come new challenges. The parents' primary responsibility to a small, helpless baby is to ensure its physical well-being around the clock. The challenge with toddlers is to strike a balance between giving them the freedom to explore and setting limits that will keep them safe and secure. As children grow toward adolescence, parents need to give them increasing independence and gradually be willing to let them risk success or failure on their own.

Marital satisfaction for most couples declines somewhat while the children are in school. Reasons include the financial and emotional pressures of a growing family and the increased job and community responsibilities of parents in their thirties, forties, and fifties. Once the last child has left

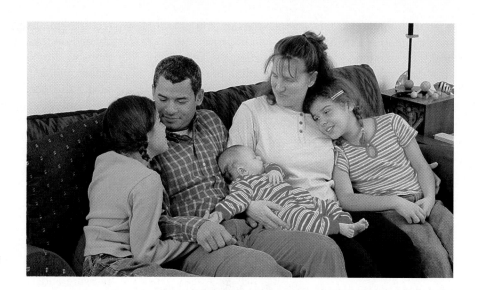

Almost one out of every five American families is a stepfamily, in which parents bring children from a previous marriage into a new family unit.

home, marital satisfaction usually increases because the couple have time to enjoy each other once more.

Single Parents

Today the family life cycle for many women is marriage, motherhood, divorce, single parenthood, remarriage, and widowhood. About 28% of all children under 18 live with only one parent. Economic difficulties are the primary problem for single mothers, especially for unmarried mothers who have not finished high school and have difficulty finding work. Divorced mothers usually experience a sharp drop in income the first few years on their own, but if they have job skills or education, they usually can eventually support themselves and their children adequately. Other problems for single mothers are the often-conflicting demands of playing both father and mother and the difficulty of satisfying their own needs for adult companionship and affection.

Financial pressures are also a complaint of single fathers, but they do not experience them to the extent that single mothers do. Because they are likely to have less practice than mothers in juggling parental and professional roles, they may worry that they do not spend enough time with their children. Because single fatherhood is not as common as single motherhood, however, the men who choose it are likely to be stable, established, and strongly motivated to be with their children.

Research about the effect on children of growing up in a single-parent family is inconclusive. Evidence seems to indicate that these children tend to have less success in school and in their careers than children from two-parent families, but these effects may be associated more strongly with low educational attainment of the single parent rather than the absence of the second parent. Two-parent families are not necessarily better if one of the parents spends little time relating to the children or is physically or emotionally abusive.

Stepfamilies

Single parenthood is usually a transitional stage; about three out of four divorced women and about four out of five divorced men will ultimately remarry. Overall, almost half the marriages in the United States are remarriages for the husband, the wife, or both. If either brings children from a previous marriage into the new family unit, a stepfamily (or "blended family") is formed.

Stepfamilies are significantly different from primary families and should not be expected to duplicate the emotions and relationships of a primary family. Research has shown that healthy stepfamilies are less cohesive and more adaptable than healthy primary families; they have a greater capacity to allow for individual differences and accept that biologically related family members will have emotionally closer relationships. Stepfamilies gradually gain more of a sense of being a family as they build a history of shared daily experiences and major life events.

Successful Families

Family life can be extremely challenging. A strong family is not a family without problems; it's a family that copes successfully with stress and crisis. Many families move through life without a clear direction. Successful families are intentionally more connected—members share experiences and meanings. An excellent way to build strong family ties is to develop family rituals—organized, repeated activities that have meaning for family members. Family rituals may include everyday activities like family meals, shared household chores, and bedtime stories; celebration of wedding anniversaries, birthdays, Father's Day, Mother's Day, and other special anniversaries; and broader family or community activities such as weddings, reunions, and graduations.

Although there is tremendous variation in American families, researchers have proposed that six major qualities or themes appear in strong families.

1. *Commitment.* The family is very important to its members; sexual fidelity between partners is included in commitment.

2. *Appreciation.* Family members care about one another and express their appreciation. The home is a positive place for family members.

3. *Communication.* Family members spend time listening to one another and enjoying one another's company. They talk about disagreements and attempt to solve problems.

4. *Time together.* Family members do things together, often simple activities that don't cost money.

5. *Spiritual wellness.* The family promotes sharing, love, and compassion for other human beings.

6. *Coping with stress and crisis.* When faced with illness, death, marital conflict, or other crises, family members pull together, seek help, and use other coping strategies to meet the challenge.

It may surprise some people that members of strong families are often seen at counseling centers. They know that the smartest thing to do in some situations is to get help. Many resources are available for individuals and families seeking counseling, including clergy, marriage and family counselors, psychologists, and other trained professionals.

Families—and intimate relationships of all kinds—are essential to our overall wellness. A fulfilling life nearly always involves other people. Whether we're single or married, young or old, heterosexual or gay, we continue to need meaningful relationships throughout life.

SUMMARY

- Successful relationships begin with a positive sense of self and reasonably high self-esteem. Personal identity, gender roles, and styles of attachment are all rooted in childhood experiences.

- Love, sex, and commitment are closely linked ideals in intimate relationships. Love includes trust, caring, respect, and loyalty.

- Common challenges in relationships relate to issues of self-disclosure, commitment, expectations, competitiveness, balancing time spent together and apart, and jealousy. Partners in successful relationships have strong communication skills and support each other in difficult times.

- The keys to good communication in relationships are self-disclosure, listening, and feedback.

- Most Americans find partners through dating or getting together in groups. Cohabitation is a growing social pattern that allows partners to get to know each other intimately without being married.

- Gay and lesbian partnerships are similar to heterosexual relationships, with some differences. Partners often don't conform to traditional gender roles, and they may experience hostility or ambivalence rather than approval from society.

- Love isn't enough to ensure a successful marriage. Partners have to be realistic, feel good about each other, have communication and conflict-resolution skills, share values, and have a balance of individual and joint interests.

- When problems can't be worked out, people often separate and divorce. Divorce is traumatic for all involved, especially children, but the negative effects are usually balanced in time by positive ones.

- Factors couples should consider when deciding whether to have children include (1) physical health and age, (2) financial circumstances, (3) relationship between partners, (4) educational, career, and child care plans, (5) emotional readiness for parenthood, (6) social support system, and (7) personal qualities.

- At each stage of the family life cycle, relationships change. Marital satisfaction may be lower during the child-rearing years and higher later. Many families today are single-parent families or stepfamilies.

- Important qualities of successful families include commitment to the family, appreciation of family members, communication, time spent together, spiritual wellness, and effective methods of dealing with stress.

Tips for Today

The fabric of human life is woven from relationships with other people. A wellness lifestyle includes ample time for nourishing relationships with friends, family, and intimate partners. Good communication is the key to keeping all these relationships on track.

Right now you can

- Seek out an acquaintance or a new friend and arrange a coffee date to get to know the person a little better.

- Call a parent, sibling, or someone else you love and let him or her know how important the relationship is to you. (Don't wait for a special occasion or a crisis!)

- Think about the last time you experienced conflict with a family member or partner. Identify some ways you might handle such situations better in the future. For example,

  - Be a better listener.

  - Communicate your feelings more clearly.

  - Avoid criticizing or blaming.

  - Be more willing to overlook minor differences.

1. Take an informal survey among your friends of what they find attractive in a member of the other sex and what they look for in a romantic partner. Are there substantial differences between people? Do men and women look for different things?

2. Ask your parents what their experiences of dating and courtship were like. How are they different from your experiences? What do your parents think of current customs?

JOURNAL ENTRY

1. What are you looking for in an intimate relationship? In your health journal, make a list of the needs you would like to have met by a partner. Are they needs that you can realistically expect to have satisfied in a relationship?

2. *Critical Thinking* What approach do you take when it comes to communicating your feelings and needs to others? Think of a particular issue that has been bothering you, and write down the statements you would make if you were discussing it. Examine

your statements to see whether unrelated feelings or issues are coming through in them. Devise a strategy for dealing with the issue, using the guidelines given in this chapter on conflict resolution.

3. Make a list of your family's strengths and weaknesses. What do you like best about your family? What would you like to change? Choose one weakness, and develop strategies for dealing with it that you and your family can work on together.

FOR MORE INFORMATION

For resources in your area, check your campus directory for a counseling center or peer counseling program, or check the agencies listed in the Mental Health section of the phone book.

Books

Amatea, E., N. M. Brown, and E. S. Amatea. 2000. *Love and Intimate Relationships: Journeys of the Heart.* New York: Brunner/Mazel. *Provides a synthesis of theoretical perspectives as well as advice for enhancing relationships.*

Christensen, A., and N. Jacobson. 2000. *Reconcilable Differences.* New York: Guilford Press. *A guide to resolving conflicts and building intimacy in relationships.*

DeGenova, M. K., and F. P. Rice. 2002. *Intimate Relationships, Marriages, and Families.* 5th ed. Mountain View, Calif.: Mayfield. *A comprehensive look at intimate relationships.*

Gottman, J. M., and N. Silver. 1999. *Seven Principles for Making Marriage Work.* New York: Crown. *Research-based advice for keeping relationships on track.*

Plante, T., and K. Sullivan. 2000. *Getting Together and Staying Together: The Stanford Course on Intimate Relationships.* Bloomington, Ind.: 1stBooks Library. *Provides a concise and practical approach to intimate relationships based on both clinical practice and scientific research.*

Organizations and Web Sites

American Association for Marriage and Family Therapy. Provides information on a variety of relationship issues and referrals to therapists.
202-452-0109
http://www.aamft.org

Association for Couples in Marriage Enrichment (ACME). An organization that promotes activities to strengthen marriage; a resource for books, tapes, and other materials.
800-634-8325
http://www.marriageenrichment.com

Family Education Network. Provides information about education, safety, health, and other family-related issues.
http://www.familyeducation.com

Go Ask Alice. Professional and peer educators provide answers to questions on many topics relating to interpersonal relationships and communication.
http://www.goaskalice.columbia.edu

Life Innovations. Provides materials for premarital counseling and marital enrichment.
800-331-1661
http://www.lifeinnovation.com

Parents Without Partners (PWP). Provides educational programs, literature, and support groups for single parents and their children. Call for a referral to a local chapter.
800-637-7974
http://www.parentswithoutpartners.org

Student Counseling Virtual Pamphlet Collection. Provides links to pamphlets produced by different student counseling centers; topics include relationships, sexual orientation, and assertiveness.
http://counseling.uchicago.edu/vpc

Yahoo/Lesbians, Gays, and Bisexuals. A Web site and search engine that contains many links to information and support for lesbians and gays.
http://dir.yahoo.com/society_and_culture/cultures_and_groups

See also the listings for Chapters 3 and 5.

Andrews, V. 1999. You've got mail: But you may want it stamped Return to Sender. *Health Scout,* February 12 (http://www.healthscout.com/cig-bin/WebObjects/af/hsaf.woa?ap=19&id=60996; retrieved February 18, 1999).

Baker, B., et al. 2000. The influence of marital adjustment on 3-year left ventricular mass and ambulatory blood pressure in mild hypertension. *Archives of Internal Medicine* 160(22): 3453–3458.

Battaglia, D. M., D. Datteri, and C. Lord. 1998. Breaking up is (relatively) easy to do: A script for the dissolutions of close relationships. *Journal of Social and Personal Relationships* 15(6): 829–845.

Bergner, R. M. 2000. Love and barriers to love. An analysis for psychotherapists and others. *American Journal of Psychotherapy* 54(1): 1–17.

Christensen, A., and N. Jacobson. 2000. *Reconcilable Differences.* New York: Guilford Press.

Columbia University Health Education Program. 1997. *Go Ask Alice: Looking for Love on the Information Superhighway* (http://www.goaskalice.columbia.edu/1185.html; retrieved September 4, 1998).

DeGenova, M. K., and F. P. Rice. 2002. *Intimate Relationships, Marriages, and Families.* 5th ed. Mountain View, Calif.: Mayfield.

Feeney, J. 1999. Issues of closeness and distance in dating relationships: Effects of sex and attachment style. *Journal of Social and Personal Relationships* 16(5): 571–590.

Fletcher, G. J., et al. 1999. Ideals in intimate relationships. *Journal of Personality and Social Psychology* 76(1): 72–89.

Grote, N. K., and M. S. Clark. 2001. Perceiving unfairness in the family: Cause or consequence of marital distress? *Journal of Personality and Social Psychology* 80(2): 281–293.

Heller, P. E., and B. Wood. 2000. The influence of religious and ethnic differences on marital intimacy: Intermarriage versus intramarriage. *Journal of Marital and Family Therapy* 26(2): 241–252.

Huston, T. L., et al. 2001. The connubial crucible: Newlywed years as predictors of marital delight, distress, and divorce. *Journal of Personality and Social Psychology* 80(2): 237–52.

Kiecolt-Glaser, J. K., et al. 1998. Marital stress: Immunologic, neuroendocrine, and autonomic correlates. *Annals of the New York Academy of Science* 840: 656–663.

Marital status and survival in prostate cancer. 1998. *Harvard Men's Health Watch,* August.

Olson, D., and J. DeFrain. 2000. *Marriage and the Family,* 3rd ed. Mountain View, Calif.: Mayfield.

Orth-Gomér, K., et al. 2000. Marital stress worsens prognosis in women with coronary heart disease. *Journal of the American Medical Association* 284(23): 3008–3014.

Payne, M. 1998. "Waiting for lightning to strike": Social support for interracial couples. In *Readings in Cultural Contexts,* ed. J. N. Martin, T. K. Nakayama, and L. A. Flores. Mountain View, Calif.: Mayfield.

Plante, T., and K. Sullivan. 2000. *Getting Together and Staying Together: The Stanford Course on Intimate Relationships.* Bloomington, Ind.: 1stBooks Library.

Roy, R., et al. 2000. Beyond intimacy: Conceptualizing sex differences in same sex friendships. *Journal of Psychology* 134(1): 93–101.

Sprecher, S. 1999. "I love you more today than yesterday." Romantic partners' perceptions of changes in love and related affect over time. *Journal of Personality and Social Psychology* 76(1): 46–53.

Strong, B., et al. 2002. *Human Sexuality: Diversity in Contemporary America,* 4th ed. Mountain View, Calif.: Mayfield.

Suler, J. 1997. *The Final Showdown Between In-Person and Cyberspace Relationships* (http://www1.rider.edu/users/suler/psycyber/showdown.html; retrieved August 28, 2000).

University of Florida Counseling Center. 2000. *Handling Common Relationship Problems* (http://www.counsel.ufl.edu/CounselNet/cnetrelprob.htm; retrieved August 26, 2000).

University of Wisconsin—Eau Claire, Counseling Services. 2000. *Building Healthy Relationships* (http://www.UWEC.EDU/admin/counsel/pubs/bhr.htm; retrieved August 26, 2000).

Watson, D., B. Hubbard, and D. Wiese. 2000. General traits of personality and affectivity as predictors of satisfaction in intimate relationships: Evidence from self- and partner-ratings. *Journal of Personality* 68(3): 413–449.

White, L., and J. G. Gilbreth. 2001. When children have two fathers: Effects of relationships with stepfathers and noncustodial fathers on adolescent outcomes. *Journal of Marriage and Family* 63(1): 155–167.

Yeung, W. J., et al. 2001. Children's time with fathers in intact families. *Journal of Marriage and Family* 63(1): 136–154.

Sexuality, Pregnancy, and Childbirth

5

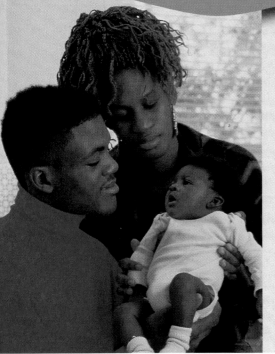

LOOKING AHEAD

After reading this chapter, you should be able to

- Describe the structure and function of the female and male sex organs
- Explain the changes in sexual functioning that occur across the life span and the various ways human sexuality can be expressed
- Describe guidelines for safe, responsible sexual behavior
- Describe the physical and emotional changes a pregnant woman typically experiences, and discuss the stages of fetal development
- List the important components of good prenatal care
- Describe the process of labor and delivery

Humans are sexual beings. Sexual activity is the source of our most intense physical pleasures, a central ingredient in many of our intimate emotional relationships, and, of course, the key to the reproduction of our species.

Sexuality is more than just sexual behavior. It includes biological sex (being biologically male or female), gender (masculine and feminine behaviors), sexual anatomy and physiology, sexual functioning and practices, and social and sexual interactions with others. Our individual sense of identity is powerfully influenced by our sexuality. We think of ourselves in very fundamental ways as male or female; as heterosexual or homosexual; as single, attached, married, or divorced. Sexuality is a complex, interacting group of inborn, biological characteristics and acquired behaviors people learn in the course of growing up in a particular family, community, and society.

Decisions about sexuality have far-reaching consequences. Understanding the basic facts about sexuality, pregnancy, and childbirth will help you make intelligent, informed decisions that are right for you.

SEXUAL ANATOMY

In spite of their different appearance, the sex organs of men and women arise from the same structures and fulfill similar functions. Each person has a pair of **gonads;** ovaries are the female gonads, and testes are the male gonads. The gonads produce **germ cells** and sex hormones. The germ cells are ova (eggs) in females and sperm in males. Ova and sperm are the basic units of reproduction; their union results in the creation of a new life.

Female Sex Organs

The external sex organs, or genitals, of the female are called the **vulva** (Figure 5-1). The mons pubis, a rounded mass of fatty tissue over the pubic bone, becomes covered

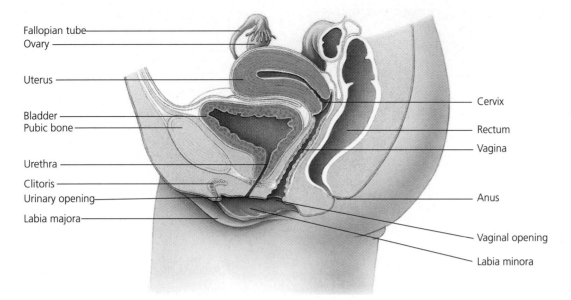

Fallopian tube
Ovary
Uterus
Bladder
Pubic bone
Urethra
Clitoris
Urinary opening
Labia majora

Cervix
Rectum
Vagina
Anus
Vaginal opening
Labia minora

Figure 5-1   The female sex organs.

with hair during puberty (biological maturation). Below it are two paired folds of skin called the labia majora (major lips) and the labia minora (minor lips). Enclosed within are the clitoris, the opening of the urethra, and the opening of the vagina. The **clitoris** is highly sensitive to touch and plays an important role in female sexual arousal and orgasm.

The female urethra leads directly from the urinary bladder to its opening between the clitoris and the opening of the vagina; it conducts urine from the bladder to the outside of the body. Unlike the male urethra, it is independent of the genitals.

The vaginal opening is partially covered by the hymen. This membrane can be stretched or torn during athletic activity or when a woman has sexual intercourse for the first time. The idea that an intact hymen is the sign of a virgin is a myth. The **vagina** is the passage that leads to the internal reproductive organs. It is the female structure for heterosexual sexual intercourse and also serves as the birth canal. Its soft, flexible walls are normally in contact with each other.

Projecting into the upper part of the vagina is the **cervix,** the neck of the uterus. Inside the pear-shaped **uterus,** which slants forward above the bladder, the fertilized egg is implanted and grows into a *fetus.* A pair of *fallopian tubes* (or *oviducts*) extends from the top of the uterus. The end of each oviduct surrounds an **ovary** and guides the mature ovum down into the uterus after the egg bursts from its follicle on the surface of the ovary.

Male Sex Organs

A man's external sex organs, or genitals, are the penis and the scrotum (Figure 5-2). The **penis** consists of spongy

tissue that becomes engorged with blood during sexual excitement, causing the organ to enlarge and become erect. The **scrotum** is a pouch that contains a pair of **testes.** The purpose of the scrotum is to maintain the testes at a temperature approximately 5°F below that of the rest of the body. The process of sperm production is extremely heat-sensitive. In hot temperatures the muscles in the scrotum relax, and the testes move away from the heat of the body. Conversely, in cold temperatures the muscles of the scrotum contract, and the testes move upward toward the body.

Terms

sexuality A dimension of personality shaped by biological, psychosocial, and cultural forces and concerning all aspects of sexual behavior.

gonads The primary reproductive organs that produce germ cells and sex hormones; the ovaries and testes.

germ cells Sperm and ova (eggs).

vulva The external female genitals, or sex organs.

clitoris The highly sensitive female genital structure.

vagina The passage leading from the female genitals to the internal reproductive organs; the birth canal.

cervix The end of the uterus opening toward the vagina.

uterus The hollow, thick-walled, muscular organ in which the fertilized egg develops; the womb.

ovary One of two female reproductive glands that produce ova (eggs) and sex hormones; ovaries are the female gonads.

penis The male genital structure consisting of spongy tissue that becomes engorged with blood during sexual excitement.

scrotum The loose sac of skin and muscle fibers that contains the testes.

testis One of two male gonads, the site of sperm production; plural, *testes*. Also called *testicle.*

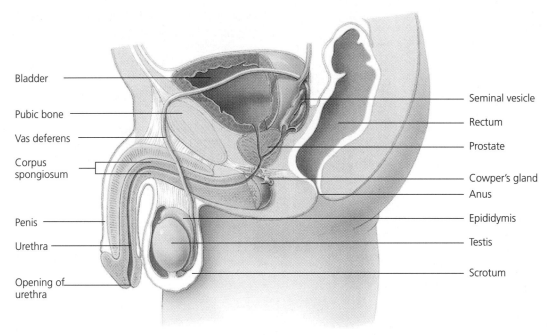

Bladder
Pubic bone
Vas deferens
Corpus spongiosum
Penis
Urethra
Opening of urethra

Seminal vesicle
Rectum
Prostate
Cowper's gland
Anus
Epididymis
Testis
Scrotum

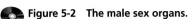 **Figure 5-2   The male sex organs.**

Through the entire length of the penis runs the urethra, which can carry both urine and *semen*, the sperm-carrying fluid, to the opening at the tip of the glans. Although urine and semen share a common passage, they are prevented from mixing together by muscles that control their entry into the urethra.

The testes contain tightly packed seminiferous tubules within which sperm are produced. These tubules end in a maze of ducts that flow into a single storage tube called the *epididymis,* on the surface of each testis. This tube leads to the *vas deferens,* a tube that rises into the abdominal cavity. Inside the prostate gland, the two vasa deferentia join the ducts of the two *seminal vesicles,* whose secretions provide nutrients to semen. The *prostate gland* produces some of the fluid in semen that nourishes and transports sperm. The tubes of the seminal vesicle and the vas deferens on each side lead to the *ejaculatory duct,* which joins the urethra. The *Cowper's glands* (bulbourethral glands) are two small structures flanking the urethra. During sexual arousal, these glands secrete a clear, mucuslike fluid that appears at the tip of the penis. The exact purpose of preejaculatory fluid is not known, but in some men, preejaculatory fluid may contain sperm, so withdrawal of the penis before ejaculation is not a reliable form of contraception.

Circumcision   The smooth, rounded tip of the penis is the highly sensitive **glans,** an important component in sexual arousal. The glans is partially covered by the foreskin, or prepuce, a retractable fold of skin that is removed by **circumcision** in about 60–70% of newborn males in

the United States. Circumcision is performed for cultural, religious, and hygienic reasons, and rates of circumcision vary widely among different groups. Worldwide, the rate is about 20%. Most Europeans, Asians, South and Central Americans, and Africans do not perform circumcision; Jews and Muslims are the major groups who circumcise for religious reasons.

The pros and cons of this simple procedure have been widely debated. Proponents argue that it promotes cleanliness and reduces the risk of urinary tract infections (UTIs) in newborns and penile cancer and sexually transmitted diseases (STDs) later in life. Research findings have been mixed; for example, a recent U.S. survey found no relationship between STD risk and circumcision, while international studies have shown a greater risk for STDs among uncircumcised males. Cultural as well as anatomical factors may explain these findings, and behavior is a far more important risk factor for STDs than circumcision status.

Opponents of circumcision state that it is an unnecessary surgical procedure that causes pain and puts a baby at risk for complications. Opponents also argue that by removing the foreskin, circumcision exposes the glans of the penis to constant irritation by clothing, thereby reducing its sensitivity; research into this issue has been inconclusive. In part because the overall risk of penile cancer and infant UTIs is low, the American Academy of Pediatrics (AAP) takes the position that although circumcision has potential medical benefits, the research is not sufficient to recommend the procedure routinely. When circumcision is performed, the AAP recommends that painkilling medication be provided.

HORMONES AND THE REPRODUCTIVE LIFE CYCLE

Many cultural and personal factors help shape the expression of your sexuality. But biology also plays an important role, particularly through the action of *hormones,* chemical messengers that are secreted directly into the bloodstream by the **endocrine glands.** The sex hormones produced by the ovaries or testes have a major influence on the development and function of the reproductive system throughout life. The sex hormones made by the testes are called **androgens,** the most important of which is *testosterone.* The female sex hormones, produced by the ovaries, belong to two groups: **estrogens** and **progestins,** the most important of which is *progesterone.* The cortex of the **adrenal glands** also produces androgens in both males and females.

The hormones produced by the testes, the ovaries, and the adrenal glands are regulated by the hormones of the **pituitary gland,** located at the base of the brain. This gland in turn is controlled by hormones produced by the **hypothalamus** in the brain. Sex hormones exert their primary developmental influences first in the embryo stage and later during adolescence.

Female Sexual Maturation

Although humans are fully sexually differentiated at birth, the differences between males and females are accentuated at **puberty,** the period during which the reproductive system matures, secondary sex characteristics develop, and the bodies of males and females come to appear more distinctive. The changes of puberty are induced by **testosterone** in the male and estrogen and **progesterone** in the female.

Physical Changes   The first sign of puberty in girls is breast development, followed by a rounding of the hips and buttocks. As the breasts develop, hair appears in the pubic region and later in the underarms. Shortly after the onset of breast development, girls show an increase in growth rate. Breast development usually begins between ages 8 and 13, and the time of rapid body growth occurs between ages 9 and 15.

The Menstrual Cycle   A major landmark of puberty for young women is the onset of the **menstrual cycle,** the monthly ovarian cycle that leads to menstruation (loss of blood and tissue lining the uterus) in the absence of pregnancy. The first *menstrual period,* or menarche, occurs at the average age of 12.8 years in the United States, but it may also normally start several years earlier or later.

The menstrual cycle consists of four phases: (1) menses, (2) the estrogenic phase, (3) ovulation, and (4) the progestational phase (Figure 5-3). Day 1 of the cycle is considered to be the day of the onset of bleeding. For the purposes of our discussion, a cycle of 28 days will be used; however, normal cycles vary in length.

During menses, characterized by the menstrual flow, hormones from the ovaries and anterior pituitary gland occur in relatively low amounts. This phase of the cycle usually lasts from day 1 to about day 5.

The estrogenic phase begins when the menstrual flow ceases, and the anterior pituitary begins to produce increasing amounts of follicle-stimulating hormone (FSH) and luteinizing hormone (LH). Under the influence of FSH, an egg-containing ovarian *follicle* begins to mature, producing increasingly higher amounts of estrogens. Stimulated by estrogen, the uterine lining, the *endometrium,* thickens with large numbers of blood vessels and uterine glands.

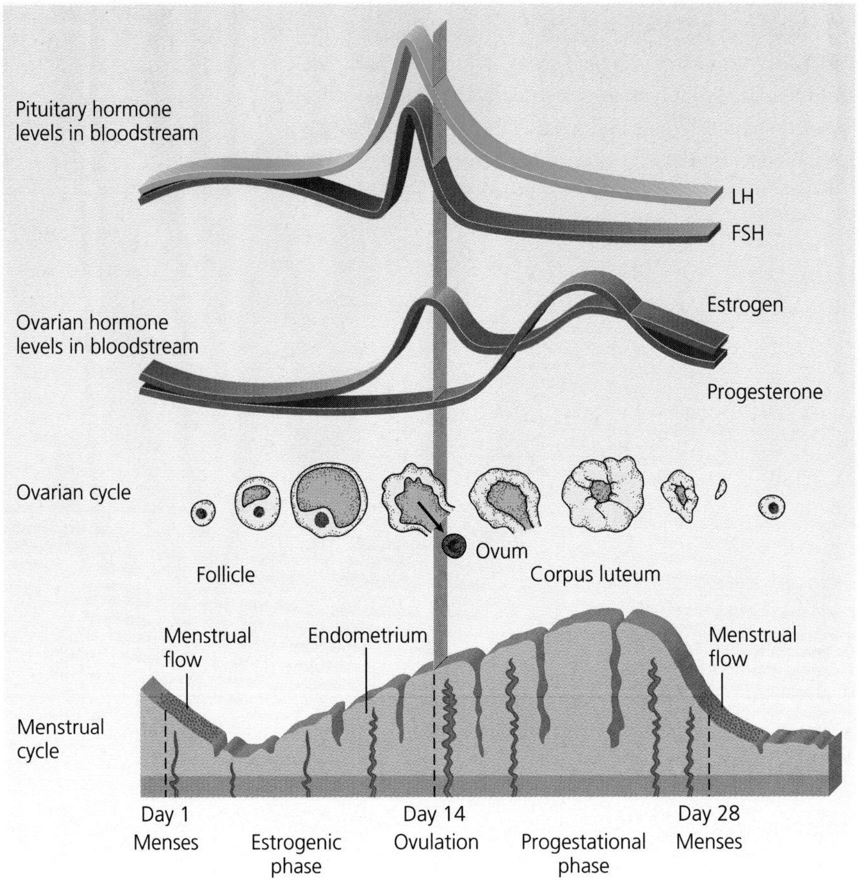

Figure 5-3 The menstrual cycle. The anterior pituitary releases FSH and LH, which stimulate the ovarian follicle to develop and release a mature egg. The ovarian follicle releases estrogen and progesterone, which stimulate the endometrium to continue to develop so that it will be ready to receive and nourish a fertilized egg. Unless pregnancy occurs, ovarian hormone levels fall and the endometrium sloughs off (menses).

A surge of a potent estrogen called estradiol from the follicle causes the anterior pituitary to release a large burst of LH and a smaller amount of FSH. The high concentration of LH stimulates the developing follicle to release its ovum. This event is known as *ovulation*. After ovulation, the follicle is transformed into the **corpus luteum**, which produces progesterone and estrogen. Ovulation usually occurs about 14 days prior to the onset of menstrual flow.

During the progestational phase of the cycle, the amount of progesterone secreted from the corpus luteum increases and remains high until the onset of the next menses. Under the influence of estrogen and progesterone, the endometrium continues to develop, readying itself to receive and nourish a fertilized ovum. When pregnancy occurs, the fertilized egg produces the hormone human chorionic gonadotropin (HCG), which maintains the corpus luteum. Thus, levels of ovarian hormones remain high and the uterine lining is preserved, preventing menses.

If pregnancy does not occur, the corpus luteum degenerates, and estrogen and progesterone levels gradually fall. Below certain hormonal levels, the endometrium can no longer be maintained, and it begins to slough off, initiating menses. As the levels of ovarian hormones fall, a rise in LH and FSH occurs, and a new cycle begins.

MENSTRUAL PROBLEMS Menstruation is a normal biological process, but it may cause physical or psychological problems. *Dysmenorrhea* is characterized by cramps in the lower abdomen, backache, vomiting, nausea, a bloated feeling, diarrhea, and loss of appetite. Some of these symptoms can be attributed to uterine muscular contractions caused by chemicals called prostaglandins. Any drug that blocks the effects of prostaglandins, such as aspirin or ibuprofen, will usually alleviate some of the symptoms of dysmenorrhea.

Many women experience transient physical and emotional symptoms prior to the onset of their menstrual flow. Depending on their severity, these symptoms may be categorized as one of three related conditions: **premenstrual tension, premenstrual syndrome (PMS),** and **premenstrual dysphoric disorder (PMDD).** Premenstrual tension symptoms are mild and may include negative mood changes and physical symptoms such as abdominal cramping and backache. More severe symptoms are classified as PMS; very severe symptoms that cause impairment in social functioning and work-related activities are classified as PMDD. All three conditions share a definite pattern: Symptoms appear prior to the onset of menses and disappear within a few days after the start of menstruation. It is estimated that as many as 75% of women report some

Many dietary supplements have been promoted for relief of the symptoms of PMS; those described below are among the most commonly advocated compounds. Only one supplement, calcium, has been shown to provide relief in rigorous clinical studies; several others show promise, but more research is needed.

- *Calcium.* Blood calcium levels are lower during the premenstrual period, and careful research studies have shown calcium supplements to be effective at relieving symptoms of PMS. The amount of calcium taken by women in these studies, 1000–1200 mg per day, is within accepted safety limits for calcium intake and may also be beneficial for building and maintaining bone density.

- *Magnesium.* Levels of magnesium in certain body cells are lower in women with PMS, and magnesium is involved in neurotransmitter activity. Results of small studies of the effects of magnesium have been promising, but larger trials are needed. Magnesium supplements can cause side effects, including diarrhea, in some people and so should be used with caution.

- *Vitamin B-6.* Vitamin B-6 plays an important role in the synthesis of neurotransmitters, so researchers have proposed that taking supplements of vitamin B-6 may help reduce mood-related symptoms of PMS. Research into the effects of vitamin B-6 has yielded mixed results, however. In addition, long-term use of high doses of vitamin B-6 can cause permanent nerve damage.

- *Vitamin E.* Although the mechanism is unclear, one study found that vitamin E supplements may improve PMS symptoms. Further research is needed.

- *Carbohydrates.* Some women with PMS report craving carbohydrate-rich foods, a change in diet that may actually improve the mood-related symptoms of PMS. Increased intake of carbohydrates may increase blood levels of tryptophan, an amino acid the body uses to produce the neurotransmitter serotonin. Although some dietary supplements containing mixtures of carbohydrates have been marketed for PMS symptoms, it is unclear whether these are any more effective than changing the diet to include more carbohydrate-rich fruits, vegetables, and grains.

Other compounds under study include evening primrose oil, black cohash, and chaste tree fruit (*vilex agnus-castus*). If you decide to try any of these or other dietary supplements for PMS, you should discuss your use of supplements with a qualified health professional. Some herbal products interact with prescription and over-the-counter drugs as well as other herbs; in addition, some may be toxic at high doses or dangerous during pregnancy (see Chapter 9).

SOURCE: Bendich, A. 2000. Review: The potential for dietary supplements to reduce premenstrual syndrome (PMS) symptoms. *Journal of the American College of Nutrition* 19(1): 3–12.

discomfort prior to the onset of menses, 20–50% of women experience PMS symptoms, and 3–10% meet the criteria for PMDD.

Many symptoms are associated with PMS and PMDD, including physical changes such as breast tenderness, water retention (bloating), headache, and fatigue; insomnia or excessive sleep; appetite changes and food cravings; irritability, anger, and increased interpersonal conflict; mood swings; depression and sadness; anxiety and tearfulness; inability to concentrate; social withdrawal; and the sense that one is out of control or overwhelmed. The key to diagnosing PMS and PMDD is to keep a daily diary of symptoms over several menstrual cycles. PMDD is distinguished from PMS by the severity of symptoms, which in PMDD interfere significantly with work or school and with usual social activities and relationships.

Despite many research studies, the causes of PMS and PMDD are still unknown, and there are no completely effective therapies. Selective serotonin reuptake inhibitors (SSRIs) such as Sarafem, which contains the same active ingredient as Prozac, have been shown to be effective at reducing symptoms. Other drug treatments include estrogen, diuretics to minimize water retention, and drugs that block the effects of prostaglandins such as aspirin, ibuprofen, and more potent prescription prostaglandin inhibitors. There are also a number of vitamins, minerals, and other dietary supplements that have been studied for PMS.

Although no universally effective treatments for PMS and PMDD have been identified, certain lifestyle changes are often recommended to help prevent or minimize symptoms:

Terms

corpus luteum The part of the ovarian follicle left after ovulation, which secretes estrogen and progesterone during the second half of the menstrual cycle.

premenstrual tension Mild physical and emotional changes associated with the time before the onset of menses; symptoms can include abdominal cramping and backache.

premenstrual syndrome (PMS) A disorder characterized by physical discomfort, psychological distress, and behavioral changes that begin after ovulation and cease when menstruation begins.

premenstrual dysphoric disorder (PMDD) Severe form of PMS, characterized by symptoms serious enough to interfere with work or school or with social activities and relationships.

- *Limit salt intake.* Salt promotes water retention and bloating. Avoid adding salt to your food, and don't eat salty snacks.
- *Exercise.* Women who exercise experience fewer symptoms both before and after their menstrual periods.
- *Don't use alcohol or tobacco.* Alcohol and tobacco may aggravate certain symptoms of PMS and PMDD.
- *Eat a nutritious diet.* Choose a low-fat diet rich in complex carbohydrates from vegetables, fruits, and whole-grain breads, cereals, and pasta. Obtain an adequate calcium intake from calcium-rich foods and, if needed, supplements. Minimize your intake of sugar and caffeine, and avoid chocolate, which is rich in both.
- *Relax.* Stress reduction is always beneficial, and stressful events can trigger PMS symptoms. Try relaxation techniques during the premenstrual time.

If symptoms persist, keep a daily diary to track both the types of symptoms you experience and their severity. See your physician for an evaluation and to learn more about treatments that are available only with a prescription.

Male Sexual Maturation

Reproductive maturation of boys occurs about 2 years later than that of girls; it usually begins at about age 10 or 11. Physical changes include enlargement of the testes, development of pubic hair, growth of the penis, the onset of ejaculation (usually at about age 11 or 12), deepening of the voice, the appearance of facial hair, and a period of rapid growth.

Aging and Human Sexuality

Changes in hormone production and sexual functioning occur as we age. As a woman approaches age 50, her ovaries gradually cease to function and she enters **menopause,** the cessation of menstruation. For some women, the associated drop in hormone production causes symptoms that are troublesome. The most common physical symptoms of menopause are hot flashes,

sensations of warmth rising to the face from the upper chest, with or without perspiration and chills. Other symptoms include headaches, dizziness, palpitations, and joint pains. Osteoporosis—decreasing bone density—can develop, making older women more vulnerable to fractures. Some menopausal women become moody, even markedly depressed, and they may also experience fatigue, irritability, and forgetfulness. As a result of decreased estrogen production, the vaginal walls become thin, and lubrication in response to sexual arousal diminishes. Hormone replacement therapy can significantly relieve most of these symptoms, but it may increase some women's risk of certain types of cancer.

Some women have a difficult time making the psychological adjustment to this stage of life, associating it with a loss of youth and sexual attractiveness. Others welcome it as a time of increased personal freedom, when the responsibilities of child rearing are over, and sex can be enjoyed without the fear of pregnancy. Menopause is seen as signaling the end of one phase of life and the beginning of another, equally meaningful, one. A recent poll of menopausal women found that more than half reported being happier now than in their younger years.

In men, testosterone production gradually decreases with age. As they get older, men depend more on direct physical stimulation for sexual arousal. They take longer to get an erection and find it more difficult to maintain; orgasmic contractions are less intense.

Many men go through a period of reassessment and readjustment in middle age, which may have repercussions for their sexuality. However, surveys have found that far from being a time of dissatisfaction and "midlife crisis," the middle years are a fulfilling time of life characterized by satisfying relationships. As with women, sexual activity can continue to be a source of pleasure and satisfaction for men as they grow older. A recent survey found that nearly half of all Americans age 60 or older engage in sexual activity at least once a month.

SEXUAL FUNCTIONING

In this section, we discuss sexual physiology—how the sex organs function during sexual activity—and problems that can occur with sexual functioning.

Sexual Stimulation

Sexual excitement can come from many sources, both physical and psychological. Although physical stimuli have an obvious and direct effect, some people believe psychological stimuli—thoughts, fantasies, desires, perceptions—are even more powerfully erotic.

Physical Stimulation Physical stimulation comes through the senses: We are aroused by things we see, hear, taste, smell, and feel. The most obvious and effective

Terms

menopause The cessation of menstruation, occurring gradually around age 50.

erogenous zone Any region of the body highly responsive to sexual stimulation.

vasocongestion The accumulation of blood in tissues and organs.

myotonia Increased muscular tension.

orgasm The discharge of accumulated sexual tension with characteristic genital and bodily manifestations and a subjective sensation of intense pleasure.

semen Seminal fluid, consisting of sperm cells and secretions from the prostate gland and seminal vesicles.

physical stimulation is touching. Even though culturally defined practices vary and individual people have different preferences, most sexual encounters eventually involve some form of touching with hands, lips, and body surfaces. Kissing, caressing, fondling, and hugging are as much a part of sexual encounters as they are of expressing affection.

The most intense form of stimulation by touching involves the genitals. Other highly responsive areas include the vaginal opening, the nipples, the breasts, the insides of the thighs, the buttocks, the anal region, the scrotum, the lips, and the earlobes. Such sexually sensitive areas, or **erogenous zones,** are especially susceptible to sexual arousal for most people, most of the time. Often, though, it's not *what* is touched but how, for how long, and by whom that determine the response. Under the right circumstances, touching any part of the body can cause sexual arousal.

Psychological Stimulation   Sexual arousal also has an important psychological component, regardless of the nature of the physical stimulation. Fantasies, ideas, memories of past experiences, and mood can all generate sexual excitement. Arousal is also powerfully influenced by emotions. How you feel about a person and how the person feels about you matter tremendously in how sexually responsive you are likely to be. Even the most direct forms of physical stimulation carry emotional overtones. Kissing, caressing, and fondling express affection and caring. The emotional charge they give to a sexual interaction is at least as significant to sexual arousal as the purely physical stimulation achieved by touching.

The Sexual Response Cycle

Noted sex researchers William Masters and Virginia Johnson were the first to describe in detail the human sexual response cycle. Men and women respond physiologically with a predictable set of reactions, regardless of the nature of the stimulation.

Two physiological mechanisms explain most genital and bodily reactions during sexual arousal and orgasm. These mechanisms are vasocongestion and myotonia. **Vasocongestion** is the engorgement of tissues that results when more blood flows into an organ than is flowing out. Thus, the penis becomes erect on the same principle that makes a garden hose become stiff when the water is turned on. **Myotonia** is increased muscular tension, which culminates in rhythmical muscular contractions during orgasm.

Four phases characterize the sexual response cycle:

1.   In the *excitement phase,* the penis becomes erect as its tissues become engorged with blood. The testes expand and are pulled upward within the scrotum. In women, the clitoris and the labia are similarly engorged with blood, and the vaginal walls become moist with lubricating fluid.

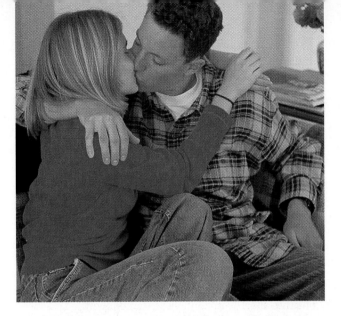

Human sexuality is not just a matter of bodies responding to each other. This couple's physical experiences together will be powerfully affected by their emotions, ideas, and values and by the quality of their relationship.

2.   The *plateau phase* is an extension of the excitement phase. Reactions become more marked: In men, the penis becomes harder, and the testes larger. In women, the lower part of the vagina swells, while its upper end expands and vaginal lubrication increases.

3.   In the *orgasmic phase,* or **orgasm,** rhythmic contractions occur along the man's penis, urethra, prostate gland, seminal vesicles, and muscles in the pelvic and anal regions. These involuntary muscular contractions lead to the ejaculation of **semen,** which consists of sperm cells from the testes and secretions from the prostate gland and seminal vesicles. In women, contractions occur in the lower part of the vagina and in the uterus, as well as in the pelvic region and the anus.

4.   In the *resolution phase,* all the changes initiated during the excitement phase are reversed. Excess blood drains from tissues, the muscles in the region relax, and the genital structures return to their unstimulated state.

More general physical reactions accompany the genital changes in both men and women. Beginning with the excitement phase, nipples become erect, the woman's breasts begin to swell, and in both sexes the skin of the chest becomes flushed; these changes are more marked in women. The heart rate doubles by the plateau phase, and respiration becomes faster. During orgasm, breathing becomes irregular and the person may moan or cry out. A feeling of warmth leads to increased sweating during the resolution phase. Deep relaxation and a sense of well-being pervade the body and the mind.

Male orgasm is marked by the ejaculation of semen. After ejaculation, men enter a *refractory period,* during which they cannot be restimulated to orgasm. Women do not have a refractory period, and immediate restimulation to orgasm is possible.

WW. Sexual Problems

Both physical and psychological factors can interfere with sexual functioning. If you are in poor physical health or experiencing high levels of stress or anxiety, sexual functioning may be negatively affected. Difficulties may be caused by infection and other sexual health problems. Disturbances in sexual desire, performance, or satisfaction are referred to as **sexual dysfunctions.**

Common Sexual Health Problems   Some problems with sexual functioning are due to treatable or preventable infections or other sexual health problems. Conditions that affect women include the following:

• *Vaginitis,* inflammation of the vagina, is caused by a variety of organisms: *Candida* (yeast infection), *Trichomonas* (trichomoniasis), and the overgrowth of a variety of bacteria (bacterial vaginosis).

• *Endometriosis* is the growth of endometrial tissue (tissue normally found lining the uterus) outside of the uterus. Endometriosis can cause serious problems if left untreated because the endometrial tissue can scar and partially or completely block the oviducts, causing infertility (difficulty conceiving) or sterility (the inability to conceive).

• *Pelvic inflammatory disease (PID)* is an infection of the uterus, oviducts, or ovaries, caused when microorganisms spread to these areas from the vagina. Approximately 50–75% of PID cases are caused by sexually transmitted organisms associated with diseases such as gonorrhea and chlamydia. PID can cause scarring of the oviducts, resulting in infertility or sterility.

Sexual health problems that affect men include the following:

• *Prostatitis* is inflammation or infection of the prostate gland.

• *Testicular cancer* occurs most commonly in men in their twenties and thirties. A rare cancer, it has a very high cure rate if detected early.

Sexual Dysfunctions   The term *sexual dysfunction* encompasses disturbances in sexual desire, performance, or satisfaction. A wide variety of physical conditions and drugs may interfere with sexual functioning.

Terms

sexual dysfunction A disturbance in sexual desire, performance, or satisfaction.

masturbation Self-stimulation for the purpose of sexual arousal and orgasm.

celibacy Continuous abstention from sexual activity.

COMMON SEXUAL DYSFUNCTIONS   Common sexual dysfunctions in men include erectile dysfunction (previously called impotence), the inability to have or maintain an erection sufficient for sexual intercourse; premature ejaculation, ejaculation before or just on penetration of the vagina or anus; and retarded ejaculation, the inability to ejaculate once an erection is achieved. Many men experience occasional difficulty achieving an erection or ejaculating because of excessive alcohol consumption, fatigue, or stress.

Two sexual dysfunctions in women are vaginismus, in which the woman experiences painful involuntary muscular spasms when sexual intercourse is attempted, and orgasmic dysfunction, the inability to experience orgasm. Vaginismus is a conditioned reflex probably related to fear of intercourse. Orgasmic dysfunction has been the subject of a great deal of discussion over the years, as people debated the nature of the female orgasm and what constitutes dysfunction in women. Many women experience orgasm but not during intercourse, or they experience orgasm during intercourse only if the clitoris is directly stimulated at the same time. In general, the inability to experience orgasm under certain circumstances is a problem only if the woman considers it so.

TREATING SEXUAL DYSFUNCTION   Most forms of sexual dysfunction are treatable. The first step is to have a thorough physical examination to identify any underlying medical condition that may be responsible for the problem. Heart disease, diabetes, smoking, drug use, and medications can all inhibit sexual response.

If physical problems continue to interfere with sexual response, many treatments are available, particularly for erectile dysfunction. Viagra (sildenafil citrate), the first-ever prescription pill for erectile dysfunction, doesn't actually cause an erection, but it enhances blood flow into the penis, thereby allowing an erection when sexual stimulation occurs. It has been shown to be effective in as many as 70% of men with erectile dysfunction, allowing them to achieve erections comparable for their age group.

If no physical problem is found, a sexual dysfunction may be psychosocial in origin. Psychosocial causes of dysfunction include troubled relationships, a lack of sexual skills, irrational attitudes and beliefs, anxiety, and psychosexual trauma, such as sexual abuse or rape. Many of these problems can be addressed by sex therapy methods that seek to modify the beliefs and behavior patterns that are interfering with satisfactory sexual relationships.

Women who seek treatment for orgasmic dysfunction often have not had the chance to learn through trial and error what types of stimulation will excite them and bring them to orgasm. Most sex therapists prefer to treat this problem with **masturbation** (genital self-stimulation). Women are taught about their own anatomy and sexual responses and then are encouraged to experiment with masturbation until they experience orgasm.

Choosing to have sex can change a relationship and an individual's life. In making decisions about sexual activity, you owe it to yourself and your partner to honestly think and talk about your choices. Consider the following issues:

- *Your background, beliefs, and goals.* What are your religious, moral, and/or personal values regarding relationships and sex? What are your priorities at this time, and how will a sexual relationship fit into your goals and plans for the future? Are you physically, emotionally, and financially ready to accept the potential consequences of the choices you make? How will you feel if you act in ways that are not consistent with your values and goals?

- *Your relationship with your partner.* How do you feel about your partner and your relationship? Do you respect and trust one another? Do you feel comfortable talking about sexual issues, and have you discussed contraception, pregnancy, and safer sex? How do you think having sex will affect your relationship and how you feel about yourself and your partner? What does having sex mean to each of you?

- *Your reasons for having sex.* Are you feeling pressured to have sex? Are you afraid of losing your partner if you say no? Are you too embarrassed, shy, or insecure to say no or discuss waiting? Are you being honest with yourself and your partner about your reasons for moving into a sexual relationship?

Personal decisions about sex should always be respected. You have the right to make your own choices and to do only what you feel comfortable with. When you make choices about sex based on self-respect, along with physical, emotional, and spiritual considerations, you'll be more likely to feel good about your decisions—now and in the future—and to enhance your health and well-being.

COMMUNICATE!   Many people have difficulty asking their physician questions about sexual matters, especially sexual functioning, yet physicians are usually an excellent resource for information and help. If you have questions you'd like answered, try writing them down as they occur to you. A week or two before you see your physician, read them out loud at home to get used to the idea of talking about them. Bring the list with you to your appointment. Try beginning with something that's easy to say, such as, "Doctor, I have a couple of questions I'd like to ask you."

WWW. SEXUAL BEHAVIOR

Many behaviors stem from sexual impulses, and sexual expression takes a variety of forms. Probably the most basic aspect of sexuality is reproduction, the process of producing offspring. As important as reproduction is, the intention of creating a child accounts for only a small measure of sexual activity; most people have sex for other reasons as well. Adult sexuality can include any of the sexual behaviors and practices described in this chapter. In mature love relationships, people ideally can integrate all the aspects of intimacy—physical, sexual, emotional—so that sexuality is a deeply meaningful part of how they express love.

Sexual Orientation

Sexual orientation is a consistent pattern of emotional and sexual attraction based on biological sex. It exists along a continuum that ranges from exclusive heterosexuality (attraction to people of the other sex) through bisexuality (attraction to people of both sexes) to exclusive homosexuality (attraction to people of one's own sex). The terms *straight* and *gay* are often used to refer to heterosexuals and homosexuals, respectively, and female homosexuals are also referred to as lesbians. Sexual orientation involves feelings and self-concept, and individuals may or may not express their sexual orientation in their behavior.

In a national survey, 2–5% of men had engaged in homosexual sex at some point in their lives, and 1–3% identified themselves as homosexuals. Of the women surveyed, 4% stated that they had engaged in homosexual sex at some point in their lives, and 1.5% identified themselves as homosexuals. Many theories have been proposed to account for the development of sexual orientation. Most scientists agree that it is most likely the result of the complex interaction of biological, psychological, and social factors, possibly different in the case of each individual.

Varieties of Human Sexual Behavior

Most people express their sexuality in a variety of ways. Some sexual behaviors are aimed at self-stimulation only, such as masturbation, while other practices involve interaction with others in behaviors such as kissing and intercourse. Some people choose not to express their sexuality and practice celibacy instead.

Celibacy   Continuous abstention from sexual activities, termed **celibacy**, can be a conscious and deliberate choice, or it can be necessitated by circumstances. Health considerations and religious and moral beliefs may lead some people to celibacy, particularly until marriage or until an acceptable partner appears. A disadvantage of the celibate life is that it may lack physical contact and affection.

Many people use the related term *abstinence* to refer to avoidance of just one sexual activity—intercourse. The use of abstinence to prevent pregnancy and sexually transmitted diseases is discussed in Chapters 6 and 13.

Autoeroticism and Masturbation The most common form of **autoeroticism** is **erotic fantasy,** creating imaginary experiences that range from fleeting thoughts to elaborate scenarios. Masturbation involves manually stimulating the genitals, rubbing them against objects (such as a pillow), or using stimulating devices such as vibrators. It may be used as a substitute for sexual intercourse or as part of sexual activity with a partner.

Touching and Foreplay Tactile stimulation, or touching, is integral to sexual experiences, whether in the form of massage, kissing, fondling, or holding. Our entire body surface is a sensory organ, and touching almost anywhere can enhance intimacy and sexual arousal. Touching can convey a variety of messages, including affection, comfort, and a desire for further sexual contact.

Oral-Genital Stimulation **Cunnilingus** (the stimulation of the female genitals with the lips and tongue) and **fellatio** (the stimulation of the penis with the mouth) are quite common practices. Oral sex may be practiced either as part of foreplay or as a sex act culminating in orgasm. Like all acts of sexual expression between two people, oral sex requires the cooperation and consent of both partners.

Anal Intercourse About 10% of heterosexuals and 50% of homosexual males regularly practice anal stimulation and penetration by the penis or a finger. Because the anus is composed of delicate tissues that tear easily under such pressure, anal intercourse is one of the riskiest of sexual behaviors associated with the transmission of HIV and the bacteria that cause gonorrhea and syphilis. The use of condoms is highly recommended for anyone engaging in anal sex. Special care and precaution should be exercised if anal sex is practiced.

Sexual Intercourse For most adults, most of the time, **sexual intercourse** is the ultimate sexual experience.

Men and women engage in coitus—make love—to fulfill both sexual and psychological needs. The most common heterosexual practice is the man inserting his erect penis into the woman's dilated and lubricated vagina after sufficient arousal. Psychological factors and the quality of the relationship are more important to overall sexual satisfaction than sophisticated or exotic sexual techniques.

Atypical and Problematic Sexual Behaviors

In American culture, many kinds of sexual behavior are accepted. However, some types of sexual expression are considered harmful; they may be against the law or classified as mental disorders, or both. Because sexual behavior occurs on a continuum, it is sometimes difficult to differentiate a behavior that is simply atypical from one that is harmful. When attempting to evaluate an unusual sexual behavior, experts consider the issues of consent between partners and whether physical or psychological harm is done to the individual or to others.

The use of force and coercion in sexual relationships is one of the most serious problems in human interactions. The most extreme manifestation of sexual coercion—forcing a person to submit to another's sexual desires—is rape, but sexual coercion occurs in many more subtle forms, such as sexual harassment. Sexual coercion—including rape, the sexual abuse of children, and sexual harassment—is discussed in detail in Chapter 16.

Commercial Sex

Conflicting feelings about sexuality are apparent in the attitudes of Americans toward commercial sex: prostitution and sexually oriented materials such as videos, magazines, and books. Our society condemns sexually explicit material and prostitution, but it also provides their customers.

Pornography Derived from the Greek word meaning "the writing of prostitutes," pornography is now often defined as obscene literature, art, or movies. A major problem in identifying pornographic material is that different people and communities have different opinions about what is obscene. Currently, the sale and rental of pornographic materials is restricted so that only adults can legally obtain them; materials depicting children in sexual contexts are illegal in any format or setting.

The appearance of thousands of sexually oriented Web sites has expanded the number of people with access to pornographic materials and has made enforcing pornography laws more difficult. People who might have hesitated to buy magazines or rent videos in person can now access sexually explicit material privately and anonymously. Of special concern is the increased availability of illegal materials such as child pornography that previously could be acquired only with great difficulty and at great legal risk.

Terms
autoeroticism Behavior aimed at sexual self-stimulation.
erotic fantasy Sexually arousing thoughts and daydreams.
cunnilingus Oral stimulation of the female genitals.
fellatio Oral stimulation of the penis.
sexual intercourse Sexual relations involving genital union; also called *coitus,* and also known as making love.

About 15% of all Internet users report visiting sexual Internet sites. Most of these sites feature pornographic images and/or sexually oriented chat rooms. A survey of nearly 10,000 users of sexual Internet sites found that about the same number of men and women visit sexual sites; men are more likely to visit sites with visual images, while women are more likely to visit chat rooms. People in chat rooms may engage in a range of behaviors, from mild flirtation with a group of chat room visitors to private, real-time discussions of explicit sexual activities with another Internet user. Many cybersex participants report feeling some degree of sexual excitement; some masturbate while viewing erotic images online or engaging in sexual chat.

Research into cybersex has identified some potential benefits of easily available online sexual material. The anonymous nature of the Internet gives people a sense of freedom and allows them to try out different identities and to seek sexual fulfillment in ways that they would not feel comfortable doing in real life. They may feel freer to talk openly about their sexual concerns or fantasies. A great deal of factual information about sexual behavior, contraception, and STDs is available for people who might not otherwise access such information; sexually oriented products such as condoms are also easily obtainable. Online sexual information may facilitate candid discussions between partners. In addition, the Internet provides opportunities for social contact and support among people with special concerns who might otherwise feel isolated; for example, rape survivors, people with herpes, or people with disabilities can meet online to share experiences and discuss sexual issues with their peers.

However, cybersex can cause problems for some people. Surveys indicate that about 5–8% of people who use the Internet for sex spend more than 11 hours per week online, with some people spending more than 50 hours per week online for sexual pursuits. This group is much more likely to report problems with work or interpersonal relationships than are people who spend lesser amounts of time online. For people who already feel isolated and lonely, cybersex may increase their social isolation as they spend more time online and less time reaching out to others in person. Online sexual encounters may offer the illusion of intimacy, but they do not have all the complexities or all the benefits of long-term, real-world intimate relationships.

For people involved in committed relationships, cybersex may be viewed as emotional infidelity and a threat to the relationship. People are likely to feel betrayed if they discover their partner has secretly been investing time and energy in online sexual interaction with others. In addition, the availability of certain types of sexual materials may reinforce abusive or problematic behaviors. For example, people have used the Internet to obtain child pornography and to contact young people and solicit meetings.

As described in Chapter 4, some people use the Internet to look for intimate partners whom they can meet face to face. Although online interaction has some special advantages for meeting people, including the opportunity to focus on interests and values before physical appearance, there are also potential dangers. Refer to Chapter 4 for more on the potential benefits and costs of looking for intimate partnerships online.

SOURCES: Cooper, A., et al. 1999. Sexuality on the Internet: From sexual exploration to pathological expression. *Professional Psychology Research and Practice.* 830(2). McClam, E. 2000. Cyber-sex addiction mushrooms in Internet climate of anonymity. *San Francisco Examiner,* May 6. Thompson, N. 2000. Sex in the digital city. *Washington Monthly,* July/August.

Much of the debate about pornography focuses on whether it is harmful. Some people argue that adults who want to view pornographic materials in the privacy of their own homes should be allowed to do so. Others feel that the exposure to explicit sexual material can lead to delinquent or criminal behavior, such as rape or the sexual abuse of children. Currently, there is no reliable evidence that pornography by itself leads to violence or harmful behavior, and debate is likely to continue.

Prostitution   The exchange of sexual services for money is prostitution. Prostitutes may be men, women, or children, and the buyer of a prostitute's services is nearly always a man. Except for parts of Nevada, prostitution is illegal in the United States. Most customers are white, middle-class, middle-aged, and married. Although they come from a wide variety of backgrounds, prostitutes are usually motivated to join the profession because of money.

AIDS is a major concern for prostitutes and their customers. Many prostitutes are injecting drug users or are involved with men who are. The rate of HIV infection among prostitutes varies widely, but in some parts of the country it is as high as 25–50%.

Responsible Sexual Behavior

Healthy sexuality is an important part of adult life. It can be a source of pleasurable experiences and emotions and an important part of intimate partnerships. But sexual behavior also carries many responsibilities, and you need to make choices about your sexuality that contribute to your well-being and that of your partner.

Open, Honest Communication   Each partner needs to clearly indicate what sexual involvement means to him or her. Does it mean love, fun, a permanent commitment, or something else? The intentions of both partners should be clear.

Agreed-On Sexual Activities   No one should pressure or coerce a partner. Sexual behaviors should be consistent

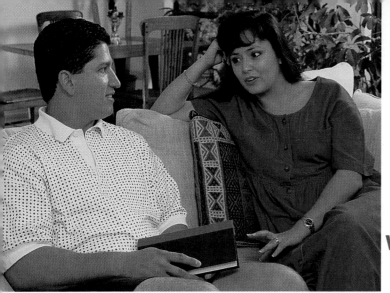

Sexual activity has many potential consequences, including pregnancy, disease, and emotional changes in the relationship. Responsible sexual behavior includes discussing these consequences openly and honestly.

with the sexual values, preferences, and comfort level of both partners. Everyone has the right to refuse sexual activity at any time.

Sexual Privacy   Intimate relationships involving sexual activity are based on trust, and that trust can be violated if partners reveal private information about the relationship to others. Sexual privacy also involves respecting other people—not engaging in activities in the presence of others that would make them uncomfortable.

Using Contraception   If pregnancy is not desired, contraception should be used during sexual intercourse. Both partners need to take responsibility for protecting against unwanted pregnancy. Partners should discuss contraception before sexual involvement begins.

Safer Sex   Both partners should be aware of and practice safer sex to guard against sexually transmitted diseases (STDs). Many sexual behaviors carry the risk of STDs, including HIV infection. Partners should be honest about their health and any medical conditions and work out a plan for protection. Behaviors that carry no risk of HIV infection are those that don't involve the exchange of body fluids (blood, semen, and vaginal secretions). Anyone who is not in a mutually monogamous relationship with an uninfected partner and who wishes to have sex should always use a condom.

Sober Sex   The use of alcohol or drugs in sexual situations increases the risk of unplanned, unprotected sexual activity. This is particularly true of young adults, many of whom engage in episodes of binge drinking during social events. Alcohol and drugs impair judgment and should not be used in association with sexual activity.

Taking Responsibility for Consequences   Individuals should be aware of the physical and emotional consequences of their sexual behavior and accept responsibility for them. Consequences include pregnancy, STDs, and emotional changes in the relationship between partners.

UNDERSTANDING FERTILITY

Conceiving a child is a highly complex process. Although many couples conceive readily, others can testify to the difficulties that can be encountered.

WW. Conception

The process of **conception** involves the **fertilization** of an egg (ovum) from a woman by a sperm from a man. Every month during a woman's fertile years, her body prepares itself for conception and pregnancy. In one of her ovaries an egg ripens and is released from its **follicle.** The egg, about the size of a pinpoint, travels through an **oviduct,** or **fallopian tube,** to the uterus, in 3–4 days. The lining of the uterus, or **endometrium,** has already thickened for the implantation of a **fertilized egg,** or zygote. If the egg is not fertilized, it lasts about 24 hours and then disintegrates. It is expelled along with the uterine lining during menstruation.

Sperm cells are produced in the man's testes and ejaculated from his penis into the woman's vagina during sexual intercourse. Sperm cells are much smaller than eggs. The typical ejaculate contains millions of sperm, but only a few complete the journey through the uterus and up the fallopian tube to the egg. As sperm approach the egg, they release enzymes that soften its hard outer layer. Enzymes from hundreds of sperm must be released in order for the egg's outer layer to soften enough to allow one sperm cell to penetrate. The first sperm cell that bumps into a spot that is soft enough can swim into the egg cell. It then merges with the nucleus of the egg, and fertilization occurs. The sperm's tail, its means of locomotion, gets stuck in the outer membrane and drops off, leaving the sperm head inside the egg. The egg then releases a chemical that makes it impenetrable by other sperm.

The ovum carries the hereditary characteristics of the mother and her ancestors; sperm cells carry the hereditary characteristics of the father and his ancestors. Each parent cell—egg or sperm—contains 23 chromosomes, each of which contains genes, packages of chemical instructions for the developing baby. Genes provide the blueprint for a unique individual.

The usual course of events is that one egg and one sperm unite to produce one fertilized egg and one baby. But if the ovaries release two (or more) eggs during ovulation, and if both eggs are fertilized, twins will develop. These twins will be no more alike than siblings from different pregnancies, because each will have come from a different fertilized egg. Twins who develop this way are referred to as **fraternal twins**; they may be the same sex or different sexes. Twins can also develop from the division of a single fertilized egg into two cells that develop separately. Because these babies share all genetic material, they will be **identical twins.**

Infertility

Although the main concern for many women and men, especially if they are young and single, is how *not* to get pregnant, the reverse is true for millions of couples who have difficulty conceiving. **Infertility** is usually defined as the inability to conceive after trying for a year or more. It affects about 6 million couples—10% of the reproductive-age population of the United States. Although the focus is often on women, up to 40% of the factors contributing to infertility are male, and in about 15% of infertile couples, both partners have problems.

Female Infertility   Female infertility usually results from one of two key causes—tubal blockage (40%) or failure to ovulate (40%). An additional 10% of cases of infertility are due to anatomical abnormalities, benign growths in the uterus, thyroid disease, and other uncommon conditions; the remaining 10% of cases are unexplained.

Blocked fallopian tubes are most commonly the result of *pelvic inflammatory disease (PID),* a serious complication of several sexually transmitted diseases. Most cases of PID are associated with untreated cases of chlamydia or gonorrhea. More than 1.5 million cases of PID are treated each year, but physicians estimate that half may go untreated because of an absence of symptoms. Other causes of PID include unsterile abortions and certain types of older IUDs. Tubal blockages can also be caused by prior surgery or by *endometriosis,* a condition in which endometrial (uterine) tissue grows outside the uterus. This tissue responds to hormones and can cause pain, bleeding, scarring, and adhesions. Endometriosis is typically treated with hormonal therapy and surgery.

Age impacts fertility; beginning around age 30, a woman's fertility naturally begins to decline. Age is probably the main factor in ovulation failure. Exposure to toxic chemicals or radiation also appears to reduce fertility, as does cigarette smoking. Daughters born to women who were given diethylstilbestrol (DES) during pregnancy are at risk for a variety of problems with conception.

Male Infertility   The leading causes of infertility among men are low sperm count, lack of sperm motility (the ability to move spontaneously), misshapen sperm, and blocked passageways between the testes and the urethra. Smoking may cause reduced sperm counts and abnormal sperm. The sons of mothers who took DES may have increased sperm abnormalities and fertility problems. Certain prescription and illegal drugs also affect the number of sperm. Large doses of marijuana, for example, cause lower sperm counts and suppress certain reproductive hormones. Other possible causes of sperm problems include injury to the testicles, infection (especially from mumps during adulthood), birth defects, subjecting the testes to high temperatures, and exposure to toxic environmental substances such as lead, radiation, or pollutants that mimic the effects of hormones.

Treating Infertility   About 90% of infertile couples receive a physical diagnosis for their condition; for the remaining 10%, the cause of the infertility remains unexplained. Most cases of infertility are treated with conventional medical therapies: Surgery can repair oviducts, clear up endometriosis, and correct anatomical problems in both men and women. Fertility drugs can help women ovulate, although they carry the risk of causing multiple births. If these conventional treatments don't work, couples can turn to more advanced techniques.

- *Intrauterine insemination:* Male infertility can sometimes be overcome collecting and concentrating the man's sperm and introducing it by syringe into the woman's vagina or uterus, a procedure known as artifical (intrauterine) insemination. The sperm can be provided by the woman's partner or, if there are severe problems with his sperm, by a donor.

- *Assisted reproduction:* Three related techniques involve removing mature eggs from a woman's ovary. With in vitro fertilzation (IVF), the harvested eggs are mixed with sperm in a laboratory dish; if fertilized, one or more of them are inserted into the woman's uterus. In gamete intrafallopian transfer (GIFT), eggs and sperm are surgically placed into the oviducts prior to fertilization. In zygote intrafallopian transfer (ZIFT), eggs are fertilized outside the woman's body and surgically introduced into the

Terms

conception The fusion of ovum and sperm, resulting in a fertilized egg.

fertilization The initiation of biological reproduction: the union of the nucleus of an egg cell with the nucleus of a sperm cell.

follicle One of many saclike structures within the ovary in which eggs mature.

oviduct (fallopian tube) One of two passages through which eggs travel from the ovaries to the uterus; the site of fertilization.

endometrium The mucous membrane that forms the inner lining of the cavity of the uterus.

fertilized egg The egg after penetration by a sperm; a zygote.

fraternal twins Twins who develop from separate fertilized eggs; not genetically identical.

identical twins Twins who develop from the division of a single zygote; genetically identical.

infertility The inability to conceive after trying for a year or more.

oviducts after they begin to divide. More advanced procedures under study include the use of cloning techniques such as nuclear transfer, in which the nucleus of an older woman's egg is transferred into an egg from a younger woman from whom the nucleus has been removed.

• *Surrogate motherhood:* This controversial approach to infertility involves a contract between an infertile couple and a fertile woman who agrees to be aritificially inseminated by the father's sperm, carry the baby to term, and give it to the couple at birth. Some people consider surrogate motherhood as essentially an arrangement to sell a baby and worry about the psychological consequences for the children. In addition, some surrogate mothers have a very difficult time giving up the baby they have carried.

Most infertility treatments are expensive and emotionally draining, and their success is uncertain. Some infertile couples choose not to try to have children, while others turn to adoption. One measure you can take now to avoid infertility is to protect yourself against STDs and to treat promptly any disease you do contract.

COMMUNICATE! Some fertility problems may be at least partly inherited, so it can be useful to know your parents' fertility history. If you don't want to approach the issue directly, you can ask such questions as, "Was there a reason that you waited so long after you got married to have children?" or "Did you plan to have me when you did?" You may learn things you didn't know about other aspects of your parents' lives as well, such as their career aspirations or their socioeconomic status when they were younger.

PREGNANCY

Pregnancy is usually discussed in terms of **trimesters**— three periods of about 3 months (or 13 weeks) each. During the first trimester, the mother experiences a few physical changes and some fairly common symptoms. During the second trimester, often the most peaceful time of pregnancy, the mother gains weight, looks noticeably pregnant, and may experience a general sense of well-being if she is happy about having a child. The third trimester is the hardest for the mother because she must breathe, digest, excrete, and circulate blood for herself and the growing **fetus.** The weight of the fetus, the pressure of its body on her organs, and its increased demands on her system cause discomfort and fatigue and may make the mother increasingly impatient to give birth.

Pregnancy Tests

The earliest tests for pregnancy are chemical tests designed to detect the presence of **human chorionic gonadotropin**

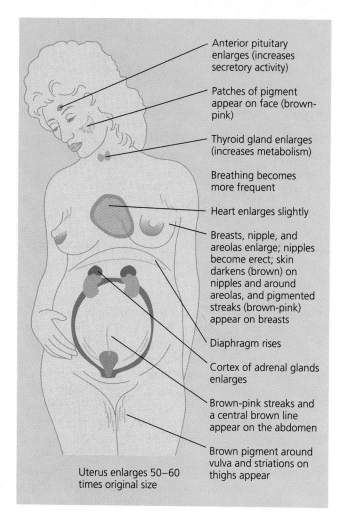

Anterior pituitary enlarges (increases secretory activity)

Patches of pigment appear on face (brown-pink)

Thyroid gland enlarges (increases metabolism)

Breathing becomes more frequent

Heart enlarges slightly

Breasts, nipple, and areolas enlarge; nipples become erect; skin darkens (brown) on nipples and around areolas, and pigmented streaks (brown-pink) appear on breasts

Diaphragm rises

Cortex of adrenal glands enlarges

Brown-pink streaks and a central brown line appear on the abdomen

Brown pigment around vulva and striations on thighs appear

Uterus enlarges 50–60 times original size

Figure 5-4   Physiological changes during pregnancy.

(HCG), a hormone produced by the implanted fertilized egg. These tests may be performed as early as 2 weeks after fertilization. Home pregnancy test kits, which are sold without a prescription in drugstores, can be very reliable if the instructions are followed carefully.

Changes in the Woman's Body

Hormonal changes begin as soon as the egg is fertilized, and for the next 9 months, the woman's body nourishes the fetus and adjusts to its growth. Let's take a closer look at the changes of early, middle, and late pregnancy (Figure 5-4).

Early Signs and Symptoms   Early recognition of pregnancy is important, especially for women with physical problems and nutritional deficiencies. The following symptoms are not absolute indications of pregnancy, but they are reasons to visit a gynecologist:

• *A missed menstrual period.* If an egg has been fertilized and implanted in the uterine wall, the endometrium is retained to nourish the embryo.

- *Slight bleeding.* Slight bleeding for a few days may follow implantation of the fertilized egg. Because this happens about the time a period is expected, the bleeding is sometimes mistaken for menstrual flow.

- *Nausea.* About two-thirds of pregnant women feel nauseated, probably as a reaction to increased levels of progesterone and other hormones. Often called morning sickness, some women have it all day long. It frequently begins during the 3rd or 4th week and disappears by the 12th week. In some cases, it can last throughout a pregnancy.

- *Breast tenderness.* Some women experience breast tenderness, swelling, and tingling, usually described as different from the tenderness experienced before menstruation.

- *Sleepiness, fatigue, and emotional upset.* These symptoms result from hormonal changes.

The first reliable physical signs of pregnancy can be distinguished about 4 weeks after a woman misses her menstrual period. A softening of the uterus just above the cervix, called *Hegar's sign,* and other changes in the cervix and pelvis are apparent during a pelvic examination. The labia minora and the cervix may take on a purple color rather than their usual pink hue.

Continuing Changes in the Woman's Body   During the first 3 months, the uterus enlarges to about three times its nonpregnant size. By the fourth month, it is large enough to make the abdomen protrude. By the seventh or eighth month, the uterus pushes up into the rib cage, which makes breathing slightly more difficult. The breasts enlarge and are sensitive; by week 8, they may tingle or throb. The pigmented area around the nipple, the areola, darkens and broadens. After the 10th week, **colostrum**, a yellowish fluid, may be squeezed from the mother's nipples.

Early in pregnancy, the muscles and ligaments attached to bones begin to soften and stretch. The joints between the pelvic bones loosen and spread, making it easier to have a baby but harder to walk. The circulatory system becomes more efficient to accommodate the blood volume, which increases by 50%, and the heart pumps it more rapidly. The mother's lungs also become more efficient, and her rib cage widens to permit her to inhale up to 40% more air.

Women of normal weight gain an average of 18–25% of their initial weight: 20–28 lb for a woman weighing 110; 23–32 lb for a woman weighing 128. About 60% of weight gained relates directly to the baby—about 6.8 lb for the baby and 7.5 lb for the placenta, amniotic fluid, heavier breasts and uterus—and 40% accumulates over the mother's entire body as fluid (blood, about 4 lb) and fat (4–8 lb).

Changes During the Later Stages of Pregnancy   By the end of the sixth month, the increased needs of the fetus place a burden on the mother's lungs, heart, and kidneys. Her back may ache from the pressure of the baby's weight and from having to throw her shoulders back to keep her balance while standing. Her body retains more water, perhaps up to 3 extra quarts of fluid. Her legs, hands, ankles, or feet may swell, and she may be bothered by leg cramps, heartburn, or constipation. Despite discomfort, both her digestion and her metabolism are working at top efficiency.

The uterus prepares for childbirth with **Braxton Hicks contractions.** Unlike true labor contractions, these are usually short, irregular, and painless. The mother may only be aware that at times her abdomen is hard to the touch. These contractions become more frequent and intense as the delivery date approaches.

In the ninth month, the baby settles into the pelvic bones, usually head down, fitting snugly. This process, called **lightening,** allows the uterus to sink down about 2 inches. Pelvic pressure increases, and pressure on the diaphragm lightens. Breathing becomes easier; urination becomes more frequent.

Fetal Development

Now that we've seen what happens to the mother's body during pregnancy, let's consider the development of the fetus (Figure 5-5).

The First Trimester   About 30 hours after the egg is fertilized, the cell divides, and this process of cell division repeats many times. On about the fourth day after fertilization, the cluster, now about 32–128 cells and hollow, arrives in the uterus; this is a **blastocyst.** On about the sixth or seventh day, the blastocyst attaches to the uterine wall; over the next few days, it becomes firmly implanted and begins to draw nourishment from the endometrium, the uterine lining.

Terms

trimester One of the three 3-month periods of pregnancy.

fetus The developmental stage of a human from the 9th week after conception to the moment of birth.

human chorionic gonadotropin (HCG) A hormone produced by the fertilized egg that can be detected in the urine or blood of the mother within a few weeks of conception.

colostrum A yellowish fluid secreted by the mammary glands around the time of childbirth until milk comes in, about the third day.

Braxton Hicks contractions Uterine contractions that occur during the third trimester of pregnancy, preparing it for labor.

lightening A process in which the uterus sinks down because the baby's head settles into the pelvic area.

blastocyst A stage of development, days 6–14, when the cell cluster becomes the embryo and placenta.

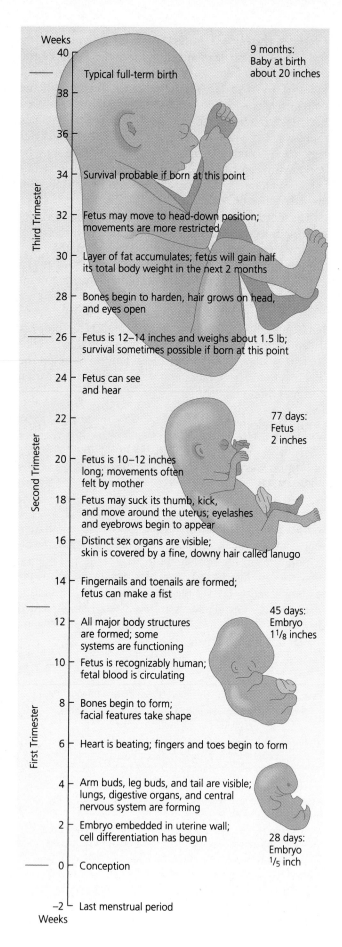

Weeks
40 — Typical full-term birth

9 months:
Baby at birth
about 20 inches

38

36

34 — Survival probable if born at this point

Third Trimester

32 — Fetus may move to head-down position;
movements are more restricted

30 — Layer of fat accumulates; fetus will gain half
its total body weight in the next 2 months

28 — Bones begin to harden, hair grows on head,
and eyes open

26 — Fetus is 12–14 inches and weighs about 1.5 lb;
survival sometimes possible if born at this point

24 — Fetus can see
and hear

22

77 days:
Fetus
2 inches

Second Trimester

20 — Fetus is 10–12 inches
long; movements often
felt by mother

18 — Fetus may suck its thumb, kick,
and move around the uterus; eyelashes
and eyebrows begin to appear

16 — Distinct sex organs are visible;
skin is covered by a fine, downy hair called lanugo

14 — Fingernails and toenails are formed;
fetus can make a fist

12 — All major body structures
are formed; some
systems are functioning

45 days:
Embryo
1 1/8 inches

10 — Fetus is recognizably human;
fetal blood is circulating

First Trimester

8 — Bones begin to form;
facial features take shape

6 — Heart is beating; fingers and toes begin to form

4 — Arm buds, leg buds, and tail are visible;
lungs, digestive organs, and central
nervous system are forming

2 — Embryo embedded in uterine wall;
cell differentiation has begun

28 days:
Embryo
1/5 inch

0 — Conception

−2 — Last menstrual period
Weeks

The blastocyst becomes an **embryo** by about the end of the second week after fertilization. The inner cells of the blastocyst separate into three layers. One layer becomes inner body parts, the digestive and respiratory systems; the middle layer becomes muscle, bone, blood, kidneys, and sex glands; and the third layer becomes the skin, hair, and nervous tissue. The outermost shell of cells becomes the **placenta, umbilical cord,** and **amniotic sac.** A network of blood vessels called chorionic villi eventually forms the placenta. The placenta brings oxygen and nutrients to the fetus and transports waste products out. The placenta does not provide a perfect barrier between the fetal circulation and the maternal circulation, however. Some blood cells are exchanged and certain substances, such as alcohol, pass freely from the maternal circulation through the placenta to the fetus.

The period between weeks 2 and 9 is a time of rapid differentiation and change. All the major body structures are formed during this time, including the heart, brain, liver, lungs, and sex organs; the eyes, nose, ears, arms, and legs also appear. Some organs begin to function—the heart begins to beat and the liver starts producing blood cells. Because body structures are forming, the developing organism is vulnerable to damage from environmental influences such as drugs and infections.

By the end of the second month, the brain sends out impulses that coordinate the functioning of other organs. The embryo is now a fetus, and most further changes will be in the size and refinement of working body parts. In the third month, the fetus begins to be quite active. By the end of the first trimester, the fetus is about 4 inches long and weighs 1 ounce.

The Second Trimester   To grow during the second trimester, to about 14 inches and 2 pounds, the fetus must have large amounts of food, oxygen, and water, which come from the mother through the placenta. All body systems are operating, and the fetal heartbeat can be heard with a stethoscope. Fetal movements can be felt by the mother beginning in the fourth or fifth month. Against great odds, a fetus born prematurely at the end of the second trimester might survive.

The Third Trimester   The fetus gains most of its birth weight during the last 3 months. Some of the weight is fatty tissue under the skin that insulates the fetus and supplies food. The fetus must obtain large amounts of calcium, iron, and nitrogen from the food the mother eats. Some 85% of the calcium and iron she consumes goes into the fetal bloodstream.

Although the fetus may live if it is born during the seventh month, it needs the fat layer acquired in the eighth month and time for the organs, especially the res-

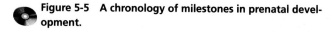 **Figure 5-5   A chronology of milestones in prenatal development.**

piratory and digestive organs, to develop. It also needs the immunity the mother's blood supplies during the final 3 months. Her blood protects the fetus against many of the diseases to which she has acquired immunity. These immunities wear off within 6 months after birth, but they can be replenished by the mother's milk if the baby is breastfed.

Diagnosing Fetal Abnormalities   Information about the health and sex of a fetus can be obtained prior to birth through prenatal testing. **Ultrasonography** (also called *ultrasound*) uses high-frequency sound waves to create a visual image, or **sonogram,** of the fetus in the uterus. Sonograms show the position of the fetus, its size and gestational age, and the presence of certain anatomical problems. Sonograms can sometimes be used to determine the sex of the fetus.

Amniocentesis involves the removal of fluid from the uterus with a long, thin needle inserted through the abdominal wall. It is usually performed between 14 and 18 weeks into the pregnancy. A genetic analysis of the fetal cells in the fluid can reveal the presence of chromosomal disorders, such as Down syndrome, and some genetic diseases, including Tay-Sachs disease. The sex of the fetus can also be determined.

A newer alternative is **chorionic villus sampling (CVS),** which can be performed earlier in pregnancy than amniocentesis, between week 10 and 12. This procedure involves removal through the cervix (by catheter) or abdomen (by needle) of a tiny section of chorionic villi, which contain fetal cells that can be analyzed.

The **triple marker screen (TMS)** is a maternal blood test that can be used to help identify fetuses with neural tube defects, Down syndrome, and other anomalies. Blood is taken from the mother at 16 to 19 weeks of pregnancy and analyzed for three hormone levels—human chorionic gonadotropin (HCG), unconjugated estriol, and alpha-fetoprotein (AFP). The three hormone levels are compared to appropriate standards, and the results are used to estimate the probability that the fetus has particular anomalies.

WW. The Importance of Prenatal Care

Adequate prenatal care—a nutritious diet, exercise, adequate rest, avoidance of drugs, and regular medical evaluation—is essential to the lifelong health of both mother and baby.

Regular Checkups and Blood Tests   In the woman's first visit to her obstetrician, she will be asked for a detailed medical history of herself and her family. The physician or midwife will note any hereditary conditions that may assume increased significance during pregnancy. The tendency to develop gestational diabetes (diabetes during pregnancy only), for example, can be inherited; appropri-

ate treatment during pregnancy reduces the risk of serious harm. A blood sample is also taken during the initial prenatal visit to determine blood type and screen for anemia. Rh factor, a blood protein, will also be checked because if a mother and fetus have incompatible Rh factors, treatment may be needed to protect the health of the fetus.

The woman is given a complete physical exam and is informed about appropriate diet. She returns for regular checkups throughout the pregnancy, during which her blood pressure and weight gain are measured, her urine is analyzed, and the size and position of the fetus are monitored. Regular prenatal visits also give the mother a chance to discuss her concerns and assure herself that everything is proceeding normally. Early advice from physicians, midwives, health educators, and teachers of childbirth classes provides the mother with invaluable information.

Prenatal Nutrition   The saying that a pregnant woman needs to "eat for two" is true. A nutritious diet throughout pregnancy is essential for both the fetus and the mother. To meet the increased nutritional demands of her body, a pregnant woman shouldn't just eat more; she should make sure that her diet is adequate in all the basic nutritional categories.

Adequate intake of the B vitamin folic acid before conception and in the early weeks of pregnancy has been shown to decrease the risk of neural tube defects, including spina bifida. It is recommended that any woman capable of becoming pregnant consume at least 400 µg (0.4 mg) of folic acid daily from fortified foods and/or supplements, in addition to folate from a varied diet. Since 1998, enriched grain products have been fortified with small amounts of folic acid; folate is found naturally in leafy green vegetables, legumes, citrus fruits, and most berries.

Terms

embryo The stage of development between blastocyst and fetus; about weeks 2–8.

placenta The organ through which the fetus receives nourishment and empties waste via the mother's circulatory system; after birth, the placenta is expelled from the uterus.

umbilical cord The cord connecting the placenta and fetus, through which nutrients pass.

amniotic sac A membranous pouch enclosing and protecting the fetus, containing amniotic fluid.

ultrasonography The use of high-frequency sound waves to view the fetus in the uterus; also known as *ultrasound*.

sonogram The visual image of the fetus produced by ultrasonography.

amniocentesis A process in which amniotic fluid is removed and analyzed to detect possible birth defects.

chorionic villus sampling (CVS) Surgical removal of a tiny section of chorionic villi to be analyzed for genetic defects.

triple marker screen (TMS) Measurement of alpha fetoprotein, esriol, and human chorionic gonadotropin to assess risk of fetal anomalies.

A healthy diet is a key part of prenatal care. To maintain her own health and help the fetus grow, a woman needs to consume about 300 extra calories per day during pregnancy. Breastfeeding an infant requires even more energy—about 500 extra calories per day.

Healthy Choices

To ensure a balanced intake of key nutrients, pregnant women should follow the U.S. Department of Agriculture's Food Guide Pyramid. The Pyramid recommends a range of servings for the following six different food groups; the number of servings in parentheses is the minimum suggested by the American College of Obstetricians and Gynecologists for pregnant women:

- Bread, cereal, rice, and pasta group: 6–11 servings (9 servings)
- Vegetables: 3–4 servings (4 servings)
- Fruits: 2–4 servings (3 servings)
- Milk, yogurt, and cheese: 2–3 servings (3 servings)
- Meat, poultry, fish, dry beans, eggs, and nuts: 2–3 servings (3 servings or 6 oz total)
- Fats, oils, and sweets: use sparingly according to total energy needs

Finally, it is also important to consume an adequate amount of fluids, the equivalent of 6–8 glasses of water per day.

Supplements

Some physicians may prescribe vitamin and mineral supplements for women who are pregnant or lactating or who are trying to get pregnant. Supplements may be for a particular nutrient, such as folic acid or iron, or may be a multivitamin and mineral supplement. It is important that a pregnant woman not supplement beyond her physician's advice because some vitamins and minerals are harmful if taken in excess. It is also important not to take herbal dietary supplements without consulting a physician; few dietary supplements have been tested for safety during pregnancy, and some have been shown to be dangerous.

Food Safety

Pregnant women should give special attention to food safety because foodborne pathogens can be particularly dangerous during pregnancy. Two such pathogens are *Listeria monocytogenes* and *Toxoplasma gondii*. *Listeria* is a bacterium most often found in undercooked or ready-to-eat meat, poultry, or seafood; soft cheeses; products made with unpasteurized milk; and unpasteurized juice. Listeriosis causes flulike symptoms in pregnant women; if the fetus is infected, the result can be miscarriage, premature birth, or birth defects.

T. gondii, a parasite carried by cats, can also contaminate food or soil. Toxoplasmosis is typically caused by eating undercooked meat or poultry or unwashed fruits and vegetables, cleaning a litter box, or handling contaminated soil. Toxoplasmosis causes few symptoms in pregnant women, but if passed to the fetus, it may cause miscarriage or mental impairment.

One further food safety recommendation for pregnant women relates to fish. Most types of fish are good choices for a healthy diet, but a few types can be contaminated with mercury or industrial pollutants. The FDA advises pregnant women not to eat swordfish, shark, king mackeral, or tilefish. Pregnant women are also advised to check with their local health departments before consuming any game fish.

For a more detailed discussion of recommended food choices, servings sizes, and food safety guidelines, see Chapter 9.

Avoiding Drugs and Other Environmental Hazards

In addition to the food the mother eats, the drugs she takes and the chemicals she is exposed to affect the fetus. Everything the mother ingests may eventually reach the fetus in some proportion. Some drugs harm the fetus but not the mother because the fetus is in the process of developing and because the proper dose for the mother is a massive dose for the fetus.

During the first trimester, when the major body structures are rapidly forming, the fetus is extremely vulnerable to environmental factors such as viral infections, radiation, drugs, and other **teratogens,** any of which can cause **congenital malformations,** or birth defects. The most susceptible body parts are those growing most rapidly at the time of exposure. The rubella (German measles) virus, for example, can cause a congenital malformation of a delicate system such as the eyes or ears, leading to blindness or deafness, if exposure occurs during the first trimester, but it does no damage later in the pregnancy. Other drugs can cause damage throughout prenatal development.

Prenatal exposure to drugs can lead to serious problems. Cigarette smoking is associated with increased risk of miscarriage, low birth weight, and infant death; in large amounts, caffeine also increases the risk of miscarriage. Getting drunk just one time during pregnancy may be enough to cause brain damage in a fetus. A high level of alcohol consumption during pregnancy is associated with miscarriages, stillbirths, and, in live babies, **fetal alcohol syndrome (FAS).** A baby born with FAS is likely to suffer from a small head and body size, unusual facial characteristics, congenital heart defects, joint problems, mental impairment, and abnormal behavior patterns. During pregnancy, total abstinence from psychoactive drugs is recommended to help ensure the health of the fetus. Prescription and nonprescription drugs, including vitamins, can also harm the fetus and should be used only under medical supervision.

Infections, including those that are sexually transmitted, are another serious problem for the fetus if contracted either before or during birth. Rubella, syphilis, gonorrhea, hepatitis B, Group B streptococcus, herpes simplex, and HIV are among the most dangerous infections for the fetus. Treatment of the mother or immunization of the baby just after birth can help prevent problems from many infections. Women at risk for HIV infection should be tested before or during pregnancy because early treatment can dramatically reduce the chance that the virus will be passed to the fetus.

Prenatal Activity and Exercise   Physical activity during pregnancy contributes to mental and physical wellness. Women can continue working at their jobs until late in their pregnancy, provided the work isn't so physically demanding that it jeopardizes their health. At the same time, pregnant women need more rest and sleep to maintain their own well-being and that of the fetus.

A moderate exercise program during pregnancy does not adversely affect pregnancy or birth; in fact, regular exercise appears to improve a woman's chance of an on-time delivery. The amniotic sac protects the fetus, and normal activities will not harm it. A woman who exercised before becoming pregnant can often continue her program, with appropriate modifications to maintain her comfort and safety. A pregnant woman who hasn't been exercising and wants to start should first consult a physician. Regular cardiorespiratory endurance exercise is recommended. Walking, swimming, and stationary cycling are all good choices; more strenuous activities that could result in a fall, such as skiing, skating, or horseback riding, are best delayed until after the birth. Recommendations for exercising safely during pregnancy include the following:

- Exercise regularly (at least three times a week) rather than intermittently.

- After 20 weeks of pregnancy, avoid exercise that requires lying on your back. Research indicates that this position restricts blood flow to the uterus. Also avoid prolonged periods of motionless standing.

- Modify the intensity of your exercise according to how you feel. Stop exercising if you feel fatigued, and don't exercise to exhaustion. You may find that non-weight-bearing exercises such as swimming and cycling are more comfortable than weight-bearing activities in the later months of pregnancy; they also minimize the risk of injury.

- Avoid any type of exercise that has the potential for even mild abdominal trauma, and take care when performing any activity in which balance is important or in which losing balance would be dangerous. Pregnancy shifts your center of gravity.

- Avoid heat stress, particularly during the first trimester, by drinking an adequate amount of fluid, wearing appropriate clothing, and avoiding activity in hot and humid weather.

- Resume prepregnancy exercise routines gradually. Many of the changes of pregnancy persist for 4–6 weeks after delivery.

- If you experience any unusual symptoms, stop exercising and consult your physician. Warning signs include pain, vaginal bleeding, dizziness, rapid heartbeat, shortness of breath, and uterine contractions.

Kegel exercises, to strengthen the pelvic floor muscles, are also recommended for pregnant women. These exercises are performed by alternately contracting and releasing the muscles used to stop the flow of urine. Each contraction should be held for about 5 seconds. Kegel exercises should be done several times a day, for a total of about 50 repetitions daily.

Preparing for Birth   Childbirth classes are almost a routine part of the prenatal experience for both mothers and fathers these days. These classes typically teach the details of the birth process as well as relaxation techniques to help deal with the discomfort of labor and delivery. The mother learns and practices a variety of techniques so she will be able to choose what works best for her during labor, when the time comes. The father typically acts as a coach, supporting his partner emotionally and helping her with her breathing and relaxing. He remains with her throughout labor and delivery, even when a cesarean section is performed. It can be an important and fulfilling time for the parents to be together.

Complications of Pregnancy and Pregnancy Loss

Pregnancy usually proceeds without major complications. Sometimes, however, complications may prevent full-term development of the fetus or affect the health of the infant at birth. As discussed earlier in the chapter, exposure to harmful substances, such as alcohol or drugs, can harm the fetus. Other complications are caused by physiological problems or genetic abnormalities.

Ectopic Pregnancy   In an **ectopic pregnancy,** the fertilized egg implants and begins to develop outside the uterus, usually in an oviduct. Ectopic pregnancies usually occur because the fallopian tube is blocked, most often as a result of pelvic inflammatory disease. The embryo may

teratogen An agent or influence that causes physical defects in a developing embryo.

congenital malformation A physical defect existing at the time of birth, either inherited or caused during gestation.

fetal alcohol syndrome (FAS) A combination of birth defects caused by excessive alcohol consumption by the mother during pregnancy.

ectopic pregnancy A pregnancy in which the embryo develops outside the uterus, usually in the fallopian tube.

Terms

spontaneously abort, or the embryo and placenta may continue to expand until they rupture the oviduct. Sharp pain on one side of the abdomen or in the lower back, usually in about the 7th or 8th week, may signal an ectopic pregnancy, and there may be irregular bleeding. If bleeding from a rupture is severe, the woman may go into shock, characterized by low blood pressure, a fast pulse, weakness, and fainting. Surgical removal of the embryo and the oviduct may be necessary to save the mother's life, although microsurgery can sometimes be used to repair the damaged oviduct. The incidence of ectopic pregnancy has more than quadrupled in the last 25 years, and it is the leading cause of pregnancy-related death in the United States.

Spontaneous Abortion   A **spontaneous abortion,** or **miscarriage,** is the termination of pregnancy before the 20th week. It is estimated that 10–40% of pregnancies end this way, some without the woman's awareness that she was even pregnant. Most miscarriages occur between the 6th and 8th weeks of pregnancy, and most—about 60%—are due to chromosomal abnormalities in the fetus. Certain occupations that involve exposure to chemicals may increase the likelihood of miscarriages.

Preeclampsia   A disease unique to human pregnancy, **preeclampsia** is characterized by high blood pressure, leaking of protein into urine, and edema (fluid retention), which typically causes swelling of the hands and face. Symptoms may include sudden weight gain, severe headache, abdominal pain, blurred vision, and swelling.

If preeclampsia is not treated, it can cause seizures, a condition called **eclampsia.** Other potential problems from preeclampsia include liver and kidney damage, internal bleeding, poor fetal growth, and fetal death. Women with mild preeclampsia may be monitored and advised to rest in bed at home. Because more severe cases can be life-threatening, patients may be hospitalized for close monitoring and treatment to prevent seizures.

Low Birth Weight   A **low-birth-weight (LBW)** baby is one that weighs less than 5.5 pounds at birth. LBW babies may be premature (born before the 37th week of pregnancy) or full-term. Babies who are born small even though they're full-term are referred to as small-for-date babies. Most LBW babies will grow normally, but some will experience problems. Although they are at greater risk than bigger babies for complications during infancy, small-for-date babies tend to have fewer problems than premature infants.

The most fundamental problem of prematurity is that many of the infant's organs are not sufficiently developed. Even mild prematurity increases an infant's risk of dying in the first month or year of life. Premature infants are subject to respiratory problems and infections. They may have difficulty eating because they may be too small to suck a breast or bottle, and their swallowing mechanism may be underdeveloped. As they get older, premature infants may have problems such as learning difficulties, poor hearing and vision, and physical awkwardness. Adequate prenatal care is the best means of preventing LBW.

Infant Mortality   The U.S. rate of infant mortality, the death of a child of less than 1 year of age, is at its lowest point ever; however, it remains far higher than that of most of the developed world.

Causes of infant death are congenital problems, infectious diseases, and injuries. In the United States, about 2800 infant deaths per years are due to **sudden infant death syndrome (SIDS),** in which an apparently healthy infant dies suddenly while sleeping. The number of SIDS deaths has decreased since 1992, when the "Back to Sleep" campaign was instituted to make people aware that putting babies to bed on their backs rather than on their stomachs significantly reduces the risk of SIDS. Other risk factors for SIDS include abnormalities in heart rhythm or in brain receptors controlling breathing; exposing a fetus or infant to tobacco smoke, alcohol, or other drugs; and putting a baby to bed on a soft mattress or with fluffy bedding, pillows, or stuffed toys. Overbundling a baby or keeping a baby's room too warm also increases the risk of SIDS.

CHILDBIRTH

By the end of the ninth month of pregnancy, most women are tired of being pregnant; both parents are eager to start a new phase of their lives. Most couples find the actual process of birth to be an exciting and positive experience.

Terms

spontaneous abortion (miscarriage) Termination of pregnancy at less than 20 weeks' gestation when the uterine contents are expelled; causes include an abnormal uterus, insufficient hormones, and genetic or physical fetal defects.

preeclampsia A condition of pregnancy characterized by high blood pressure, edema, and protein in the urine.

eclampsia A severe, potentially life-threatening form of preeclampsia, characterized by convulsions and coma.

low birth weight (LBW) Weighing less than 5.5 lb at birth, often the result of prematurity.

sudden infant death syndrome (SIDS) The sudden death of an apparently healthy infant during sleep.

electronic fetal monitoring (EFM) The use of an external or internal electronic monitor during labor to measure uterine contractions and fetal heart rate.

episiotomy An incision made to widen the vaginal opening to facilitate childbirth and prevent uncontrolled tearing during delivery.

rooming-in The practice of allowing the mother and baby to remain together in the hospital or birth center after delivery.

labor The act or process of giving birth to a child, expelling it with the placenta from the mother's body by means of uterine contractions.

contraction Shortening of the muscles in the uterine wall, which causes effacement and dilation of the cervix and assists in expelling the fetus.

A variety of birth situations can have positive physical and psychological outcomes. Parents should discuss their preferences in the following areas with their physician or midwife:

1. Who will be present at the birth? The father? Friends? Children and other relatives? Will young siblings be allowed to visit the mother and new baby?

2. What type of room will the mother be in during labor, delivery, and recovery? How many times will she be moved?

3. What type of tables, beds, or birthing chairs are available? What type of environment can be created for the birth? Can specific music be played?

4. Will the mother receive any routine preparation, such as an enema or intravenous feeding?

5. What is the policy regarding food and drink during labor? Will the mother have the option of walking around or taking a shower or bath during labor?

6. Under what circumstances does the physician or midwife administer drugs to induce or augment labor? The use of these drugs tends to change the course of labor and carries a small risk.

7. Is **electronic fetal monitoring (EFM)** typically used during labor? About 75% of all births are electronically monitored, but there is disagreement among medical authorities about the risks or benefits of EFM. The American College of Obstetricians and Gynecologists recommends periodic monitoring using a stethoscope rather than EFM for low-risk pregnancies.

8. Under what circumstances will an **episiotomy,** an incision at the base of the vaginal opening, be performed? Are any steps taken to avoid it?

9. Under what circumstances will forceps or vacuum extraction be used? In some cases of fetal distress, the use of forceps or vacuum extraction may be necessary to save the infant's life, but some authorities believe these techniques are overused.

10. What types of medications are typically used during labor and delivery? Different types of anesthetics, including short-acting narcotics, regional nerve blocks, and local anesthetics, may be available; each has different effects on the mother and the fetus.

11. Under what conditions or circumstances does the physician perform a cesarean section? If prospective parents are concerned, they should research the cesarean frequency rates of different physicians before they make their final choice.

12. Who will "catch" the baby as she or he is born? Who will cut the umbilical cord?

13. What will be done to the baby immediately after birth? What kinds of tests and procedures will be done on the baby, and when?

14. How often will the baby be brought to the mother while they remain in the hospital or birthing center? Can the baby stay in the mother's room rather than in the nursery? This practice is known as **rooming-in**.

15. How will the baby be fed—by breast or bottle? Will feeding be on a schedule or "on demand"? Is there someone with breastfeeding experience available to answer questions if necessary?

Choices in Childbirth

Many couples today can choose the type of practitioner and the environment they want for the birth of their child. A high-risk pregnancy is probably best handled by a specialist physician in a hospital with a nursery, but for low-risk births, many options are available.

Parents can choose to have their baby delivered by a physician (an obstetrician or family practitioner) or by a certified nurse-midwife (a registered nurse with special obstetrical training). Most babies in the United States are delivered in hospitals or in freestanding alternative birth centers; only about 2% of women choose to have their babies at home. Many hospitals have introduced alternative birth centers in response to criticisms of traditional hospital routines. Alternative birth centers provide a comfortable, emotionally supportive environment in close proximity to up-to-date medical equipment.

Labor and Delivery

The birth process occurs in three stages (Figure 5-6). **Labor** begins when hormonal changes in both the mother and the baby cause strong, rhythmic uterine **contractions** to begin. These contractions exert pressure on the cervix and cause the lengthwise muscles of the uterus to pull on the circular muscles around the cervix, causing effacement (thinning) and dilation (opening) of the cervix. The contractions also pressure the baby to descend into the mother's pelvis, if it hasn't already. The entire process of labor and delivery usually takes between 2 and 36 hours, depending on the size of the baby, the baby's position in the uterus, the size of the mother's pelvis, and other factors. The length of labor is generally shorter for second and subsequent births.

The First Stage of Labor   The first stage of labor averages 13 hours for a first birth, although there is a wide variation among women. It begins with cervical effacement and dila-

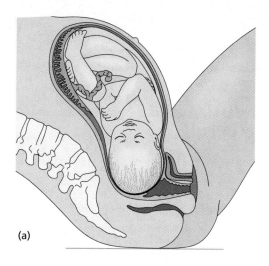

(a)

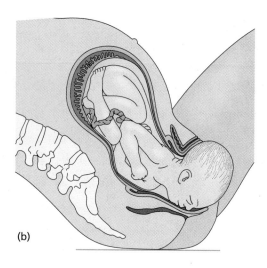

(b)

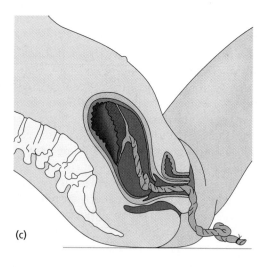

(c)

Figure 5-6 Birth: labor and delivery. (a) The first stage of labor; (b) the second stage of labor: delivery of the baby; (c) the third stage of labor: expulsion of the placenta.

tion and continues until the cervix is completely dilated (10 centimeters). Contractions usually last about 30 seconds and occur every 15–20 minutes at first, more often later. Early in the first stage, a small amount of bleeding may occur as a plug of slightly bloody mucus that blocked the opening of the cervix during pregnancy is expelled. In some women, the amniotic sac ruptures and the fluid rushes out; this is sometimes referred to as "breaking of the waters."

The last part of the first stage of labor, called **transition,** is characterized by strong and frequent contractions, much more intense than in the early stages of labor. Contractions may last 60–90 seconds and occur every 1–3 minutes. During transition the cervix opens completely, to a diameter of about 10 centimeters. Since the head of the fetus usually measures 9–10 centimeters, once the cervix has dilated completely, the head can pass through. Many women report that transition, which normally lasts about 30 minutes to an hour, is the most difficult part of labor.

The Second Stage of Labor   The second stage of labor begins with complete cervical dilation and ends with the delivery of the baby. The baby is slowly pushed down, through the bones of the pelvic ring, past the cervix, and into the vagina, which it stretches open. The mother bears down with the contractions to help push the baby down and out. Some women find this the most difficult part of labor, while others find that the contractions and bearing down bring a sense of euphoria. The baby's back bends, the head turns to fit through the narrowest parts of the passageway, and the soft bones of the baby's skull move together and overlap as it is squeezed through the pelvis. When the top of the head appears at the vaginal opening, the baby is said to be crowning.

As the head of the baby emerges, the physician or midwife will remove any mucus from the mouth and nose, wipe the baby's face, and check to ensure that the umbilical cord is not around the neck. As the baby is squeezed through the pelvis, cervix, and vagina, the fluid in the lungs is forced out by the pressure on the baby's chest. Once this pressure is released as the baby emerges from the vagina, the chest expands and the lungs fill with air for the first time. The baby will still be connected to the mother via the umbilical cord, which is not cut until it stops pulsating. The baby's head may be oddly shaped at first, due to the molding of the soft plates of bone during birth, but it usually takes on a normal appearance within 24 hours.

The Third Stage of Labor   In the third stage of labor, the uterus continues to contract until the placenta is expelled. This stage usually takes 5–20 minutes. If the placenta does not come out on its own, the physician or midwife may exert gentle pressure on the abdomen to help with its delivery. It is important that the entire placenta be expelled; if part remains in the uterus, it may

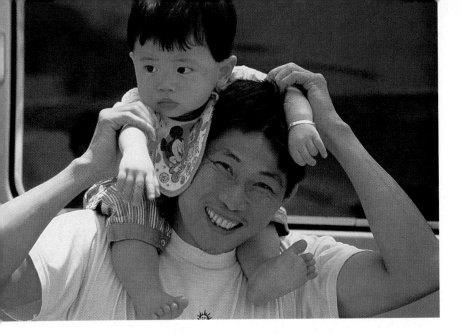

Having a child is one of the most important and rewarding experiences a person can undertake. Careful preparation can help maximize the benefits for both parents and children.

cause infection or bleeding. Breastfeeding soon after delivery helps control uterine bleeding because it stimulates the secretion of a hormone that makes the uterus contract; massaging the abdomen may also help.

In the meantime, the physical condition of the baby will be assessed with the **Apgar score,** a formalized system for assessing the baby's need for medical assistance during the first few minutes of life. Heart rate, respiration, color, reflexes, and muscle tone are individually rated with a score of 0–2, and a total score between 0 and 10 is given at 1 and 5 minutes after birth. A score of 7–10 at 5 minutes is considered normal. The baby is then usually wrapped tightly in a blanket and returned to the mother, who may begin to nurse the baby right away.

Cesarean Deliveries About 22% of the babies born in the United States are delivered by **cesarean section,** in which the baby is removed through a surgical incision in the abdominal wall and uterus. Cesarean sections are necessary when a baby cannot be delivered vaginally—for example, if the baby's head is bigger than the mother's pelvic girdle or if the baby is in an unusual position. If the mother has a serious health condition such as high blood pressure, a cesarean may be safer for her than labor and a vaginal delivery. Other reasons for cesarean delivery include abnormal or difficult labor, fetal distress, and the presence of a dangerous infection like herpes that can be passed to the baby during delivery. Repeat cesarean deliveries are also very common; about 75% of American women who have had one child by cesarean have subsequent children delivered the same way.

A cesarean section is major surgery and carries some risk, but it is relatively safe. A regional anesthetic may be used so the woman can remain conscious during the operation, and the father may be present.

The Postpartum Period

The **postpartum period,** a stage of about 3 months following childbirth, is a time of critical family adjustments. Parenthood—a job that goes on around the clock without relief—begins literally overnight, and the transition can cause considerable physical and emotional stress.

Currently, just over 60% of mothers breastfeed their infants, up from about 10% in 1970. **Lactation,** the production of milk, begins about 3 days after childbirth. Prior to that time (sometimes as early as the second trimester), colostrum is secreted by the nipples. Colostrum contains antibodies that help protect the newborn from infectious diseases and is also high in protein.

The American Academy of Pediatricians recommends breastfeeding for at least the first year of a baby's life and for as long after that as a mother and baby desire. Human milk is perfectly suited to the baby's nutritional needs and digestive capabilities, and it supplies the baby with anti-

transition The last part of the first stage of labor, during which the cervix becomes fully dilated; characterized by intense and frequent contractions.

Apgar score A formalized system for assessing a newborn's need for medical assistance.

cesarean section A surgical incision through the abdominal wall and uterus, performed to extract a fetus.

postpartum period The period of about 3 months after delivering a baby.

lactation The production of milk.

Terms

bodies. Breastfeeding decreases the incidence of infant ear infections, allergies, anemia, diarrhea, and bacterial meningitis. One study has even suggested that children who are breastfed do better in school and score higher on standardized tests. Breastfeeding is also beneficial to the mother: It stimulates contractions that help the uterus return to normal more rapidly, contributes to postpregnancy weight loss, and may reduce the risk of ovarian cancer, breast cancer, and postmenopausal hip fracture.

For some women, physical problems such as tenderness or infection of the nipples can make breastfeeding difficult. If a woman has an illness or requires drug treatment, she may have to bottlefeed her baby because drugs and infectious agents may show up in breast milk. Breastfeeding can be restrictive, making it especially difficult for working mothers. Employers rarely provide nursing breaks, so bottlefeeding or the use of a breast pump (to express milk for use while the mother is away from her infant) may be the only practical alternatives. Bottlefeeding makes it easier to tell how much milk an infant is taking in, and bottlefed infants tend to sleep longer. Bottlefeeding also allows the father or other caregiver to share in the nurturing process. Both breastfeeding and bottlefeeding can be part of loving, secure parent-child relationships.

Many women experience fluctuating emotions during the postpartum period as hormone levels change. The physical stress of labor, as well as dehydration, blood loss, and other physical factors, contribute to lowering the woman's stamina. About 50–80% of new mothers experience "baby blues," characterized by episodes of sadness, weeping, anxiety, headache, sleep disturbances, and irritability. A mother may feel lonely and anxious about caring for her infant. About 10% of new mothers experience **postpartum depression,** a more disabling syndrome characterized by despondency, mood swings, guilt, and occasional hostility. Rest, sharing feelings with others, and relying on relatives and friends for assistance are usually helpful in dealing with mild cases of postpartum depression, which generally lasts only a few weeks. If the depression is serious, professional treatment may be needed.

Another feature of the postpartum period is the development of attachment—the strong emotional tie that grows between the baby and the adult who cares for the baby. Parents can foster secure attachment relationships in the early months by responding sensitively to the baby's needs. Parents who respond appropriately to the baby's signals of gazing, looking away, smiling, and crying establish feelings of trust in their child. They feed the baby when she's hungry, for example; respond when she cries; interact with her when she gazes, smiles, or babbles; and stop stimulating her when she frowns or looks away. A se-

cure attachment relationship helps the child develop and function well socially, emotionally, and mentally.

For most people, the arrival of a child is one of life's most important events, providing a deep sense of joy and accomplishment. However, adjusting to parenthood requires effort and energy. Talking with friends and relatives about their experiences during the first few weeks or months with a baby can help prepare new parents for the period when the baby's needs may require all the energy that both parents have to expend. But the pleasures of nurturing a new baby are substantial, and many parents look back on this time as one of the most significant and joyful of their lives.

Tips for Today

Wellness includes understanding and enjoying your own sexuality. This means understanding your sexual anatomy, physiology, and functioning; your sexual orientation; and the various ways of expressing your sexuality and of interacting sexually with others. Preparation for being a parent begins long before pregnancy; it includes healthy lifestyle choices in all areas of wellness.

Right now you can

- Take a few moments to reflect on and articulate to yourself exactly what your beliefs are about sexual relationships at this point in your life. Consider your values, emotions, plans, and resources; also consider whether you are acting in accordance with your beliefs.

- If you are in a sexual relationship, ask yourself whether you are acting responsibly and in the best interest of yourself and your partner 100% of the time. For example, do you always respect each other's wishes and limits when it comes to sexual activity? Do you always avoid mixing sex and alcohol or drugs? If the answer to these or any similar questions is no, resolve to change that behavior.

- Take some time to think about whether *you* want to have children; try to cut through the cultural, societal, family, and personal expectations that may stand in the way of your making the decision you really want to make.

- Think of one thing your mother or father did as a parent that you particularly disliked; if you become a parent, how can you keep from repeating that behavior with your own children?

- Think of one thing your mother or father did as a parent that you particularly liked; if you become a parent, how can you make sure you do the same thing with your own children?

Terms   **postpartum depression** An emotional low that may be experienced by the mother following childbirth.

SUMMARY

- The female external sex organs are called the vulva; the clitoris plays an important role in sexual arousal and orgasm. The vagina leads to the internal sex organs, including the uterus, oviducts, and ovaries.

- The male external sex organs are the penis and the scrotum; the glans of the penis is an important site of sexual arousal. Internal sexual structures include the testes, vasa deferentia, seminal vesicles, and prostate gland.

- The menstrual cycle consists of four phases: menses, the estrogenic phase, ovulation, and the progestational phase.

- The ovaries gradually cease to function as women approach age 50 and enter menopause. The pattern of male sexual responses changes with age, and testosterone production gradually decreases.

- The sexual response cycle has four stages: excitement, plateau, orgasm, and resolution.

- Physical and psychological problems can both interfere with sexual functioning. A treatment for sexual dysfunction first addresses any underlying medical conditions and then looks at psychosocial problems.

- Human sexual behaviors include celibacy, erotic fantasy, masturbation, touching, cunnilingus, fellatio, anal intercourse, and coitus.

- Responsible sexuality includes open, honest communication; agreed-on sexual activities; sexual privacy; using contraception; safer sex practices; sober sex; and taking responsibility for consequences.

- Fertilization is a complex process culminating when a sperm penetrates the membrane of the egg released from the woman's ovary. Infertility affects about 10% of the reproductive-age population of the United States.

- During pregnancy, the uterus enlarges until it pushes up into the rib cage; the breasts enlarge and may secrete colostrum; the muscles and ligaments soften and stretch; and the circulatory system, lungs, and kidneys become more efficient.

- The fetal anatomy is almost completely formed in the first trimester and is refined in the second; during the third trimester, the fetus grows and gains most of its weight, storing nutrients in fatty tissues.

- Information about the health and sex of a fetus can be obtained through prenatal tests such as ultrasound, amniocentesis, chorionic villus sampling, and triple marker screening.

- Important elements of prenatal care include regular checkups; good nutrition; avoiding drugs, alcohol, tobacco, infections, and other harmful environmental agents or conditions; regular physical activity; and childbirth classes.

- Pregnancy usually proceeds without major complications. Problems that can occur include ectopic pregnancy, spontaneous abortion, preeclampsia, and low birth weight.

- The first stage of labor begins with contractions that exert pressure on the cervix, causing effacement and dilation. The second stage begins with complete cervical dilation and ends when the baby emerges. The third stage of labor is expulsion of the placenta.

- During the postpartum period, the mother's body begins to return to its prepregnancy state, and she may begin to breastfeed. Both mother and father must adjust to their new roles as parents.

TAKE ACTION

1. Many reputable self-help books about sexual functioning are available in libraries and bookstores. If you're not satisfied with your level of knowledge and understanding, consider consulting some other sources.

2. Interview your parents to find out what your birth was like. What were the cultural conditions like at the time, and what were their personal preferences? Find out as much as you can about hospital procedure, the use of anesthetics, length of hospital stay, and so on. Did your father have a role in your birth? If possible, interview your grandparents or someone of their generation. How was their experience different from that of your parents?

JOURNAL ENTRY

1. *Critical Thinking* Consider one or two of your favorite television shows or movies. How are sexuality and sexual behavior presented? How many sexual references occur? What types of sexual behaviors are shown or alluded to? What impression would a viewer have about the typical sexual behaviors of the characters? Are any of the potential emotional or physical consequences of sexual behavior shown?

Write a short essay outlining your findings, and state whether you think the depiction of sexuality is accurate. In your opinion, can the presentation of sexuality in the programs or movies you chose influence the behavior of viewers? Explain your reasoning.

2. Sexual myths and misconceptions are common in our culture. In your health journal, make a list of statements about sexuality that you've heard but are not sure are accurate. Find out the facts by consulting books and pamphlets mentioned here or available through your school health center or library.

3. Do you think you are ready to become a parent? Make a list of the qualities you possess that you think would make you a good parent. Then list those qualities that might be a hindrance to good parenting. Do you think your partner (if you have one) is ready to become a parent? Create the same type of lists based on his or her personal qualities.

FOR MORE INFORMATION

Books

American College of Obstetricians and Gynecologists. 2000. *Planning Your Pregnancy and Birth*, 3rd ed. Washington, D.C.: ACOG. *An excellent guide to conception, pregnancy, and birth.*

Ammer, C. 2000. *The New A to Z of Women's Health: A Concise Encyclopedia.* New York: Facts on File. *Topics include the reproductive system, sexuality, STDs, and contraception.*

Dalton, K., and W. Holton. 2000. *Once a Month: Understanding and Treating PMS*, 6th ed. Alameda, Calif.: Hunter House. *An up-to-date discussion of symptoms and self-help strategies for PMS.*

Men's Health Books. 2000. *The Complete Book of Men's Health.* Emmaus, Penn.: Rodale. *A comprehensive guide to a healthy lifestyle, including information on communication and sexuality.*

Strong, B., et al. 2002. *Human Sexuality: Diversity in Contemporary America*, 4th ed. New York: McGraw-Hill. *A comprehensive introduction to human sexuality.*

WWW. Organizations and Web Sites

American College of Obstetricians and Gynecologists (ACOG). Provides written materials relating to many aspects of preconception care, pregnancy, and childbirth.
202-863-2518
http://www.acog.org

The American Society for Reproductive Medicine. Provides up-to-date information on all aspects of infertility.
205-978-5000
http://www.asrm.org

Dr. Drew. Provides answers to frequently asked questions about sexuality and relationships, geared toward young adults.
http://www.drDrew.com

Generational Health. Helps you create a family health tree online and provides information about detection and screening for any conditions that are common in your family history.
http://healthygenerations.com

La Leche League International. Provides advice and support for breastfeeding mothers.
800-LaLeche
http://www.lalecheleague.org

Male Health Center. A commercial site that provides a variety of information on male sexual health topics.
http://www.malehealthcenter.com

The March of Dimes. Provides public education materials on many pregnancy-related topics, including preconception care, genetic screening, diet and exercise, and the effects of smoking and drinking during pregnancy.
888-MODIMES; 914-428-7100
http://www.modimes.org

National Institute of Child Health and Human Development. Provides information about reproductive and genetic problems; sponsors the "Back to Sleep" campaign to fight SIDS.
800-505-CRIB (Back to Sleep hotline)
http://www.nichd.nih.gov

National Maternal and Child Health Clearinghouse. Distributes publications, posters, and videos relating to maternal, infant, and family health; most items are available free-of-charge.
888-434-4MCH; 703-356-1964
http://www.nmchc.org

New York University Sexual Disorders Screening. Provides interactive online screening tests for common sexual disorders.
http://www.med.nyu.edu/Psych/screens/sdsm.html (men)
http://www.med.nyu.edu/Psych/screens/sdsf.html (women)

ParentsPlace.com Pregnancy Department. Includes a pregnancy calendar, a due date calculator, and lots of advice on preparing a birth plan and other pregnancy topics.
http://www.parentsplace.com/pregnancy

PMS Access/Women's Health America Group. Provides information about PMS and links to other sites dealing with PMS and women's health issues.
800-222-4767; 800-558-7046
http://www.womenshealth.com

San Jose Marital and Sexuality Centre. Provides articles on issues relating to cybersex and an online sexual compulsion assessment.
http://www.sex-centre.com

Sexuality Information and Education Council of the United States (SIECUS). Provides information on many aspects of sexuality and has an extensive library and numerous publications.
http://www.siecus.org

The following sites include information, graphics, and video clips of fetal development:

Nova/Odyssey of Life
http://www.pbs.org/wgbh/nova/odyssey/clips
University of Pennsylvania Basic Embryology Review
http://www.med.upenn.edu/meded/public/berp
Visible Embryo
http://visembryo.com

See also the listings for Chapters 4, 6, and 13.

Adler, R., M. S. Ottaway, and S. Gould. 2001. Circumcision: We have heard from the experts; now let's hear from the parents. *Pediatrics* 107(2): E20.

American Academy of Pediatrics. 2000. *Circumcision: Information for Parents* (http://www.aap.org/family/circ.htm; retrieved September 5, 2000).

American Academy of Pediatrics Task Force on Circumcision. 1999. Circumcision. Policy Statement. *Pediatrics* 103(3): 686–693.

American College of Obstetricians and Gynecologists. 2000. *HIV Tests Urged for All Pregnant Women* (http://www.acog.org/from_home/publications/press_releases/nr05-23-00-2.htm; retrieved September 27, 2000).

American College of Obstetricians and Gynecologists. 2000. *Premenstrual Syndrome*. Washington, D.C.: American College of Obstetricians and Gynecologists.

Baeten, J. M., E. A. Bukusi, and M. Lambe. 2001. Pregnancy complications and outcomes among overweight and obese nulliparous women. *American Journal of Public Health* 91(3): 436–440.

Breastfeeding. 2001. *Journal of the American Medical Association* 285(4): 490.

Campbell, M. K., and M. F. Mottola. 2001. Recreational exercise and occupational activity during pregnancy and birth weight: A case-control study. *American Journal of Obstetrics and Gynecology* 184(3): 403–408.

Centers for Disease Control and Prevention. 2000. Alcohol policy and sexually transmitted disease rates—United States, 1981–1995. *Morbidity and Mortality Weekly Report* 49(16): 346–349.

Centers for Disease Control and Prevention. 2000. Entry into prenatal care—United States, 1989–1997. *Morbidity and Mortality Weekly Report* 49(18): 393–398.

Centers for Disease Control and Prevention, Division of Birth Defects and Developmental Disabilities. 2000. *Preventing Neural Tube Birth Defects: A Prevention Model and Resource Guide*. Atlanta, Ga.: CDC.

Centers for Disease Control and Prevention. 2001. Knowledge and use of folic acid among women of reproductive age. *Morbidity and Mortality Weekly Report* 50(10): 185–189.

Feeding your newborn. 2000. *Journal of the American Medical Association Patient Page* 283(9).

Food and Drug Administration. 2000. *FDA Approves Fluoxetine to Treat Premenstrual Dysphoric Disorder* (http://www.fda.gov/bbs/topics/ANSWERS/ANS01024.html; retrieved September 9, 2000).

Goldstein, I. 2000. Male sexual circuitry. *Scientific American* 283(2): 70–75.

Ikonomidou, C., et al. 2000. Ethanol-induced apoptotic neurodegeneration and fetal alcohol syndrome. *Science* 287(5455): 1056–1060.

Joint United Nations Programme on HIV/AIDS (UNAIDS). 2000. Male circumcision and HIV infection. *Report on the Global HIV/AIDS Epidemic—June 2000* (http://www.unaids.org/epidemic_update/report/Epi_report_chap_prevention.htm; retrieved September 5, 2000).

Klebanoff, M. A., et al. 1999. Maternal serum paraxanthine, a caffeine metabolite, and the risk of spontaneous abortion. *New England Journal of Medicine* 341(22): 1639–1644.

Kraemer, G. R., and R. R. Kraemer. 1998. Premenstrual syndrome: Diagnosis and treatment experiences. *Journal of Women's Health* 7(7): 893–907.

Kramer, M. S., et al. 2000. The contribution of mild and moderate preterm birth to infant mortality. *Journal of the American Medical Association* 284(7): 843–849.

Laumann, E. O., A. Paik, and R. C. Rosen. 1999. Sexual dysfunction in the United States: Prevalence and predictors. *Journal of the American Medical Association* 281: 537–544.

Leiblum, S. R. 2001. Critical overview of the new consensus-based definitions and classification of female sexual dysfunction. *Journal of Sex and Marital Therapy* 27(2): 159–67.

March of Dimes. 1999. *Food-borne Risks in Pregnancy* (http://www.modimes.org/HealthLibrary2/FactSheets/Food_Born_Risks.htm; retrieved September 25, 2000).

National Center for Health Statistics. 2000. Births: Preliminary data for 1999. *National Vital Statistics Reports* 48(14).

National Council on Aging. 1998. *Half of Older Americans Report They Are Sexually Active; 4 in 10 Want More Sex, Says New Survey* (http://www.ncoa.org/press/sexsurvey.htm; retrieved September 28, 1998).

Newman, R. B., et al. 2001. Occupational fatigue and preterm premature rupture of membranes. *American Journal of Obstetrics and Gynecology* 184(3): 438–446.

Nielsen, G. L., et al. 2001. Risk of adverse birth outcome and miscarriage in pregnant users of non-steroidal anti-inflammatory drugs. *British Medical Journal* 322: 266–270.

North American Menopause Society. 1998. *Menopause Is the Beginning of a New, Fulfilling Stage of Life* (http://www.menopause.org/news.htm#anchor10312017; retrieved October 26, 1998).

Paz Galupo, M., and S. St. John. 2001. Benefits of cross-sexual orientation friendships among adolescent females. *Journal of Adolescence* 24(1): 83–93.

Schrag, S. J., et al. 2000. Group B streptococcal disease in the era of intrapartum antibiotic prophylaxis. *New England Journal of Medicine* 342: 15–20.

Silence about sexual problems can hurt relationships. 1999. *Journal of the American Medical Association* 281:210.

Steinberg, S., et al. 1999. A placebo-controlled clinical trial of L-tryptophan in premenstrual dysphoria. *Biological Psychiatry* 45(3): 313–320.

Strong, B., et al. 2002. *Human Sexuality: Diversity in Contemporary America*, 4th ed. New York: McGraw-Hill.

Thys-Jacobs, S., et al. 1998. Calcium carbonate and the premenstrual syndrome: Effects on premenstrual and menstrual symptoms. Premenstrual Syndrome Study Group. *American Journal of Obstetrics and Gynecology* 179(2): 444–452.

Wisborg, K., et al. 2000. A prospective study of smoking during pregnancy and SIDS. *Archives of Disease in Childhood* 83(3): 203–206.

Contraception and Abortion

In her lifetime, the ovaries of an average woman release over 400 eggs, one a month for about 35 years. Each egg is capable of developing into a human embryo if fertilized by one of the millions of sperm a man produces in every ejaculate. Furthermore, unlike most other mammals, humans are capable of sexual activity at any time of the month or year. These facts help explain why people have always had a compelling interest in controlling fertility and in preventing unwanted pregnancies.

Today, people have many options when it comes to making decisions about their sexual and **contraceptive** behavior. In addition to the primary purpose of preventing pregnancy, many types of contraception play an important role in protecting against **sexually transmitted diseases (STDs).** Being informed about the realities and risks and making responsible decisions about sexual and contraceptive behavior are crucial components of lifelong wellness. Among the most important choices of your life will be deciding what type of sexual involvement is best

for you; equally critical is the commitment to always protect yourself against unwanted pregnancy and STDs.

 ## PRINCIPLES OF CONTRACEPTION

The underlying principle of contraceptives used today is to block the female's egg from uniting with the male's sperm (conception), thereby preventing pregnancy. A variety of effective approaches in preventing conception are based on different principles of birth control. *Barrier methods* work by physically blocking the sperm from reaching the egg. Diaphragms, condoms, and several other methods are based on this principle. *Hormonal methods,* such as oral contraceptives (birth control pills), alter the biochemistry of the woman's body, preventing ovulation (the release of the egg) and producing changes that make it more difficult for the sperm to reach the egg if ovulation does occur. So-called *natural methods* of contraception are based on the fact that egg and sperm have to be present at the same time if fertilization is to occur. Finally, *surgical methods*—female and male sterilization—more or less permanently prevent transport of the sperm or eggs to the site of conception.

All contraceptive methods have advantages and disadvantages that make them appropriate for some people but not for others or the best choice at one period of life but not at another. Factors that affect the choice of method include effectiveness, convenience, cost, reversibility, side effects and risks, and protection against STDs. Later in this chapter, we help you sort through these factors to decide on the method that's best for you.

Contraceptive effectiveness is partly determined by the reliability of the method itself—the failure rate if it were always used exactly as directed ("perfect use"). Effectiveness is also determined by characteristics of the user, including fertility of the individual, frequency of intercourse, and, more important, how consistently and correctly the method is used. This "typical use" **contraceptive failure rate** is based on studies that directly measure the percentage of women experiencing an unintended pregnancy. For example, the 5% failure rate of oral contraceptives means 5 out of 100 typical users will become pregnant in the first year. This failure rate is likely to be lower for women who are consistently careful in following instructions and higher for those who are frequently careless.

Another measure of effectiveness is the **continuation rate**—the percentage of people who continue to use the method after a specified period of time. This measure is important because many unintended pregnancies occur when a method is stopped and not immediately replaced with another. Thus, a contraceptive with a high continuation rate would be more effective at preventing pregnancy than one with a low continuation rate.

REVERSIBLE CONTRACEPTIVES

Reversibility is an important consideration for young adults when they choose a contraceptive method, because most people either plan to have children or at least want to keep their options open until they're older. In this section we discuss the reversible contraceptives, beginning with the hormonal methods, then moving to the barrier methods, and finally covering the natural methods.

WW Oral Contraceptives: The Pill

During pregnancy, the corpus luteum secretes progesterone and estrogen in amounts high enough to suppress ovulation. **Oral contraceptives (OCs),** or birth control pills, prevent ovulation by mimicking the hormonal activity of the corpus luteum. The active ingredients in OCs

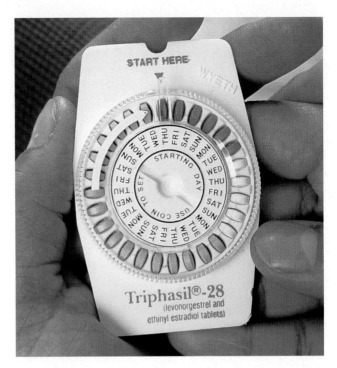

Oral contraceptives are the most popular reversible method of contraception among American women. When used correctly, oral contraceptives are highly effective.

are estrogen and progestins, laboratory-made compounds that are closely related to progesterone.

In addition to preventing ovulation, the birth control pill has other backup contraceptive effects. It inhibits the movement of sperm by thickening the cervical mucus, alters the rate of ovum transport by means of its hormonal effects on the oviducts, and may prevent implantation by changing the lining of the uterus, in the unlikely event that a fertilized ovum reaches that area.

The most common type of OC is the combination pill. Each 1-month packet contains 3 weeks of pills that combine varying types and amounts of estrogen and progestin.

Terms

contraceptive Any agent that can prevent conception; condoms, diaphragms, intrauterine devices, and oral contraceptives are examples.

sexually transmitted disease (STD) Any of several contagious diseases contracted through intimate sexual contact.

contraceptive failure rate The percentage of women using a particular contraceptive method who experience an unintended pregnancy in the first year of use.

continuation rate The percentage of women who continue to use a particular contraceptive after a specified period of time.

oral contraceptive (OC) Any of various hormone compounds (estrogen and progestins) in pill form that prevent conception by preventing ovulation.

Most packets also include a 1-week supply of inactive pills to be taken following the hormone pills; others instruct the woman to simply take no pills at all for 1 week before starting the next cycle. During the week in which no hormones are taken, a light menstrual period occurs.

A second, much less common, type of OC is the minipill, a small dose of a synthetic progesterone taken every day of the month. Because the minipill contains no estrogen, it has fewer side effects and health risks, but it also carries a higher risk of pregnancy and irregular bleeding.

A user must take each month's pills completely and according to instructions. Taking a few pills just prior to having sexual intercourse will not provide effective contraception. A backup method is recommended during the first week and any subsequent cycle in which the woman forgets to take any pills.

Advantages The main advantage of the oral contraceptive is its high degree of effectiveness in preventing pregnancy. Nearly all unplanned pregnancies result because the pills were not taken as directed. The pill is relatively simple to use and does not require any interruptions that could hinder sexual spontaneity. Most women also enjoy the predictable regularity of periods, as well as the decrease in cramps and blood loss. For young women, the reversibility of the pill is especially important; **fertility**—the ability to reproduce—returns after the pill is discontinued (although not always immediately). Medical advantages include a decreased incidence or severity of benign breast disease, iron-deficiency anemia, pelvic inflammatory disease (PID), ectopic pregnancy, endometrial cancer (of the lining of the uterus), and ovarian cancer.

Disadvantages Oral contraceptives do not protect against HIV infection or other STDs in the lower reproductive tract and have been associated with increased cervical chlamydia. Regular condom use is recommended for an OC user, unless she is in a long-term, mutually monogamous relationship with an uninfected partner.

OCs can cause a variety of minor side effects, including nausea, weight gain, and swollen breasts during the first few months of use. Other possible effects include depression, nervousness, migraine, and changes in vaginal discharge. Serious but uncommon side effects, including blood clots, stroke, and heart attack, have been reported in a small number of users, mostly older women who smoke or have a history of circulatory disease. OC users may be slightly more prone to high blood pressure, blood

clots in the legs and arms, and benign liver tumors. Most adverse effects of OCs disappear after pill use is discontinued, and studies show no long-term effect on mortality.

Birth control pills are not recommended for women with a history of blood clots, heart disease or stroke, any form of cancer or liver tumor, or impaired liver function. Women with certain other health conditions or behaviors, including migraines, high blood pressure, cigarette smoking, and sickle-cell disease, require close monitoring.

In trying to decide whether to use oral contraceptives, each woman needs to weigh the benefits against the risks with the help of a health care professional. A woman can take several steps to decrease her risk from OC use:

1. Request a low-dosage pill.
2. Stop smoking.
3. Follow the dosage carefully and consistently.
4. Be alert to preliminary danger signals, which can be remembered with the word ACHES:

   Abdominal pain (severe)

   Chest pain (severe), cough, shortness of breath or sharp pain on breathing in

   Headaches (severe), dizziness, weakness, or numbness, especially if one-sided

   Eye problems (vision loss or blurring) and/or speech problems

   Severe leg pain (calf or thigh)
5. Have regular checkups to monitor blood pressure, weight, and urine, and have an annual examination of the thyroid, breasts, abdomen, and pelvis.
6. Have regular **Pap tests** to check for early cervical changes. Because OC use may temporarily increase some women's susceptibility to the STDs chlamydia and gonorrhea, regular screening for those diseases is also recommended, especially when condoms aren't being used.

For most women, the known, directly associated risk of death from taking birth control pills is much lower than the risk of death from pregnancy (Table 6-1).

Effectiveness If taken exactly as directed, the failure rate of OCs is extremely low (0.1%). However, among average users, lapses such as forgetting to take a pill do occur, and a typical first-year failure rate of OCs is 5%. The continuation rate for OCs also varies; the average rate is 71% after 1 year.

Contraceptive Implants

Contraceptive implants are placed under the skin and deliver a small but steady dose of hormones over a period of several years. In 1990, the Norplant contraceptive implant became available in the United States. Norplant consists of six flexible, matchstick-sized capsules that contain

Terms **fertility** The ability to reproduce.

Pap test A scraping of cells from the cervix for examination under a microscope to detect cancer.

Table 6-1	Contraceptive Risks

Contraceptive Method	Risk of Death in Any Given Year
Oral contraceptives	
Nonsmoker	1 in 66,700
Age less than 35	1 in 200,000
Age 35–44	1 in 28,600
Heavy smoker (25 or more cigarettes/day)	1 in 1,700
Age less than 35	1 in 5,300
Age 35–44	1 in 700
IUDs	1 in 10,000,000
Barrier methods, spermicides	none
Fertility awareness methods, withdrawal	none
Sterilization	
Laparoscopic tubal ligation	1 in 38,500
Hysterectomy	1 in 1,600
Vasectomy	1 in 1,000,000
Legal abortion	
Before 9 weeks	1 in 262,800
9–12 weeks	1 in 100,100
13–15 weeks	1 in 34,400
After 15 weeks	1 in 10,200
Illegal abortion	1 in 3,000
Pregnancy and childbirth	1 in 10,000

SOURCES: Hatcher, R. A., et al. 1998. *Contraceptive Technology*, 17th rev. ed. New York: Ardent Media. Carlson, K. J., S. A. Eisenstat, and T. Ziporyn. 1996. *The Harvard Guide to Women's Health*. Cambridge, Mass.: Harvard University Press.

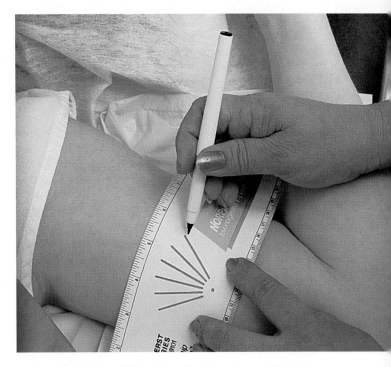

Contraceptive implants, filled with synthetic hormones and inserted under the skin on the arm or leg, can provide 5 years of protection against pregnancy.

progestin, a synthetic progesterone. The capsules are placed under the skin, usually on the inside of a woman's upper arm in a fan-shaped configuration. The procedure can be done in less than 15 minutes. The progestin in Norplant has several contraceptive effects: Hormonal shifts may inhibit ovulation and affect development of the uterine lining, thickening of cervical mucus inhibits the movement of sperm, and transport of the egg through the fallopian tubes may be slowed.

Other types of contraceptive implants are available in other countries and may soon be available in the United States; these include a single capsule device, Implanon, and the two-capsule Norplant 2. In studies, these implants have been easier to insert and remove than the six-capsule Norplant; Implanon comes preloaded in a dis-

posable applicator. Contraceptive implants are best suited for women who wish to have continuous and long-term protection against pregnancy.

Advantages Norplant implants are the most effective reversible method of contraception now available. After insertion of the implants, no further action is required for up to 5 years of protection; at the same time, contraceptive effects are quickly reversed upon removal. Because Norplant, unlike the combination pill, contains no estrogen, it carries a lower risk of certain side effects, such as blood clots and other cardiovascular complications. In addition, the progestin is released at a steady rate, in smaller quantities than are found in oral contraceptives. The thickened cervical mucus resulting from Norplant use has a protective effect against PID.

Disadvantages As with the pill, Norplant gives no protection against HIV infection and STDs in the lower reproductive tract. Although the implants are barely visible, their appearance may bother some women. The initial cost can be substantial (but protection is provided for 5 years). Only specially trained practitioners can insert or remove the implants, and removal is sometimes difficult. Lawsuits filed against the manufacturer of Norplant have focused on removal difficulties and inadequate warnings about side effects. A further problem with Norplant has been the discovery of certain product lots with low hormone levels and reduced effectiveness. To help address some of the problems with Norplant, the manufacturer offers a consumer information hotline (800-934-5556).

The most common side effects of contraceptive implants are menstrual irregularities, including longer menstrual periods, spotting between periods, or having no bleeding at all. Less common side effects include headaches, weight gain, breast tenderness, nausea, acne, and mood swings. Cautions and more serious health concerns are similar to those associated with oral contraceptives but are less common.

Effectiveness Typical failure rates are very low (0.05%) in the first year, increasing slowly with each additional year of use. The cumulative failure rate at the end of 5 years is about 3.7%; the continuation rate is about 88%.

Injectable Contraceptives

The first injectable contraceptive approved for use in the United States was Depo-Provera, which uses long-acting progestins. Injected in the arm or buttocks, Depo-Provera is usually given every 12 weeks, although it actually provides effective contraception for a few weeks beyond that. As another progestin-only contraceptive, it prevents pregnancy in the same ways as Norplant.

Lunelle, an injectable containing both estrogen and progestin, was approved for use in the United States in 2000. Lunelle injections are given every month rather than every 3 months as with Depo-Provera. Lunelle prevents pregnancy in the same way as OCs.

Advantages Injectable contraceptives are highly effective and require little action on the part of the user. Because the injections leave no trace and involve no ongoing supplies, injectables allow women almost total privacy in their decision to use contraception. Like Norplant, Depo-Provera has no estrogen-related side effects; it requires only periodic injections rather than the minor surgical procedures of implant insertion and removal. Lunelle, which does contain estrogen, has many of the same benefits as oral contraceptives and may be preferred by women who do not want to take a pill every day.

Disadvantages Injectable contraceptives provide no protection against HIV infection and STDs in the lower reproductive tract. A woman must visit a health care facility every month (Lunelle) or every 3 months (Depo-Provera) to receive the injections. The side effects of

Depo-Provera are similar to those of Norplant; menstrual irregularities are the most common, and after 1 year of using Depo-Provera, many women have no menstrual bleeding at all. Lunelle causes less menstrual irregularity than Depo-Provera. Weight gain is a common side effect of both Depo-Provera and Lunelle. After discontinuing the use of Depo-Provera, women may experience temporary infertility for up to 12 months. Reasons for not using Depo-Provera are similar to those for not using Norplant; contraindications for Lunelle are similar to those for OCs.

Effectiveness Typical failure rates with Depo-Provera are 0.3%; those reported for Lunelle are 0.2–0.4%. The 1-year continuation rate for Depo-Provera is 42%.

Emergency Contraception

Emergency contraception refers to postcoital methods— those used after unprotected sexual intercourse. An emergency contraceptive may be appropriate if a regularly used method has failed (for example, if a condom breaks) or if unprotected sex has occurred. Emergency contraceptives are designed only for emergency use and should not be relied on as a regular method.

The most frequently used emergency contraceptive is a two-dose regimen of certain combination oral contraceptives. In 1996, an FDA advisory panel concluded that six brands of OCs already available in the United States are safe and effective for emergency contraception, reducing the risk of pregnancy by 75%. Postcoital pills appear to act by inhibiting or delaying ovulation and altering the transport of sperm and/or eggs.

By 2000, two FDA-approved products specifically designed for emergency contraception were available in the United States—Preven, which contains both estrogen and progestin, and Plan B, which contains only progestin. These and other regimens for emergency contraception involve taking two doses of hormones 12 hours apart. The first dose must be taken within 72 hours after intercourse (the sooner, the better). The most common side effects are nausea, vomiting, and breast tenderness. Early indications are that Plan B may be more effective than Preven and cause less nausea and vomiting; if taken within 24 hours after intercourse, Plan B may prevent as many as 95% of expected pregnancies.

Other emergency contraceptives that are available or under study include mifepristone (also known as RU-486 or the "abortion pill") and intrauterine devices.

The Intrauterine Device (IUD)

The **intrauterine device (IUD)** is a small plastic device placed in the uterus as a contraceptive. IUD use has declined since the 1970s, mostly as a result of publicity about the increased risk of serious infections associated with the popular Dalkon Shield and its withdrawal

Terms   **intrauterine device (IUD)** A plastic device inserted into the uterus as a contraceptive.

      male condom A sheath, usually made of thin latex (synthetic rubber), that covers the penis during sexual intercourse; used for contraception and to prevent STDs.

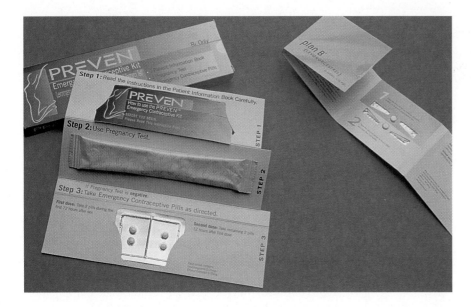

Emergency hormonal contraceptives reduce the risk of pregnancy by about 75% if taken within 72 hours of unprotected intercourse. The most commonly used regimens for emergency contraception involve taking two doses of hormones about 12 hours apart.

from the market. Three IUDs are now available in the United States: the hormone-releasing Progestasert, which requires replacement every year; the Copper T-380A (also known as the ParaGard), which gives protection for up to 10 years; and the Levonorgestral IUD (Mirena), approved in 2000, which releases small amounts of progestin and is effective for up to 5 years.

Researchers do not know exactly how IUDs prevent pregnancy. They may cause biochemical changes in the uterus and affect the movement of sperm and eggs; although less likely, they may also interfere with implantation of fertilized eggs. Progestasert and Mirena slowly release very small amounts of hormones, which impede fertilization or implantation.

Advantages   Intrauterine devices are highly reliable and are simple and convenient to use. They do not require the woman to anticipate or interrupt sexual activity. Usually IUDs have only localized side effects, and in the absence of complications, they are considered a fully reversible contraceptive.

Disadvantages   IUDs must be inserted and removed by a trained professional. Most side effects of IUD use are limited to the genital tract. Heavy menstrual flow and bleeding and spotting between periods may occur, although with Mirena, menstrual periods tend to become shorter and lighter over time. Another side effect is pain, particularly uterine cramps and backache, which seem to occur most often in women who have never been pregnant. Spontaneous expulsion of the IUD happens to 5–6% of women within the first year, most commonly during the first months after insertion.

A serious but rare complication of IUD use is pelvic inflammatory disease (PID). Most pelvic infections among IUD users are relatively mild and can be treated successfully with antibiotics. However, early and adequate treatment is critical, for a lingering infection can lead to tubal scarring and subsequent infertility.

Some physicians advise against the use of IUDs by young women who have never been pregnant because of the increased incidence of side effects in this group and the risk of infection with the possibility of subsequent infertility. Early IUD danger signals are abdominal pain, fever, chills, foul-smelling vaginal discharge, irregular menstrual periods, and other unusual vaginal bleeding. A change in string length should also be noted. An annual checkup is important for IUD users.

Effectiveness   The typical failure rate of IUDs during the first year of use is 1–2%. Effectiveness can be increased by periodically checking to see that the device is in place and by using a backup method for the first few months after IUD insertion. The continuation rate of IUDs is about 80% after 1 year of use.

Ww. Male Condoms

The **male condom** is a thin sheath designed to cover the penis during sexual intercourse. Most brands sold in the United States are made of latex, although condoms made of polyurethane are also now available. Condoms prevent sperm from entering the vagina and provide protection against disease. Condom sales have increased dramatically in recent years, primarily because they provide some protection against all STDs and are the only method that provides substantial protection against HIV infection. At least one-third of all male condoms are bought by women. Women are more likely to contract an STD from an infected partner than men are. Women also face additional

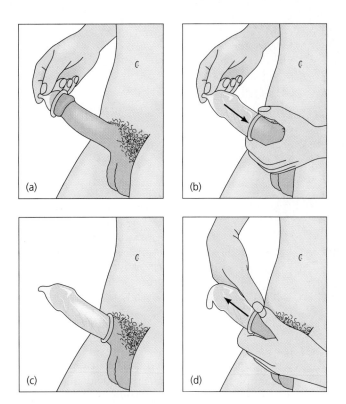

Figure 6-1 Use of the male condom. (a) Place the rolled-up condom over the head of the erect penis. Hold the top half-inch of the condom (with air squeezed out) to leave room for semen. (b) While holding the tip, unroll the condom onto the penis. Gently smooth out any air bubbles. (c) Unroll the condom down to the base of the penis. (d) To avoid spilling semen after ejaculation, hold the condom around the base of the penis as the penis is withdrawn. Remove the condom away from your partner, taking care not to spill any semen.

health risks from STDs, including cervical cancer, PID, ectopic pregnancy (which is potentially life-threatening), and infertility.

The man or his partner must put the condom on the penis before it is inserted into the vagina, because the small amounts of fluid that may be secreted unnoticed prior to **ejaculation** often contain sperm capable of causing pregnancy. The rolled-up condom is placed over the head of the erect penis and unrolled down to the base of the penis, leaving a half-inch space (without air) at the tip to collect semen (Figure 6-1). Some brands of condoms have a reservoir tip designed for this purpose. Uncircumcised men must first pull back the foreskin of the penis. Partners must be careful not to damage the condom with fingernails, rings, or other rough objects.

Terms

ejaculation An abrupt discharge of semen from the penis after sexual stimulation.

spermicide A chemical agent that kills sperm.

Prelubricated condoms are available containing **spermicide**; these condoms may decrease the risk of pregnancy, but the extent of decreased risk has not been established. If desired, users can lubricate their own condoms with contraceptive foam, creams, or jelly or with water-based preparations such as K-Y Jelly. Any product that contains mineral or vegetable oil—including baby oil, many lotions, regular Vaseline petroleum jelly, cooking oils (corn oil, Crisco, butter, and so on), and some vaginal lubricants and anti-fungal or anti-itch creams—should never be used with latex condoms; they can cause latex to begin to disintegrate within 60 seconds, thus greatly increasing the chance of condom breakage. (Polyurethane is not affected by oil-based products.)

Advantages Condoms are easy to purchase and are available without prescription or medical supervision. Simple to use, they provide for greater male participation in contraception. Their effects are immediately and completely reversible. In addition to being free of medical side effects (other than occasional allergic reactions), latex condoms help protect against STDs. Condoms made of polyurethane are appropriate for people who are allergic to latex; they also provide STD protection, but they are not as well studied as latex condoms, so their exact effectiveness is unknown. (Lambskin condoms permit the passage of HIV and other disease-causing organisms, so they can be used only for pregnancy prevention, not the prevention of STDs.) Except for abstinence, correct and consistent use of latex male condoms offers the most reliable available protection against the transmission of HIV.

Disadvantages The two most common complaints about condoms are that they diminish sensation and interfere with spontaneity. Although some people find these drawbacks serious, others consider them only minor disadvantages.

Effectiveness First-year rates among typical users average about 14%. At least some pregnancies happen because the condom is carelessly removed after ejaculation. Some may also occur because of a break or a tear, which may happen 1–2 times in every 100 instances of use for latex condoms; some studies have found higher breakage and slippage rates for polyurethane condoms. Breakage is more common among inexperienced users. Other contributing factors include poorly fitting condoms, insufficient lubrication, and excessively vigorous sex. Because heat destroys rubber, latex condoms should not be stored for long periods in a wallet or a car's glove compartment. It is important to note, however, that most condom failures are due to inconsistent or improper use, not problems with condom quality.

If a condom breaks or is carelessly removed, the risk of pregnancy can be reduced somewhat by the immediate use of a vaginal spermicide. If postcoital (emergency)

You can buy several types of contraceptives without a prescription. These have several advantages—they are readily accessible and relatively inexpensive, they are moderately effective at preventing pregnancy, and some offer some protection against HIV infection and other STDs. But like all methods, over-the-counter contraceptives work only if they are used correctly. The following guidelines can help you maximize the effectiveness of your method of choice.

Male Condoms

- *Buy latex condoms.* If you're allergic to latex, use a polyurethane condom or wear a lambskin condom under a latex one. Lambskin condoms provide no STD protection; polyurethane condoms may provide protection against pregnancy and STDs comparable to latex condoms, but more studies are needed.

- *Buy and use condoms while they are fresh.* Packages have an expiration date or a manufacturing date. Don't use a condom after the expiration date or more than 5 years after the manufacturing date (2 years if it contains spermicide).

- *Try different styles and sizes.* Male condoms come in a variety of textures, colors, shapes, lubricants, and sizes. Shop around until you find a brand that's right for you. Condom widths and lengths vary by about 10–20%. A condom that is too tight may be uncomfortable and more likely to break; one that is too loose may slip off.

- *Use "thinner" condoms with caution.* Condoms advertised as "thinner" are often no thinner than others, and those that really are the thinnest tend to break more easily.

- *Don't remove the condom from an individual sealed wrapper until you're ready to use it.* Open the packet carefully. Don't use a condom if it's gummy, dried out, or discolored. Keep extra condoms on hand.

- *Store condoms correctly.* Don't leave condoms in extreme heat or cold, and don't carry them in a pocket wallet.

- *Use only water-based lubricants.* Never use oil-based lubricants like Vaseline or hand lotion, as they may cause a latex condom to break. Avoid oil-based vaginal products.

- *Use male condoms correctly* (see Figure 6-1). Use a new condom every time you have intercourse. Misuse is by far the leading reason that condoms fail.

Female Condoms

- *Make sure your condom comes with the necessary supplies and information.* The Reality female condom comes individually wrapped. With your condom, you should receive a leaflet containing instructions and a small bottle of additional lubricant.

- *Buy and use female condoms while they are fresh.* Check the expiration dates on the condom packet and the lubricant bottle.

- *Buy several condoms.* Buy one or more for practice before using one during sex. Have a backup in case you have a problem with insertion or use.

- *Read the leaflet instructions carefully.* Practice inserting the condom and checking that it's in the proper position.

- *Use the female condom correctly.* Make sure the penis is inserted into the pouch and that the outer ring is not pushed into the vagina. Add lubricant around the outer ring if needed.

Contraceptive Sponges

- *Buy and use contraceptive sponges when they are fresh.* Check the expiration date on each package.

- *Read and follow the package instructions carefully.* Moisten the sponge with water and place high in the vagina.

- *Use each sponge only once.* The sponge may be left in place for up to 24 hours without the addition of spermicide for repeated intercourse.

Spermicides

- *Try different types of spermicides.* You may find one type easier or more convenient to use. Foams come in aerosol cans and are similar to shaving cream in consistency. Foams are thicker than creams, which are thicker than jellies. Foams, creams, and jellies usually require applicators; spermicidal suppositories and films do not.

- *Read and follow the package directions carefully.* Cans of foam must be shaken before use. Jellies and creams are often inserted with an applicator just outside the entrance to the cervix. Suppositories and film must be placed with the finger.

- *Pay close attention to the timing of use.* Follow the package instructions for inserting the spermicide at the appropriate time before intercourse actually occurs. Spermicides have a fairly narrow window of effectiveness. Be sure to also allow the recommended amount of time for suppositories and films to dissolve.

- *Use an additional full dose for each additional act of intercourse.*

- *Leave the spermicide in place for 8 hours after the last act of intercourse.*

- *Consider using spermicides with another form of birth control.* These include a condom, diaphragm, or cervical cap. Combined use provides greater protection against pregnancy.

More than 60 medical, public health, and women's groups have filed petitions with the FDA urging the agency to change the status of emergency contraceptive pills from prescription to over the counter; several state legislatures are considering measures that would allow women to obtain the pills from a pharmacist without a prescription. If emergency contraceptive pills do become available over the counter, it will be important for users to follow the instructions carefully.

contraception is an appropriate option, a health care provider should be consulted as soon as possible. The effectiveness of the condom can be greatly improved if a spermicidal foam is also inserted just *before* intercourse.

COMMUNICATE!   Couples sometimes fail to use condoms or other contraceptive methods because they feel it reduces the spontaneity of sex or destroys a romantic atmosphere. If you are in a relationship and find yourself facing this problem, think about what you will do and practice what you will say. Talk with your partner ahead of time, and be confident about your right to control your own fertility. You might begin by saying something like, "I know you think using a condom is unromantic, but not using one means taking a chance on getting pregnant—and I'm not ready for that right now. Being worried doesn't make me feel very romantic. Let's talk about how we can use condoms and still stay in the mood."

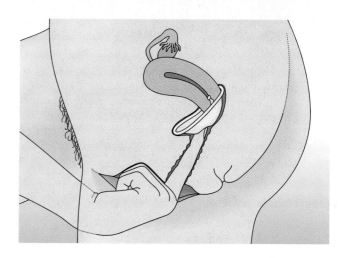

Figure 6-2   The diaphragm properly positioned to cover the cervix.

Female Condoms

A female condom is a latex or polyurethane pouch that a woman or her partner inserts into her vagina. One brand, Reality, was approved in May 1993 for use in the United States. Reality is a disposable device that comes in one size and consists of a soft, loose-fitting polyurethane sheath with two flexible rings. The ring at the closed end is inserted into the vagina and placed at the cervix much like a diaphragm. The ring at the open end remains outside the vagina.

The condom can be inserted up to 8 hours before intercourse and should be used with the supplied lubricant or a spermicide. Following intercourse, the woman should remove the condom immediately, before standing up. By twisting and squeezing the outer ring, she can prevent the spilling of semen.

Advantages   Female condoms can be inserted before sexual activity and are thus less disruptive than male condoms. Because the outer part of the condom covers the

area around the vaginal opening as well as the base of the penis during intercourse, it offers potentially better protection against genital warts or herpes. The polyurethane pouch can be used by people who are allergic to latex. When used correctly, the female condom should theoretically provide protection against HIV transmission and STDs comparable to that of the latex male condom. However, in research involving typical users, the female condom was less effective in preventing both pregnancy and STDs.

Disadvantages   As with the traditional condom, interference with spontaneity is likely to be a common complaint. Female condoms, like male condoms, are made for one-time use. A single female condom costs about four times as much as a single male condom.

Effectiveness   The typical first-year failure rate of the female condom is 21%.

The Diaphragm with Spermicide

The **diaphragm** is a dome-shaped cup of thin rubber stretched over a collapsible metal ring. When correctly used with spermicidal cream or jelly, the diaphragm covers the cervix, blocking sperm from entering the uterus (Figure 6-2). A diaphragm can be obtained only by prescription. Because of individual anatomical differences, a diaphragm must be carefully fitted by a trained clinician to ensure both comfort and effectiveness. The fitting should be checked with each routine annual medical examination, as well as after childbirth, abortion, or a weight change of more than 10 pounds.

The woman spreads spermicidal jelly or cream on the diaphragm, squeezing it into a long narrow shape with

Terms

diaphragm   A contraceptive device consisting of a flexible, dome-shaped cup that covers the cervix and prevents sperm from entering the uterus.

toxic shock syndrome (TSS)   A bacterial disease usually associated with tampon use; can also occur in men; symptoms include weakness, cold and clammy hands, fever, nausea, and headache. TSS can progress to life-threatening complications, including very low blood pressure (shock) and kidney and liver failure.

cervical cap   A thimble-shaped cup that fits over the cervix, to be used with spermicide.

the thumb and forefinger, inserting it into the vagina, and pushing it up along the back wall of the vagina as far as it will go. The cervix should be completely covered, and the front rim of the diaphragm should be tucked behind the pubic bone. If more than 6 hours elapse between the time of insertion and the time of intercourse, additional spermicide must be applied. The diaphragm must be left in place for at least 6 hours after the last act of coitus to give the spermicide enough time to kill all the sperm.

To remove the diaphragm, the woman simply hooks the front rim down from the pubic bone with one finger and pulls it out. She should wash it with mild soap and water, rinse it, pat it dry, and then examine it for holes or cracks. After inspecting the diaphragm, she should dust it with cornstarch and store it in its case.

Advantages A diaphragm can be inserted up to 6 hours before intercourse, and it allows for immediate and total reversibility. The diaphragm is free of medical side effects (other than rare allergic reactions). When used along with spermicidal jelly or cream, it offers significant protection against gonorrhea and possibly chlamydia, STDs that are transmitted only by semen and for which the cervix is the sole site of entry. Diaphragm use can also protect the cervix from semen infected with the human papillomavirus, which has been implicated as an important factor in cellular changes in the cervix that can lead to cancer. However, the diaphragm is unlikely to protect against STDs that can be transmitted through vaginal or vulvar surfaces (in addition to the cervix), including HIV infection, genital herpes, and syphilis.

Disadvantages Diaphragms must always be used with a spermicide, so a woman must keep both of these somewhat bulky supplies with her whenever she anticipates sexual activity. Diaphragms require extra attention, since they must be cleaned and stored with care to preserve their effectiveness. Some women cannot wear a diaphragm because of their vaginal or uterine anatomy or because of frequent bladder infections. It has also been associated with a slightly increased risk of **toxic shock syndrome (TSS)**, an occasionally fatal bacterial infection. To diminish the risk of TSS, a woman should wash her hands carefully with soap and water before inserting or removing the diaphragm, should not use the diaphragm during menstruation or in the presence of an abnormal vaginal discharge, and should never leave the device in place for more than 24 hours.

Effectiveness Typical failure rates are 20% during the first year of use. The main causes of failure are incorrect insertion, inconsistent use, and inaccurate fitting. If a diaphragm slips during intercourse, a woman may choose to contact her physician to discuss use of emergency contraception.

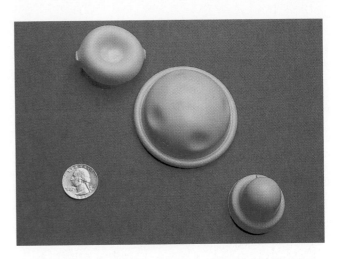

The diaphragm and cervical cap work by covering the mouth of the cervix, blocking sperm from entering the cervix; both require professional fitting. The sponge acts as a barrier, a spermicide, and a seminal fluid absorbent.

The Cervical Cap

The **cervical cap**, another barrier device, is a thimble-shaped rubber or plastic cup that fits snugly over the cervix and is held in place by suction. The cap comes in various sizes and must be fitted by a trained clinician. It is used in a manner similar to that of the diaphragm, a small amount of spermicide being placed in the cup before each insertion.

Advantages Advantages of the cervical cap are similar to those associated with diaphragm use and include partial STD protection. It is an alternative for women who cannot use a diaphragm because of anatomical reasons or recurrent urinary tract infections. Because the cap fits tightly, it does not require a fresh dose of spermicide with repeated intercourse. It may be left in place for up to 48 hours (compared with 24 hours for the diaphragm).

Disadvantages Along with most of the disadvantages associated with the diaphragm, difficulty with insertion and removal is more common for cervical cap users. In addition, some studies have indicated that women who use the cap rather than the diaphragm initially have a higher rate of abnormal Pap test results. Because there may be a slightly increased risk of TSS with prolonged use, the cap should not be left in place for more than 48 hours.

Effectiveness For women who have never had children, the cervical cap failure rate is about 20%, similar to that of the diaphragm. For women who have given birth, the failure rate goes up to about 40%.

The Contraceptive Sponge

The **sponge** was sold in the United States between 1983 and 1995, at which time the original manufacturer decided to withdraw the contraceptive rather than to bring its manufacturing plant up to FDA standards. The safety or effectiveness of the sponge itself was never in question, and FDA approval of the product was never rescinded. A new company has bought the rights to the sponge and expects to have it on the market in the near future.

The sponge is a round, absorbent device about 2 inches in diameter with a polyester loop on one side (for removal) and a concave dimple on the other side, which helps it fit snugly over the cervix. The sponge is made of polyurethane and is presaturated with the same spermicide that is used in contraceptive creams and foams. The sponge acts as a barrier, as a spermicide, and as a seminal fluid absorbent.

Advantages The sponge offers advantages similar to those of the diaphragm and cervical cap, including partial STD protection. In addition, sponges can be obtained without a professional fitting, and they may be safely left in place for 24 hours without the addition of spermicide for repeated intercourse.

Disadvantages Reported disadvantages include difficulty with removal and an unpleasant odor if left in place for more than 18 hours. Allergic reactions, such as irritation of the labia, are more common with the sponge than with other spermicide products, probably because the overall dose contained in each sponge is significantly higher than that used with other methods. Because the sponge has also been associated with TSS, the same precautions must be taken as described for diaphragm use.

Effectiveness The typical effectiveness of the sponge is similar to that of the diaphragm (20% failure rate during the first year of use) for women who have never experienced childbirth. For women who have had a child, however, sponge effectiveness is significantly lower than diaphragm effectiveness.

Vaginal Spermicides

Spermicidal compounds developed for use with a diaphragm have been adapted for use without a diaphragm by combining them with a bulky base. Foams, creams, and jellies must be placed deep in the vagina near the cervical entrance and must be inserted no more than 30 minutes before intercourse. Suppositories, which are inserted like tampons, must be inserted at least 15 minutes before intercourse. The same is true for the vaginal contraceptive film (VCF), a paper-thin 2-inch square of spermicide-containing film that can be folded and placed high in the vagina. After an hour, the effectiveness of spermicides is drastically reduced, and a new dose must be inserted. Another application is also required before each repeated act of coitus. If the woman wants to **douche,** she should wait for at least 6 hours after the last intercourse to make sure that there has been time for the spermicide to kill all the sperm; douching is not recommended, however, because it can irritate vaginal tissue and increase the risk of various infections.

Advantages The use of vaginal spermicides is relatively simple and can be limited to times of sexual activity. They are readily available in most drugstores and do not require a prescription or a pelvic examination. Spermicides allow for complete and immediate reversibility, and the only medical side effects are occasional allergic reactions. Vaginal spermicides may provide limited protection against some STDs but should never be used instead of condoms for reliable protection.

Disadvantages When used alone, vaginal spermicides must be inserted shortly before intercourse, so their use may be seen as an annoying disruption. Spermicides can alter the balance of bacteria in the vagina and increase the risk of urinary tract infections. Overuse of spermicides can irritate vaginal tissues; if this occurs, the risk of HIV transmission may actually increase.

Terms

sponge A contraceptive device about 2 inches in diameter that fits over the cervix and acts as a barrier, spermicide, and seminal fluid absorbent.

douche To apply a stream of water or other solutions to a body part or cavity such as the vagina; not a contraceptive technique.

abstinence Avoidance of sexual intercourse; a method of contraception.

fertility awareness method (FAM) A method of preventing conception based on avoiding intercourse during the fertile phase of a woman's cycle.

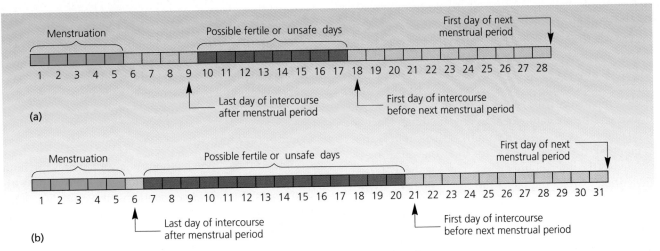

Figure 6-3 The fertility awareness method of contraception. This chart shows the safe and unsafe days for (a) a woman with a regular 28-day cycle and (b) a woman with an irregular cycle, ranging from 25 to 31 days.

Effectiveness The typical failure rate is about 26%. Spermicide use is generally recommended only in combination with other barrier methods or as a backup with other contraceptives.

Abstinence, Fertility Awareness, and Withdrawal

Millions of people throughout the world do not use any of the contraceptive methods we have described because of religious conviction or cultural prohibitions or because of poverty or lack of information and supplies. If they use any method at all, they are likely to use one of the following relatively "natural" methods of attempting to prevent conception.

Abstinence The decision not to engage in sexual intercourse for a chosen period of time, or **abstinence**, has been practiced throughout history for a variety of reasons. Until relatively recently, many people abstained because they had no other contraceptive measures. Today, with other methods available, about 1.5% of all American women rely on periodic abstinence as a contraceptive method. To some, other methods simply seem unsuitable. Concern about possible side effects, STDs, and unwanted pregnancy may be factors. For others, the most important reason for choosing abstinence is a moral one, based on cultural or religious beliefs or strongly held personal values. Individuals may feel that sexual intercourse is appropriate only for married couples or for people in serious, committed relationships. Abstinence may also be considered the wisest choice in terms of an individual's emotional needs. A period of abstinence may be useful as a time to focus energies on other aspects of interpersonal or personal growth.

Anyone can practice abstinence at any time, including people who are not yet sexually active, those who are be-

ginning a relationship with a new partner, and those who are not currently in a relationship. Couples may choose abstinence to allow time for their relationship to grow. A period of abstinence allows partners to get to know each other better and to develop trust and respect for one another. Many couples who do choose to abstain from sexual intercourse in the traditional sense turn to other mutually satisfying alternatives. When open communication between partners exists, many new avenues may be explored. These may include dancing, massage, hugging, kissing, petting, mutual masturbation, and oral-genital sex. Sexual feelings and intimacy may be expressed and satisfied through a wide range of activities.

The Fertility Awareness Method The basis for the **fertility awareness method (FAM)** is abstinence from coitus during the fertile phase of a woman's menstrual cycle. Ordinarily only one egg is released by the ovaries each month, and it lives about 24 hours unless it is fertilized. Sperm deposited in the vagina are on average capable of fertilizing an egg for about 6–7 days, so conception can theoretically occur only during 8 days of any cycle. Predicting which 8 days is difficult. It is done by either the calendar method or the temperature method. Information on cyclical changes of the cervical mucus can also help determine the time of ovulation.

The *calendar method* is based on the knowledge that the average woman releases an egg 14–16 days before her next period begins. Few women menstruate with complete regularity, so a record of the menstrual cycle must be kept for 12 months, during which time some other method of contraception must be used. The first day of each period is counted as day 1. To determine the first fertile, or "unsafe," day of the cycle, subtract 18 from the number of days in the shortest cycle (Figure 6-3). To determine the last unsafe day of the cycle, subtract 11 from the number of days in the longest cycle.

The *temperature method* is based on the knowledge that a woman's body temperature drops slightly just before ovulation and rises slightly after ovulation. A woman using the temperature method records her basal (resting) body temperature (BBT) every morning before getting out of bed and before eating or drinking anything. Once the temperature pattern is apparent (usually after about 3 months), the unsafe period for intercourse can be calculated as the interval from day 5 (day 1 is the first day of the period) until 3 days after the rise in BBT. To arrive at a shorter unsafe period, some women combine the calendar and temperature methods, calculating the first unsafe day from the shortest cycle of the calendar chart and the last unsafe day as the third day after a rise in BBT.

The *mucus method* (or Billings method) is based on changes in the cervical secretions throughout the menstrual cycle. During the estrogenic phase, cervical mucus increases and is clear and slippery. At the time of ovulation, some women can detect a slight change in the texture of the mucus and find that it is more likely to form an elastic thread when stretched between thumb and finger. After ovulation, these secretions become cloudy and sticky and decrease in quantity. Infertile, safe days are likely to occur during the relatively dry days just before and after menstruation. These additional clues have been found to be helpful by some couples who rely on the fertility awareness method.

FAM is not recommended for women who have very irregular cycles—about 15% of all menstruating women. Any woman for whom pregnancy would be a serious problem should not rely on FAM alone, because the failure rate is high—approximately 25% during the first year of use. FAM offers no protection against STDs.

Withdrawal In withdrawal, or coitus interruptus, the male removes his penis from the vagina just before he ejaculates. Withdrawal has a relatively high failure rate because the male has to overcome a powerful biological urge. In addition, because preejaculatory fluid may contain viable sperm, pregnancy can occur even if the man withdraws prior to ejaculation. Sexual pleasure is often affected because the man must remain in control and the sexual experience of both partners is interrupted.

Withdrawal is probably about as effective as the diaphragm and cervical cap. Men who are less experienced with sexual intercourse and withdrawal or who have difficulty foretelling when ejaculation will occur have higher failure rates. Withdrawal does not protect against STDs.

Combining Methods

Couples can combine methods in a variety of ways, both to add STD protection and/or to increase contraceptive effectiveness. For example, condoms are strongly recommended along with OCs whenever there is a risk of STDs (Table 6-2). Foam may be added to condom use to increase protection against both STDs and pregnancy. For many couples, and especially for women, the added benefits will far outweigh the extra effort and expense.

Table 6-3 summarizes the effectiveness of available contraceptive methods.

PERMANENT CONTRACEPTION: STERILIZATION

Sterilization is permanent, and it is highly effective at preventing pregnancy. For these reasons, it is becoming an increasingly popular method of contraception. At present it is the most commonly used method in the United States and in the world. It is especially popular among couples who have been married 10 or more years, as well as those who have had all the children they intend. Sterilization provides no protection against STDs.

An important consideration in choosing sterilization is that, in most cases, it cannot be reversed and should be considered permanent. Some couples choosing male sterilization store sperm as a way of extending the option of childbearing. Male sterilization may be preferable to female sterilization in several ways. The overall cost of a female procedure is about four times that of a male procedure, and women are much more likely than men to experience both minor and major complications following the operation. Furthermore, feelings of regret seem to be somewhat more prevalent in women than in men after sterilization.

Male Sterilization: Vasectomy

The procedure for male sterilization, **vasectomy**, involves severing the *vasa deferentia*, two tiny ducts that transport sperm from the testes to the seminal vesicles. The testes continue to produce sperm, but the sperm are absorbed into the body. Because the testes contribute only about 10% of the total seminal fluid, the actual quantity of ejaculate is only slightly reduced. Hormone production from the testes continues with very little change, and secondary sex characteristics are not altered.

Vasectomy is ordinarily performed in a physician's office and takes about 30 minutes. A local anesthetic is in-

Terms

sterilization Surgically altering the reproductive system to prevent pregnancy. Vasectomy is the procedure in males; tubal sterilization or hysterectomy is the procedure in females.

vasectomy The surgical severing of the ducts that carry sperm to the ejaculatory duct.

tubal sterilization Severing or in some manner blocking the oviducts, preventing eggs from reaching the uterus.

laparoscopy Examining the internal organs by inserting a tube containing a small light through an abdominal incision.

hysterectomy Total or partial surgical removal of the uterus.

Table 6-2 — Contraceptive Methods and STD Protection

Method	Level of Protection
Hormonal methods	Do not protect against HIV or STDs in lower reproductive tract; increase risk of cervical chlamydia; may reduce severity of PID symptoms.
IUD	Does not protect against STDs; associated with PID in first month after insertion.
Latex male condom	Best method for protection against STDs (if used correctly); does not protect against infections from lesions that are not covered by the condom. (Polyurethane condoms should provide protection, but definitive findings are not yet available; lambskin condoms do not protect against STDs.)
Female condom	Theoretically should reduce the risk of STDs, but research results are not yet available.
Diaphragm, sponge, or cervical cap	May protect against cervical infections. Research results regarding HIV and PID protection are contradictory, but diaphragms, sponges, and cervical caps are not as effective as male condoms.
Spermicide	Modestly reduces the risk of cervical gonorrhea and chlamydia: effectiveness against other STDs is uncertain. If vaginal irritation occurs, infection risk may increase.
FAM	Does not protect against STDs.
Sterilization	Does not protect against STDs.
Abstinence	Complete protection against STDs (as long as all activities that involve the exchange of body fluids are avoided).

Abstinence or sex with a mutually monogamous, uninfected partner is the surest way to protect yourself against HIV and other STDs. Barring this, correct and consistent use of latex male condoms provides the best protection against STDs.

jected into the skin of the scrotum near the vasa. Small incisions are made at the upper end of the scrotum where it joins the body, and the vas deferens on each side is exposed, severed, and tied off or sealed by electrocautery. Bleeding and infection occasionally develop but are usually easily treated. Fewer complications occur with an alternative procedure involving a midline puncture rather than incisions; this "no-scalpel" technique is used in about 30% of vasectomies performed in the United States.

Vasectomy is highly effective. In a small number of cases, a severed vas rejoins itself, so some physicians advise yearly examination of a semen sample. The overall failure rate for vasectomy is 0.15%. Some surgeons report pregnancy rates of about 80% for partners of men who have their vasectomies reversed within 10 years of the original procedure, most studies report figures in the 50% range.

Female Sterilization

The most common method of female sterilization involves severing, or in some manner blocking, the oviducts, thereby preventing the egg from reaching the uterus and the sperm from entering the fallopian tubes. Ovulation and menstruation continue, but the unfertilized eggs are released into the abdominal cavity and absorbed. Although progesterone levels in the blood may decline slightly, hormone production by the ovaries and secondary sex characteristics are generally not affected.

Tubal sterilization is most commonly performed by a method called **laparoscopy.** A laparoscope, a tube containing a small light, is inserted through a small abdominal incision, and the surgeon looks through it to locate the fallopian tubes. Instruments are passed either through the laparoscope or through a second small incision, and the two fallopian tubes are sealed off with ties or staples or by electrocautery. Either a local or a general anesthetic can be used; the operation takes about 15 minutes. Tubal sterilization can also be performed shortly after a vaginal delivery, or in the case of cesarean section immediately after the uterine incision is repaired. **Hysterectomy,** removal of the uterus, is the preferred method of sterilization for only a small number of women, usually those with preexisting menstrual problems.

Female sterilization is somewhat riskier than male sterilization, with a complication rate of about 0.1–7%. Potential problems include bowel injury, wound infection, and bleeding. Serious complications are rare, and the death rate is low.

The failure rate for tubal sterilization is about 0.5%. When pregnancies do occur, an increased percentage of them are ectopic. Reversibility rates of current methods are about 50–70%

Table 6-3	Contraceptive Effectiveness	
	Percentage of Women Experiencing an Unintended Pregnancy in the First Year of Use	
Method	**Typical Use**	**Perfect Use**
Norplant	0.05%	0.05%
Male sterilization (vasectomy)	0.15	0.10
Depo-Provera	0.30	0.30
Female sterilization	0.50	0.50
Copper T IUD	0.8	0.6
Progestasert IUD	2.0	1.5
Oral contraceptives	5	
Combination		0.1
Progestin only		0.5
Male condom (latex)	14	3
Withdrawal	19	4
Diaphragm with spermicide	20	6
Sponge*	20	9
Cervical cap*	20	9
Female condom	21	5
Fertility awareness method	25	
Calendar alone		9
Combination of FAM methods		2
Spermicides	26	6
Chance	85	85

* For women who have given birth, the rates of unintended pregnancy increase to 40% for typical use and 26% (cervical cap) and 20% (sponge) for perfect use.

SOURCE: Hatcher, R. A., et al. 1998. *Contraceptive Technology*, 17th rev. ed. New York: Ardent Media.

WWW. WHICH CONTRACEPTIVE METHOD IS RIGHT FOR YOU?

Each person must consider many variables in deciding which contraceptive method is most acceptable and appropriate for her or him:

1. *Health risks.* Is there anything in your personal or family medical history that would affect your choice of method? For each method you consider, what are the potential health risks that apply to you? For example, hormonal methods should be used only after a clinical evaluation of your medical history. Other methods have only minor and local side effects. If necessary, talk with your physician about the potential health effects of different methods for you.

2. *The implications of an unplanned pregnancy.* How would an unplanned pregnancy affect you and your future? What are your feelings regarding the options—abortion, adoption, or raising a child? If effectiveness is of critical importance to you, carefully consider the ways the effectiveness of each method can be improved. Abstinence is 100% effective, if maintained. If used correctly, hormonal methods offer very good protection against pregnancy. Barrier methods can be combined with spermicides to improve their effectiveness.

3. *STD risk.* How likely are you to be exposed to any sexually transmitted diseases? Have you and your partner been screened for STDs recently? Have you openly and honestly discussed your past sexual behavior? Condom use is of critical importance whenever any risk of STDs is present. This is especially true when you are not in an exclusive, long-term relationship or when you are taking the pill, because cervical changes that occur during hormone use may increase vulnerability to certain diseases. Abstinence or activities that don't involve intercourse or any other exchange of body fluids can be a satisfactory alternative for some people.

4. *Convenience and comfort level.* How do your partner and you view each of the methods? Which would you most likely use consistently? The hormonal methods are generally ranked high in this category, unless there are negative side effects and health risks or forgetting to take pills is a problem for you. Some people think condom use disrupts spontaneity and lowers penile sensitivity. (Creative approaches to condom use and improved quality can decrease these concerns.) The diaphragm, cervical cap, sponge, female condom, and spermicides can be inserted before intercourse begins but are still considered a significant inconvenience by some.

5. *Type of relationship.* How easy is it for you to talk with your partner about contraception? How willing is he or she to be involved? Barrier methods require more motivation and a sense of responsibility from *each* partner than hormonal methods do. When the method depends on the cooperation of one's partner, assertiveness is necessary, no matter how difficult. This is especially true in new relationships, when condom use is most important. When sexual activity is infrequent, a barrier method may make more sense than an IUD or one of the hormonal methods.

6. *Ease and cost of obtaining and maintaining each method.* If a physical exam and clinic follow-up is required, how readily accessible is this to you? Can you and your partner afford the associated expenses of the

About 60 million women in the United States are in their child-bearing years (15–44) and thus face decisions about contraception. Overall, about 64% of American women use some form of contraception, and most of the remaining 36% are either sterile, pregnant or trying to become pregnant, or not sexually active. Only 5% of American women are fertile, sexually active, and not seeking pregnancy; this small group accounts for almost half of the 3 million unintended pregnancies that occur each year. The unintended pregnancies that occur among contraceptive users are usually the result of inconsistent or incorrect use of methods. For example, in a large-scale survey asking women about their use of contraception in the previous 3 months, 13% of pill users reported missing two or more pills, and 20% of barrier method users reported that they actually used their method of choice only half the time—or less.

Female sterilization and oral contraceptives are the two most popular methods among American women (see figure). However, choice of contraceptive method and consistency of use vary with age, marital status, and other factors:

- *Age:* Sterilization is much more common among older women, particularly those who are over 35 years of age and/or who have had children. Older women are also much more likely to use reversible methods consistently—they are least likely to miss pills and most likely to use barrier methods during every act of intercourse. Young women between the ages of 15 and 17 years who use OCs are more likely by far to miss pills than women in any other age group.

- *Marital status:* Women who are or have been married have much higher rates of sterilization than women who have never been married. Those who have never been married have high rates of OC and condom usage.

- *Ethnicity:* Overall rates of contraceptive use and use of female sterilization and OCs are highest among white women. Implants and injectables are more often used by African American women and Latinas, and IUD use is highest among Latinas. Condom use is highest among Asian American women and similar across other ethnic groups. Male sterilization is much more common among white men than among men of other ethnic groups.

- *Socioeconomic status and educational attainment:* Low socioeconomic status and low educational attainment are associated with high rates of female sterilization and low rates of pill and condom use. However, women who are poor or have low educational attainment and who do use OCs have higher rates of consistent use than women who are wealthier or have more education.

Some trends in contraceptive use may also reflect the differing priorities and experiences of women and men. For example, female sterilization is more expensive and carries greater health risks than male sterilization—yet it is more than twice as common. (Worldwide, female sterilization is more than four times as common as male sterilization.) This pattern may reflect culturally defined gender roles and the fact that women are more directly affected by unintended pregnancy. In surveys, women rate pregnancy prevention as the single most important factor when choosing a contraceptive method; in contrast, men rate STD prevention as equally important.

SOURCES: Alan Guttmacher Institute. 2000. *Facts in Brief: Contraceptive Use* (http://www.agi-usa.org/ pubs/fb_contr_use.html; retrieved March 24, 2001). Grady, W. R., D. H. Klepinger, and A. Nelson-Wally. 1999. Contraceptive characteristics: The perceptions and priorities of men and women. *Family Planning Perspectives* 31(4): 168–175. National Center for Health Statistics. 1997. Fertility, family planning, and women's health: New data from the 1995 survey of family growth. *Vital and Health Statistics* 23(19).

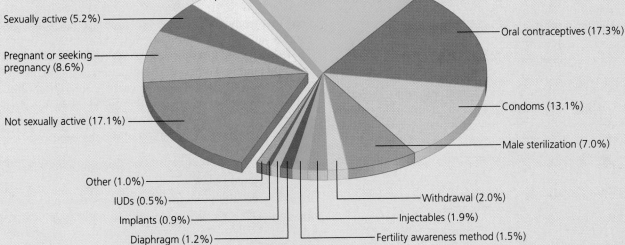

Women not using contraception (35.8% of U.S. women)

Sterile for noncontraceptive reasons or with sterile male partner (4.9%)
Sexually active (5.2%)
Pregnant or seeking pregnancy (8.6%)
Not sexually active (17.1%)
Other (1.0%)
IUDs (0.5%)
Implants (0.9%)
Diaphragm (1.2%)

Method reported by women using contraception (64.2% of U.S. women)

Female sterilization (17.8%)
Oral contraceptives (17.3%)
Condoms (13.1%)
Male sterilization (7.0%)
Withdrawal (2.0%)
Injectables (1.9%)
Fertility awareness method (1.5%)

Contraceptive use among American women age 15–44 years.

Many people have a difficult time talking about contraception with a potential sex partner. How should you bring it up? And whose responsibility is it, anyway? Talking about the subject may be embarrassing at first, but imagine the possible consequences of *not* talking about it. An unintended pregnancy or a sexually transmitted disease could profoundly affect you for the rest of your life. Talking about contraception is one way of showing that you care about yourself, your partner, and your future.

Before you talk with your partner, explore your own thoughts and feelings. Find out the facts about different methods of contraception, and decide which one you think would be most appropriate for you. If you're nervous about having this discussion with your partner, it may help to practice with a friend.

Pick a good time to bring up the subject. Don't wait until you've started to have sex. A time when you're both feeling comfortable and relaxed will maximize your chances of having

a good discussion. Tell your partner what you know about contraception and how you feel about using it, and talk about what steps you both need to take to get and use a method you can live with. Listen to what your partner has to say, and try to understand his or her point of view. You may need to have more than one discussion, and it may take some time for both of you to feel comfortable with the subject. *But don't have sex until this issue is resolved.*

If you want your partner to be involved but he or she isn't interested in talking about contraception, or if he or she leaves all the responsibility for it up to you, consider whether this is really a person you want to be sexually involved with. If you decide to go ahead with the involvement, you may want to enlist the support of a friend, family member, or health care worker to help you make and implement decisions about the essential issue of contraception.

---

method? Investigate the costs of different methods. Find out if your insurance covers any of the costs.

7. *Religious or philosophical beliefs.* Are any of the methods unacceptable to you because of your personal beliefs? For some, abstinence and/or FAM may be the only permissible contraceptive methods.

Whatever your needs, circumstances, or beliefs, *do* make a choice about contraception. Not choosing anything is the one method known *not* to work. This is an area in which taking charge of your health has immediate and profound implications for your future.

THE ABORTION ISSUE

In the United States today, few issues are as complex and emotion-filled as abortion. While most public attention has focused on legal definitions and restrictions, the most difficult aspects of abortion actually take place at a much more personal level. Because the majority of women having abortions are young, many college students have had some type of direct exposure to these more personal experiences of abortion.

The word **abortion,** by strict definition, means the expulsion of an embryo or fetus from the uterus before it is sufficiently developed to survive. As commonly used, however, *abortion* refers only to expulsions that are artificially induced by mechanical means or drugs, and *miscar-*

riage is generally used for a spontaneous abortion, one that occurs naturally with no causal intervention. In this chapter, *abortion* will mean a deliberately induced expulsion.

 The History of Abortion in the United States

For more than two centuries, abortion policy in the United States followed English common law, which made the practice a crime only when performed after "quickening" (fetal movement that begins at about 20 weeks). There was little public objection to this policy until the early 1800s, when an anti-abortion movement began, led primarily by physicians who questioned the doctrine of quickening and who objected to the growing practice of abortion by untrained persons (in part because it weakened their control of medical services).

This anti-abortion drive gained minimal attention until the mid-1800s, when newspaper advertisements for abortion preparations became common and concern grew that women were using abortion as a means of birth control (and perhaps to cover up extramarital activity). There was much discussion about the corruption of morality among women in the United States, and by the 1900s, abortion was illegal in every state. These anti-abortion laws stayed in effect until the 1960s, when courts began to invalidate them on the grounds of constitutional vagueness and violation of the right to privacy.

WW. Current Legal Status

In 1973, the U.S. Supreme Court made abortion legal in the landmark case of *Roe v. Wade.* To replace the restrictions most states still imposed at that time, the justices devised new standards to govern abortion decisions. They

Terms   **abortion** The expulsion or removal of an embryo or fetus from the uterus.

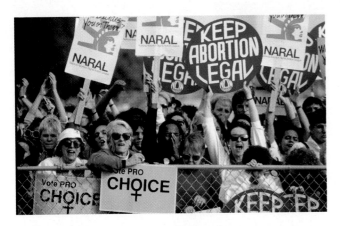
Pro-choice groups believe that the decision to end or continue a pregnancy is a personal matter that should be left up to the individual.

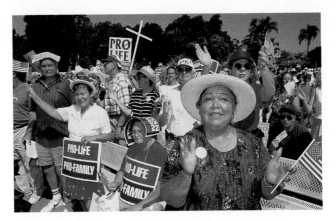
Pro-life groups oppose abortion on the basis of their belief that life begins at the moment of conception.

divided pregnancy into three parts, or trimesters, giving a pregnant woman less choice about abortion as she advances toward full term. In the first trimester, the abortion decision must be left to the judgment of the pregnant woman and her physician. During the second trimester, similar rights remain but a state may regulate factors that protect the health of the woman, such as type of facility where an abortion may be performed. In the third trimester, when the fetus is viable (capable of survival outside of the uterus), a state may regulate and even bar all abortions except those considered necessary to preserve the mother's life or health.

Additional rulings by the Supreme Court in 1989 (*Webster v. Reproductive Health Services*) and 1992 (*Planned Parenthood of Southeastern Pennsylvania v. Casey*) allow states to regulate abortion throughout pregnancy as long as an "undue burden" is not imposed on women seeking the procedure. As a result, states have passed a variety of laws that have had the effect of reducing women's access to abortion. These laws include bans on the use of public funding, employees, and facilities for abortion services; mandatory counseling and waiting periods; insurance prohibitions; and requirements for parental consent for minors.

In addition to state abortion restrictions, the U.S. Congress has barred the use of federal Medicaid funds to pay for abortions, except when a woman's life is in danger or in cases of rape or incest. Currently, only 18 states provide nonfederal public money to assist poor women seeking abortions. Concerns have been raised that a two-tiered system has been created—one for women with means and another for those without.

Opponents of abortion have recently focused on specific methods of abortion. For example, many states have passed legislation outlawing a particular method of late-term abortion referred to by abortion opponents as "partial birth abortion." (*Partial birth abortion* is a nonmedical term for a rarely used late abortion method.) However, a Nebraska ban on "partial birth abortion" was struck down in a 5 to 4 decision by the Supreme Court in June 2000 (*Stenberg v. Carhart*); the judges in the majority view found that the ban placed an undue burden on women seeking abortion and that it failed to take into consideration the need to protect women's health.

Legal and legislative efforts have also targeted medications that can be used to induce abortion. The drug mifepristone (RU-486) was used extensively in other countries to perform nonsurgical early abortions for years before being approved for use in the United States.

Both pro-choice and pro-life groups are likely to remain active, seeking to advance their positions both by promoting legislation and by supporting political candidates who share their views.

COMMUNICATE! What are your government representatives' views on abortion? Contact their offices or go to their Web pages to find out their positions. Do they present clearly thought-out and articulated views? Do you see any fallacies in their thinking, such as false dilemma (presenting only two options when more are available), ad hominem (attacking the person making a claim rather than the claim itself), slippery slope (arguing that one action or event leads inevitably to a progression of additional actions or events), or false analogy (claiming that two things that are alike in one way are also alike in other ways)? If you see these or other flaws in logic, consider communicating with the representatives to seek clarification. If their views are not in line with your own, also consider letting them know where you stand.

Moral Considerations

Along with the legal debates are ongoing arguments between pro-life and pro-choice groups regarding the ethics of abortion. Central to the pro-life position is the belief that the fertilized egg must be valued as a human being from the moment of conception and that abortion at any time is equivalent to murder. This group holds that any woman who has sexual intercourse knows that pregnancy is a possibility, and should she willingly have intercourse and get pregnant, she is morally obligated to carry the pregnancy through. Pro-life followers encourage adoption for women who feel they are unable to raise the child and point out how many couples are seeking babies for adoption. Pro-life individuals do not consider the availability of legal abortion essential to women's well-being but view it instead as having an overall destructive effect on our traditional morals and values.

By contrast, the pro-choice viewpoint holds that distinctions must be made between the stages of fetal development and that preserving the fetus early in pregnancy (or *gestation*) is not always the ultimate moral concern. Members of this group maintain that women must have the freedom to decide whether and when to have children; they argue that pregnancy can result from contraceptive failure or other factors out of a woman's control. When pregnancy does occur, pro-choice individuals believe that the most moral decision possible must be determined according to each situation and that, in some cases, greater injustice would result if abortion were not an option. If legal abortions were not available, pro-choice supporters say, "back-alley shops" and do-it-yourself techniques, with their many health risks, as well as the births of unplanned children, would again grow in number. Others argue that discrimination in health care would result, since wealthy women could more easily make the travel arrangements necessary for a legal abortion elsewhere.

Some people strongly identify exclusively with either the pro-life or the pro-choice stance, but many have moral beliefs that are blurred, less defined, and in some cases a mixture of the two. Although the most vocal groups in the abortion debate tend to paint a black-and-white picture, the majority of Americans view abortion as a complex issue without any easy answers.

Public Opinion

In general, U.S. public opinion on abortion seems to change, depending on the specific situation. Many individuals approve of legal abortion as an option when destructive health or welfare consequences could result from continuing pregnancy, but they do not advocate abortion as a simple way out of an inconvenient situation. Overall, most adults in the United States continue to approve of legal abortion and are opposed to overturning the basic right to abortion established in *Roe v. Wade* (Figure 6-4). But the amount of public support varies considerably, depending on the circumstances surrounding the abortion request (Table 6-4).

VITAL STATISTICS

Table 6-4   Views on Abortion

1. Should a pregnant woman be able to obtain an abortion in the following circumstances?

	Yes
Her life is endangered.	84%
Her physical health is endangered.	81%
The pregnancy was caused by rape or incest.	78%
Her mental health is endangered.	64%
The baby is physically or mentally impaired.	53%
The woman or family cannot afford to raise the child.	34%

2. Should a woman be permitted to have an abortion during the following stages of pregnancy?

	Yes
In the first 3 months	65%
In the second 3 months	24%
In the last 3 months	8%

SOURCE: Gallup Organization. 2000. *Abortion Issues* (http://www.gallup.com/poll/Indicators/indabortion.asp; retrieved September 22, 2000).

Although opinions vary as to whether, or when, abortion rights should be tightly regulated by law, most people agree that abortions done later in pregnancy present more difficulties in personal, medical, philosophical, and social terms. Of all abortions done after the 12th week of gestation, more than 35% are performed on teenagers. Possible explanations include teenagers' ignorance, denial, fear, and lack of supportive family or friends, as well as state regulatory hurdles faced by teenagers. Other typical recipients of late abortions include low-income women, who may have more difficulty finding suitable facilities as well as necessary funds, and premenopausal women who fail to recognize a delayed period as pregnancy. Another small group of women who may seek late abortion are those who have learned through genetic tests that the fetus has a specific abnormality.

Current Trends

With the increased accessibility to legalized abortion following the mid-1970s, the rate of late abortions dropped steadily, until fewer than 1% of all abortions were performed at more than 20 weeks and fewer than 12% at more than 12 weeks by the 1990s (Figure 6-5). The overall abortion *rate* rose during most of the 1970s, leveled off around 1980, and decreased in the 1990s (Figure 6-6). Possible future influences on the number, rate, and timing of abortions in the United States include legal decisions,

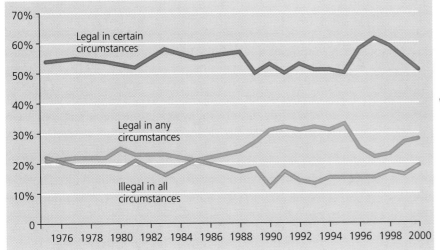

Figure 6-4 Public opinion about abortion. This graph represents responses to the question: Do you think abortions should be legal under any circumstances, legal only under certain circumstances, or illegal in all circumstances? SOURCE: Gallup Organization. 2001. *Majority of Americans Say* Roe v. Wade *Decision Should Stand.* (http://www.gallup.com/poll/releases/pr010122.asp; retrieved January 24, 2001).

more widespread availability of emergency contraceptives, and the increasing use of medical abortion.

Since the 1989 *Webster* and 1992 *Casey* decisions, many states have imposed additional restrictions on abortion. By 2001, 30 states required mandatory counseling, followed in 19 states by a waiting period; 42 states required parental consent or notification for minors; more than half of the states banned certain abortion procedures; and 32 states restricted the use of public funds for abortion. Overall, the number of laws restricting abortion in the states has more than quadrupled since 1995. Research into the effects of these restrictions has been mixed. Parental consent and notification laws may result in minors traveling out of state to obtain abortions. Mandatory delay laws have been found to influence the number and timing of abortions.

Adding to the legal restrictions is the growing scarcity of physicians willing to provide abortion services. Currently, 86% of all U.S. counties, 90% of rural counties, and about 30% of metropolitan areas have no abortion providers. It is unclear whether the approval of mifepristone for medical abortion will significantly affect these numbers. The diminishing number of providers is due in part to increased anti-abortion protests and violence, including arson, bombings, and the murders of several physicians and clinic workers. Women living in areas that have restrictive laws and few abortion providers may continue to obtain abortions, but they are likely to face significant increases in expense and time delays.

Unless accompanied by a greater effort at preventing unwanted pregnancy, especially among the young single women who make up the majority of those seeking abortions, legal changes alone will probably not dramatically reduce the number of abortions. At current rates, about 43% of American women will have at least one abortion by the time they are 45 years old.

Methods of Abortion

Abortion methods can be divided into two categories: surgical and medical. Surgical abortion is by far the most common, accounting for about 98% of all abortions performed in the United States. Medical abortion, in which medications are used to induce abortion, may become more common following the approval in 2000 of mifepristone (Mifeprex).

Suction curettage, also called vacuum aspiration, is the most common method of abortion from the 6th to the 12th week of pregnancy; it is used in about 90% of all abortions performed in the United States. In this procedure, the cervix is dilated and a suction curette, a hollow tube attached to an electric pump, is inserted into the uterus. Suction is applied to empty the uterus, and the uterine lining is usually scraped with a metal curette to remove any remaining tissue. The procedure takes about 5–10 minutes and has a low risk of complications.

Because suction curettage is believed to be more effective if performed at least 6 or 7 weeks after the last menstrual period, pregnant women seeking abortion early in pregnancy are sometimes told to wait several weeks. A relatively new option available at some clinics for women at the very earliest stages of pregnancy is a surgical procedure called **manual vacuum aspiration (MVA).** In MVA, the cervix is dilated and a plastic tube attached to a handheld syringe is inserted into the uterus, which is then emptied with gentle suction provided by the syringe.

---

suction curettage Removal of the embryo or fetus by means of suction; also called *vacuum aspiration.*

manual vacuum aspiration (MVA) The vacuum aspiration of uterine contents shortly after a missed period using a handheld syringe.

Terms

By woman's age

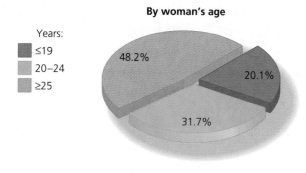

Years:
- ■ ≤19
- ■ 20–24
- ■ ≥25

48.2%
20.1%
31.7%

By gestation period

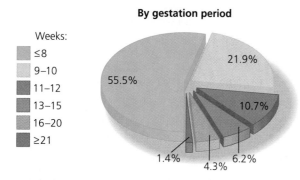

Weeks:
- ■ ≤8
- ■ 9–10
- ■ 11–12
- ■ 13–15
- ■ 16–20
- ■ ≥21

55.5%
21.9%
10.7%
1.4%
4.3%
6.2%

VITAL STATISTICS

Figure 6-5   Distribution of abortions by the woman's age and by the weeks of gestation.   SOURCE: Centers for Disease Control and Prevention. 2000. Abortion surveillance—United States, 1997. *Morbidity and Mortality Weekly Report* 49(SS–11).

Medical abortion, ending a pregnancy with medications rather than surgery, is an option for women who are in the early phase of pregnancy. The drug mifepristone, also called RU-486 or the "abortion pill," can be administered under medical supervision up to 49 days following the last menstrual period. A woman takes a dose of mifepristone and follows it up two days later with a second drug, misprostol, which induces contractions. Abortion can take anywhere from a few hours to several weeks; about 75% of abortions occur within 24 hours. Two weeks after taking mifepristone, a woman must return to her health care provider for a follow-up visit. The two-drug regimen has a rate of completed abortion of about 92–95%. A second drug, methotrexate, can also be used with misoprostol for early medical abortion; however, methotrexate is slightly less effective than mifepristone.

Only about 1 in 10 abortions is performed after the 12th week of pregnancy. The method most commonly used for abortion from 13 to 24 weeks of pregnancy is **dilation and evacuation (D & E).** The cervix is gradually opened overnight using dilators; the next day, the uterus is emptied using surgical instruments and an aspirating machine. *Partial birth abortion* is a nonmedical term for a particular type of D & E in which the fetal limbs and body are delivered first and then the skull is collapsed to allow it to pass more easily through the cervix. This procedure is performed only rarely, but it can be useful in the presence of fetal anomalies such as severe hydrocephalus (a condition in which fluid collects around the brain, causing brain damage and an enlarged head). Chemically inducing labor is another infrequently used method of late abortion.

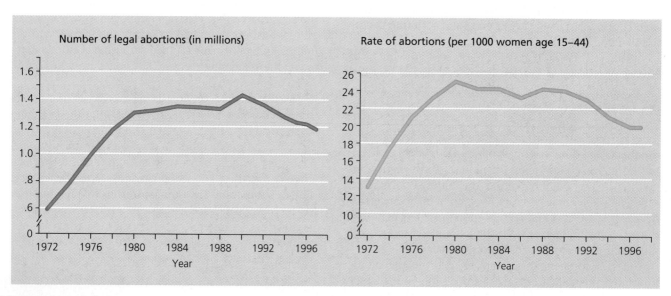

VITAL STATISTICS

Figure 6-6   Abortion rates in the United States.   SOURCE: Centers for Disease Control and Prevention. 2000. Abortion surveillance—United States, 1997. *Morbidity and Mortality Weekly Report* 49(SS–11).

One of the options available to a woman facing an unplanned pregnancy is adoption. Between 1952 and 1972, nearly 9% of unmarried pregnant women gave their children up for adoption; currently, however, only about 2% of women choose to place a child for adoption. This decline is probably due to a variety of factors, including increased rates of contraceptive use and an easing of the social stigma of single parenthood. The drop in adoption rates in the 1970s probably reflected an increase in the abortion rate following the 1973 legalization of abortion; however, since 1990 adoption rates have remained steady, while the abortion rate has declined, indicating that women are not choosing abortion over adoption.

If you are pregnant and considering adoption, make sure you explore all possibilities before you make a final choice. The decision to go through an unwanted pregnancy and then give the baby to another family is difficult and takes tremendous love, maturity, and courage. Adoption is permanent: The adoptive parents will raise your child and have legal authority for his or her welfare. Think about your life now and in the future as you weigh alternatives. There are many people who can help you consider your options, including your partner, friends, family members, or a professional counselor at a crisis pregnancy center, family planning clinic, or family services, social services, or adoption agency. A counselor should always treat you with respect and be willing to discuss all your options with you—keeping the baby, having an abortion, or arranging an adoption. If you aren't comfortable with a particular counselor, find a different one.

There are two types of adoptions, confidential and open. In confidential adoption, the birth parents and the adoptive parents never know each other. Adoptive parents will be given any information, such as medical information, that they would need to help take care of the child. A later meeting between the child and birth parents is possible in confidential adoption, however, if the birth parents leave information with the agency or lawyer who handled the adoption and/or in a national adoption registry. In an open adoption, the birth parents and adoptive parents know something about each other. There are different levels of openness, ranging from reading a brief description of prospective adoptive parents to meeting them and sharing full information. Birth parents may also be able to arrange to stay in touch with the family over the years, by visiting, calling, or writing. Some women feel that an open adoption enables them to keep in touch with a baby they will always love; others feel that this would be too difficult and decide against contact with the adoptive family.

In all states, you can work with a licensed child-placing (adoption) agency. In most, you can also work directly with an adopting couple or their attorney; this is called a private or independent adoption. Prospective adoptive parents can be located through personal ads, a physician, adoptive parent support groups, national matching services, and family members and friends.

You will also need to consider the reaction and rights of the birth father. A woman can choose to have an abortion without the consent or knowledge of the father, but once the baby is born, the father has certain rights. If you are considering placing a child for adoption, it is important to find out about birth fathers' rights in your state and to make appropriate arrangements.

As with abortion, there are emotional and physical risks associated with pregnancy, childbirth, and adoption. Throughout the adoption process, make sure that you have the help you need and that you carefully consider all your options. Deciding how to handle an unplanned pregnancy is important, and you have the power to make your own decisions.

SOURCES: National Adoption Information Clearinghouse. 2000. *Are You Pregnant and Thinking About Adoption?* (http://www.calib.com/naic/ pubs/ f_pregna.htm; retrieved September 21, 2000). National Adoption Information Clearinghouse. 2000. *Placing Children for Adoption* (http://www.calib. com/naic/pubs/s_place.htm; retrieved September 21, 2000).

Complications of Abortion

Along with questions regarding the actual procedure of abortion, many people have concerns about possible aftereffects. More information is gradually being gathered on this important subject.

Possible Physical Effects   The incidence of immediate problems following an abortion (infection, bleeding, trauma to the cervix or uterus, and incomplete abortion requiring repeat curettage) varies widely. The potential for problems is significantly reduced by a woman's good health, early timing of the abortion, use of the suction method and local anesthetic, performance by a well-trained clinician, and the availability and use of prompt follow-up care. Studies on long-term complications—subsequent infertility, spontaneous second abortions, pre-mature delivery, and babies of low birth weight—have not revealed any major risks with the most common abortion methods.

Problems related specifically to infection can be minimized through preabortion testing and treatment for gonorrhea, chlamydia, and other infections. Postabortion danger signs are fever above 100°F; abdominal pain or swelling, cramping, or backache; abdominal tenderness; prolonged or heavy bleeding; foul-smelling vaginal discharge; vomiting or fainting; and a delay in resuming menstrual periods (6 weeks or more).

dilation and evacuation (D & E) The method of abortion most commonly used between 13 and 15 weeks of pregnancy. Following dilation of the cervix, both vacuum aspiration and curettage instruments are used as needed.

Terms

In September 2000, the FDA approved the use of mifepristone (trade name Mifeprex) in the United States for the termination of early pregnancy. Mifepristone, also known as RU-486 or the "abortion pill," has been mired in controversy for the past two decades. It was first approved for use for medical abortion in France in 1988. Protests in the United States, France, and Germany led the manufacturer to temporarily take the drug off the market, but distribution was resumed by the order of the French minister of health in the interests of public health. Since then, more than 600,000 women in Europe have had medical abortions using mifepristone. The drug has also been approved for use in the United Kingdom, China, Russia, Israel, and much of Europe.

Despite political opposition, clinical trials of the drug were allowed in the United States during the mid-1990s. In 1996, the FDA stated that mifepristone is safe and effective for abortion in early pregnancy and that it could be approved for use if concerns regarding manufacturing and labeling were resolved. However, political and manufacturing issues delayed final approval until 2000.

Pro-life groups in the United States have strongly opposed the approval of mifepristone, at least in part because of concerns that it would make abortion easier to obtain and more common. Groups that target abortion clinics and providers would have a more difficult time organizing protests if medical abortion were widely available in the privacy of a physician's office. Opponents of mifepristone also point to the drug's side effects and potential health risks.

Those in favor of the drug's approval argue that ready access to very early medical abortion would help decrease the need for riskier late abortions. Widespread availability of mifepristone could also help ensure access to abortion services for poor women and women who live in areas with no providers of surgical abortion. Surveys indicate that some physicians who do not currently provide surgical abortions would be willing to prescribe mifepristone. There are some special requirements, however: Physicians who distribute mifepristone must be able to accurately determine the duration of a pregnancy and to detect an ectopic pregnancy; they must also be able to either provide surgical intervention in cases of incomplete abortion or severe bleeding or arrange in advance to provide such care through others.

The FDA approval of mifepristone is unlikely to end the controversy. Individuals and groups opposed to abortion have promised to work through legislative and legal channels in an effort to have the drug removed from the market or its use restricted. Changes in the makeup of the U.S. Supreme Court or Cabinet could also affect the status of mifepristone. It is also unclear how the use of mifepristone will fit into current legal requirements in some states for such things as waiting periods and parental notification; states may also pass additional laws specifically related to mifepristone.

On the national level, legislation has been introduced to ban all drugs that can be used to induce abortion. If passed, such a law could have effects far beyond a ban on mifepristone, because some medications used to treat serious illnesses also induce abortion. For example, methotrexate is widely used to treat both cancer and rheumatoid arthritis. Mifepristone itself may have potential medical uses besides pregnancy termination, including treatment of breast cancer, endometriosis, and glaucoma. Banning all drugs that can be used to induce abortion could limit the development of new therapies for a variety of diseases. Other proposed legislation would require formal training and certification for any physician who plans to prescribe mifepristone.

Even if the drug remains available and is offered by a significant number of physicians, it is unclear what effect it will have on patterns and rates of abortion in the United States. In France, where the drug has been used extensively, the abortion rate has actually declined since the drug was introduced. Mifepristone is used in about 20–30% of all abortions performed in France; as in the United States, surgical abortion is still used in the majority of cases.

Possible Psychological Effects   After an exhaustive review completed in 1988, the then surgeon general, C. Everett Koop, concluded that the available evidence failed to demonstrate either a negative or a positive long-term impact of abortion on mental health. More recent research has resulted in the same general conclusion. The psychological side effects of abortion are less clearly defined than the physical ones. Responses vary and depend on the individual woman's psychological makeup, family background, current personal and social relationships, cultural attitudes, and many other factors. A woman who has specific goals with a somewhat structured life pattern may be able to incorporate her decision to have an abortion as the unequivocally "best" and acceptable course more easily than a woman who feels uncertain about her future.

Although many women experience great relief after an abortion and virtually no negative feelings, some go through a period of ambivalence. Along with relief, they often feel a mixture of other responses, such as guilt, regret, loss, sadness, and/or anger.

For a woman who does experience psychological or emotional effects after an abortion, talking with a close friend or family member can be very helpful. Supportive people can help her feel positive about herself and her decision. In a few cases, unresolved emotions may persist, and a woman should seek professional counseling.

Your decisions about contraception and abortion are among the most important you will make in your life. They affect your physical and emotional health, your relationship and family choices, and your career and life plans. You may never have to face an unintended pregnancy, but you should know what choices you would have—abortion, adoption, parenthood—as well as where you stand on the issue. Take time out now to consider your personal views on contraception and abortion.

Right now you can

- Close your eyes and visualize the life you hope to have in 5 years, 10 years, and 15 years. Does it include a relationship, a family, children? Are you doing anything right now— such as taking a chance on an unintended pregnancy— that could prevent you from realizing your dreams?

- If you are sexually active or considering becoming so, make an appointment with a physician or health care practitioner to discuss which contraceptive method is right for you.

- Take time to consider your views on the morality of abortion. If you are sexually active, talk to your partner about abortion—do you have similar views and feelings, or are they different? How would you resolve a conflict?

SUMMARY

- Barrier methods of contraception physically prevent sperm from reaching the egg; hormonal methods are designed to prevent ovulation, fertilization, and/or implantation; and surgical methods permanently block the movement of sperm or eggs to the site of conception.

- In oral contraceptives (OCs), a combination of estrogen and progestins prevents ovulation, inhibits the movement of sperm, and affects the uterine lining so that implantation is prevented.

- Contraceptive implants consist of hormone-filled capsules inserted under the skin that release steady doses of synthetic progesterone.

- Depo-Provera injections contain a long-acting progestin that protects against pregnancy for a period of 3 months. Lunelle injections contain both estrogen and progestin and must be repeated every month.

- The most commonly used emergency contraceptives are two-dose regimens of combined or progesterone-only oral contraceptives.

- How IUDs work is not clearly understood; they may cause biochemical changes in the uterus, affect movement of sperm and eggs, or interfere with the implantation of the egg in the uterus.

- Advantages of male condoms include availability and ease of purchase, simplicity of use, immediate reversibility, STD protection, and freedom from side effects. Female condoms consist of a polyurethane sheath that can be inserted well before intercourse.

- A diaphragm or cervical cap covers the cervix and blocks sperm from entering. The contraceptive sponge is a round device that is saturated with spermicide.

- Vaginal spermicides come in the form of foams, creams, jellies, suppositories, and film.

- The so-called natural methods include abstinence, the fertility awareness methods, and withdrawal.

- Vasectomy—male sterilization—involves severing the vasa deferentia. Female sterilization involves severing or blocking the oviducts so that the egg cannot reach the uterus.

- Issues to be considered in choosing a contraceptive include the health risks of each method, the implications of an unplanned pregnancy, STD risk, convenience and comfort level, type of relationship, the cost and ease of obtaining and maintaining each method, and religious or philosophical beliefs.

- The 1973 *Roe v. Wade* Supreme Court case devised new standards to govern abortion decisions; based on the trimesters of pregnancy, it limited a woman's choices as her pregnancy advanced.

- Although the Supreme Court continued to uphold its 1973 decision, it gave states further power to regulate abortion in *Webster v. Reproductive Health Services* and *Planned Parenthood of Southeastern Pennsylvania v. Casey*.

- The controversy between pro-life and pro-choice viewpoints focuses on the issue of when life begins. Overall public opinion in the United States supports legal abortion in at least some circumstances and opposes overturning *Roe v. Wade*.

- Methods of abortion include suction curettage, manual vacuum aspiration, dilation and evacuation, and medical abortion using mifepristone and misoprostol.

- Physical complications following abortion can be minimized by good patient care. Psychological aftereffects of abortion vary with the individual; having a supportive partner, friend, and/or family member can be helpful.

1. Make an appointment with a physician or other health care provider to review the health risks of different contraceptive methods as they apply to you. For each method, determine whether any risk factors associated with its use apply to you or your partner.

2. Visit a local drugstore and make a list of the contraceptives they sell, along with their prices. Next, investigate the costs of prescription contraceptive methods by contacting your physician, medical clinic, and/or phar-

macy. Estimate the annual cost of regular use for each method, and rank the methods from most to least expensive.

3. Survey your classmates about their position on the abortion issue. How many people consider themselves pro-choice and how many pro-life? How strong are their opinions? What, if anything, might cause them to change their minds? Do opinions seem to depend on age, gender, or any other factor?

WW. JOURNAL ENTRY

1. Consider the different methods of contraception described in this chapter. In your health journal, rank the methods according to how they suit your particular lifestyle. Take into account such considerations as convenience, cost, and how often you have sexual intercourse.

2. In your health journal, list the positive behaviors and attitudes that help you adhere to your beliefs about contraception. (For example, not getting drunk would probably help prevent you from making an unwise choice.) Are there ways you can strengthen these behav-

iors? Then list behaviors and attitudes that might interfere with your effective use of contraception. Can you do anything to change or improve any of these?

3. ***Critical Thinking*** Write a one-page essay presenting your personal opinion on the abortion issue. Include arguments to refute the points typically made by the opposing side. Then write an essay presenting a convincing case for the opposite position. Make sure your arguments are clearly stated and that you can defend them, where appropriate, with facts.

FOR MORE INFORMATION

Books

Boston Women's Health Book Collective. 1998. *Our Bodies, Ourselves for the New Century.* New York: Simon & Schuster. *Broad coverage of many women's health concerns, with extensive coverage of contraception.*

Glasier, A., and B. Winikoff. 2000. *Fast Facts: Contraception.* Oxford: Health Press. *Basic facts and figures related to contraceptive methods, including future trends. Succinct and easy to read.*

Hatcher, R. A., et al. 1998. *Contraceptive Technology,* 17th rev. ed. New York: Ardent Media. *A reliable source of up-to-date information on contraception.*

Hatcher, R. A., et al. 2000. *Safely Sexual.* New York: Ardent Media. *Realistic recommendations on the prevention of unplanned pregnancy, as well as HIV infection and other STDs.*

National Abortion and Reproductive Rights Action League Foundation. 2001. *Who Decides: A State-by-State Review of Abortion and Reproductive Rights.* Washington, D.C.: NARAL Foundations. *An in-depth annual review of the legal status of reproductive rights in the United States.*

Rein, M. L., et al., eds. 2000. *Abortion 2000: An Eternal Social and Moral Issue.* Wylie, Tex.: Information Plus. *A brief reference outlining the legal, political, and ethical issues relating to abortion.*

Tone, A. 2001. *Devices and Desires: Men, Women, and the Commercialization of Contraception in the United States.* New York: Hill and Wang. *An engaging history of contraception in America.*

WW. Organizations, Hotlines, and Web Sites

Abortion Law Homepage. Includes an overview of the background and state of U.S abortion law, including the text of major legal decisions.

http://hometown.aol.com/abtrbng

The Alan Guttmacher Institute. A nonprofit institute for reproductive health research, policy analysis, and public education.

212-248-1111

http://www.agi-usa.org

Ann Rose's Ultimate Birth Control Links Page. A Web site with information on methods of birth control and decision-making strategies.

http://gynpages.com/ultimate

Association of Reproductive Health Professionals. Offers educational materials about family planning, contraception, and other reproductive health issues; the Web site includes an interactive questionnaire to help people choose contraceptive methods.

202-466-3825

http://www.arhp.org

Emergency Contraception Hotline. Provides information and referrals.

888-NOT-2-LATE

Emergency Contraception Web Site. Provides extensive information about emergency contraception; sponsored by the Office of Population Research at Princeton University.

http://ec.princeton.edu

It's Your Sex Life. Provides information about sexuality, relationships, contraceptives, and STDs; geared toward teenagers and young adults.

> http://www.itsyoursexlife.com

Managing Contraception. Provides brief descriptions and tips for using many forms of contraception.

> http://www.managingcontraception.com

National Abortion and Reproductive Rights Action League. Provides information on the politics of the pro-choice movement.

> 202-973-3000
>
> http://www.naral.org

National Adoption Information Clearinghouse. Provides resources on all aspects of adoption.

> 888-251-0075
>
> http://www.calib.com/naic

National Right to Life Committee. Provides information on alternatives to abortion and the politics of the pro-life movement.

> 202-626-8800
>
> http://www.nrlc.org

Planned Parenthood Federation of America. Provides information on family planning, contraception, and abortion and provides counseling services.

> 800-669-0156 (to order publications)
>
> 800-230-PLAN (for a list of health centers)
>
> http://www.plannedparenthood.org

Reproductive Health Online (Reproline). Presents information on contraceptive methods currently available and those under study for future use.

> http://www.reproline.jhu.edu

U.S. Food and Drug Administration: Mifepristone. Provides information on the testing, labeling, and use of mifepristone.

> http://www.fda.gov/cder/drug/infopage/mifepristone

See also the listings for Chapters 5 and 13.

SELECTED BIBLIOGRAPHY

Alan Guttmacher Institute. 2000. *Facts in Brief: Induced Abortion* (http://www.agi-usa.org/pubs/fb_induced_abortion.html; retrieved September 22, 2000).

American College of Obstetricians and Gynecologists. 2000. *Statement of the American College of Obstetricians and Gynecologists on the U.S. Supreme Court Abortion Case* Stenberg v. Carhart, *April 21, 2000* (http://www.acog.com/from_home/publications/press-releases/nr04-21-00.htm; retrieved July 5, 2000).

Annas G. J. 2001. Partial-birth abortion and the Supreme Court. *New England Journal of Medicine* 344(2):152–156.

Burkman, R. T. 2001. Oral contraceptives: Current status. *Clinical Obstetrics and Gynecology* 44(1): 62–72.

Centers for Disease Control and Prevention. 2000. Abortion surveillance—United States, 1997. *Morbidity and Mortality Weekly Report* 49(SS-11).

Centers for Disease Control and Prevention. 2000. National and state-specific pregnancy rates among adolescents—United States, 1995–1997. *Morbidity and Mortality Weekly Report* 49(27): 605–611.

Christin-Maitre, S., P. Bouchar, and I. Spitz. 2000. Drug therapy: Medical termination of pregnancy. *New England Journal of Medicine* 342(13): 946–956.

Croxatto, H. B. 2000. Progestagen implants. *International Planned Parenthood Federation Medical Bulletin* 34(1): 1–3.

Dunn, N., et al. 2000. Oral contraceptives and myocardial infarction: A meta-analysis. *Journal of the American Medical Association* 284(1): 72–78.

International Medical Advisory Panel (IMAP). 2000. IMAP statement on the non-latex condom. 2000. *International Planned Parenthood Federation Medical Bulletin* 34(1): 3.

Le, J., and C. Tsourounis. 2001. Implanon: A critical review. *Annals of Pharmacotherapy* 35(3): 329–36.

Major, B., et al. 2000. Psychological responses of women after first-trimester abortion. *Archives of General Psychiatry* 57(8): 777–784.

McClanahan, P., et al. 2000. Characteristics of Norplant users. *Journal of Obstetric, Gynecologic, and Neonatal Nursing* 29(3): 275–281.

Melbye, M., et al. 1997. Induced abortion and the risk of breast cancer. *New England Journal of Medicine* 336(2): 81–85.

National Abortion and Reproductive Rights Action League. 2001. *Who Decides: A State-by-State Review of Abortion and Reproductive Rights* (http://www.naral.org; retrieved February 12, 2001).

Perlman, S. E., et al. 2001. Contraception. Myths, facts and methods. *Journal of Reproductive Medicine* 46(2 Suppl): 169–77.

Princeton University Office of Population Research: Emergency Contraception World Wide Web Site. 2000. *Emergency Contraception* (http://ec.princeton.edu/info/ecp.html; retrieved July 19, 2000).

Rodrigues, I., F. Grou, and J. Joly. 2001. Effectiveness of emergency contraceptive pills between 72 and 120 hours after unprotected sexual intercourse. *American Journal of Obstetrics and Gynecology* 184(4): 531–537.

Rosen, A. D., and T. Rosen. 1999. Study of condom integrity after brief exposure to over-the-counter vaginal preparations. *Southern Medical Journal* 92(3): 305–307.

Schwingl, P. J., and H. A. Guess. 2000. Safety and effectiveness of vasectomy. *Fertility and Sterility* 73(5): 923–936.

Shelton, J. D. 2001. Risk of clinical pelvic inflammatory disease attributable to an intrauterine device. *Lancet* 357(9254): 443.

Skegg, D. C. G. 1999. Oral contraception and health: Long term study of mortality shows no overall effect in a developed country. *British Medical Journal* 318: 69–70.

Stephenson, J. 2000. Widely used spermicide may increase, not decrease, risk of HIV transmission. *Journal of the American Medical Association* 284(8): 949.

Supreme Court of the United States. 2000. *Stenberg, Attorney General of Nebraska, et al. v. Carhart* (http://www.supremecourtus.gov/opinions/99pdf/99-830.pdf; retrieved September 22, 2000).

Tan, J. K., and H. Degreef. 2001. Oral contraceptives in the treatment of acne. *Skin Therapy Letter* 6(5): 1–3.

U.S. Food and Drug Administration, Center for Drug Evaluation and Research. 2000. *Mifepristone Questions and Answers* (http://www.fda.gov/cder/drug/infopage/mifepristone/mifepristone-qa.htm; retrieved September 28, 2000).

Wiebe, E. R. 2001. Misoprostol administration in medical abortion. A comparison of three regimens. *Journal of Reproductive Medicine* 46(2): 125–129.

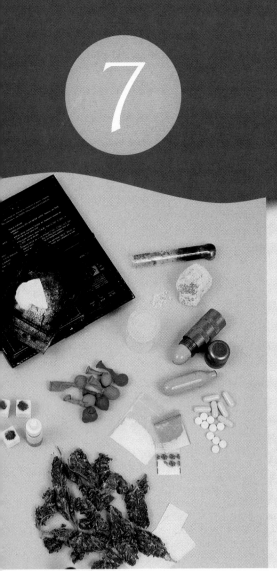

7

The Use and Abuse of Psychoactive Drugs

LOOKING AHEAD

After reading this chapter, you should be able to

- Define and discuss the concepts of addictive behavior, substance abuse, and substance dependence
- Explain factors contributing to drug use and dependence
- List the major categories of psychoactive drugs and describe their effects, methods of use, and potential for abuse and dependence
- Discuss social issues related to psychoactive drug use and its prevention and treatment
- Evaluate the role of drugs and other addictive behaviors in your life and identify your risk factors for abuse or dependence

The use of **drugs** for both medical and social purposes is widespread in American society (Table 7-1). Many people believe that every problem, no matter how large or small, has or should have chemical solutions. For fatigue, many of us turn to caffeine; for insomnia, sleeping pills; for anxiety or boredom, alcohol or other recreational drugs. Advertisements, social pressures, and the human desire for quick fixes to life's difficult problems all contribute to the prevailing attitude that drugs can ease all pain. Unfortunately, using drugs can—and often does—have serious consequences.

The most serious consequences are abuse and addiction. The drugs most often associated with abuse are **psychoactive drugs**—those designed to alter a person's experiences or consciousness. In the short term, psychoactive drugs can cause **intoxication.** A person who is intoxicated may experience unpredictable and potentially serious changes in physical functioning; his or her emotions and judgment may be affected in ways that lead to un-

characteristic and unsafe behavior. In the long term, recurrent drug use can have profound physical, emotional, and social effects.

ADDICTIVE BEHAVIOR

Although addiction is most often associated with drug use, many experts now extend the concept of addiction to other areas. **Addictive behaviors** are habits that have gotten out of control, with a resulting negative impact on a person's health. Looking at the nature of addiction and a range of addictive behaviors can help us understand similar behaviors when they involve drugs.

What Is Addiction?

The word *addiction* tends to be a highly charged one for most people. We may jokingly say we're "addicted to" fudge swirl ice cream or our morning jog, but most of us

Table 7-1	Nonmedical Drug Use Among Americans	
	Percentage Using Substance in the Past 30 Days	
	College Students	All Americans
Alcohol	63.2	47.3
Tobacco (all forms)*	39.6	30.2
Cigarettes	*33.8*	*25.8*
Cigars	*11.4*	*5.5*
Spit tobacco	*5.4*	*3.4*
Pipes	*1.4*	*1.1*
Marijuana/hashish	17.3	5.1
Pain relievers	2.5	1.2
Hallucinogens	2.3	0.4
Cocaine	1.4	0.7
Stimulants	1.2	0.4
Inhalants	1.1	0.5
Tranquilizers	0.9	0.5
Sedatives	0.1	0.1
Heroin	0.0	0.1

*Some people use more than one form of tobacco, so the sum of the percentages for different forms of tobacco exceeds the total percentage of tobacco users.

SOURCE: Substance Abuse and Mental Health Services Administration. 2000. *National Household Survey on Drug Abuse, 1999—Appendix G: Detailed National Tables* (http://www.samhsa.gov/oas/NHSDA/1999/Appendixg.htm; retrieved October 4, 2000).

think of true addiction as a habitual and uncontrollable behavior, usually involving the use of a drug. Some people think of addiction as a moral flaw or a personal weakness. Others think addictions arise from certain personality traits, genetic factors, or socioeconomic influences. Views on the causes of addictions have an impact on our attitudes toward people with addictive disorders, as well as on the approaches to treatment.

Historically, the term *addiction* was applied only when the habitual use of a drug produced chemical changes in the user's body. One such change is physical tolerance, in which the body adapts to a drug so that the initial dose no longer produces the original emotional or psychological effects. This process, caused by chemical changes, means the user has to take larger and larger doses of the drug to achieve the same "high." (Tolerance will be discussed in greater detail later in the chapter.) The concept of addiction as a disease process, one based in brain chemistry, rather than a moral failing, has led to many advances in the understanding and treatment of drug addiction.

Some scientists think that other behaviors may share some of the chemistry of drug addiction. Activities like gambling, eating, exercising, and sex may trigger the release of brain chemicals that cause a pleasurable "rush" in much the same way that psychoactive drugs do. The brain's own chemicals thus become the "drug" that can cause addiction. These theorists suggest that drug addiction and addiction to other pleasurable behaviors have a common mechanism in the brain. In this view, addiction is partly the result of our own natural "wiring."

However, and very importantly, the view that addiction is based in our own brain chemistry does *not* imply that an individual bears no responsibility for his or her addictive behavior. Many experts believe that it is inaccurate and counterproductive to think of all bad habits and excessive behaviors as diseases. They point to other factors, especially lifestyle and personality traits, that play key roles in the development of addictive behaviors.

Characteristics of Addictive Behavior

It is often difficult to distinguish between a healthy habit and one that has become an addiction. Experts have identified some general characteristics typically associated with addictive behaviors:

- *Reinforcement.* Addictive behaviors are physically and/or psychologically reinforcing. Some aspect of the behavior produces pleasurable physical and/or emotional states or relieves negative ones.

- *Compulsion or craving.* The individual feels a strong compulsion—a compelling need—to engage in the behavior, often accompanied by obsessive planning for the next opportunity to perform it.

- *Loss of control.* The individual loses control over the behavior and cannot block the impulse to engage in it. He or she may deny that the behavior is problematic or may have tried but failed to control it.

- *Escalation.* Addiction often involves a pattern of escalation, in which more and more of a particular substance or activity is required to produce its desired effects. This escalation typically means that a person must give an increasing amount of his or her time, attention, and resources to the behavior.

- *Negative consequences.* The behavior has serious negative consequences, such as problems with academic or job performance, personal relationships, and health; legal or financial troubles are also typical.

drug Any chemical other than food intended to affect the structure or function of the body.

psychoactive drug A drug that can alter a person's consciousness or experience.

intoxication The state of being mentally affected by a chemical (literally, a state of being poisoned).

addictive behavior Any habit that has gotten out of control, resulting in a negative effect on one's health.

Terms

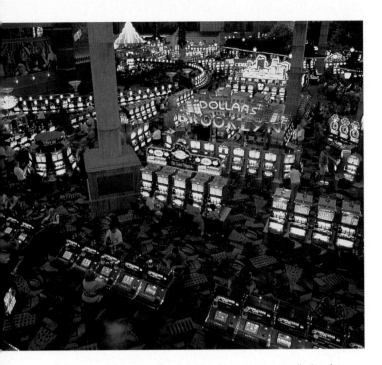

Most people who gamble do so casually and occasionally, but for a few, the habit spins out of control and becomes the central focus of their life. A variety of factors appear to influence whether a habit becomes an addiction, including personality, lifestyle, heredity, social environment, and the nature of the activity.

The Development of Addiction

There is no single cause of addiction. Instead, characteristics of an individual person, of the environment in which the person lives, and of the substance or behavior he or she abuses combine in an addictive behavior.

We all engage in activities that are potentially addictive. Some of these activities can be part of a wellness lifestyle if they are done appropriately and in moderation, but if a behavior starts to be excessive, it may become an addiction. An addiction often starts when a person does something he or she thinks will bring pleasure or help avoid pain. The activity may be drinking a beer, going on the Internet, playing the lottery, or going shopping. If it works, and the behavior does bring pleasure or dull pain, the person is likely to repeat it. He or she becomes increasingly dependent on the behavior, and tolerance develops—that is, the person needs more of the behavior to feel the same effect. Eventually, the behavior becomes a central focus of the person's life, and there is a deterioration in other areas, such as school performance or relationships. The behavior no longer brings pleasure, but it is necessary to avoid the pain of going without it.

Many common behaviors are potentially addictive, but most people who engage in them do not develop problems. The reason, again, lies in the combination of factors that are involved in the development of addiction, including personality, lifestyle, heredity, the social and physical environment, and the nature of the substance or behavior in question. For a behavior to become an addiction, these diverse factors must come together in a certain way. For example, nicotine, the psychoactive drug in tobacco, has a very high potential for physical addiction; but a person who doesn't choose to try cigarettes, perhaps because of family influence or a tendency to develop asthma, will never develop nicotine addiction.

Characteristics of People with Addictions

The causes and course of an addiction are extremely varied, but people with addictions do seem to share some characteristics. Many use the substance or activity as a substitute for other, healthier, coping strategies. People vary in their ability to manage their lives, and those who have the most trouble dealing with stress and painful emotions may be more susceptible to addiction.

Some people may have a genetic predisposition to addiction to a particular substance; such predispositions may involve variations in brain chemistry. People with addictive disorders usually have a distinct preference for a particular addictive behavior, and they typically expect to have a positive experience with it even before they try it. They also often have problems with impulse control and self-regulation and tend to be risk takers.

WWW. Examples of Addictive Behaviors

The use and abuse of psychoactive drugs will be explored in detail later in the chapter. In this section, we'll examine some behaviors that are not related to drugs and that can become addictive for some people.

Compulsive or Pathological Gambling Many people gamble casually by putting a dollar in the office football pool, buying a lottery ticket, or going to the races. But a few become compulsive gamblers, unable to resist or control the urge to gamble, even in the face of financial and personal ruin. Most compulsive gamblers say they are seeking excitement even more than money. Increasingly larger bets are necessary to produce the desired level of excitement. A series of losses can lead to a perceived need to keep placing bets to win back the money. When financial resources become strained, the person may lie or steal to pay off debts. The consequences of compulsive gambling are not just financial; the suicide rate of compulsive gamblers is 20 times higher than that of the general population.

Compulsive gamblers may gamble to relieve negative feelings and become restless and irritable when they are unable to gamble. As with many addictive behaviors, compulsive gambling may begin or flare up in times of stress. Many compulsive gamblers also have drug and alcohol abuse problems.

The American Psychiatric Association (APA) recognizes pathological gambling as a mental disorder and lists ten characteristic behaviors, including preoccupation with gambling, unsuccessful efforts to cut back or quit, using gambling to escape problems, and lying to family members to conceal the extent of involvement with gambling. Compulsive gambling shares many of these traits with other addictive behaviors, including drug use. An estimated 1.1 million adolescents and 1.9 million adults in the United States may be compulsive gamblers. These numbers may increase due to the spread of legalized gambling, both on the Internet and on American Indian tribal reservations.

Compulsive Spending or Shopping A compulsive spender repeatedly gives in to the impulse to buy much more than he or she needs or can afford. For the compulsive shopper, spending may serve to relieve painful feelings like depression or anxiety, or it may produce positive emotions like excitement or happiness. Compulsive spenders usually buy luxury items rather than daily necessities. Men tend to buy cars, exercise equipment, and sporting gear; women are more likely to buy clothes, jewelry, and perfume. Some experts link compulsive shopping with neglect or abuse during childhood; it also seems to be associated with eating disorders, depression, and bipolar disorder. Some compulsive shoppers are helped by antidepressant medications.

Compulsive shoppers are usually significantly distressed by their behavior and its social, personal, and financial consequences. Characteristics of out-of-control spending include shopping in order to "feel better," using money or time that had been set aside for other purposes, hiding spending from others, and spending so much that one goes into debt or engages in illegal activities such as shoplifting or writing bad checks. Like other addictive behaviors, compulsive shopping is characterized by a loss of control over the behavior and significant negative consequences.

Internet Addiction Some recent research has indicated that surfing the World Wide Web can also be addictive. In order to spend more time online, Internet addicts skip important social, school, or recreational activities, thereby damaging personal relationships and jeopardizing academic and job performance. Despite the negative consequences they are experiencing, they don't feel able to stop. The Internet addicts identified in one study averaged 38 online hours per week. Internet addicts may feel uncomfortable or be moody when they are not online. They may be preoccupied with getting back online and may stay there longer than they intend. As with other addictive behaviors, online addicts may be using their behavior to alleviate stress or avoid painful emotions.

Activities by Internet addicts may take many forms, some of which, such as e-mail and chat rooms, are specific to the online format. However, widespread access to the Internet may expose many more people to other potentially addictive behaviors, including gambling, shopping,

and sex. There are thousands of online gambling sites and millions of online stores that allow people to gamble or shop from their homes at all times of the day or night; in addition, sites featuring online auctions or stock trading offer activities that are very similar to gambling. It remains to be seen whether increasing access to the Internet among Americans will lead to more problems with many types of addictive behaviors.

Other behaviors that can become addictive include eating, watching TV, and working. Any substance or activity that becomes the focus of a person's life at the expense of other needs and interests can be damaging to health.

We turn now to the substances most commonly associated with addiction: psychoactive drugs.

> **COMMUNICATE!** Ample opportunities for "addiction" are offered by computers in general and the Internet in particular, through games, gambling, shopping, stock trading, pornography, and chat rooms. Many people "binge" on computer activities once or twice and then never do it again, while others seem to lose control. If a friend or roommate is spending more and more time online and doesn't seem to be able to set limits, you might want to talk to him or her about it. For example, "You've been spending so much time online that I'm getting worried about you. You seem to feel more connected to your online friends and activities than your real-life ones. I wonder if you'd consider cutting back on your computer time—I miss your company! If you can't do it, maybe you should talk to a counselor about it."

DRUG USE, ABUSE, AND DEPENDENCE

Drugs are chemicals other than food that are intended to affect the structure or function of the body. They include prescription medicines such as antibiotics; nonprescription, or over-the-counter (OTC), substances, such as alcohol, tobacco, and caffeine products; and illegal substances, such as cocaine and heroin.

The APA's *Diagnostic and Statistical Manual of Mental Disorders* is the authoritative reference for defining all sorts of behavioral disorders, including those related to drugs. The APA has chosen not to use the term *addiction*, in part because it is so broad and has so many connotations. Instead, the APA refers to two forms of substance (drug) disorders: substance abuse and substance dependence. Both are maladaptive patterns of substance use that lead to significant impairment or distress. Although the APA's definitions are more precise and more directly related to drug use, they clearly encompass the general characteristics of addictive behavior described in the last section.

Drug Abuse

As defined by the APA, **substance abuse** involves one or more of the following:

- Recurrent drug use, resulting in a failure to fulfill major responsibilities at work, school, or home
- Recurrent drug use in situations in which it is physically hazardous, such as before driving a car
- Recurrent drug-related legal problems
- Continued drug use despite persistent social or interpersonal problems caused or exacerbated by the effects of the drug

The pattern of use may be constant or intermittent, and **physical dependence** may or may not be present. For example, a person who smokes marijuana once a week but cuts classes because he or she is high is abusing marijuana, even though he or she is not physically dependent.

Drug Dependence

Substance dependence is a more complex disorder and is what many people associate with the idea of addiction. The seven specific criteria the APA uses to diagnose substance dependence are listed below. The first two are associated with physical dependence; the final five are associated with compulsive use. To be considered dependent, an individual must experience a cluster of three or more of these seven symptoms during a 12-month period.

1. *Developing tolerance to the substance.* When a person requires increased amounts of a substance to achieve the desired effect or notices a markedly diminished effect with continued use of the same amount, he or she has developed **tolerance.** For example, heavy heroin users may need to take ten times the amount they took at the beginning in order to achieve the desired effect.

2. *Experiencing withdrawal.* In an individual who has maintained prolonged, heavy use of a substance, a drop in its concentration within the body can result in unpleasant physical and cognitive **withdrawal** symptoms. For example, nausea, vomiting, and tremors are common withdrawal symptons for alcohol, opioids, and sedatives.

3. *Taking the substance in larger amounts or over a longer period than was originally intended.*

4. *Expressing a persistent desire to cut down or regulate substance use.* This desire is often accompanied by many unsuccessful efforts to reduce or discontinue use of the substance.

5. *Spending a great deal of time obtaining the substance, using the substance, or recovering from its effects.*

6. *Giving up or reducing important social, school, work, or recreational activities because of substance use.* A dependent person may withdraw from family activities and hobbies to use the substance or to spend more time with substance-using friends.

7. *Continuing to use the substance in spite of recognizing that it is contributing to a psychological or physical problem.*

If a drug-dependent person experiences either tolerance or withdrawal, he or she is considered physically dependent. However, dependence can occur without a physical component, based solely on compulsive use.

Who Uses Drugs?

The use and abuse of drugs occur at all income and education levels, among all ethnic groups, and at all ages. One reason for our society's concern with the casual use of drugs is that it is not really possible to know when drug use will lead to abuse or dependence. Some casual users develop substance-related problems; others do not. Some drugs are more likely than others to lead to dependence (Table 7-2). People who begin to use drugs at very young ages have a greater risk for dependence and serious health consequences.

Although we can't accurately predict which drug users will become drug abusers, researchers have identified some characteristics that place young people at higher-than-average risk for *trying* illicit drugs. An adolescent who is male; has a poor self-image; lacks self-control; is aggressive, impulsive, or moody; or suffers from attention-deficit hyperactivity disorder (ADHD) may be at increased risk for trying drugs. A thrill-seeking or risk-taking personality is another factor. People who drive too fast or who don't wear safety belts may have this personality type, which is characterized by a sense of invincibility.

Belonging to a peer group or family that accepts or rewards drug use is a significant risk factor for trying illicit drugs. Chaotic home environments, dysfunctional families, lack of parental supervision, and parental abuse also

---

Terms

substance abuse A maladaptive pattern of use of any substance that persists despite adverse social, psychological, or medical consequences. The pattern may be intermittent, with or without tolerance and physical dependence.

physical dependence The result of physiological adaptation that occurs in response to the frequent presence of a drug; typically associated with tolerance and withdrawal.

substance dependence A cluster of cognitive, behavioral, and physiological symptoms that occur in an individual who continues to use a substance despite suffering significant substance-related problems, leading to significant impairment or distress; also known as *addiction.*

tolerance Lower sensitivity to a drug so that a given dose no longer exerts the usual effect and larger doses are needed.

withdrawal Physical and psychological symptoms that follow the interrupted use of a drug on which a user is physically dependent; symptoms may be mild or life-threatening.

| Table 7-2 | Psychoactive Drugs and Their Potential for Producing Dependence |

	Potential for Dependence	
Drug	Physical	Psychological
Nicotine	Very high	Very high
Heroin	Very high	Very high
Methamphetamine smoked ("ice")	Very high	Very high
Crack cocaine	Possible	Very high
Alcohol	High	High
Barbiturates	High	High
Methaqualone (Quaalude)	High	High
Amphetamine	Possible	High
Cocaine	Possible	High
Diazepam (Valium)	Low	High
PCP	Unknown	High
Chloral hydrate ("mickey")	Moderate	Moderate
Codeine	Moderate	Moderate
Marijuana/ hashish	Unknown	Moderate
Inhalants	Unknown	Moderate
Steroids	Possible	Possible
LSD	None	Unknown

SOURCES: National Clearinghouse for Alcohol and Drug Information. 2000. *Drugs of Abuse* (http://www.health.org/govpubs/rpo926; retrieved October 3, 2000). Beers, M. H., and R. Berkow, eds. 1999. *Merck Manual of Diagnosis and Therapy*, 17th ed. Rahway, N. J.: Merck. Food and Drug Administration. 1995. Nicotine in cigarettes and smokeless tobacco products is a drug and these products are nicotine delivery devices under the Federal Food, Drug, and Cosmetic Act. *Federal Register* 60(155): 41454–41459.

increase risk. Young people who live in disadvantaged areas are more likely to be offered drugs at a young age, thereby increasing their risk of drug use. However, drug use rates among middle-class youths with college-educated parents tend to catch up with, and in some cases outstrip, those of other groups by the time students reach the twelfth grade.

What about people who *don't* use drugs? People who perceive drug use as risky and who disapprove of it are less likely to use drugs than those who believe otherwise. Drug use is less common among people who have positive self-esteem and self-concept and who are assertive, independent thinkers who are not controlled by peer pressure. Self-control, social competence, optimism, academic achievement, and regular church attendance are also linked to lower rates of drug use.

Home environments are also influential: Coming from a strong family, one that has a clear policy on drug use, is another characteristic of people who don't use drugs. Although parents may feel they have little effect on their children's drug-related attitudes and behaviors, evidence suggests that they can be a major influence. Some parents may wait too long to express a clear drug policy. Recent surveys indicate that attitudes about drugs and access and exposure to drugs change most dramatically between the ages of 12 and 13. Compared to a 12-year-old, a 13-year-old is about three times more likely to know teens who use and sell drugs and to know where and how to buy drugs. Yet nearly half of 13-year-olds report that their parents have never seriously discussed the dangers of illegal drugs with them.

Why Do People Use Drugs?

Young people, especially those from middle-class backgrounds, are frequently drawn to drugs by the allure of the exciting and illegal. They may be curious, rebellious, or vulnerable to peer pressure. Young people may want to appear to be daring and to be part of the group. They may want to imitate adult models in their lives or in the movies. Most people who have taken illicit drugs have done so on an experimental basis, typically trying the drug one or more times but not continuing. The main factors in the initial choice of a drug are whether it is available and whether other people around are already using it.

Although some people use drugs because they have a desire to alter their mood or are seeking a spiritual experience, others are motivated primarily by a desire to escape boredom, anxiety, depression, feelings of worthlessness, or other distressing symptoms of psychological problems. They use drugs as a way to cope with the difficulties they are experiencing in life. The common practice in our society of seeking a drug solution to every problem is a factor in the widespread reliance on both illicit and prescription drugs.

For people living in poverty in the inner cities, many of these reasons for using drugs are magnified. The problems are more devastating, the need for escape more compelling. Furthermore, the buying and selling of drugs provide access to an unofficial, alternative economy that may seem like an opportunity for success.

Risk Factors for Dependence

Why do some people use psychoactive drugs without becoming dependent, while others aren't as lucky? The answer seems to be a combination of physical, psychological, and social factors. Research indicates that some people may be born with certain characteristics of brain chemistry or metabolism that make them more vulnerable to drug dependence. Psychological risk factors for drug dependence include difficulty in controlling impulses and a strong need for excitement, stimulation, and immediate gratification. Feelings of rejection, hostility, aggression, anxiety, or depression are also associated with

The use of alcohol and other drugs is intertwined with spirituality and religion. Some religions use drugs in the quest for spiritual transcendence: American Indian, Polynesian, African, and other indigenous religions have used psychoactive drugs such as peyote, khat, alcohol, and hashish for expanding consciousness and developing personal spirituality. For other religions, the use of psychoactive drugs is seen as a threat to spirituality. In Islam, for example, the consumption of alcohol and certain other drugs is strictly forbidden. Although there are diverse religious viewpoints on drug use, many religions infer some link between psychoactive drugs and spirituality.

In studies of American teens and adults, spiritual or religious involvement is generally associated with a lower risk of trying psychoactive drugs and, for those who do use drugs, a lower risk of heavy use and dependence. The mechanism for this protective effect is unclear; possibilities include the adoption of a strict code of behavior or set of principles that forbids drug use; the presence of a social support system for abstinence or moderation; and the promotion of a large, complex set of values that includes avoidance of drug use. Overall, people who spend time regularly engaging in spiritual practices such as prayer and transcendental meditation have lower rates of drug abuse.

People with current substance abuse problems tend to have lower rates of religious affiliation and involvement and lower levels of spiritual wellness. One of the hallmarks of drug dependence is spending increasing amounts of time and energy obtaining and using drugs; such a pattern of behavior inevitably reduces the resources an individual puts toward developing physical, emotional, and spiritual wellness.

What about those seeking to break their dependence on drugs? Among people in treatment for substance abuse, higher levels of religious faith and spirituality may contribute to the recovery process. A study of people recovering from alcohol or other drug abuse found that spirituality and religiosity were associated with increased coping skills, greater optimism about life, greater resilience to stress, and greater perceived social support. If, for a particular individual, there is a spiritual aspect to his or her substance abuse problem, then it is likely that spirituality may also play a role in recovery.

More research is needed to clarify the relationship among spirituality, religion, drug use, and recovery. One of the difficulties in conducting research in this area is the difficulty in defining and measuring spirituality and religious involvement. Spirituality is a complex part of human nature, involving behavior, belief, and experience. And although behaviors such as the spiritual practices of prayer or meditation can be measured, it is more difficult to determine what such practices mean to an individual and her or his overall sense of self.

SOURCES: Plante, T. G., and D. A. Pardini. 2000. Religious denomination affiliation and psychological health: Results from a substance abuse population. Presented at the American Psychological Association Annual Convention, August 7. Miller, L., M. Davies, and S. Greenwald. 2000. Religiosity and substance use and abuse among adolescents in the national comorbidity survey. *Journal of the American Academy of Child and Adolescent Psychiatry* 39(9): 1190–1197. Miller, W. R. 1998. Researching the spiritual dimensions of alcohol and other drug problems. *Addiction* 93(7): 979–990.

drug dependence. People may turn to drugs to blot out their emotional pain. People with mental illnesses have a very high risk of substance dependence.

Other Risks of Drug Use

Dependence is not the only serious potential consequence of drug use. People who are under the influence of drugs—intoxicated—may act in uncharacteristic and unsafe ways because both their physical and mental functioning are impaired. They are more likely to be injured from a variety of causes, including falls, drowning, and automobile crashes; to engage in unsafe sex, increasing their risk for sexually transmitted diseases and unintended pregnancy; and to be involved in incidents of aggression and violence, including sexual assault.

Psychoactive drugs have many physical and psychological effects beyond the alteration of consciousness. These effects range from nausea and constipation to paranoia, depression, and heart failure; some drugs also carry the risk of potentially fatal overdose. Certain methods of drug administration are inherently dangerous; injecting drugs, for example, increases one's risk of HIV infection, hepatitis

C, and gangrene. There is no quality control in the illegal drug market, so the composition, dosage, and toxicity of street drugs is highly variable. Finally, many psychoactive drugs are illegal, so using them can result in large fines and/or imprisonment.

HOW DRUGS AFFECT THE BODY

The psychoactive drugs discussed in this chapter have complex and variable effects. The same drug may affect different people differently or the same person in different ways under different circumstances. Beyond a fairly predictable general change in brain chemistry, the effects of a drug may vary depending on three general categories of factors: drug factors, user factors, and social factors.

Changes in Brain Chemistry

Psychoactive drugs produce most of their key effects by acting on brain chemistry in a characteristic fashion. Before any changes in brain chemistry can occur, however,

Different methods of administering drugs are associated with different risks—dangers beyond the actual effects of the drug being used. The method of drug use most frequently linked to serious health problems is injection drug use. Many injection drug users (IDUs) share or reuse needles, syringes, and other injection equipment, which can easily become contaminated with the user's blood. In addition, IDUs typically prepare drugs using unsterile water and equipment, and they do not clean injection sites before injecting drugs, giving disease-causing microorganisms easy access to the body.

Small amounts of blood can carry enough human immunodeficiency virus (HIV) and hepatitis C virus (HCV) to be infectious, and injection drug use accounts for almost a third of all AIDS cases and half of all hepatitis C cases reported in the United States. It's estimated that about 15% of current IDUs are infected with HIV, and as many as 80% may carry HCV. Unsterile injection practices can cause skin and soft tissue infections, which can progress to gangrene and be fatal if untreated. IDUs are also at greater risk for endocarditis (microbial infection of the heart valves), tuberculosis, human herpesvirus 8, tetanus, the collapse of veins, and scarring at the site of injections.

Heroin and other injectable opiates are the drugs most often used by IDUs, but cocaine, amphetamines, and other drugs may also be injected. Concerns have also recently been raised about steroids: Steroid users who inject the drug face the same health risks as other IDUs, and steroids have been found to be a gateway to the use of other drugs. A study of steroid users who progressed to heroin use found that the steroid users typically obtained heroin from the same dealer who provided the steroids; they also originally used heroin in an effort to blunt some of the side effects of steroid use and withdrawal, including insomnia, irritability, and depression.

The surest way to prevent diseases related to injection drug use is never to inject drugs. Those who do inject drugs should use a new needle and syringe with each injection and should use sterile water and other equipment to prepare drugs. Bleach or boiling water may kill some viruses and bacteria, but they are not foolproof sterilization methods. Many viruses can survive in a syringe for a month or more.

Some public health experts believe free syringe exchange programs (SEPs)—in which IDUs can turn in a used syringe and get a new, clean one back—could help slow the spread of HIV and reduce the rates of other health problems associated with injection drug use. Opponents of SEPs argue that supplying addicts with syringes gives them the message that illegal drug use is acceptable and could thus exacerbate the nation's drug program. However, studies have shown that well-implemented programs do not increase the use of illegal drugs. Other strategies include distribution of new syringes through physician prescriptions or through local pharmacies. Getting people off drugs is clearly the best solution, but there are far more IDUs than treatment facilities can currently handle.

SOURCES: Centers for Disease Control and Prevention. 2000. *Fact Sheet: Access to Sterile Syringes.* Washington, D.C.: Academy for Educational Development. Arvary, D., and H. G. Pope. 2000. Anabolic-androgenic steroids as a gateway to opioid dependence. *New England Journal of Medicine* 342(20): 1532. Centers for Disease Control and Prevention. 1998. Update: Syringe-exchange programs. *Morbidity and Mortality Weekly Report* 47(31): 652–655.

molecules of the drug have to be carried to the brain through the bloodstream. A drug that is taken by mouth has to dissolve in the stomach, be absorbed into the bloodstream through the lining of the small intestine, and then pass through the liver, heart, and lungs before returning to the heart to be carried via arteries to the brain. A drug that is already dissolved and is injected directly into the bloodstream will reach the brain in much less time, and drugs that are inhaled and absorbed by the lungs travel to the brain even more rapidly.

Once a psychoactive drug reaches the brain, it acts on one or more neurotransmitters, either increasing or decreasing their concentration and actions. Cocaine, for example, affects dopamine, a neurotransmitter thought to play a key role in the process of reinforcement—the brain's way of telling itself, "that's good; do the same thing again." Heroin, nicotine, and amphetamines also affect dopamine levels.

The duration of a drug's effect depends on many factors and may range from 5 minutes (crack cocaine) to 12 or more hours (peyote). As drugs circulate through the body, they are metabolized by the liver and eventually excreted by the kidneys in urine. Small amounts may also be eliminated in other ways, including in sweat, in breast milk, and via the lungs.

Drug Factors

When different drugs or dosages produce different effects, the differences are usually caused by one or more of five different drug factors:

1. The **pharmacological properties** of a drug are its overall effects on a person's body chemistry, behavior, and psychology. The pharmacological properties also include the amount of a drug required to exert various effects, the time course of these effects, and other characteristics, such as a drug's chemical composition.

pharmacological properties The overall effects of a drug on a person's behavior, psychology, and chemistry.   Terms

2. The **dose-response function** is the relationship between the amount of drug taken and the type and intensity of the resulting effect. Many psychological effects of drugs reach a plateau in the dose-response function, so that increasing the dose does not increase the effect any further. However, all drugs have more than one effect, and the dose-response functions usually are different for different effects. This means that increasing the dose of any drug may begin to result in additional effects, which are likely to be increasingly unpleasant or dangerous at high doses.

3. The **time-action function** is the relationship between the time elapsed since a drug was taken and the intensity of its effect. The effects of a drug are greatest when concentrations of the drug in body tissues are changing the fastest, especially if they are increasing.

4. The person's *drug use history* may influence the effects of a drug. A given amount of alcohol, for example, will generally affect a habitual drinker less than an occasional drinker. Tolerance to some drugs, such as LSD, builds rapidly. To experience the same effect, a user has to abstain from the drug for a period of time before that dosage will again exert its original effects.

5. The *method of use* has a direct effect on how strong a response a drug produces. Methods of use include ingestion, inhalation, injection, and absorption through the skin or tissue linings. Drugs are usually injected one of three ways: intravenously (IV, or mainlining), intramuscularly (IM), or subcutaneously (SC, or "skin popping"). If a drug is taken by a method that allows the drug to enter the bloodstream and reach the brain rapidly, the effects are usually stronger and the potential for dependence greater than when the method involves slower absorption. For example, injecting a drug intravenously produces stronger effects than swallowing the same drug. Inhaling a drug, such as when tobacco or crack cocaine is smoked, produces very rapid effects on the brain.

Terms

dose-response function   The relationship between the amount of a drug taken and the intensity or type of the resulting effect.

time-action function   The relationship between the time elapsed since a drug was taken and the intensity of its effect.

high   The subjectively pleasing effects of a drug, usually felt quite soon after the drug is taken.

placebo effect   A response to an inert or innocuous medication given in place of an active drug.

opioid   Any of several natural or synthetic drugs that relieve pain and cause drowsiness and/or euphoria; examples are opium, morphine, and heroin; also called *narcotic*.

euphoria   An exaggerated feeling of well-being.

User Factors

The second category of factors that determine how a person will respond to a particular drug involves certain physical and psychological characteristics. Body mass is one variable. The effects of a certain dose of a drug on a 100-pound person will be twice as great as on a 200-pound person. Other variables include general health and genetic factors. For example, some people have an inherited ability to rapidly metabolize a cough suppressant called dextromethorphan, which also has psychoactive properties. These people must take a higher-than-normal dose to get a given cough-suppressant effect.

If a person's biochemical state is already altered by another drug, this too can make a difference. Some drugs intensify the effects of other drugs, as is the case with alcohol and sedatives. Some drugs block the effects of other drugs, such as when a tranquilizer is used to relieve anxiety caused by cocaine. Interactions between drugs, including many prescription and OTC medications, can be unpredictable and dangerous.

One physical condition that requires special precautions is pregnancy. It can be risky for a woman to use any drugs at all during pregnancy, including alcohol and common OTC preparations like cough medicine. The risks are greatest during the first trimester, when the fetus's body is rapidly forming and even small biochemical alterations in the mother can have a devastating effect on fetal development. Even later, the fetus is more susceptible than the mother to the adverse effects of any drugs she takes. The fetus may even become physically dependent on a drug being taken by the mother and suffer withdrawal symptoms after birth.

Sometimes a person's response to a drug is strongly influenced by the user's expectations about how he or she will react. With large doses, the drug's chemical properties do seem to have the strongest effect on the user's response. But with small doses, psychological (and social) factors are often more important. When people strongly believe that a given drug will affect them a certain way, they are likely to experience those effects regardless of the drug's pharmacological properties. In one study, regular users of marijuana reported a moderate level of intoxication (**high**) after using a cigarette that smelled and tasted like marijuana but contained no THC, the active ingredient in marijuana. This is an example of the **placebo effect**—when a person receives an inert substance yet responds as if it were an active drug. In other studies, subjects who smoked low doses of real marijuana that they believed to be a placebo experienced no effects from the drug. Clearly, the user's expectations had greater effects on the smokers than the drug itself.

Social Factors

The *setting* is the physical and social environment surrounding the drug use. If a person uses marijuana at home with trusted friends and pleasant music, the effects are likely to be different from the effects if the same dose is taken in an austere experimental laboratory with an impassive research technician. Similarly, the dose of alcohol that produces mild euphoria and stimulation at a noisy, active cocktail party might induce sleepiness and slight depression when taken at home while alone.

COMMUNICATE! As a college student, you will probably sooner or later find yourself in a situation where drugs are being used or abused. Anticipate such situations and think ahead about how you will respond. Remember that you are entitled to make your own decisions about your life, even in the face of peer pressure. Sometimes, all you have to do is say, "No, thanks." Other times, it's best to use nonverbal communication—leave the situation as soon as you can and go home.

W. REPRESENTATIVE PSYCHOACTIVE DRUGS

What are the major psychoactive drugs, and how do they produce their effects? We discuss six different representative groups in this chapter: (1) opioids, (2) central nervous system depressants, (3) central nervous system stimulants, (4) marijuana and other cannabis products, (5) hallucinogens, and (6) inhalants. (For the sources of selected psychoactive drugs, see Figure 7-1.)

Opioids

Also called *narcotics,* **opioids** are natural or synthetic (laboratory-made) drugs that relieve pain, cause drowsiness, and induce **euphoria.** Opium, morphine, heroin, methadone, codeine, meperidine, and fentanyl are examples of drugs in this category. Opioids tend to reduce anxiety and produce lethargy, apathy, and an inability to concentrate. Opioid users become less active and less responsive to frustration, hunger, and sexual stimulation. These effects are more pronounced in novice users; with repeated use, many effects diminish.

Opioids are typically injected or absorbed into the body from the stomach, intestines, nasal membranes (from snorting or sniffing), or lungs (from smoking). Although the euphoria associated with opioids is an important factor in their abuse, many people experience a feeling of uneasiness when they first use these drugs. Users also often feel nauseated and vomit, and they may have other unpleasant sensations. Even so, the abuse of opioids often results in dependence. Tolerance can develop rapidly and be pronounced. Withdrawal symptoms include cramps, chills, sweating, nausea, tremors, irritability, and feelings of panic.

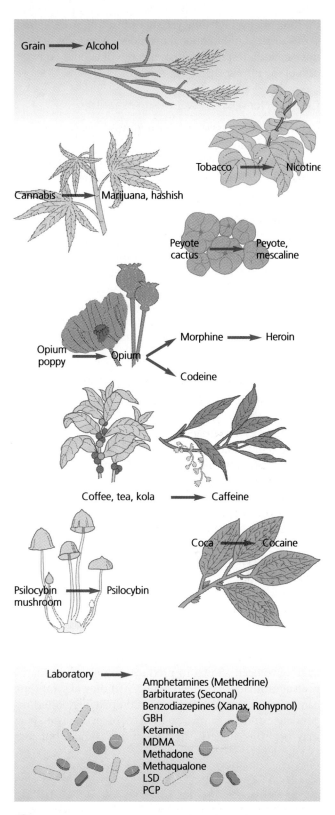

🔴 **Figure 7-1   Sources of selected psychoactive drugs.**

Users who sniff or smoke heroin avoid the special disease risks of injection drug use, but dependence can readily result from sniffing and smoking heroin. In addition, the potentially high but variable purity of street heroin poses a risk of unintentional overdose. Symptoms of overdose include respiratory depression, coma, and constriction of the pupils; death can result.

Central Nervous System Depressants

Central nervous system **depressants,** also known as **sedative-hypnotics,** slow down the overall activity of the **central nervous system (CNS).** The result can range from mild **sedation** to death. CNS depressants include alcohol (discussed in Chapter 8), barbiturates, and other sedatives.

Types The various types of barbiturates ("downers" or "downs") are similar in chemical composition and action, but they differ in how quickly and how long they act. People usually take barbiturates in capsules, but they may also inject them. Antianxiety agents, also called sedatives or **tranquilizers,** include the benzodiazepines such as Xanax, Valium, Librium, clonazepam (Klonopin), and flunitrazepam (Rohypnol, also called "roofies"). Other CNS depressants include methaqualone (Quaalude), ethchlorvynol (Placidyl), chloral hydrate ("mickey"), and gamma hydroxy butyrate (GHB, or "liquid ecstasy").

Effects CNS depressants reduce anxiety and cause mood changes, impaired muscular coordination, slurring of speech, and drowsiness or sleep. Mental functioning is also affected, but the degree varies from person to person and also depends on the kind of task the person is trying to do. Most people become drowsy with small doses, although a few become more active.

From Use to Abuse People are usually introduced to CNS depressants either through a medical prescription or through drug-using peers. The use of Rohypnol and GHB is often associated with dance clubs and raves. Most CNS depressants, including alcohol, can lead to classical physical dependence. Tolerance, sometimes for up to 15 times the usual dose, can develop with repeated use. Tranquilizers have been shown to produce physical dependence even at ordinary prescribed doses. Withdrawal symptoms can be more severe than those accompanying opioid dependence and are similar to the DTs of alcoholism. They may begin as anxiety, shaking, and weakness but may turn into convulsions and possibly cardiovascular collapse and death.

While intoxicated, people on depressants cannot function very well. They are mentally confused and are frequently obstinate, irritable, and abusive. Even prescription use of benzodiazepines has been associated with an increased risk of automobile crashes. After long-term use, depressants like alcohol can lead to generally poor health and brain damage, with impaired ability to reason and make judgments.

Too much depression of the central nervous system slows respiration and may stop it entirely. CNS depressants are particularly dangerous in combination with another depressant, such as alcohol. Rohypnol is ten times more potent than Valium and can be fatal if combined with alcohol. GHB is often produced clandestinely, resulting in widely varying degrees of purity; it has been responsible for many poisonings and several deaths.

Central Nervous System Stimulants

CNS **stimulants** speed up the activity of the nervous or muscular system. Under their influence, the heart rate accelerates, blood pressure rises, blood vessels constrict, the pupils of the eyes and the bronchial tubes dilate, and gastric and adrenal secretions increase. There is greater muscular tension and sometimes an increase in motor activity. Small doses usually make people feel more awake and alert, less fatigued and bored. Common CNS stimulants are cocaine, amphetamine, nicotine (discussed in Chapter 8), ephedrine, and caffeine.

Cocaine Usually derived from the leaves of coca shrubs that grow high in the Andes Mountains in South America, cocaine—also known as "coke" or "snow"—is a potent CNS stimulant. For centuries, natives of the Andes have chewed coca leaves both for pleasure and to increase their endurance.

METHODS OF USE Cocaine is usually inhaled or injected intravenously, providing rapid increases of the drug's concentration in the blood and therefore fast, intense effects. Another method of use involves processing cocaine with baking soda and water, yielding the ready-to-smoke form known as crack. Crack is typically available as small beads or pellets smokable in glass pipes.

EFFECTS The effects of cocaine are usually intense but short-lived. The euphoria lasts from 5 to 20 minutes and ends abruptly, to be replaced by irritability, anxiety, or slight depression. When cocaine is absorbed via the lungs, by either smoking or inhalation, it reaches the brain in about 10 seconds, and the effects are particularly intense. The effects from IV injections occur almost as quickly—in about 20 seconds. Since the mucous membranes in the nose briefly slow absorption, the onset of ef-

Terms

depressant or sedative-hypnotic A drug that decreases nervous or muscular activity, causing drowsiness or sleep.

central nervous system (CNS) The brain and spinal cord.

sedation The induction of a calm, relaxed, often sleepy state.

tranquilizer A CNS depressant that reduces tension and anxiety.

stimulant A drug that increases nervous or muscular activity.

In the United States and elsewhere, euphoria-inducing drugs known as club drugs have gained popularity in recent years. Club drugs include a variety of very different drugs that are part of the popular dance culture of clubs and "raves"—all-night dance parties held in fields or abandoned buildings. Some people refer to club drugs as "soft" drugs because they see them as recreational—more for the casual, weekend user—rather than as addictive. But club drugs have many potential negative effects and are particularly potent and unpredictable when mixed with alcohol. Substitute drugs are often sold in place of club drugs, putting users at risk for taking dangerous combinations of unknown drugs.

MDMA (ecstasy, E, X, XTC, Adam, clarity, lover's speed): Taken in pill form, MDMA (methylenedioxymethamphetamine) is a stimulant with mildly hallucinogenic and amphetamine-like effects. In club settings, using it can produce dangerously high body temperature and potentially fatal dehydration; some users experience confusion, depression, anxiety, or paranoia. Even low doses may affect concentration and driving ability. Chronic use of MDMA may produce long-lasting, perhaps permanent, damage to the neurons that release serotonin; this may explain why heavy use is associated with persistent problems with verbal and visual memory. At high doses or mixed with other drugs, MDMA is extremely dangerous; several deaths in 2000 were traced to pills containing a combination of MDMA and the related drug PMA or PMAA. Research suggests that pregnant women who use MDMA are at increased risk for having a baby with congenital malformations.

LSD (acid, boomers, yellow sunshines, red dragon): A popular and potent hallucinogen, LSD (lysergic acid diethylamide) is sold in tablets or capsules, in liquid form, or on small squares of paper called blotters. LSD increases heart rate and body temperature and may cause nausea, tremors, sweating, numbness, and weakness. (See p. 144 for more on LSD.)

Ketamine (special K, vitamin K, K, cat valium): A veterinary anesthetic that can be taken in powdered or liquid form, ketamine may cause hallucinations and impaired attention and memory. At higher doses, ketamine can cause delirium, amnesia, high blood pressure, and potentially fatal respiratory problems. Tolerance to ketamine develops rapidly.

GHB (Georgia home boy, G, grievous bodily harm, liquid ecstasy): GHB (gamma hydroxybutyrate) can be produced in clear liquid, white powder, tablet, and capsule form; it is often made in basement chemistry labs, where toxic substances may unintentionally be added or produced. GHB is a CNS depressant that in large doses can cause sedation, loss of consciousness, respiratory arrest, and death. In 2000, three teens were convicted of manslaughter after they gave a female party guest a soda laced with GHB; the young woman lost consciousness and died from choking on her own vomit. Evidence suggests that GHB is addictive and that it may cause prolonged and potentially life-threatening withdrawal symptoms. Some products sold as dietary supplements for bodybuilding, weight loss, or insomnia contain the chemically similar compounds GBL (gamma butyrolactone) or BD (butanediol); the FDA considers these products dangerous and is working to remove them from the market.

Rohypnol (roofies, roche, forget-me pill): Taken in tablet form, Rohypnol (flunitrazepam) is a sedative that is 10 times more potent than Valium. Its effects, which are magnified by alcohol, include reduced blood pressure, dizziness, confusion, gastrointestinal disturbances, and loss of consciousness. Users of Rohypnol may develop physical and psychological dependence on the drug.

An additional problem associated with Rohypnol, GHB, and several other club drugs is their potential use as "date rape drugs." Because they can be added to beverages surreptitiously, these drugs may be unknowingly consumed by intended rape victims. In addition to depressant effects, some drugs also cause *anterograde amnesia,* the loss of memory of things occurring while under the influence of the drug. Because of concern about Rohypnol, GHB, and other similarly abused drugs, Congress passed the "Drug-Induced Rape Prevention and Punishment Act," which increased federal penalties for use of any controlled substance to aid in sexual assault.

---

fects from snorting takes 2–3 minutes. Heavy users may inject cocaine intravenously every 10–20 minutes to maintain the effects.

The larger the cocaine dose and the more rapidly it is absorbed into the bloodstream, the greater the immediate—and sometimes lethal—effects. Sudden death from cocaine is most commonly the result of excessive CNS stimulation that causes convulsions and respiratory collapse, irregular heartbeat, blood clots, and possibly heart attack or stroke. Although rare, fatalities can occur in healthy young people; among people ages 18–59, cocaine users are seven times more likely than nonusers to have a heart attack. Chronic cocaine use produces inflammation of the nasal mucosa, which can lead to persistent bleeding and ulceration of the septum between the nostrils. The use of cocaine may also cause paranoia and/or aggressiveness.

COCAINE USE DURING PREGNANCY   A woman who uses cocaine during pregnancy is at higher risk for miscarriage, premature labor, and stillbirth. She is more likely to deliver a low-birth-weight baby who has a small head circumference. Her infant may be at increased risk for defects of the genitourinary tract, cardiovascular system, central nervous system, and extremities. It is difficult to pinpoint the effects of cocaine because many women who use cocaine also use tobacco and/or alcohol. Infants whose mothers use cocaine may also be born intoxicated; cocaine also passes into breast milk, from where it can intoxicate a breastfeeding infant.

Research on the long-term effects of prenatal exposure to cocaine has been inconclusive. Recent studies suggest that prenatal cocaine exposure may cause subtle changes in the brain that affect IQ, language skill, and motor development; behavioral problems—disorganization, poor social skills, and hyperactivity—have also been reported. Although fetal cocaine exposure is an important issue, the type and magnitude of effects produced by nicotine are similar, and there are nearly 20 times more infants exposed to cigarettes than to cocaine.

Amphetamines   Amphetamines are a group of synthetic chemicals that are potent CNS stimulants. Some common drugs in this family are amphetamine (Benzedrine), dextroamphetamine (Dexedrine), and methamphetamine (Methedrine). Popular names for these drugs include "speed," "crank," "chalk," "crystal," ""ice," and "meth," and users refer to them all as "uppers."

EFFECTS   Small doses of amphetamines usually make people feel more alert and wide-awake and less fatigued or bored. Amphetamines generally increase motor activity but do not measurably alter a normal, rested person's ability to perform tasks calling for challenging motor skills or complex thinking. When amphetamines do improve performance, it is primarily by counteracting fatigue and boredom. Amphetamines in small doses also increase heart rate and blood pressure and change sleep patterns.

Amphetamines are sometimes used to curb appetite, but after a few weeks the user develops tolerance, and higher doses are necessary. When people stop taking the drug, their appetite usually returns, and they gain back the weight they lost unless they have made permanent changes in eating behavior.

FROM USE TO ABUSE   Much amphetamine abuse begins as an attempt to cope with a temporary situation. A student cramming for an exam or an exhausted long-haul truck driver can go a little longer by taking amphetamines, but the results can be disastrous. The likelihood of making bad decisions significantly increases. An additional danger is that the stimulating effects may wear off suddenly, and the user may precipitously feel exhausted or fall asleep ("crash"). Another problem is **state dependence**, the phenomenon whereby information learned in a drug-induced state is difficult to recall when the person is not in that same physiological state. Test performance may deteriorate when students use drugs to study and then take tests in their normal, nondrug state.

Terms
state dependence A situation in which information learned in a drug-induced state is difficult to recall when the effect of the drug wears off.

psychosis A severe mental disorder characterized by a distortion of reality; symptoms might include delusions or hallucinations.

DEPENDENCE   If injected in large doses, amphetamines produce a feeling of intense pleasure, followed by sensations of vigor and euphoria that last for several hours. As these feelings wear off, they are replaced by feelings of irritability and vague uneasiness. Long-term use of amphetamines at high doses can cause paranoia, hallucinations, delusions, and incoherence. Researchers have also identified signs of brain damage in methamphetamine users that appear to persist even after drug use ceases, causing impaired memory and motor coordination. Withdrawal symptoms may include muscle aches and tremors, along with profound fatigue, deep depression, despair, and apathy. Chronic high-dose amphetamine use is often associated with pronounced psychological cravings and obsessive drug-seeking behavior.

Women who use amphetamines during pregnancy risk premature birth, stillbirth, and early infant death. Babies born to amphetamine-using mothers have a higher incidence of cleft palate, cleft lip, and deformed limbs. They may also be born dependent on amphetamines.

Ritalin   A stimulant with effects similar to amphetamines, Ritalin (methylphenidate) is used to treat attention-deficit/hyperactivity disorder. When taken orally at prescribed levels, it has little potential for abuse. When injected or snorted, however, dependence and tolerance can rapidly result.

Ephedrine   Amphetamine was made in the 1920s by modifying the chemical ephedrine, which was originally isolated from a Chinese herbal tea. Although somewhat less potent than amphetamine, ephedrine does produce stimulant effects. It is found in OTC weight-loss preparations, energy-boosting supplements, and a product known as "herbal ecstasy." Uncontrolled use of ephedrine has been associated with some deaths. The FDA recently banned the chemically similar compound phenylpropanolamine (PPA) because it increases the risk of stroke.

Caffeine   Caffeine is probably the most popular psychoactive drug and also one of the most ancient. It is found in coffee, tea, cocoa, soft drinks, headache remedies, and OTC preparations like No-Dōz. In ordinary doses, caffeine produces greater alertness and a sense of well-being. It also decreases feelings of fatigue or boredom, and using caffeine may enable a person to keep at physically exhausting or repetitive tasks longer. Such use is usually followed, however, by a sudden letdown. Caffeine does not noticeably influence a person's ability to perform complex intellectual tasks unless fatigue, boredom, alcohol, or other factors have already affected normal performance.

Caffeine mildly stimulates the heart and respiratory system, increases muscular tremor, and enhances gastric secretion. Higher doses may cause nervousness, anxiety,

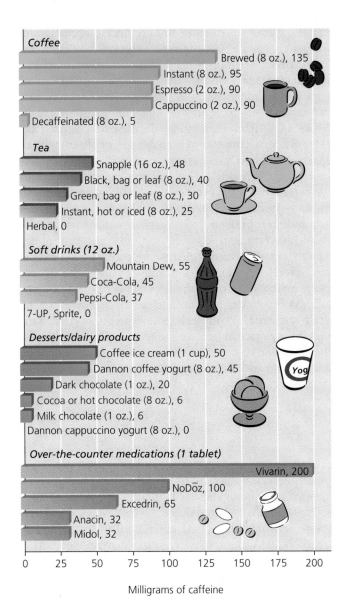

Coffee
- Brewed (8 oz.), 135
- Instant (8 oz.), 95
- Espresso (2 oz.), 90
- Cappuccino (2 oz.), 90
- Decaffeinated (8 oz.), 5

Tea
- Snapple (16 oz.), 48
- Black, bag or leaf (8 oz.), 40
- Green, bag or leaf (8 oz.), 30
- Instant, hot or iced (8 oz.), 25
- Herbal, 0

Soft drinks (12 oz.)
- Mountain Dew, 55
- Coca-Cola, 45
- Pepsi-Cola, 37
- 7-UP, Sprite, 0

Desserts/dairy products
- Coffee ice cream (1 cup), 50
- Dannon coffee yogurt (8 oz.), 45
- Dark chocolate (1 oz.), 20
- Cocoa or hot chocolate (8 oz.), 6
- Milk chocolate (1 oz.), 6
- Dannon cappuccino yogurt (8 oz.), 0

Over-the-counter medications (1 tablet)
- Vivarin, 200
- NoDōz, 100
- Excedrin, 65
- Anacin, 32
- Midol, 32

0   25   50   75   100   125   150   175   200

Milligrams of caffeine

Figure 7-2 Common sources of caffeine. The caffeine content of products varies with the brand and preparation method; the values shown here are averages. Among Americans, the average daily intake of caffeine is about 230 milligrams. SOURCES: Become a bean counter. 2000. *Prevention*, July. International Food Information Council. 1998. *IFIC Review: Caffeine and Health* (http://ificinfo.health.org/review/ircaffh.htm; retrieved October 8, 2000). Caffeine content of foods and drugs. 1996. *Nutrition Action Healthletter*, December.

irritability, headache, disturbed sleep, and gastric irritation or peptic ulcers. In people with high blood pressure, caffeine can cause blood pressure to rise even further above normal. Some people, especially children, are quite vulnerable to the adverse effects of caffeine. They become "wired"—hyperactive and overly sensitive to any stimulation in their environment. In rare instances, the disturbance is so severe that there is misperception of their surroundings—a toxic **psychosis.**

Drinks containing caffeine are rarely harmful for most individuals, but some tolerance develops, and withdrawal

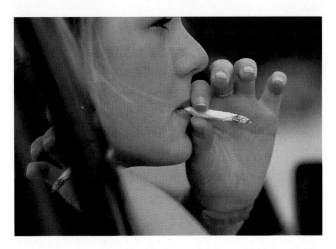

Marijuana is the most widely used illegal drug in the United States. At low doses, marijuana users typically experience euphoria and a relaxed attitude. Further research is needed to determine its precise physiological and psychological effects, particularly for chronic use.

symptoms of irritability, headaches, and even mild depression do occur. Thus, although we don't usually think of caffeine as a dependence-producing drug, for some people it is. People can usually avoid problems by simply decreasing their daily intake of caffeine (Figure 7-2).

Marijuana and Other Cannabis Products

Marijuana is the most widely used illegal drug in the United States (cocaine is second). More than 30% of Americans—more than 70 million—have tried marijuana at least once; among 18–25-year-olds, more than 45% have tried marijuana.

Marijuana is a crude preparation of various parts of the Indian hemp plant *Cannabis sativa*, which grows in most parts of the world. THC (tetrahydrocannabinol) is the main active ingredient in marijuana. Based on THC content, the potency of marijuana preparations varies widely. Marijuana plants that grow wild often have less than 1% THC in their leaves, whereas when selected strains are cultivated by separation of male and female plants (*sinsemilla*), the bud leaves from the flowering tops may contain 7–8% THC. Hashish, a potent preparation made from the thick resin that exudes from the leaves, may contain up to 14% THC. Marijuana is usually smoked, but it can also be ingested.

Short-Term Effects and Uses As is true with most psychoactive drugs, the effects of a low dose of marijuana are strongly influenced both by the user's expectations and by past experiences. At low doses, marijuana users typically experience euphoria, a heightening of subjective sensory experiences, a slowing down of the perception of passing time, and a relaxed, "laid-back" attitude. These pleasant effects are the reason this drug is so widely used.

With moderate doses, these effects become stronger, and the user can also expect to have impaired memory function, disturbed thought patterns, lapses of attention, and feelings of **depersonalization,** in which the mind seems to be separated from the body. Decreased driving and workplace safety can also be expected.

The effects of marijuana in higher doses are determined mostly by the drug itself rather than by the user's expectations and setting. Very high doses produce feelings of depersonalization, as well as marked sensory distortion and changes in body image (such as a feeling that the body is very light). Inexperienced users sometimes think these sensations mean they are going crazy and become anxious or even panicky. Such reactions resemble a bad trip on LSD, but they happen much less often, are less severe, and do not last as long. Physiologically, marijuana increases heart rate and dilates certain blood vessels in the eyes, which creates the characteristic bloodshot eyes. The user also feels less inclined toward physical exertion.

The question of whether marijuana has any medical uses has been hotly debated. A legal, prescription form of THC called dronabinol has been available in a capsule for some patients since 1985; however, many patients argue that oral THC is not as effective as smoked marijuana. A 1999 government-commissioned report from the Institute of Medicine concluded that substances in marijuana have potential therapeutic value for pain relief, for control of nausea and vomiting in chemotherapy patients, and for stimulating appetite in people with AIDS-related wasting. Although effective drugs already exist for these conditions, marijuana may be suitable for patients who do not respond to other therapies. The report recommends further studies and the development of alternative methods of drug delivery—inhalers or patches—that would safely deliver set doses of specific compounds in marijuana.

Long-Term Effects The most probable long-term effect of smoking marijuana is respiratory damage, including chronic bronchial irritation and precancerous changes in the lungs. People who smoke marijuana may be at increased risk for emphysema and cancer of the head and neck. Heavy users who are frequently intoxicated experience subtle impairments of attention and memory that may or may not be reversible following long-term abstinence. Long-term use may also decrease testosterone levels and sperm counts and increase sperm abnormalities. Heavy marijuana use during pregnancy may cause impaired fetal growth and development and low birth weight. Marijuana may act synergistically with alcohol to increase the damaging effects of alcohol on the fetus. THC rapidly enters breast milk and may impair an infant's early motor development.

Regular users of marijuana can develop tolerance; a few develop dependence. Withdrawal symptoms are generally mild and short-lived; they include restlessness, irritability, insomnia, nausea, and cramping. As with all drugs that relieve "bad" feelings and produce "good" feelings, marijuana can become the focus of the user's life, to the exclusion of other activities. Drug uses appear to be related, and the chronic marijuana user is more likely to be a heavy user of tobacco, alcohol, and other dangerous drugs.

Hallucinogens

Hallucinogens are a group of drugs whose predominant pharmacological effect is to alter the user's perceptions, feelings, and thoughts. Hallucinogens include LSD (lysergic acid diethylamide), mescaline, psilocybin, STP (dimethoxymethyl amphetamine), DMT (dimethyltryptamine), MDMA (3,4-methylene-dioxymethamphetamine), ketamine, and PCP (phencyclidine). These drugs are most commonly ingested or smoked.

LSD LSD is one of the most powerful psychoactive drugs. Tiny doses will produce noticeable effects in most people, such as an altered sense of time, visual disturbances, an improved sense of hearing, mood changes, and distortions in how people perceive their bodies. Dilation of the pupils and slight dizziness, weakness, and nausea may also occur. With larger doses, users may experience a phenomenon known as **synesthesia**, feelings of depersonalization, and other alterations in the perceived relationship between self and external reality.

Many hallucinogens induce tolerance so quickly that after only one or two doses, their effects decrease substantially. The user must then stop taking the drug for several days before his or her system can be receptive to it again. These drugs cause little drug-seeking behavior and no physical dependence or withdrawal symptoms.

The immediate effects of low doses of hallucinogens are largely determined by expectations and setting. Many effects are hard to describe because they involve subjective and unusual dimensions of awareness—the **altered states**

of consciousness for which these drugs are famous. For this reason, hallucinogens have acquired a certain aura not associated with other drugs. People have taken LSD in search of a religious or mystical experience or in the hope of exploring new worlds.

A severe panic reaction, which can be terrifying in the extreme, can result from taking any dose of LSD. It is impossible to predict when a panic reaction will occur. Some LSD users report having hundreds of pleasurable and ecstatic experiences before having a "bad trip," or "bummer." Even after the drug's chemical effects have worn off, spontaneous flashbacks and other psychological disturbances can occur. **Flashbacks** are perceptual distortions and bizarre thoughts that occur after the drug has been entirely eliminated from the body.

Other Hallucinogens   Most other hallucinogens have the same general effects as LSD, but there are some variations. For example, a DMT or ketamine high does not last as long as an LSD high; an STP high lasts longer. MDMA has both hallucinogenic and amphetamine-like properties. Tolerance to MDMA develops quickly, and high doses can cause anxiety, delusions, and paranoia.

PCP, also known as "angel dust," "hog," and "peace pill," reduces and distorts sensory input, especially **proprioception,** the sensation of body position and movement; it creates a state of sensory deprivation. Because it can be easily made, PCP is often available illegally and is sometimes used as an inexpensive replacement for other psychoactive drugs. The effects of ketamine are similar to those of PCP—confusion, agitation, aggression, and lack of coordination—but tend to be less predictable. Tolerance to either drug can develop rapidly.

Mescaline (peyote), the ceremonial drug of the Native North American Church, produces an experience different from that caused by LSD. Obtaining mescaline costs far more than making LSD, however, so most street mescaline is LSD that has been highly diluted. Hallucinogenic effects can be obtained from certain mushrooms (*Psilocybe mexicana,* or "magic mushrooms"), certain morning glory seeds, nutmeg, jimsonweed, and other botanical products, but unpleasant side effects, such as dizziness, have limited the popularity of these products.

Inhalants

Inhaling certain chemicals can produce effects ranging from heightened pleasure to delirium. Inhalants fall into three major groups: (1) volatile solvents, which include adhesives and aerosols; (2) nitrites, such as butyl nitrite and amyl nitrite; and (3) anesthetics, which include nitrous oxide, or "laughing gas." Inhalant use is difficult to control because inhalants are easy to obtain. They are present in a variety of seemingly harmless products, from dessert-topping sprays to underarm deodorants, that are both inexpensive and legal. Using the drugs also requires

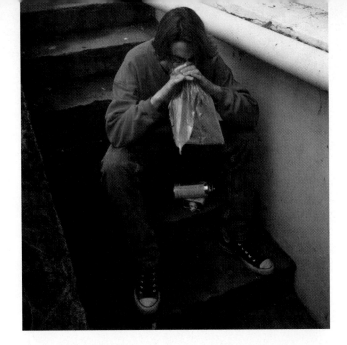

Inhalant use is difficult to monitor and control because inhalants are found in many inexpensive and legal products. Low doses of inhalants may cause a user to feel slightly stimulated; higher concentrations can cause a loss of consciousness, heart failure, and death.

no illegal or suspicious paraphernalia. Inhalant users get high by "sniffing," "snorting," "bagging" (inhaling fumes from a plastic bag), or "huffing" (placing an inhalant-soaked rag in the mouth).

Although different in makeup, nearly all inhalants produce effects similar to those of anesthetics, which slow down body functions. Low doses may cause users to feel slightly stimulated; at higher doses, users may feel less inhibited and less in control. Sniffing high concentrations of the chemicals in solvents or aerosol sprays can cause a loss of consciousness, heart failure, and death. High concentrations of any inhalant can also cause death from suffocation by displacing the oxygen in the lungs and central nervous system. Deliberately inhaling from a bag or in a closed area greatly increases the chances of suffocation. Other possible effects of the excessive or long-term use of inhalants include damage to the nervous system (impaired perception, reasoning, memory, and muscular coordination); hearing loss; and damage to the liver, kidneys, and bone marrow.

DRUG USE: THE DECADES AHEAD

Drug research will undoubtedly provide new information, new treatments, and new chemical combinations in the decades ahead. Although the use of some drugs, both legal and illegal, has declined dramatically since the 1970s, the use of others has held steady or increased. Mounting

Most people associate drug abuse problems with big cities. However, a recent report that examined drug use patterns in the United States found that small cities and rural areas have rates of drug abuse and related problems that are as high as or even higher than the rates in large cities. Adults in rural areas are just as likely as those in urban centers to use and abuse illegal drugs, alcohol, and tobacco. Young teens in small cities and rural areas are even more likely to abuse substances than teens in large metropolitan areas. Eighth-graders living in rural America are

- 104% more likely to use amphetamines

- 83% more likely to use crack

- 50% more likely to use cocaine

- 34% more likely to smoke marijuana

- 29% more likely to drink alcohol and 70% more likely to get drunk

In addition, rural eighth-graders are more than twice as likely to smoke cigarettes and nearly five times as likely to use spit tobacco. The trend continues for older teens: Among tenth-graders living in rural areas, rates of drug use exceed those for tenth-graders in large urban areas for every drug except MDMA (ecstasy) and marijuana. One group at particular risk for drug use and related problems is Native American teens living on reservations. A high rate of drug use among young teens is of particular concern because the earlier people begin to use drugs, the more likely they are to suffer serious medical and social consequences.

Along with higher rates of drug use come higher rates of drug-related problems—legal, medical, and social. In the

1990s, the smaller the community, the faster the rate of increase in drug-related crimes. Arrest rates for DUIs in small cities and rural areas are more than double those of large cities. The proportion of teens and young adults who have used drugs intravenously is greatest in rural areas; related to this, AIDS cases since 1994 have increased at a greater rate in rural areas (82%) than in large metropolitan areas (59%). In addition, more workers in rural areas test positive for drugs, which can lead to higher rates of absenteeism, unemployment, and job-related injuries.

Small cities and rural areas also face greater challenges in dealing with substance abuse problems. Drugs are equally available in all areas of the United States: In surveys, the percentage of people in rural towns, small cities, and large urban areas who report that drugs are "very easy" or "fairly easy" to obtain is essentially the same. However, rural areas must tackle drug-related problems with less information and fewer resources. Due to stereotypes about drug abuse patterns in the United States, there has been little research examining the drug problem in rural areas. Rural communities have a smaller tax base, making it difficult for substance abuse service providers to achieve the economies of scale needed to provide effective treatment services. Thus, most people in rural areas who need services must travel long distances for treatment or go without help. Smaller cities and rural areas also lack the money, personnel, and expertise to deal with drug trafficking organizations.

SOURCE: National Center on Addiction and Substance Abuse. 2000. *No Place to Hide: Substance Abuse in Mid-Size Cities and Rural America.* New York: National Center on Addiction and Substance Abuse.

public concern has led to great debate and a wide range of opinions about what should be done. Efforts to combat the problem include workplace drug testing, tougher law enforcement and prosecution, and treatment and education.

Drugs, Society, and Families

The economic cost of drug use is staggering. Each year, Americans spend over $50 billion on illegal drugs, with an additional $100 billion going to cover enforcement, prevention, treatment, lost wages, and drug-related injuries and crime. But the costs are more than just financial; they are also paid in human pain and suffering

The relationship between drugs and crime is complex. The criminal justice system is inundated with people accused of crimes related to drug possession, sale, or use. More than 2 million arrests are made each year for drug and alcohol violations, and more than 100,000 people are in jail for violating drug laws. Violence and the use of guns are more common in neighborhoods where drug

trafficking is prevalent. Addicts commit more robberies and burglaries than criminals not on drugs. People under the influence of drugs, especially alcohol, are more likely to commit violent crimes like rape and murder than people who do not use drugs.

Drug use is also a health care issue for society. In the United States, illegal drug use leads to more than 500,000 emergency room admissions and about 20,000 deaths annually. While it is in the best interest of society to treat addicts who want help, there is not nearly enough space in treatment facilities to help the estimated 5 million Americans in need of immediate treatment. Drug addicts who want to quit, especially those among the urban poor, often have to wait a year or more for acceptance into a residential care or other treatment program.

Drug abuse also takes a toll on individuals and families. Children born to women who use drugs like alcohol, tobacco, or cocaine may have long-term health problems. Drug use in families can become a vicious cycle. Observing adults around them using drugs, children assume it is an acceptable way to deal with problems. Other problems like abuse, neglect, lack of opportunity, and unemployment become contributing factors to drug use and serve to perpetuate the cycle.

Legalizing Drugs

Pointing out that many of the social problems associated with drugs are related to prohibition rather than to the effects of the drugs themselves, some people have argued for various forms of drug legalization. Proposals range from making such drugs as marijuana and heroin available by prescription to allowing licensed dealers to sell some of these drugs to adults. Proponents argue that crimes by drug users are usually committed to buy drugs that cost relatively more than alcohol and tobacco because they are produced illegally. By making some currently illicit drugs legal—but putting controls on them similar to those used for alcohol, tobacco, and prescription drugs—many of the problems related to drug use could be eliminated.

Opponents of drug legalization argue that allowing easier access to drugs would expose many more people to possible abuse and dependence. Drugs would be cheaper and easier to obtain, and drug use would be more socially acceptable. Legalizing drugs could cause an increase in drug use among children and teenagers. Opponents point out that alcohol and tobacco are major causes of disease and death in our society and that they should not be used as models for other practices.

Drug Testing

One of the most controversial issues in American politics is drug testing in the workplace. It has been estimated that as many as 10% of workers use psychoactive drugs on the job. For some occupations, such as air traffic controllers, truck drivers, and train engineers, drug use can create significant hazards, sometimes involving hundreds of people. Some people believe that the dangers are so great that all workers should be tested and that anyone found with traces of drugs in the blood or urine should be either fired or treated. Others insist that this would violate people's right to privacy and to freedom from unreasonable search, guaranteed by the Fourth Amendment. Opponents point out that most jobs do not involve hazards, so employees who take drugs are not any more dangerous than employees who do not.

Despite the expense, many employers now test their employees, and the U.S. armed forces test military personnel regularly. People in jobs involving transportation are required by federal law to be tested regularly to ensure public safety. The primary criterion leading most companies to use drug testing is the company's liability if an employee under the influence of a drug makes a mistake that could potentially harm others. If a person tests positive for drugs, the employer may provide drug counseling or treatment, suspend the employee until he or she tests

negative, or fire the individual. There are also several FDA-approved over-the-counter home drug testing kits designed to allow parents to check their children for drug use.

Treatment for Drug Dependence

A variety of programs are available to help people break their drug habits, but there is no single best method of treatment. The relapse rate is high for all types of treatment but is similar to the rate of relapse seen in people being treated for diabetes, high blood pressure, and asthma. Numerous studies have shown that being treated is better than not being treated. To be successful, a treatment program must deal with the reasons behind people's drug abuse and help them develop behaviors, attitudes, and a social support system that will help them remain drug-free.

Drug Substitution Programs   Sometimes a less debilitating drug can be substituted for one with many damaging effects, thus reducing the risks of the drug use. Methadone is a synthetic drug used as a substitute for heroin. When methadone is used, addicts can stop taking heroin without experiencing severe withdrawal reactions. Although methadone is addictive, it decreases the craving for heroin and enables the individual to function normally in social and vocational activities. Methadone maintenance treatment allows many former heroin abusers to live more useful lives. Other heroin substitutes in use or being studied include LAAM (levo-alpha-acetylmethadol), buprenorphine, and naltrexone.

Because they are relatively inexpensive to administer, drug substitution programs are a popular form of treatment. However, the relapse rate is high. Combining drug substitution with psychological and social services improves success rates, underscoring the importance of psychological factors in drug dependence.

Treatment Centers   Treatment centers offer a variety of short-term and long-term services, including hospitalization, detoxification, counseling, and other mental health services. A specific type of center is the therapeutic community, a residential program run in a completely drug-free atmosphere. Administered by ex-addicts, these programs use confrontation, strict discipline, and unrelenting peer pressure to attempt to resocialize the addict with a different set of values. "Halfway houses," transitional settings between a 24-hour-a-day program and independent living, are an important phase of treatment for some people.

Self-Help Groups and Peer Counseling   Groups such as Alcoholics Anonymous (AA) and Narcotics Anonymous (NA) have helped many people. These groups follow a 12-step program. Group members' first step is to acknowledge that they have a problem over which they

If you notice changes in behavior and mood in someone you know, they may signal a growing dependence on drugs. Signs that a person's life is beginning to focus on drugs include the following:

- Sudden withdrawal or emotional distance
- Rebellious or unusually irritable behavior
- A loss of interest in usual activities or hobbies
- A decline in school performance
- A sudden change in the chosen group of friends
- Changes in sleeping or eating habits
- Frequent borrowing of money or stealing
- Secretive behavior about personal possessions, such as a backpack or the contents of a drawer
- Deterioration of physical appearance

If you believe a family member or friend has a drug problem, obtain information about resources for drug treatment available on your campus or in your community. Communicate your concern, provide him or her with information about treatment options, and offer your support during treatment. If the person continues to deny having a problem, you may want to talk with an experienced counselor about setting up an "intervention"— a formal, structured confrontation designed to end denial by having family, friends, and other caring individuals present their concerns to the drug user. Participants in an intervention would indicate the ways in which the individual is hurting others as well as himself or herself. If your friend or family member agrees to treatment, encourage him or her to attend a support group such as Narcotics Anonymous or Alcoholics Anonymous. And finally, examine your relationship with the abuser for signs of codependency. If necessary, get help for yourself; friends and family of drug users can often benefit from counseling.

---

have no control. Peer support is a critical ingredient of these programs, and members usually meet at least once a week. Each member is paired with a sponsor to call on for advice and support if the temptation to relapse becomes overwhelming. Chapters of AA and NA meet on some college campuses; community-based chapters are listed in the phone book and local newspapers.

Many colleges also have peer counseling programs, in which students are trained to help other students who have drug problems. A peer counselor's role may be as limited as referring a student to a professional with expertise in substance dependence for an evaluation or as involved as helping arrange a leave of absence from school for participation in a drug-treatment program. Most peer counseling programs are founded on principles of strict confidentiality. Peer counselors may also be able to help students who are concerned about a classmate or loved one with an apparent drug problem.

Codependency   Many treatment programs also offer counseling for those who are close to drug abusers. Drug abuse takes a toll on friends and family members, and counseling can help people work through painful feelings

of guilt and powerlessness. Sometimes people close to a drug abuser develop patterns of behavior, known as **codependency,** that help or enable the person to remain drug dependent. Codependency, also called *enabling,* removes or softens the effects of the drug use on the user. People often become enablers spontaneously and naturally. When someone they love becomes dependent on a drug, they want to help, and they may assume that their good intentions will persuade the drug user to stop. However, the habit of enabling may actually inhibit a drug-dependent person's recovery because the person never has to experience the consequences of his or her behavior.

Have you ever been an enabler in a relationship? You may have, if you've ever done any of the following:

- Given someone one more chance to stop abusing drugs, then another, and another . . .
- Made excuses or lied for someone to his or her friends, teachers, or employer
- Joined someone in drug use and blamed others for your behavior
- Loaned money to someone to continue drug use
- Stayed up late waiting for or gone out searching for someone who uses drugs
- Felt embarrassed or angry about the actions of someone who uses drugs
- Ignored the drug use because the person got defensive when you brought it up
- Not confronted a friend or relative who was obviously intoxicated or high on a drug

Terms   **codependency** A relationship in which a non–substance-abusing partner or family member enables the other's substance abuse.

If you come from a codependent family or see yourself developing codependency relationships, consider acting now to make changes in your patterns of interaction.

Preventing Drug Abuse

Obviously, the best solution to drug abuse is prevention. Government attempts at controlling the drug problem tend to focus on stopping the production, importation, and distribution of illegal drugs. Creative effort also has to be put into stopping the demand for drugs. Developing persuasive antidrug educational programs offers the best hope for solving the drug problem in the future. Indirect approaches to prevention involve building young people's self-esteem, improving their academic skills, and increasing their recreational opportunities. Direct approaches involve giving information about the adverse effects of drugs and teaching tactics that help students resist peer pressure to use drugs in various situations. Developing strategies for resisting peer pressure is one of the more effective techniques.

Prevention efforts need to focus on the different motivations individuals have for using and abusing specific drugs at different ages. For example, adolescents are often responsive to peer counselors. Many young adults tend to be influenced by efforts that focus on health education. For all ages, it is important to provide nondrug alternatives that speak to people's reasons for using drugs, such as recreational facilities, counseling, greater opportunities for leisure activities, and places to socialize. Reminding young people that most people, no matter what age, are *not* users of illegal drugs, do *not* smoke cigarettes, and do *not* get drunk frequently, is a critical part of preventing substance abuse.

The Role of Drugs in Your Life

Where do you fit into this complex picture of drug use and abuse? Chances are that you've had experience with OTC and prescription drugs, and you may or may not have had experience with one or more of the drugs described in this chapter. You probably know someone who has used or abused a psychoactive drug. Whatever your experience has been up to now, it's likely that you will encounter drugs at some point in your life. To make sure you'll have the inner resources to resist peer pressure and make your own decision, cultivate a variety of activities you enjoy doing, realize that you are entitled to have your own opinion, and don't neglect your self-esteem.

Issues to Consider Before you try a psychoactive drug, consider the following questions:

- *What are the risks involved?* Many drugs carry a immediate risk of injury or death. Almost all involve the longer-term risk of abuse and dependence.
- *Is using the drug compatible with your goals?* Consider how drug use will affect your education and career objectives, your relationships, your future happiness, and the happiness of those who love you.
- *What are your ethical beliefs about drug use?* Consider whether using a drug would cause you to go against your personal ethics, religious beliefs, social values, or family responsibilities.
- *What are the financial costs?* Many drugs are expensive, especially if you become dependent on them.
- *Are you trying to solve a deeper problem?* Drugs will not make emotional pain go away; in the long run, they will only make it worse. If you are feeling depressed or anxious, seek help from a mental health professional instead of self-medicating with drugs.

Like all aspects of health-related behavior, making responsible decisions about drug use depends on information, knowledge, and insight into yourself. Many choices are possible; making the ones that are right for you is what counts.

What to Do Instead of Drugs If you have used or considered using drugs, think carefully about your reasons for doing so. Consider trying healthier strategies for dealing with difficult emotions and peer pressure. For ideas, look over the following list of reasons for drug use and suggested alternative activities:

- *Bored?* Go for a walk or a run; stimulate your senses at a museum; challenge your mind with a new game or book; introduce yourself to someone new.
- *Stressed?* Practice relaxation or visualization; try to slow down and open your senses to the natural world; get some exercise.
- *Shy or lonely?* Talk to a counselor; enroll in a shyness clinic; practice communication techniques.
- *Feeling low on self-esteem?* Give yourself credit for the things you do well. A program of regular exercise can also enhance self-esteem.
- *Depressed or anxious?* Talk to a friend, parent, or counselor.
- *Apathetic or lethargic?* Force yourself to get up and get some exercise to energize yourself; assume responsibility for someone or something outside yourself; volunteer.
- *Searching for meaning?* Try yoga or meditation; explore spiritual experiences through religious groups, church, prayer, or reading.
- *Afraid to say no?* Take a course in assertiveness training; get support from others who don't want to use drugs; remind yourself that you have the right and the responsibility to make your own decisions.
- *Still feeling peer pressure?* Begin to look for new friends or roommates. Take a class or join an organization that attracts other health-conscious people.

The essence of wellness is taking charge of your life. Dependence on drugs or compulsive activities is the very opposite of wellness, since it involves relinquishing control over your life to chemical substances or forces outside yourself. The best treatment for dependence is prevention—not starting in the first place—but it's never too late to regain control of your life.

Right now you can

- Go outside and sit on a park bench, or walk around outside at half your normal pace, opening all your senses to the beauty of nature. If you can't get to a beautiful place, close your eyes and visualize one. See if you can experience a "natural high."

- Substitute some bottled water for your caffeinated soda, and make your next cup of coffee half decaf.

- Consider whether someone you love has a drug problem; if so, consider how you can best help that person face and solve the problem.

- Plan to get enough sleep this week, so you won't feel the need for stimulants to be awake and alert.

- Examine what you've been doing lately to see if you are truly making your own decisions—or if some substance or out-of-control behavior has you in its power; if so, start thinking about how to regain control.

SUMMARY

- Addictive behaviors are reinforcing. Addicts experience a strong compulsion for the behavior and a loss of control over it; an escalating pattern of abuse with serious negative consequences may result.

- The sources or causes of addiction include heredity, personality, lifestyle, and environmental factors. People may use an addictive behavior as a means of alleviating stress or painful emotions.

- Many common behaviors are potentially addictive, including gambling, shopping, sexual activity, Internet use, eating, and working.

- Drug abuse is a maladaptive pattern of drug use that persists despite adverse social, psychological, or medical consequences.

- Drug dependence involves taking a drug compulsively, which includes neglecting constructive activities because of it and continuing to use it despite experiencing adverse effects. Tolerance and withdrawal symptoms are often present.

- The effect of a drug depends on the properties of the drug and how it's used (drug factors), the physical and psychological characteristics of the user (user factors), and the physical and social environment surrounding drug use (social factors).

- Opioids relieve pain, cause drowsiness, and induce euphoria; they reduce anxiety and produce lethargy, apathy, and an inability to concentrate.

- CNS depressants slow down the overall activity of the nerves; they reduce anxiety and cause mood changes, impaired muscular coordination, slurring of speech, and drowsiness or sleep.

- CNS stimulants speed up the activity of the nerves, causing acceleration of the heart rate and a rise in blood pressure.

- Marijuana usually causes euphoria and a relaxed attitude at low doses; very high doses produce feelings of depersonalization and sensory distortion.

- Hallucinogens alter perception, feelings, and thought and may cause an altered sense of time, visual disturbances, and mood changes.

- Inhalants are present in a variety of harmless products. Their use can lead to loss of consciousness, heart failure, suffocation, and death.

- Economic and social costs of drug abuse include the financial costs of law enforcement, treatment, and health care and the social costs of crime, violence, and family problems.

- Approaches to treatment include drug substitution programs, treatment centers, self-help groups, and peer counseling; many programs also offer counseling to family members.

Behavior Change Strategy   Changing Your Drug Habits

This behavior change strategy focuses on one of the most commonly used drugs—caffeine. If you are concerned about your use of a different drug or another type of addictive behavior, you can devise your own plan based on this one and on the steps outlined in Chapter 1.

Because caffeine supports certain behaviors that are characteristic of our culture, such as sedentary, stressful work, you may find yourself relying on coffee (or tea, chocolate, or cola) to get through a busy schedule. Such habits often begin in college. Fortunately, it's easier to break a habit before it becomes entrenched as a lifelong dependency.

When you are studying for exams, the forced physical inactivity and the need to concentrate even when fatigued may lead you to overuse caffeine. But caffeine doesn't "help" unless you are already sleepy. And it does not relieve any underlying condition (you are just more tired when it wears off). How can you change this pattern?

Self-Monitoring

Keep a log of how much caffeine you eat or drink. Use a measuring cup to measure coffee or tea. Using Figure 7-2, convert the amounts you eat or drink into an estimate expressed in milligrams of caffeine. Be sure to include all forms, such as chocolate bars and OTC medications, as well as caffeine candy, colas, cocoa or hot chocolate, chocolate cake, tea, and coffee.

Self-Assessment

At the end of the week, add up your daily totals and divide by 7 to get your daily average in milligrams. How much is too much? At more than 250 mg per day, you may well be experiencing some adverse symptoms. If you are experiencing at least five of the following symptoms, you may want to cut down.

- Restlessness
- Nervousness
- Excitement
- Insomnia
- Flushed face
- Excessive sweating
- Gastrointestinal problems
- Muscle twitching
- Rambling thoughts and speech
- Irregular heartbeat
- Periods of inexhaustibility
- Excessive pacing or movement

Set Limits

Can you restrict your caffeine intake to a daily total, and stick to this contract? If so, set a cutoff point, such as one cup of coffee. Pegging it to a specific time of day can be helpful, because then you won't confront a decision at any other point (and possibly fail). If you find you cannot stick to your limit, you may want to cut out caffeine altogether; abstinence can be easier than moderation for some people. If you experience caffeine withdrawal symptoms (headache, fatigue), you may want to cut your intake more gradually.

Find Other Ways to Keep Your Energy Up

If you are fatigued, it makes sense to get enough sleep or exercise more, rather than drowning the problem in coffee or tea. Different people need different amounts of sleep; you may also need more sleep at different times, such as during a personal crisis or an illness. Also, exercise raises your metabolic rate for hours afterward—a handy fact to exploit when you want to feel more awake and want to avoid an irritable caffeine jag. And if you've been compounding your fatigue by not eating properly, try filling up on complex carbohydrates such as whole-grain bread or crackers instead of candy bars.

Tips on Cutting Out Caffeine   Here are some more ways to decrease your consumption of caffeine:

- Keep some noncaffeinated drinks on hand, such as decaffeinated coffee, herbal teas, mineral water, bouillon, or hot water.
- Alternate between hot and very cold liquids.
- Fill your coffee cup only halfway.
- Avoid the office or school lunchroom or cafeteria and the chocolate sections of the grocery store. (Often people drink coffee or tea and eat chocolate simply because they're available.)
- Read labels of over-the-counter medications to check for hidden sources of caffeine.

TAKE ACTION

1. Find out what types of services are available on your campus or in your community to handle drug dependence and other addictive behaviors. If there are none, what services are needed? Locate the school official and public health agency responsible for your campus and community, and ask why these needs aren't being met.

2. Survey three older adults and three young students about their attitudes toward legalizing marijuana. Are there any differences? If so, what accounts for these differences? What kinds of reasons do they give for their positions?

3. Look at a current movie or television program, paying special attention to how drug use is portrayed. What messages are being conveyed? If possible, compare a recent movie with a movie made 10–20 years ago. Has the presentation of drug use changed? If so, how?

JOURNAL ENTRY

1. Keep track of your own drug use for a week, noting in your health journal the name of the drug, the approximate dosage, the time of day, and what you think your reasons were for taking each dose. Don't forget to include coffee, soft drinks, and OTC medications. What types of drugs are you taking? Are there any patterns? Are there any signs of abuse or dependence? If you'd like to cut down, begin by making a list of alternative behaviors you could substitute for drug use.

2. Critical Thinking Does a woman have an obligation to avoid alcohol and other drugs during pregnancy? What about smoking cigarettes and eating junk food? If she doesn't follow her physician's advice, should she be held legally responsible for the effects on her child? What rights do the mother and child have in this situation? In your health journal, write an essay stating your opinion; be sure to defend your position.

3. Critical Thinking Do you think there is such a thing as the responsible use of illegal psychoactive drugs? Are they a legitimate recreational activity? Would you change any of the current laws governing drugs? If so, how would you draw the line between legitimate and illegitimate use? Write an essay explaining your position.

FOR MORE INFORMATION

Books

Dupont, R. L. 2000. *The Selfish Brain: Learning from Addiction*. Center City, Minn.: Hazelden Information and Educational Services. *Explores the biological roots of addiction and various approaches to treatment.*

Escohotado, A. 1999. *A Brief History of Drugs: From the Stone Age to the Stoned Age*. Rochester, Vt.: Inner Traditions. *A history of human involvement with psychoactive plants and drugs that explores the cultural, spiritual, and social effects of drug use.*

Hardiman, M., and M. Russell. 2000. *Overcoming Addiction: A Common Sense Approach*. Freedom, Calif.: Crossing Press. *A practical guide to the nature of addiction and how to find help.*

Hurley, J. A. 2000. *Addiction: Opposing Viewpoints*. San Diego: Greenhaven Press. *Explores contrasting views about the roots, contributory factors, and treatment of addiction.*

Julien, R. M. 2001. *A Primer of Drug Action*, 9th ed. New York: Freeman. *A guide to the actions, uses, and side effects of psychoactive drugs.*

Kuhn, C., et al. 1998. *Buzzed: The Straight Facts About the Most Used and Abused Drugs from Alcohol to Ecstasy*. New York: Norton. *An accurate, straightforward guide to commonly used drugs.*

Weinberg, B. A., and B. K. Bealer. 2001. *The World of Caffeine: The Science and Culture of the World's Most Popular Drug*. New York: Routledge. *An interesting history of the use of caffeine.*

W.W. Organizations, Hotlines, and Web Sites

Center for On-Line Addiction. Contains information about Internet and cybersex addiction.
http://netaddiction.com

ClubDrugs.Org. Provides information on drugs commonly classified as "club drugs."
http://www.clubdrugs.org

Do It Now Foundation. Provides youth-oriented information about drugs.
http://www.doitnow.org

Drug Enforcement Administration: Drugs of Abuse. Provides basic facts about major drugs of abuse, including penalties for drug trafficking.
http://www.usdoj.gov/dea/concern/abuse/contents.htm

DrugHelp Hotlines. A 24-hour service that provides confidential information and referrals.

800-DRUGHELP; 800-COCAINE; 800-HEROIN; MARIJUANA; 800-RELAPSE
http://www.drughelp.org

Gamblers Anonymous. Includes questions to help diagnose gambling problems and resources for getting help.
http://www.gamblersanonymous.org

Habitsmart. Contains information about addictive behavior, including tips for effectively managing problematic habitual behaviors, a self-scoring alcohol check-up, and links.
http://www.habitsmart.com

Higher Eduction Center for Alcohol and Other Drug Prevention. Gives information about alcohol and drug abuse on campus and links to related sites; it includes an area designed specifically for students.
http://www.edc.org/hec

Indiana Prevention Resource Center. A clearinghouse of information and links on substance-abuse topics, including specific psychoactive drugs and issues such as drug testing and drug legalization.
http://www.drugs.indiana.edu

Narcotics Anonymous (NA). Similar to Alcoholics Anonymous, NA sponsors 12-step meetings and provides other support services for drug abusers.
818-773-9999
http://www.na.org

There are also 12-step programs that focus on specific drugs:
Cocaine Anonymous
http://www.ca.org
Marijuana Anonymous
http://www.marijuana-anonymous.org

National Center on Addiction and Substance Abuse (CASA) at Columbia University. Provides information about the costs of substance abuse to individuals and society.
http://www.casacolumbia.org

National Clearinghouse for Alcohol and Drug Information. Provides statistics, information, and publications on substance abuse, including resources for people who want to help friends and family members overcome substance-abuse problems.
800-729-6686; 301-468-2600
http://www.health.org

National Drug Information, Treatment, and Referral Hotlines. Sponsored by the SAMHSA Center for Substance Abuse Treatment, these hotlines provide information on drug abuse and on HIV infection as it relates to substance abuse; referrals to support groups and treatment programs are available.

800-662-HELP
800-729-6686 (Spanish)
800-487-4889 (TDD for hearing impaired)

National Institute on Drug Abuse. Develops and supports research on drug abuse prevention programs; fact sheets on drugs of abuse are available on the Web site or via recorded phone messages, fax, or mail.

888-644-6432 (Infofax)

http://www.nida.nih.gov; http://www.drugabuse.gov

Office of National Drug Control Policy (ONDCP). Provides information on national and international drug-related topics, including U.S. policies relating to prevention, education, treatment, and enforcement.

http://www.whitehousedrugpolicy.gov

Substance Abuse and Mental Health Services Administration (SAMHSA). Provides statistics, information, and other resources relating to substance-abuse prevention and treatment.

301-443-8956

http://www.samhsa.gov

Web of Addictions. Provides a wealth of information about substance abuse and dependence, including fact sheets, contact information for relevant agencies and organizations, and links to related sites.

http://www.well.com/user/woa

See also the listing for Chapter 8.

SELECTED BIBLIOGRAPHY

American Psychiatric Association. 2000. *Diagnostic and Statistical Manual of Mental Disorders,* Fourth Edition, Text Revision (*DSM-IV-TR*). Washington, D.C.: American Psychiatric Association.

Ashton, C. H. 2001. Pharmacology and effects of cannabis: A brief review. *British Journal of Psychiatry* 178: 101–106.

Cannon, M. J., et al. 2001. Blood-borne and sexual transmission of human herpesvirus 8 in women with or at risk for human immunodeficiency virus infection. *New England Journal of Medicine* 344(9): 637–643.

Centers for Disease Control and Prevention. 2000. *A Comprehensive Approach to Preventing Blood-Borne Infections Among IDUs* (http://www.cdc.gov/hiv/projects/idu-ta/idu.htm; retrieved October 5, 2000).

Coke, crack, pot, speed, et al. 2001. *Scientific American,* January, p. 26.

Dyer, J. E., B. Roth, and B. A. Hyma. 2001. Gamma-hydroxybutyrate withdrawal syndrome. *American College of Emergency Physicians* 37: 147–153.

Ernst, T., et al. 2000. Evidence for long-term neurotoxicity associated with methamphetamine abuse. *Neurology* 54(6): 1344–1349.

Frank, D. A., et al. 2001. Growth, development, and behavior in early childhood following prenatal cocaine exposure. *Journal of the American Medical Association* 285(12): 1613–1625.

Hartley, T. R., et al. 2000. Hypertension risk status and effect of caffeine on blood pressure. *Hypertension* 36(1): 137–141.

Institute of Medicine. 1999. *Marijuana and Medicine: Assessing the Science Base.* Washington, D.C.: National Academy Press.

Johnson, M. K., et al. 2000. Large lung bullae in marijuana smokers. *Thorax* 55(4): 340–342.

Johnson, R. E., et al. 2000. A comparison of levomethadyl acetate, buprenorphine, and methadone for opioid dependence. *New England Journal of Medicine* 343(18): 1290–1297.

Kish, S. J., et al. 2000. Striatal serotonin is depleted in brain of a human MDMA (Ecstasy) user. *Neurology* 55(2): 294–296.

McElhatton, P. R., et al. 1999. Congenital anomalies after prenatal ecstasy exposure. *Lancet* 354(9188): 1441–1442.

McLellan, A. T., et al. 2000. Drug dependence, a chronic medical illness: Implications for treatment, insurance, and outcomes evaluation. *Journal of the American Medical Association* 284(13): 1689–1695.

Meyer, G., et al. 2000. Casino gambling increases heart rate and salivary cortisol in regular gamblers. *Biological Psychiatry* 48(9): 948–953.

Miller, T. R., D. C. Lestina, and G. S. Smith. 2001. Injury risk among medically identified alcohol and drug abusers. *Alcoholism: Clinical and Experimental Research* 25(1): 58.

Monitoring the Future Study. 2000. *Trends in Lifetime Prevalence of Use of Various Drugs for Eighth, Tenth, and Twelfth Graders* (http://monitoringthefuture.org; retrieved December 15, 2000).

National Clearinghouse for Alcohol and Drug Information. 2000. *Drugs of Abuse* (http://www.health.org/govpubs/rpo926; retrieved October 3, 2000).

National Institute on Drug Abuse. 2000. *Community Drug Alert Bulletin: Club Drugs* (http://www.nida.nih.gov/ClubAlert/Clubdrugalert.html; retrieved October 5, 2000).

National Institute on Drug Abuse. 2000. *Community Drug Alert Bulletin: Hepatitis C* (http://www.nida.nih.gov/HepatitisAlert/HepatitisAlert.html; retrieved October 4, 2000).

National Research Council. 1999. *Pathological Gambling.* Washington, D.C.: National Academy Press.

Office of National Drug Control Policy. 2001. *National Drug Control Strategy, 2001 Annual Report.* Rockville, Md.: Office of National Drug Control Policy.

Parker, J. 2000. *Heroin: The Junk Equation.* Tempe, Az.: Do It Now Foundation.

Qureshi, A. I., et al. 2001. Cocaine use and the likelihood of nonfatal myocardial infarction and stroke: Data from the Third National Health and Nutrition Examination Survey. *Circulation* 103: 502–506.

Substance Abuse and Mental Health Services Administration. 2000. *Drug Abuse Warning Network: Annual Medical Examiner Data, 1998.* Rockville, Md.: Substance Abuse and Mental Health Services Administration.

Substance Abuse and Mental Health Services Administration. 2000. *National Household Survey on Drug Abuse. 1999.* Rockville, Md.: Substance Abuse and Mental Health Services Administration.

U.S. Drug Enforcement Administration. 2000. *Drug Intelligence Brief: An Overview of Club Drugs.* Arlington, Va.: Drug Enforcement Administration.

Volkow, N. D., et al. 2001. Association of dopamine transporter reduction with psychomotor impairment in methamphetamine abusers. *American Journal of Psychiatry* 158(3): 377–382.

Zakzanis, K. K., and D. A. Young. 2001. Memory impairment in abstinent MDMA ("ecstasy") users: A longitudinal investigation. *Neurology* 56: 966–969.

Zvosec, D. L., et al. 2001. Adverse events, including death, associated with the use of 1,4-butanediol. *New England Journal of Medicine* 344(2): 87–94.

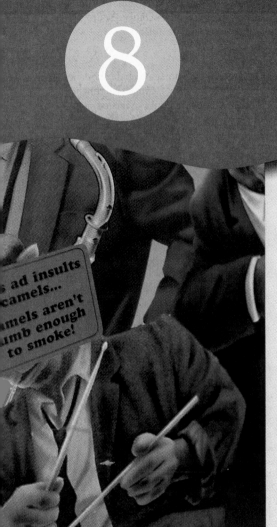

Alcohol and Tobacco

8

LOOKING AHEAD

After reading this chapter, you should be able to

- Explain how alcohol is absorbed and metabolized by the body

- Describe the immediate and long-term effects of drinking alcohol

- Define alcohol abuse, binge drinking, and alcoholism and discuss their effects on the drinker and others

- List the reasons people start using tobacco and why they continue to use it

- Explain the short- and long-term health risks associated with tobacco use and exposure to environmental tobacco smoke

- Describe strategies for using alcohol responsibly, for quitting tobacco use, and for avoiding environmental tobacco smoke

When we hear about the dangers of drugs, most of us think of illicit drugs like marijuana, cocaine, heroin, and ecstasy. Stories of violence and deaths related to the sale and use of illegal drugs often appear in the news. Far less attention is given to the drugs that are actually responsible for the most injuries and deaths in the United States—**alcohol** and **tobacco**. Indeed, alcohol and tobacco are seldom even thought of as drugs. The truth is that both alcohol and **nicotine** (the psychoactive drug in tobacco) are powerful drugs that can have a devastating impact on health.

About 64% of Americans over the age of 12 drink alcohol in some form. Many people think of alcohol the way it's portrayed in advertisements, on television, and in movies—as part of a good time, an integral ingredient of celebrations. However, like other drugs, alcohol can impair functioning in the short term and cause devastating damage in the long term. Through automobile crashes and other injuries, alcohol is the leading cause of death among people between the ages of 15 and 24.

Although the proportion of cigarette smokers among Americans has dropped over the last four decades, tobacco use remains widespread and 24% of American adults smoke. Smoking is the leading preventable cause of death in this country, killing more than 400,000 people each year. Nonsmokers subjected to the smoke of others also suffer. Exposure to **environmental tobacco smoke (ETS)** causes more than 60,000 deaths each year, and smoking by pregnant women is responsible for up to 10% of all infant deaths in this country.

Avoiding tobacco and using alcohol wisely, if at all, are important parts of a healthy lifestyle. This chapter explores the reasons people use alcohol and tobacco, how these drugs affect health, and how people can make healthy and responsible choices about the role of alcohol and tobacco in their lives.

THE NATURE OF ALCOHOL

How does alcohol affect people? Does it affect some people differently than others? Can some people "handle" alcohol? Is it possible to drink a safe amount of alcohol? Misconceptions about the effects of alcohol can be cleared up by taking a closer look at the chemistry of alcohol and how it is absorbed and metabolized by the body.

The Chemistry of Alcohol

Ethyl alcohol is the psychoactive ingredient in all alcoholic beverages. Beer, a mild intoxicant brewed from a mixture of grains, usually contains 3–6% alcohol by volume. Ales and malt liquors are 6–8% alcohol by volume. Wines are made by *fermenting* the juices of grapes or other fruits. The concentration of alcohol in table wines is about 9–14%. *Fortified wines,* so named because alcohol has been added to them, contain about 20% alcohol; these include sherry, port, and Madeira. Stronger alcoholic beverages, called *hard liquors,* are made by *distilling* brewed or fermented grains or other products. These beverages, including gin, whiskey, brandy, rum, tequila, vodka, and liqueurs, usually contain 35–50% alcohol.

The concentration of alcohol in a beverage is indicated by the **proof value,** which is two times the percentage concentration. For example, if a beverage is 100 proof, it contains 50% alcohol. Two ounces of 100-proof whiskey contain 1 ounce of pure alcohol. The proof value of hard liquors can usually be found on the bottle labels. When alcohol consumption is discussed, "one drink" refers to a 12-ounce bottle of beer, a 5-ounce glass of table wine, or a cocktail with 1.5 ounces of 80-proof liquor. Each of these different drinks contains approximately the same amount of alcohol: 0.6 ounce.

Absorption

When a person ingests alcohol, about 20% is rapidly absorbed from the stomach into the bloodstream. About 75% is absorbed through the upper part of the small intestine. Any remaining alcohol enters the bloodstream further along the gastrointestinal tract. The rate of absorption is affected by a variety of factors. For example, the carbonation in a beverage like champagne increases the rate of alcohol absorption. Food in the stomach slows the rate of absorption, as does the drinking of highly concentrated alcoholic beverages such as hard liquor. But remember: *All* alcohol a person consumes is eventually absorbed.

Metabolism and Excretion

Alcohol is quickly transported throughout the body by the blood. Because alcohol easily moves through most biological membranes, it is rapidly distributed throughout most body tissues. The main site of alcohol **metabolism** is the liver, though a small amount of alcohol is metabolized

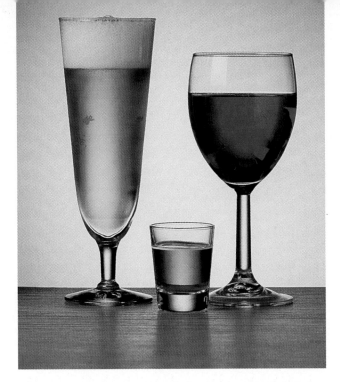

Ethyl alcohol is the common psychoactive drug found in all alcoholic beverages. One drink—a 12-ounce beer, a 1.5-ounce cocktail, or a 5-ounce glass of wine—contains about 0.6 ounce of ethyl alcohol.

in the stomach. About 2–10% of ingested alcohol is not metabolized in the liver or other tissues, but is excreted unchanged by the lungs, kidneys, and sweat glands. Excreted alcohol causes the telltale smell on a drinker's breath and is the basis of breath and urine analyses for alcohol levels.

There are some genetic differences in alcohol metabolism that are associated with gender and ethnicity. Women metabolize less alcohol in the stomach than men do, so they release more unmetabolized alcohol into the bloodstream. (The stomach enzyme that breaks down alcohol is

alcohol The intoxicating ingredient in fermented liquors; a colorless, pungent liquid.

tobacco The leaves of cultivated tobacco plants prepared for smoking, chewing, or use as snuff.

nicotine A poisonous, addictive substance found in tobacco and responsible for many of the effects of tobacco.

environmental tobacco smoke (ETS) Smoke that enters the atmosphere from the burning end of a cigarette, cigar, or pipe, as well as smoke that is exhaled by smokers; also called *secondhand smoke.*

proof value Two times the percentage of alcohol by volume; a beverage that is 50% alcohol by volume is 100 proof.

metabolism The chemical transformation of food and other substances in the body into energy and waste.

Terms

Table 8-1	The Effects of Alcohol	
BAC (%)	**Common Behavioral Effects**	**Hours Required to Metabolize Alcohol**
0.00–0.05	Slight change in feelings, usually relaxation and euphoria. Decreased alertness.	2–3
0.05–0.10	Emotional instability, with exaggerated feelings and behavior. Reduced social inhibitions. Impairment of reaction time and fine motor coordination. Increasingly impaired during driving. Legally drunk at 0.08% in many states and 0.10% in others.	3–6
0.10–0.15	Unsteadiness in standing and walking. Loss of peripheral vision. Driving is extremely dangerous.	6–10
0.15–0.30	Staggering gait. Slurred speech. Pain and other sensory perceptions greatly impaired.	10–24
More than 0.30	Stupor or unconsciousness. Anesthesia. Death possible at 0.35% and above. Can result from rapid or binge drinking with few earlier effects.	More than 24

less active in women than in men.) The same amount of alcohol will thus have more effect on a woman than on a man—she will feel the effects sooner and more strongly.

Some people, including many of Asian descent, have different forms of the two enzymes that metabolize alcohol. When this group drinks alcohol, they experience a physiological reaction referred to as *flushing syndrome*. Their skin feels hot, their heart and respiration rates increase, and they may get a headache, vomit, or break out in hives. Because of these unpleasant symptoms, people who experience flushing syndrome rarely become addicted to alcohol.

Alcohol Intake and Blood Alcohol Concentration

Blood alcohol concentration (BAC), a measure of intoxication, is determined by the amount of alcohol consumed in a given amount of time and by individual factors such as body weight and amount of body fat. In most cases, a smaller person develops a higher BAC than a larger person after drinking the same amount of alcohol. This is because a smaller person has less overall body tissue into which alcohol can be distributed. A person with a higher percentage of body fat will usually develop a higher BAC than a more muscular person who weighs the same. This is because alcohol does not concentrate as much in fatty tissue as in muscle and most other tissues, in part because fat has fewer blood vessels. Women generally have higher BACs than men after consuming the same amount of alcohol because they usually have a higher percentage of body fat than men and because the stomach enzyme that breaks down alcohol is more active in men than in women.

BAC also depends on the balance between the rate of alcohol absorption and the rate of alcohol metabolism. A man who weighs 154 pounds and has normal liver function metabolizes about 0.3–0.5 ounce of alcohol per hour, the equivalent of slightly less than a 12-ounce bottle of beer or a 5-ounce glass of wine. The rate of alcohol metabolism varies among individuals and is largely determined by genetic factors and drinking behavior. Contrary to popular myths, this metabolic rate cannot be influenced by exercise, breathing deeply, eating, drinking coffee, or taking other drugs. The rate of alcohol metabolism is the same whether a person is asleep or awake.

If a person absorbs slightly less alcohol each hour than he or she can metabolize in an hour, the BAC remains low. People can drink large amounts of alcohol this way over a long period of time without becoming noticeably intoxicated; however, they do run the risk of significant long-term health hazards (described later in the chapter). If a person is absorbing alcohol more quickly than it can be metabolized, the BAC will steadily increase, and he or she will become more and more drunk (Table 8-1). How fast you drink makes a big difference in how high your BAC will be. Consuming several drinks over a period of 2 or 3 hours is likely to cause intoxication, followed on the next day by a hangover; chugging the same amount of alcohol in an hour or less could be lethal.

ALCOHOL AND HEALTH

The effects of alcohol consumption on health depend on the individual, the circumstances, and the amount of alcohol consumed.

Remember: Being very drunk is potentially life-threatening. Helping a drunken friend could save a life.

- Be firm but calm. Don't engage the person in an argument or discuss her drinking behavior while she is intoxicated.

- Get the person out of harm's way—don't let her drive or wander outside. Don't let her drink any more alcohol.

- If the person is unconscious, don't assume she is just "sleeping it off." Place her on her side with her knees up. This position will help prevent choking if the person should vomit.

- Stay with the person—you need to be ready to help if she vomits or stops breathing.

- Don't try to give the person anything to eat or drink, including coffee or other drugs. Don't give cold showers or try to make her walk around. None of these things help sober someone up, and they can be dangerous.

Call 911 immediately in any of the following instances:

- You can't wake the person up even with shouting or shaking.

- The person is taking fewer than 8 breaths per minute or her breathing seems shallow or irregular.

- You think the person took other drugs in addition to alcohol.

- The person has had an injury, especially a blow to the head.

- The person drank a large amount of alcohol within a short period of time and then became unconscious. Death due to alcohol poisoning most often occurs when the blood alcohol level rises very quickly due to rapid ingestion of alcohol.

If you aren't sure what to do, call 911. You may be saving a life.

The Immediate Effects of Alcohol

BAC is a primary factor determining the effects of alcohol (see Table 8-1). At low concentrations, alcohol tends to make people feel relaxed and jovial, but at higher concentrations people are more likely to feel angry, sedated, or sleepy. Alcohol is a CNS depressant, and its effects vary because body systems are affected to different degrees at different BACs. At any given BAC, the effects of alcohol are more pronounced when the BAC is rapidly increasing compared to when it is slowly increasing, steady, or decreasing. The effects of alcohol are more pronounced if a person drinks on an empty stomach, because alcohol is absorbed more quickly and the BAC rises more quickly.

Low Concentrations of Alcohol
The effects of alcohol can first be felt at a BAC of about 0.03–0.05%. These effects may include light-headedness, relaxation, and a release of inhibitions. Most drinkers experience mild euphoria and become more sociable. When people drink in social settings, alcohol often seems to act as a stimulant, enhancing conviviality or assertiveness. This apparent stimulation occurs because alcohol depresses inhibitory centers in the brain.

Higher Concentrations of Alcohol
At higher concentrations, the pleasant effects tend to be replaced by more negative ones: interference with motor coordination, verbal performance, and intellectual functions. The drinker often becomes irritable and may be easily angered or given to crying. When the BAC reaches 0.1%, most sensory and motor functioning is reduced, and many people become sleepy. Vision, smell, taste, and hearing become less acute. At 0.2%, most drinkers are completely unable to function, either physically or psychologically, because of the pronounced depression of the central nervous system, muscles, and other body systems. Coma usually occurs at a BAC of 0.35%, and any higher level can be fatal.

Alcohol causes flushing and sweating, which lower internal body temperature. Drinking alcohol to keep warm in cold weather does not work, and it can even be dangerous. Alcohol use also disturbs normal sleep patterns.

Alcohol Hangover
Despite all the jokes about hangovers, anyone who has experienced a severe hangover knows they are no laughing matter. The symptoms include headache, shakiness, nausea, diarrhea, fatigue, and impaired mental functioning. During a hangover, heart rate and blood pressure increase, making some individuals more vulnerable to heart attack. Brain wave testing shows diffuse slowing of brain waves for up to 16 hours after BAC drops to zero. Studies of pilots, drivers, and skiers all indicate that coordination and cognition are impaired in a person with a hangover, increasing the risk of injury.

The best treatment for hangover is prevention. Nearly all men can expect a hangover if they drink more than 5 or 6 drinks; for women, the number is 3 to 4 drinks. Drinking less, drinking more slowly, and consuming plenty of nonalcoholic liquids decrease the risk of hangover. If you do get a hangover, remember that your ability to drive is impaired, even after your BAC has returned to zero.

blood alcohol concentration (BAC) The amount of alcohol in the blood in terms of weight per unit volume; used as a measurement of intoxication.

Terms

Alcohol Poisoning Drinking large amounts of alcohol over a short period of time can rapidly raise the BAC into the lethal range. A common scenario for alcohol poisoning occurs when inexperienced drinkers try to outdo each other by consuming glass after glass of alcohol as rapidly as possible. Death from alcohol poisoning may be caused either by central nervous system and respiratory depression or by inhaling fluid or vomit into the lungs. The amount of alcohol it takes to make a person unconscious is dangerously close to a fatal dose. Children are at especially high risk for alcohol poisoning. Even a partially empty glass of liquor carelessly left out after a party can result in serious poisoning, or even death, if consumed by a toddler or small child.

Using Alcohol with Other Drugs Alcohol-drug combinations are the number one cause of drug-related deaths in this country. Using alcohol while taking any other drug that can cause CNS depression increases the effects of both drugs, potentially leading to coma, respiratory depression, and death. Examples of common drugs that can result in oversedation when combined with alcohol include barbiturates, Valium-like drugs, narcotics such as codeine, antidepressants such as Prozac, and OTC antihistamines like Benadryl. For people who consume three or more drinks per day, use of OTC pain relievers like aspirin, ibuprofen, or acetaminophen increases the risk of stomach bleeding or liver damage. Some antibiotics and diabetes medications can also interact dangerously with alcohol. Many illegal drugs are especially dangerous when combined with alcohol. Life-threatening overdoses occur at much lower doses when heroin and other narcotics are combined with alcohol.

The safest strategy is to avoid combining alcohol with any other drug—prescription, over-the-counter, or illegal. If in doubt, ask your pharmacist or physician before using any drug in combination with alcohol, or just don't do it.

Alcohol-Related Injuries and Violence The combination of impaired judgment, weakened sensory perception, reduced inhibitions, impaired motor coordination, and, often, increased aggressiveness and hostility that characterize alcohol intoxication can be dangerous or even deadly. Through homicide, suicide, automobile crashes (discussed in the next section), and other incidents, alcohol kills over 100,000 Americans each year. Alcohol use contributes to over 50% of all murders, assaults, and rapes, and alcohol is frequently found in the bloodstream of both perpetrators and victims. Nearly 80% of people who attempt suicide have been drinking, and about half of all successful suicides are alcoholics. Alcohol use more than triples the chances of fatal injuries during leisure activities such as swimming and boating, and more than half of all fatal falls and serious burns happen to people who have been drinking. Being drunk is clearly hazardous to your health.

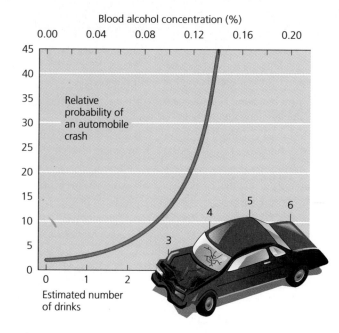

Figure 8-1 The dose-response relationship between BAC and automobile crashes.

Alcohol and Sexual Decision Making Alcohol seriously affects a person's ability to make wise decisions about sex. Heavy drinkers are more likely to engage in unplanned, unprotected sex; to have multiple sex partners; and to engage in other forms of high-risk sexual behavior. For all these reasons, rates of sexually transmitted diseases and unwanted pregnancy are higher among people who drink heavily than among people who drink moderately or not at all.

Women who binge-drink are at increased risk for rape and other forms of nonconsensual sex. The laws regarding sexual consent are clear: A person who is very drunk or passed out cannot consent to sex. If you have sex with a person who is drunk or unconscious, you are committing sexual assault. Claiming that you were drunk at the time won't absolve you of your legal and moral responsibility for this serious crime.

Drinking and Driving

Every year, more than 800,000 Americans are injured in alcohol-related automobile crashes—an average of *one person every 40 seconds*. About 40% of the more than 40,000 crash fatalities each year are alcohol-related. Even low doses of alcohol increase the risk of automobile crashes, but as the dose increases, the risk goes up at a spectacular rate (Figure 8-1). Still, in surveys, more than 1 in 4 of U.S. drivers admit to having used alcohol or another drug within 2 hours before driving a vehicle.

In addition to an increased risk of injury and death, driving while intoxicated can have serious legal conse-

BAC Zones: 90–109 lb								110–129 lb								130–149 lb								150–169 lb								170–189 lb								190–209 lb								210 lb & Over							
Time from First Drink	Total Drinks								Total Drinks								Total Drinks								Total Drinks								Total Drinks								Total Drinks								Total Drinks							
	1	2	3	4	5	6	7	8	1	2	3	4	5	6	7	8	1	2	3	4	5	6	7	8	1	2	3	4	5	6	7	8	1	2	3	4	5	6	7	8	1	2	3	4	5	6	7	8	1	2	3	4	5	6	7	8
1 hr																																																								
2 hr																																																								
3 hr																																																								
4 hr																																																								

□ (0.00%) Not impaired ■ (0.05–0.07%) Usually impaired

□ (0.01–0.04%) Sometimes impaired ■ (0.08% and up) Always impaired

Figure 8-2 Approximate blood alcohol concentration and body weight. This chart illustrates the BAC an average person of a given weight would reach after drinking the specified number of drinks in the time shown. The legal limit for BAC is 0.08% in some states and 0.10% in others. For drivers under 21 years of age, many states have "zero tolerance" laws that set BAC limits of 0.01% or 0.02%.

quences. Drunk driving is against the law. In 2000, the legal limit for BAC was 0.08% in 18 states and the District of Columbia and 0.10% in 31 other states (in Massachusetts, a BAC of 0.08% is evidence of alcohol impairment but not illegal per se). Under a law signed in 2000, states must lower their BAC limits to 0.08% by 2004 to avoid federal penalties. Under current "zero tolerance" laws in many states, drivers under age 21 who have consumed *any* alcohol may have their licenses suspended. There are stiff penalties for drunk driving, including fines, loss of license, confiscation of vehicle, and jail time.

People who drink and drive are unable to drive safely because their judgment is impaired, their reaction time is slower, and their coordination is reduced. The number of drinks it takes the average person to reach various BACs is shown in Figure 8-2. However, any amount of alcohol impairs your ability to drive safely, and fatigue augments alcohol's effects. If you are out of your home and drinking, find an alternative means of transportation or follow the practice of having a *designated driver,* an individual who refrains from drinking in order to provide safe transportation home for others in the group.

It's more difficult to protect yourself against someone else who drinks and drives. Learn to be alert to the erratic driving that signals an impaired driver. Warning signs include wide, abrupt, and illegal turns; straddling the center line or lane marker; driving on the shoulder; weaving, swerving, or nearly striking an object or another vehicle; following too closely; erratic speed; driving with headlights off at night; and driving with the window down in very cold weather. If you see any of these signs, try the following strategies:

- If the driver is ahead of you, maintain a safe following distance. Don't try to pass.

- If the driver is behind you, turn right at the nearest intersection, and let the driver pass.

- If the driver is approaching your car, move to the shoulder and stop. Avoid a head-on collision by sounding your horn or flashing your lights.

- When approaching an intersection, slow down and stay alert for vehicles that don't appear to be slowing in preparation for stopping at a stop sign or red light.

- Make sure your safety belt is fastened and children are in approved safety seats.

- Report suspected impaired drivers to the nearest police station by phone. Give a description of the vehicle, license number, location, and direction the vehicle is headed.

COMMUNICATE! To avoid dangerous alcohol-related situations, such as riding with a driver who has been drinking, you may need to use assertive communication. Try stating specifically what you want, using a firm but neutral tone. For example, "I don't feel comfortable riding with you after you've been drinking, and I don't think it's safe for you either. I'd feel better if we used a designated driver. I'll volunteer for tonight, and in the future we can all take turns."

The Effects of Chronic Use

Because alcohol is distributed throughout most of the body, it can affect many different organs and tissues (Figure 8-3).

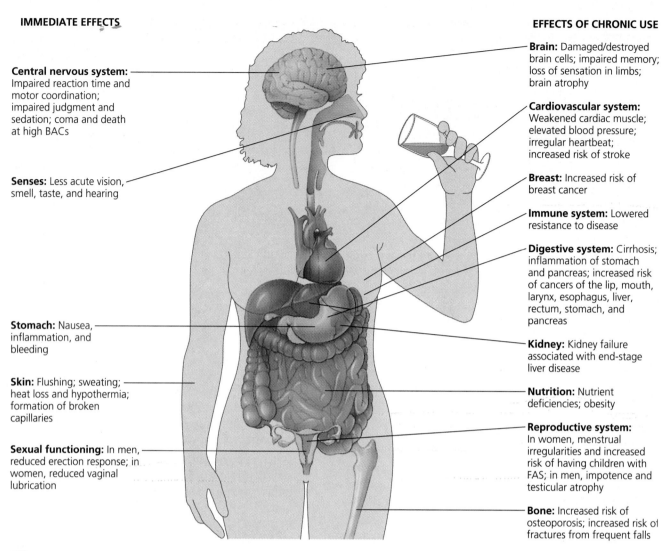

Central nervous system: Impaired reaction time and motor coordination; impaired judgment and sedation; coma and death at high BACs

Senses: Less acute vision, smell, taste, and hearing

Stomach: Nausea, inflammation, and bleeding

Skin: Flushing; sweating; heat loss and hypothermia; formation of broken capillaries

Sexual functioning: In men, reduced erection response; in women, reduced vaginal lubrication

Brain: Damaged/destroyed brain cells; impaired memory; loss of sensation in limbs; brain atrophy

Cardiovascular system: Weakened cardiac muscle; elevated blood pressure; irregular heartbeat; increased risk of stroke

Breast: Increased risk of breast cancer

Immune system: Lowered resistance to disease

Digestive system: Cirrhosis; inflammation of stomach and pancreas; increased risk of cancers of the lip, mouth, larynx, esophagus, liver, rectum, stomach, and pancreas

Kidney: Kidney failure associated with end-stage liver disease

Nutrition: Nutrient deficiencies; obesity

Reproductive system: In women, menstrual irregularities and increased risk of having children with FAS; in men, impotence and testicular atrophy

Bone: Increased risk of osteoporosis; increased risk of fractures from frequent falls

Figure 8-3   The immediate and long-term effects of alcohol use.

The Digestive System   Even in relatively small amounts, alcohol can alter the normal functioning of the liver. With continued use, liver cells are progressively damaged and then permanently destroyed. The destroyed cells are replaced by fibrous scar tissue, a condition known as **cirrhosis.** Alcohol-precipitated cirrhosis is the tenth leading cause of death in the United States.

Alcohol can inflame the pancreas, causing nausea, vomiting, abnormal digestion, and severe pain. Unlike cirrhosis, which usually occurs after years of fairly heavy alcohol use, pancreatitis can occur after just one or two severe binge-drinking episodes. Acute pancreatitis is often fatal and can also develop into a chronic condition. Overuse of alcohol can also cause bleeding in the gastrointestinal tract and painful irritation of the lining of the stomach.

The Cardiovascular System   The effects of alcohol on the cardiovascular system depend on the amount of alcohol consumed. Moderate doses of alcohol—less than one

drink a day for women and two drinks a day for men—may reduce the risk of heart disease and heart attack in some people. However, higher doses of alcohol have harmful effects on the cardiovascular system. In some people, more than two drinks a day will elevate blood pressure, making stroke and heart attack more likely. Some alcoholics show a weakening of the heart muscle, a condition known as **cardiac myopathy.** Binge drinking can cause "holiday heart," a syndrome characterized by serious abnormal heart rhythms, which usually appear within 24 hours of a binge episode.

Cancer   Alcoholics have a cancer rate about ten times higher than that of the general population. They are particularly vulnerable to cancers of the throat, larynx, esophagus, upper stomach, liver, and pancreas. Drinking three or more alcoholic beverages per day doubles a woman's risk of developing breast cancer. Some studies have linked even moderate drinking to increased risk for cancers of the breast, mouth, throat, and esophagus. The

U.S. Department of Health and Human Services has classified alcoholic beverages as known human carcinogens.

Mortality   As an ancient proverb states, "Those who worship Bacchus [the god of wine] die young." Excessive alcohol consumption is a factor in five of the ten leading causes of death for Americans. Average life expectancy among alcoholics is about 58 years; heavy drinkers may die in their 20s or 30s.

The Effects of Alcohol Use During Pregnancy

Alcohol ingested during pregnancy is harmful to the developing fetus, the damage depends on the stage of pregnancy and the amount of alcohol consumed. Alcohol use in early pregnancy can cause a miscarriage. Moderate to heavy alcohol use in pregnancy can cause a collection of birth defects known as **fetal alcohol syndrome (FAS).** Children with FAS have a characteristic mixture of deformities that include a small head, abnormal facial structure, heart defects, and other physical abnormalities; most are mentally impaired and their physical and mental growth is slower than normal.

FAS is a permanent, incurable condition that causes lifelong disability; it is by far the most common preventable cause of mental retardation in the Western world. Full-blown FAS occurs in about 1 or 2 out of every 1000 live births in the United States. Many more babies are born with **alcohol-related neurodevelopmental disorder (ARND).** Children with ARND appear physically normal, but they often have significant learning and behavioral disorders. Getting drunk just one time during the final 3 months of pregnancy, when brain cells are developing rapidly, can cause fetal brain damage. Experts agree that the safest course of action is complete abstinence from alcohol during pregnancy.

Any alcohol consumed by a nursing mother quickly enters the breast milk. What impact this has on the child or on the mother's milk production is a matter of controversy. However, many physicians advise nursing mothers to abstain from drinking because any amount may have negative effects on the baby's brain development.

Possible Health Benefits of Alcohol

According to the *Dietary Guidelines for Americans,* published by the U.S. Department of Agriculture, drinking in moderation may lower risk of coronary heart disease, mainly among men over age 45 and women over age 55. Moderate drinking provides little if any health benefits for younger people, and it is not without risk. It increases the risk of dying from unintentional injuries, violence, and certain types of cancer. There is also a risk that moderate drinking will not stay moderate. People who avoid alcohol because they or family members have had problems with dependence in the past should not start drinking for their health. People with conditions such as diabetes or depression that are worsened by alcohol use should probably avoid even moderate drinking. Nor should drinkers use this information as an excuse to overindulge; any health benefits of alcohol are negated by heavy use. In addition, there are many situations in which consuming any amount of alcohol is unwise, including during pregnancy, while taking medication that may interact with alcohol, and when driving or engaging in another activity that requires alertness.

The bottom line is that limited, regular consumption of alcohol appears to be beneficial for some adults, but there is a narrow window of benefit, and excessive drinking causes serious health problems. The *Dietary Guidelines for Americans* recommend that if you drink alcoholic beverages, do it in moderation, with meals, at times when consumption does not put you or others at risk.

ALCOHOL ABUSE AND DEPENDENCE

Abuse and dependence on alcohol affect more than just the drinker. Friends, family members, coworkers, strangers that drinkers encounter on the road, and society as a whole pay the physical, emotional, and financial costs of the misuse of alcohol.

Alcohol Abuse

As explained in Chapter 7, the APA's *Diagnostic and Statistical Manual of Mental Disorders* makes a distinction between substance abuse and substance dependence. **Alcohol abuse** is recurrent alcohol use that has negative consequences, such as drinking in dangerous situations (before driving, for instance), or drinking patterns that result in academic, professional, interpersonal, or legal difficulties. **Alcohol dependence,** or **alcoholism,** involves

cirrhosis A disease in which the liver is severely damaged by alcohol, other toxins, or infection.

cardiac myopathy Weakening of the heart muscle through disease.

fetal alcohol syndrome (FAS) A characteristic group of birth defects caused by excessive alcohol consumption by the mother, including facial deformities, heart defects, and physical and mental impairments.

alcohol-related neurodevelopmental disorder (ARND) Cognitive and behavioral problems seen in people whose mothers drank alcohol during pregnancy.

alcohol abuse The use of alcohol to a degree that causes physical damage, impairs functioning, or results in behavior harmful to others.

alcohol dependence A pathological use of alcohol or impairment in functioning due to alcohol; characterized by tolerance and withdrawal symptoms; alcoholism.

alcoholism A chronic psychological disorder characterized by excessive and compulsive drinking.

Terms

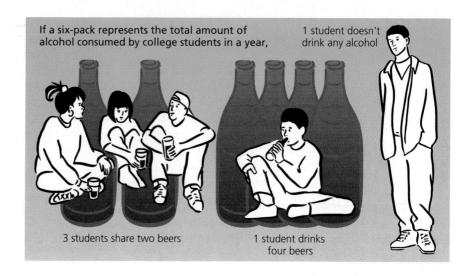

Figure 8-4 Alcohol consumption by college students. Alcohol consumption by students varies considerably, with some abstaining and some drinking large amounts. Only one in five college students is a frequent binge drinker, but this group accounts for two-thirds of all the alcohol consumed by college students each year and causes or experiences the majority of alcohol-related problems. SOURCE: Wechsler, H., et al. 2000. *From Knowledge to Action: How Harvard's College Alcohol Study Can Help Your Campus Design a Campaign Against Student Alcohol Abuse* (http://www.hsph.harvard.edu/cas/test/articles/change2.html; retrieved July 17, 2000).

If a six-pack represents the total amount of alcohol consumed by college students in a year,

3 students share two beers

1 student drinks four beers

1 student doesn't drink any alcohol

more extensive problems with alcohol use, usually involving physical tolerance and withdrawal. Alcoholism is discussed in greater detail later in the chapter.

Other authorities use different definitions to describe problems associated with drinking. The important point is that one does not have to be an alcoholic to have problems with alcohol. The person who drinks only once a month, perhaps after an exam, but then drives while intoxicated is an alcohol abuser.

How can you tell if you are beginning to abuse alcohol or if someone you know is doing so? Look for the following warning signs:

- Drinking alone or secretively
- Using alcohol deliberately and repeatedly to perform or get through difficult situations
- Feeling uncomfortable on certain occasions when alcohol is not available
- Escalating alcohol consumption beyond an already established drinking pattern
- Consuming alcohol heavily in risky situations, such as before driving
- Getting drunk regularly or more frequently than in the past
- Drinking in the morning or at other unusual times

Binge Drinking

A common form of alcohol abuse on college campuses is known as **binge drinking.** In surveys of students on over 100 college campuses, 44% reported binge drinking, defined as having five drinks in a row for men or four in a row for women on at least one occasion in the 2 weeks prior to the survey. Some 23% of all students were found to be frequent binge drinkers, defined as having at least three binges during the 2-week period. Students living at fraternity or sorority houses had the highest rate of binge drinking, 80%. Men were more likely to binge than women, and white students had higher rates of binge drinking than students of other ethnicities. Nineteen percent of students abstained from alcohol (Figure 8-4).

Binge drinking has a profound effect on students' lives. Frequent binge drinkers were found to be 3–7 times more likely than non–binge drinkers to engage in unplanned or unprotected sex, to drive after drinking, and to get hurt or injured (Table 8-2). Binge drinkers were also more likely to miss classes, get behind in schoolwork, and argue with friends. The more frequent the binges, the more problems the students encountered. Despite their experiences, fewer than 1% of the binge drinkers identified themselves as problem drinkers.

Binge drinking kills dozens of American college students each year. Some die from acute alcohol poisoning. The typical scenario involves a hazing ritual, a competition, or a bet that involves drinking a large amount of alcohol very quickly. This kind of fast, heavy drinking can result in unconsciousness and death very quickly, before anyone realizes that something is seriously wrong. Many other students die from alcohol-related injuries, including those from motor vehicle crashes.

Binge drinking also affects nonbingeing students. At schools with high rates of binge drinking, the nonbingers were up to twice as likely to report being bothered by the alcohol-related behaviors of others than students at

Terms

binge drinking Periodically drinking alcohol to the point of severe intoxication.

DTs (delirium tremens) A state of confusion brought on by the reduction of alcohol intake in an alcohol-dependent person; other symptoms are sweating, trembling, anxiety, hallucinations, and seizures.

Table 8-2	The Effects of Binge Drinking on College Students

	Percentage of Students Experiencing Problems	
Alcohol-Related Problem	Non–Binge Drinkers	Frequent Binge Drinkers
Drove after drinking alcohol	19	57
Did something they regretted	18	62
Got behind in schoolwork	10	46
Argued with friends	10	43
Missed a class	9	63
Engaged in unplanned sex	8	42
Had unprotected sex	4	20
Got hurt or injured	4	27
Got into trouble with police	1	13
Had five or more of these problems since school year began	4	48

SOURCE: Wechsler, H. et al. 2000. College binge drinking in the 1990s: A continuing problem. *Journal of American College Health* 48: 199–210.

schools with lower rates of binge drinking. These problems included having sleep or studying disrupted; having to take care of a drunken student; being insulted or humiliated; experiencing unwanted sexual advances; and being pushed, hit, or assaulted.

COMMUNICATE! Responsible drinking typically involves saying no to alcoholic beverages—either because you choose not to drink at all or because you want to limit your drinks. Because it's much more difficult to say no once you're in a social situation, it's a good idea to plan ahead and even rehearse what you'll say. Some possible responses are "No thanks—I've had enough for now," "I'm going to wait for a while," "I have to get up early," and "I think I'll switch to soda." Develop responses that are comfortable for you and that work in your social situations.

Alcoholism

As mentioned earlier, alcoholism, or alcohol dependence, is usually characterized by tolerance to alcohol and withdrawal symptoms. Everyone who drinks—even nonalcoholics—develops tolerance after repeated alcohol use. As described in Chapter 7, *tolerance* means that a drinker needs more alcohol to achieve intoxication or the desired effect, that the effects of continued use of the same amount of alcohol are diminished, or that the drinker can function adequately at doses or a BAC that would produce significant impairment in a casual user. Heavy users of alcohol may need to consume about 50% more than they originally needed in order to experience the same degree of intoxication.

Withdrawal occurs when someone who has been using alcohol heavily for several days or more suddenly stops drinking or markedly reduces her or his intake. Symptoms of withdrawal include trembling and nervousness and sometimes even hallucinations and seizures.

Patterns and Prevalence Alcoholism occurs among people of all ethnic groups and at all socioeconomic levels. There are different patterns of alcohol dependence, including these four common ones: (1) regular daily intake of large amounts, (2) regular heavy drinking limited to weekends, (3) long periods of sobriety interspersed with binges of daily heavy drinking lasting for weeks or months, (4) heavy drinking limited to periods of stress. Once established, alcoholism often exhibits a pattern of exacerbations and remissions.

According to the 1999 National Household Survey on Drug Abuse, about 12.4 million Americans are heavy drinkers and 45 million are binge drinkers. Studies suggest that the lifetime risk of alcoholism in the United States is about 10% for men and about 3% for women.

Health Effects Tolerance and withdrawal can have a serious impact on health. Symptoms of withdrawal include trembling hands ("shakes" or "jitters"), a rapid pulse and accelerated breathing rate, insomnia, nightmares, anxiety, and gastrointestinal upset. These symptoms usually begin 5–10 hours after alcohol intake is decreased and improve after 4–5 days; occasionally anxiety, insomnia, and other symptoms can persist for 6 months or more.

More severe withdrawal symptoms occur in about 5% of alcoholics. These include seizures (sometimes called "rum fits"), confusion, and hallucinations. Still less common is **DTs (delirium tremens)**, a medical emergency characterized by severe disorientation, confusion, multiple seizures, and vivid hallucinations, often of vermin. The mortality rate from DTs can be as high as 15%.

Alcoholics face all the physical health risks associated with intoxication and chronic drinking described earlier in the chapter. Some of the damage is worsened by nutritional deficiencies that often accompany alcoholism. Some people develop alcoholic paranoia, characterized by delusions, jealousy, suspicion, and mistrust. Other mental problems associated with alcoholism include profound memory gaps (commonly known as "blackouts").

Gender Differences Among American men, excessive drinking often begins in the teens or twenties and progresses gradually through the thirties, until the individual is clearly identifiable as an alcoholic by the time he is in

- About 20% of students do not use any alcohol, and a large majority (66%) do not binge-drink. About 23% of college students are frequent binge drinkers.

- Students who do well academically tend to drink less than those who do poorly. About 40% of students' academic problems and 28% of dropouts are related to alcohol use.

- Among students at two-year colleges, those with an A average have about 2.5 drinks per week; B students have 3.5; C students, 4; and D or F students, 6. A similar pattern is seen among students at four-year colleges.

- Students who drink moderately or not at all are less likely to be victims of crime. Between 50% and 80% of all violence on college campuses is alcohol-related, with both perpetrators and victims likely to have been drinking. Nearly 70% of perpetrators and 80% of victims of sexual assault are under the influence of alcohol at the time of the attack.

- College students who abstain or drink moderately are less likely to acquire sexually transmitted diseases or have an unwanted pregnancy.

- One in ten female frequent binge drinkers reports having engaged in nonconsensual sexual intercourse while drunk.

- Binge drinking is especially common in fraternities and sororities and among athletes. Enrollment in Greek organizations has been flat or down during the past few years on most campuses, in part due to negative publicity about alcohol abuse, hazing, violence, and poor academics.

- Seven in eight nonbingeing students have been negatively affected by the drinking of others. In surveys, more than half of all students favor more college intervention to stop excessive student drinking.

- Nearly 90% of college students support the policy of providing alcohol-free dormitories on campus. Three of five non–binge drinkers either currently live in an alcohol-free dorm or would like to live in one.

- College students sometimes turn to alcohol because it is one of the least expensive forms of "entertainment" available. A recent survey of college communities showed that students could binge-drink for well under five dollars, making drinking much cheaper than going to the movies or to a concert. Many large campuses are surrounded by a high density of stores and bars that sell alcohol at very low cost.

SOURCES: Wechsler, H., et al. 2000. College binge drinking in the 1990s: A continuing problem. *Journal of American College Health* 48: 199–210. Wechsler, H., et al. 2000. Environmental correlates of underage alcohol use and related problems of college students. *American Journal of Preventive Medicine* 19(1): 24–29. Elgin, L. D. 1991. *Alcohol Practices, Policies, and Potentials of American Colleges and Universities*. Washington, D.C.: U.S. Department of Health and Human Services.

his late thirties or early forties. Other men remain controlled drinkers until later in life, sometimes becoming alcoholic in association with retirement, illness, or psychological disorders.

The progression of alcoholism in women is usually different. Women tend to become alcoholic at a later age and with fewer years of heavy drinking. It is not unusual for women in their forties or fifties to become alcoholic after years of controlled drinking. Women alcoholics develop cirrhosis and other medical complications somewhat more often than men. Women alcoholics may have more medical problems because they are less likely to seek early treatment. In addition, there may be an inherently greater biological risk for women who drink.

Social and Psychological Effects   Alcohol use causes more serious social and psychological problems than all other forms of substance abuse combined. For every person who is an alcoholic, another three or four people are directly affected.

Alcoholics frequently suffer from *dual disorders,* mental disorders in addition to their substance dependence. Alcoholics are much more likely than nonalcoholics to suffer from clinical depression, panic disorder, schizophrenia, and antisocial personality disorders. People with anxiety or panic attacks may try to use alcohol to lessen their anxiety, even though alcohol often makes these disorders worse.

An estimated 3 million Americans age 14–17 show signs of potential alcohol dependence. These numbers are far greater than those associated with cocaine, heroin, or marijuana use. The social and psychological consequences of excessive drinking in young people are more difficult to measure than the risks to physical health. One of the consequences is that excessive drinking interferes with learning the interpersonal and job-related skills required for adult life. Perhaps most important is that people who were excessive drinkers in college are more likely to have social, occupational, and health problems 20 years later. Despite media attention on cocaine and other drugs, alcohol abuse remains our society's number one drug problem.

Causes of Alcoholism   The precise causes of alcoholism are unknown, but many factors are probably involved. Recent studies of twins and adopted children clearly demonstrate the importance of genetics. However, not all children of alcoholics become alcoholic, and it is clear that other factors are involved. A person's risk of developing alcoholism may be increased by certain person-

Examine Your Attitudes and Behavior

Think about how you really feel about drinking: Is it of little consequence to you or perhaps even an intrusion into your college experience? Or is alcohol the key ingredient for any and all fun activities? How do you perceive nondrinkers at a party where others are drinking?

Also consider the sources of your ideas about alcohol. How was alcohol used in your family when you were growing up? How is it used—or how do you think it's used—by students at your school? And how is alcohol use portrayed in advertisements you're exposed to? Try examining some alcohol ads to determine what messages they convey, what audiences they target, and what effect they may have on you and your attitudes about drinking.

Finally, carefully examine your drinking behavior. If you drink alcohol, what are your reasons for doing so? Is your drinking behavior moderate and responsible? Or do you frequently overindulge and suffer negative consequences? Try tracking your alcohol use in your health journal for a week or two to help evaluate your drinking behavior.

Drink Moderately and Responsibly

- *Drink slowly and space your drinks.* Sip your drinks, and alternate them with nonalcoholic choices. Don't drink alcoholic beverages to quench your thirst, and avoid drinks made with carbonated mixers.

- *Eat before and while drinking.* Don't drink on an empty stomach. Food in your stomach will slow the rate at which alcohol is absorbed and thus often lower the peak BAC.

- *Know your limits and your drinks.* Learn how different BACs affect you and how to keep your BAC and behavior under control.

- *Be aware of the setting.* In dangerous situations, such as driving or operating complicated machinery, abstinence is the only appropriate choice.

- *Use designated drivers.* Arrange carpools to and from parties or events where alcohol will be served. Rotate the responsibility for acting as a designated driver.

- *Learn to enjoy activities without alcohol.* If you can't have fun without drinking, you may have a problem with alcohol.

Encourage Responsible Drinking in Others

- *Encourage responsible attitudes.* Learn to express disapproval about someone who has drunk too much. Don't treat the choice to abstain as strange. The majority of American adults drink moderately or not at all.

- *Be a responsible host.* Serve only enough alcohol for each guest to have a moderate number of drinks, and serve lots of nonalcoholic choices. Always serve food along with alcohol, and stop serving alcohol an hour or more before people will leave. Insist that a guest who drank too much take a taxi, ride with someone else, or stay overnight rather than drive.

- *Hold drinkers fully responsible for their behavior.* Pardoning unacceptable behavior fosters the attitude that the behavior is due to the drug rather than the person.

- *Take community action.* Find out about prevention programs on your campus or in your community. Consider joining an action group such as Students Against Destructive Decisions (SADD) or Mothers Against Drunk Driving (MADD).

---

ality disorders, having been subjected as a child to destructive child-rearing practices, and imitating the alcohol abuse of peers and other role models. People who begin drinking excessively in their teens are especially prone to alcoholism later in life. Certain social factors have also been linked with alcoholism, including urbanization, disappearance of the extended family, a general loosening of kinship ties, increased mobility, and changing values.

Treatment   Some alcoholics recover without professional help. How often this occurs is unknown, but possibly as many as 25% stop drinking on their own or reduce their drinking enough to eliminate problems. Often these spontaneous recoveries are linked to an alcohol-related crisis, such as a health problem or the threat of being fired. Most alcoholics, however, require a treatment program of some kind in order to stop drinking. Many different kinds of programs exist. No single treatment works for everyone, so a person may have to try several

before finding the right one. Over 1 million Americans enter treatment for alcoholism every year.

One of the oldest and best-known recovery programs is Alcoholics Anonymous (AA). AA consists of self-help groups that meet several times each week in most communities and follow a 12-step program. Important steps for people in these programs include recognizing that they are "powerless over alcohol" and must seek help from a "higher power" in order to regain control of their lives. By verbalizing these steps, the alcoholic directly addresses the denial that is often prominent in alcoholism and other addictions. Many AA members have a sponsor of their choosing who is available by phone 24 hours a day for individual support and crisis intervention.

Alcoholics Anonymous is generally recognized as an effective mutual help program, but not everyone responds to its style and message, and other recovery approaches are available. Some, like Rational Recovery and Women for Sobriety, deliberately avoid any emphasis on higher spiritual powers. A more controversial approach to problem drinking is offered by the group Moderation Management, which encourages people to manage their drinking behavior by limiting intake or abstaining.

A companion program to AA is Al-Anon, which consists of groups for families and friends of alcoholics. In Al-Anon, spouses and others explore how they enabled the alcoholic to drink by denying, rationalizing, or covering up his or her drinking and how they can change this codependent behavior.

Other types of programs include inpatient hospital rehabilitation, employee-assistance programs, and school-based programs. Pharmacological treatments for alcoholism include the use of disulfiram (Antabuse), which makes a person violently ill if she or he drinks; and naltrexone, which reduces the pleasant effects of alcohol. For people with depression or anxiety, antidepressant or antianxiety medications can improve both psychological health and drinking behavior. Drug therapy is usually combined with psychosocial treatment.

Helping Someone with an Alcohol Problem

Helping a friend or relative with an alcohol problem requires skill and tact. One of the first steps is making sure you are not an enabler or codependent, perhaps unknowingly allowing someone to continue excessively using alcohol. Enabling takes many forms. One of the most common is making excuses or covering up for the alcohol abuser—for example, saying "he has the flu" when it is really a hangover. Whenever you find yourself minimizing or lying about someone's drinking behavior, a warning bell should sound. Another important step is open, honest labeling—"I think you have a problem with alcohol." Such explicit statements usually elicit emotional rebuttals and may endanger a relationship. In the long run, however, you are not helping your friends by allowing them to deny their problems with alcohol or other drugs. Even when problems are acknowledged, there may be reluctance to get help. Your best role might be to obtain information about the available resources and persistently encourage their use.

WHY PEOPLE USE TOBACCO

About 48 million American adults and 4 million adolescents smoke. About 80% of adult smokers believe that they'll die of tobacco-related causes if they don't quit. Yet each day, 6000 young people try cigarettes and 3000 become regular smokers. This section examines the personal and societal forces that induce people to start smoking and encourage them to continue.

Nicotine Addiction

The primary reason people continue to use tobacco despite the health risks is that they have become addicted to a powerful psychoactive drug: nicotine. Many researchers consider nicotine to be the most physically addictive of all the psychoactive drugs. Recent neurological studies indicate that nicotine acts on the brain in much the same way as cocaine and heroin. Nicotine reaches the brain via the bloodstream seconds after it is inhaled or, in the case of spit tobacco, absorbed through membranes of the mouth or nose. It triggers the release of powerful chemical messengers in the brain, including epinephrine, norepinephrine, and dopamine. But unlike street drugs, most of which are used to achieve a high, nicotine's primary attraction seems to lie in its ability to modulate everyday emotions.

At low doses, nicotine acts as a stimulant: It increases heart rate and blood pressure and can enhance alertness, concentration, rapid information processing, memory, and learning. People type faster on nicotine, for instance. At high doses, on the other hand, nicotine appears to act as a sedative; it can reduce aggressiveness and alleviate the stress response. Tobacco users may be able to fine-tune nicotine's effects and regulate their moods by increasing or decreasing their intake of the drug.

All tobacco products contain nicotine, and the use of any of them can lead to addiction. Nicotine addiction fulfills the criteria for substance dependence described in Chapter 7, including loss of control, tolerance, and withdrawal.

Loss of Control Three out of four smokers want to quit but find they cannot. Of the 60–80% of people who kick cigarettes at stop-smoking clinics, 75% start smoking again within a year—a relapse rate similar to rates for alcoholics and heroin addicts.

Regular tobacco users live according to a rigid cycle of need and gratification. On average, they can go no more than 40 minutes between doses of nicotine; otherwise, they begin feeling edgy and irritable and have trouble concentrating. If ignored, nicotine cravings build until getting a cigarette or some spit tobacco becomes a paramount concern, crowding out other thoughts. Tobacco users become adept, therefore, at keeping a steady amount of nicotine circulating in the blood and going to the brain.

Tolerance and Withdrawal Using tobacco builds up tolerance. Where one cigarette may make a beginning smoker nauseated and dizzy, a long-term smoker may have to chain-smoke a pack or more to experience the same effects. For most regular tobacco users, sudden abstinence from nicotine produces predictable withdrawal symptoms as well. These symptoms, which come on several hours after the last dose of nicotine, can include severe cravings, insomnia, confusion, tremors, difficulty concentrating, fatigue, muscle pains, headache, nausea, irritability, anger, and depression. While most of these symptoms pass in 2–3 days, many ex-smokers report intermittent, intense urges to smoke for years after quitting.

What contributions can the world's religions make to efforts to limit tobacco use? This was the question behind a meeting attended by representatives of the major religions of the world at the headquarters of the World Health Organization (WHO).

Tobacco Use as a Violation of Religious Principles

A primary thread among all the religions is a condemnation of tobacco use for its damaging effects on the body. Most religions regard the human body as the dwelling place of the spirit; as such, it deserves care and respect. The Baha'i faith, for example, strongly discourages smoking as unclean and unhealthy. The Roman Catholic Church endorses the age-old adage "a sound mind in a sound body." For Muslims, one of the five essential principles on which religious law is based is the protection of the integrity of the individual. Buddhists believe that the body doesn't belong to the person at all—even suicide is considered murder—and one must do nothing to harm it.

A second thread common to most religions is the notion that dependence and addiction run counter to ideas of freedom, choice, and human dignity. Hindus regard tobacco use as a *vyasana,* a dependence that is not necessary for the preservation of health. Protestant churches caution that any form of dependence is contrary to the notion of Christian freedom. A third argument against tobacco use is the immorality of harming others by imposing secondhand smoke on nonsmokers. In Hinduism, harming others is sinful. In the Jewish tradition, those who force nonsmokers to breathe smoke jeopardize the lives of others, and to do so is to jeopardize the whole universe.

The Role of Individual Responsibility

Most religions focus on the role of individual responsibility in overcoming dependence on tobacco. For example, Baha'is support the use of strategies that encourage individuals to find solutions to their problems within themselves, often with the help of a supportive group. In Buddhism, people must assume responsibility for their habits; they practice introspection to understand the cause of problems within themselves and the effects of their actions on others. A fundamental message of Islam is that you are personally responsible for your body and for your health.

Religion and Tobacco Control

Common threads also emerged in discussions of how the problem of tobacco use should be approached. The Islamic view is that the campaign to control tobacco use must be based on awareness, responsibility, and justice. Developing awareness means providing information on the global tobacco problem, from cultivation to marketing, from consumption to its effects. Fostering responsibility means helping people understand what they need to do to attain well-being. Emphasizing social and human justice means helping the farmers and societies that depend on tobacco cultivation to find alternative crops.

According to the representative from the Geneva Inter-religious Platform (a project involving Hindus, Buddhists, Muslims, Christians, Jews, and Baha'is), the best approach is prevention. Here, the rights of nonsmokers must be protected because they clearly prevail over the freedom of smokers. In support of this position, the common religious exhortation not to do unto others what you would not have them do unto you can be invoked. Further, adequate information should be provided to counter the deceptive images projected by tobacco advertising, especially where minors are concerned. Protection of the weak and denunciation of dishonesty are underlying values of all religious traditions. The religious traditions may best assist adult smokers by reminding them of two principles: one, the value of liberation from any form of slavery, and two, respect for life out of deference to the source of all life, which religions call by different names—God, ultimate reality, and so on—but which is the supreme value of any religious commitment.

SOURCE: World Health Organization Tobacco Free Initiative. 1999. *Meeting Report: Meeting on Tobacco and Religion* (3 May 1999). Geneva: World Health Organization.

Addiction occurs at an early age, despite many teenagers' beliefs that they will be able to stop when they wish to. Nicotine addiction can start within a few days of smoking and after just a few cigarettes. Over half of teenagers who try cigarettes progress to daily use, and about half of those who ever smoke daily progress to nicotine dependence. In polls, about 75% of smoking teens state they wish they had never started.

Social and Psychological Factors

Why do tobacco users have such a hard time quitting even when they want to? Social and psychological forces combine with physiological addiction to maintain the tobacco habit. Many people, for example, have established habits of smoking while doing something else—while talking, working, drinking, and so on. The spit tobacco habit is also associated with certain situations—studying or playing sports. It is difficult for these people to break their habits because the activities they associate with tobacco use continue to trigger their urge.

Why Start in the First Place?

A junior high school girl takes up smoking in an attempt to appear older. A high school boy uses spit tobacco in the bullpen, emulating the major league ball players he admires. An overweight first-year college student turns to

A common misconception among smokers is that a few cigarettes a day aren't enough to cause harm. Perhaps this is why a recent survey showed that among college students who smoke, 75% smoke 10 or fewer cigarettes a day. These smokers are ignoring the very real health risks of even one cigarette. The U.S. Public Health Service suggests a "5 R's" strategy to enhance movitation to quit. If you are a smoker, think about these areas of concern and see if they help develop a desire and readiness to make a real attempt at quitting.

Relevance: Think about the personal relevance of quitting tobacco use. What would the effects be on your family and friends? How would your daily life improve? What is the most important way that quitting would change your life?

Risks: There are immediate risks, such as shortness of breath, infertility, and impotence, and long-term risks, including cancer, heart disease, and respiratory problems. Remember, smoking is harmful both to you and to anyone exposed to your smoke.

Rewards: The list of rewards of quitting is almost endless, including improving immediate and long-term health, saving money, and feeling better about yourself. You can also stop worrying about quitting and set a good example for others.

Roadblocks: What are the potential obstacles to quitting? Are you worried about withdrawal symptoms, weight gain, or lack of support? How can these barriers be overcome?

Repetition: Revisit your reasons for quitting and strengthen your resolve until you are ready to prepare a plan. Most people make several attempts to quit before they succeed. Relapsing once does not mean that you will never succeed.

If someone you care about uses tobacco, you can try the following strategies to help them quit.

1. **Ask** about tobacco use. How many cigarettes does your girlfriend smoke each day? How long has your roommate being dipping snuff?

2. **Advise** tobacco users to stop. Express your concern over the tobacco user's habit. "When we're close, the smell of smoke on your hair and breath bothers me. I've noticed you cough a lot and your voice is raspy. I'm worried about your health. You should stop."

3. **Assess** the tobacco user's willingness to quit. "Next week would be a good time to try to quit. Would you be willing to give it a try?"

4. **Assist** the tobacco user who is willing to stop. To coincide with your partner's quit date, take him away for a romantic weekend far from the places he associates with smoking. Offer to be an exercise partner. Call once a day to offer support and help. Bring gifts of low-calorie snacks or projects that occupy the hands. If the quitter lapses, be encouraging. A lapse doesn't have to become a relapse.

5. **Arrange** follow-up. Maintaining abstinence is an ongoing process. Celebrate milestones of one week, one month, one year without tobacco. Note how much better your friend or partner's car, room, and person smell, how much healthier he or she is, and how much you appreciate not having to breathe tobacco smoke.

SOURCES: Rigotti, N. A., J. E. Lee, and H. Wechsler. 2000. U.S. college students' use of tobacco products. *Journal of the American Medical Association* 284(6):699–705. Fiore, M. C., et al. 2000. *Treating Tobacco Use and Dependence.* Clinical Practice Guidelines. Rockville, Md.: U.S. Department of Health and Human Services.

cigarettes, hoping they will curb her appetite. Smoking rates among American youth declined throughout the 1980s, but rose steadily during the 1990s. Children and teenagers constitute 90% of all new smokers in this country: Every day, an estimated 3000 adolescents become regular cigarette smokers, while hundreds of others take up snuff or chewing tobacco. The average age for starting smokers is 13; for spit tobacco users, 10. The earlier people begin smoking, the more likely they are to become heavy smokers—and to die of tobacco-related disease.

Making the decision to smoke requires minimizing or denying both the health risks of tobacco use and the tremendous pain, disability, emotional trauma, family stress, and financial expense involved in tobacco-related diseases such as cancer and emphysema. A sense of invincibility, characteristic of many adolescents and young adults, also contributes to the decision to use tobacco.

Advertising is another influence. The tobacco industry spends more than $6 billion each year on ads—more than the entire annual budget for Puerto Rico. These ads link tobacco products with desirable traits such as confidence, popularity, sexual attractiveness, and slenderness. Young people are a prime target of these ads. One measure of the effectiveness of advertising can be seen in the fact that 86% of teens prefer the three most heavily advertised brands (Marlboro, Camel, Newport); these three are preferred by just 32% of adults, who tend to favor cheap generic brands. New regulations issued recently may help reduce the exposure of minors to tobacco advertising, but it will be many years before the positive image of smoking promoted in tobacco ads fades from the public's mind.

COMMUNICATE!   Many people are not aware of the power advertising has to influence their attitudes toward smoking or drinking. A good way to resist the influence of ads is to critically evaluate them. Try analyzing an ad, looking at the image

Who Uses Tobacco?

About 26% of men and 22% of women smoke cigarettes. Adults with less than a twelfth-grade education are three times as likely to smoke cigarettes as those with a college degree. The reverse is true for cigars: Cigar smoking is most common among the affluent and those with high educational attainment.

Although all states ban the sale of tobacco to anyone under 18 years of age, at least 500 million packs of cigarettes and 26 million containers of chewing tobacco are consumed by minors each year. About 13% of middle school students use some form of tobacco. Among high school students, about 28% smoke cigarettes at least occasionally and 15% smoke cigars. An estimated 7%, including 19% of white male students, use spit tobacco. Male college athletes and professional baseball players report even higher rates of spit tobacco use.

HEALTH HAZARDS

Tobacco adversely affects nearly every part of the body, including the brain, stomach, mouth, and reproductive organs.

Tobacco Smoke: A Poisonous Mix

Tobacco smoke contains hundreds of damaging chemical substances, including acetone (nail polish remover), ammonia, hexamine (lighter fluid), and toluene (industrial solvent). Smoke from a typical unfiltered cigarette contains about 5 billion particles per cubic millimeter—50,000 times as many as are found in an equal volume of smoggy urban air. These particles, when condensed, form the brown, sticky mass called **cigarette tar.** At least 43 chemicals in tobacco smoke are linked to the development of cancer. Other substances in tobacco cause health problems because they damage the lining of the respiratory tract or decrease the lungs' ability to fight off infection.

Tobacco also contains poisonous substances, including arsenic. In addition to being an addictive psychoactive drug, nicotine is also a poison and can be fatal in high doses. Many cases of nicotine poisoning occur each year in toddlers and infants who pick up and eat cigarette butts they find at home or on the playground. Cigarette smoke contains carbon monoxide, the deadly gas in automobile exhaust, in concentrations 400 times greater than

is considered safe in industrial workplaces. Carbon monoxide displaces oxygen in red blood cells, depleting the body's supply of life-giving oxygen.

Some smokers switch to low-tar, low-nicotine, or filtered cigarettes because they believe them to be healthier alternatives. But there is no such thing as a "safe" cigarette, and smoking behavior is a more important factor in tar and nicotine intake than the type of cigarette smoked. Smokers who switch to a low-nicotine brand often compensate by smoking more cigarettes, inhaling more deeply, taking larger or more frequent puffs, or blocking ventilation holes with lips or fingers to offset the effects of filters. Studies have found that people who smoke "light" cigarettes inhale up to eight times as much tar and nicotine as printed on the label.

Concerns have also been raised about menthol cigarettes. About 76% of African American smokers smoke these cigarettes, as compared to 23% of whites. Studies have found that blacks absorb more nicotine than other groups and metabolize it more slowly. The anesthetizing effect of menthol, which may allow smokers to inhale more deeply and hold smoke in their lungs for a longer period, may be partly responsible for this difference.

The Immediate Effects of Smoking

The beginning smoker often has symptoms of mild nicotine poisoning: dizziness; faintness; rapid pulse; cold, clammy skin; and sometimes nausea, vomiting, and diarrhea. The effects of nicotine on smokers vary, depending greatly on the size of the nicotine dose and how much tolerance previous smoking has built up. Nicotine can either excite or tranquilize the nervous system, depending on dosage.

Nicotine has many other immediate effects (Figure 8-5). It stimulates the part of the brain called the **cerebral cortex.** It also stimulates the adrenal glands to discharge adrenaline. And it inhibits the formation of urine; constricts the blood vessels, especially in the skin; accelerates the heart rate; and elevates blood pressure. Higher blood pressure, faster heart rate, and constricted blood vessels require the heart to pump more blood. Smoking also depresses hunger contractions and dulls the taste buds. Smoking is not useful for weight loss, however. (Smoking for decades may lessen or prevent age-associated weight gain for some smokers; but for people under 30, smoking is not associated with weight loss.)

cigarette tar A brown, sticky mass created when the chemical particles in tobacco smoke condense.   Terms

cerebral cortex The outer layer of the brain, which controls complex behavior and mental activity.

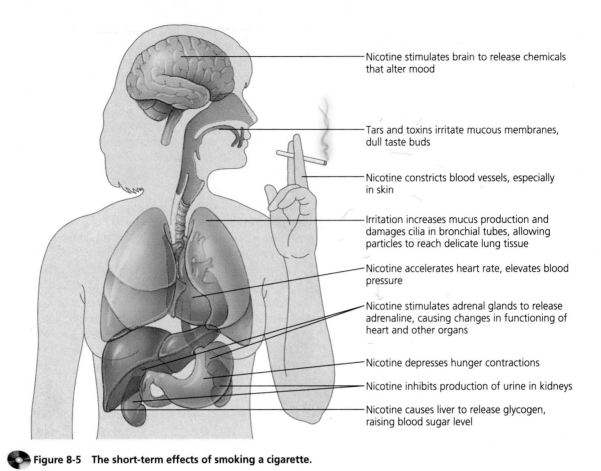

Nicotine stimulates brain to release chemicals that alter mood

Tars and toxins irritate mucous membranes, dull taste buds

Nicotine constricts blood vessels, especially in skin

Irritation increases mucus production and damages cilia in bronchial tubes, allowing particles to reach delicate lung tissue

Nicotine accelerates heart rate, elevates blood pressure

Nicotine stimulates adrenal glands to release adrenaline, causing changes in functioning of heart and other organs

Nicotine depresses hunger contractions

Nicotine inhibits production of urine in kidneys

Nicotine causes liver to release glycogen, raising blood sugar level

Figure 8-5   The short-term effects of smoking a cigarette.

The Long-Term Effects of Smoking

Smoking is a dangerous habit that is linked to many deadly and disabling diseases (Figure 8-6). Research indicates that the total amount of tobacco smoke inhaled is a key factor contributing to disease. People who smoke more cigarettes per day, inhale deeply, puff frequently, smoke cigarettes down to the butts, or begin smoking at an early age run a greater risk of disease than do those who smoke more moderately or who do not smoke at all.

Cardiovascular Disease   Although cancer tends to receive the most publicity, one form of cardiovascular disease, **coronary heart disease (CHD),** is actually the most widespread single cause of death for cigarette smokers. CHD often results from *atherosclerosis,* a condition in which fatty deposits called *plaques* form on the inner walls of heart arteries, causing them to narrow and stiffen. Smoking and exposure to environmental tobacco smoke (ETS) permanently accelerate the rate of plaque accumulation in the coronary arteries—50% for smokers, 25% for ex-smokers, and 20% for people regularly exposed to ETS. If the plaque completely blocks the flow of blood to

a portion of the heart, a heart attack occurs. CHD can also interfere with the heart's electrical activity, resulting in disturbances of the normal heartbeat rhythm.

Smokers have a death rate from CHD that is 70% higher than that of nonsmokers. The risks of CHD decrease rapidly when a person stops smoking; this is particularly true for younger smokers, whose coronary arteries have not yet been extensively damaged. Cigarette smoking has also been linked to other cardiovascular diseases, including

- *Stroke,* a sudden interference with the circulation of blood in a part of the brain, resulting in the destruction of brain cells
- *Aortic aneurysm,* a bulge in the aorta caused by a weakening in its walls
- *Pulmonary heart disease,* a disorder of the right side of the heart, caused by changes in the blood vessels of the lungs

Lung Cancer and Other Cancers   Cigarette smoking is the primary cause of lung cancer. Benzo(a)pyrene, a chemical found in tobacco smoke, causes genetic muta-

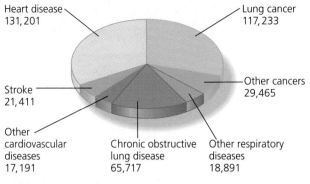

Heart disease
131,201

Lung cancer
117,233

Other cancers
29,465

Stroke
21,411

Other
cardiovascular
diseases
17,191

Chronic obstructive
lung disease
65,717

Other respiratory
diseases
18,891

VITAL STATISTICS

Figure 8-6 Annual deaths among smokers attributable to smoking-related diseases. SOURCE: Thun, M. J., L. F. Apicella, and S. J. Henley. 2000. Smoking vs. other risk factors as the cause of smoking-attributable deaths. *Journal of the American Medical Association* 284(6): 706–712.

tions in lung cells. Those who smoke two or more packs of cigarettes a day have lung cancer death rates 12–25 times greater than nonsmokers. The dramatic rise in lung cancer rates among women in the past 40 years clearly parallels the increase of smoking in this group; lung cancer now exceeds breast cancer as the leading cause of cancer deaths among women. The risk of developing lung cancer increases with the number of cigarettes smoked each day, the number of years smoking, and the age at which the person started smoking.

Evidence suggests that after 1 year without smoking, the risk of lung cancer decreases substantially. After 10 years, the risk of lung cancer among ex-smokers is 50% of that of continuing smokers. The sooner one quits, the better: If smoking is stopped before cancer has started, lung tissue tends to repair itself, even if cellular changes that can lead to cancer are already present.

Research has also linked smoking to cancers of the trachea, mouth, pharynx, esophagus, larynx, pancreas, bladder, kidney, cervix, stomach, liver, and colon.

Chronic Obstructive Lung Disease The lungs of a smoker are constantly exposed to dangerous chemicals and irritants, and they must work harder to function adequately. The stresses placed on the lungs by smoking can permanently damage lung function and lead to *chronic obstructive lung disease (COLD)*, also known as chronic obstructive pulmonary disease. COLD is the fourth leading cause of death in the United States. This progressive and disabling disorder consists of several different but related diseases; emphysema and chronic bronchitis are two of the most common.

EMPHYSEMA Smoking is the primary cause of **emphysema,** a particularly disabling condition in which the walls of the air sacs in the lungs lose their elasticity and

are gradually destroyed. The lungs' ability to obtain oxygen and remove carbon dioxide is impaired. A person with emphysema is breathless, is constantly gasping for air, and has the feeling of drowning. The heart must pump harder and may become enlarged. People with emphysema often die from a damaged heart. There is no known way to reverse this disease. In its advanced stage, the victim is bedridden and severely disabled.

CHRONIC BRONCHITIS Persistent, recurrent inflammation of the bronchial tubes characterizes **chronic bronchitis.** When the cell lining of the bronchial tubes is irritated, it secretes excess mucus. Bronchial congestion is followed by a chronic cough, which makes breathing more and more difficult. If smokers have chronic bronchitis, they face a greater risk of lung cancer.

Other Respiratory Damage Even when the smoker shows no signs of lung impairment or disease, cigarette smoking damages the respiratory system. Normally the cells lining the bronchial tubes secrete mucus, a sticky fluid that collects particles of soot, dust, and other substances in inhaled air. Mucus is carried up to the mouth by the continuous motion of the cilia, hairlike structures that protrude from the inner surface of the bronchial tubes. If the cilia are destroyed or impaired, or if the pollution of inhaled air is more than the system can remove, the protection provided by cilia is lost.

Cigarette smoke first slows, then stops the action of the cilia. Eventually it destroys them, leaving delicate membranes exposed to injury from substances inhaled in cigarette smoke or from polluted air. This interference with the functioning of the respiratory system often leads rapidly to the conditions known as smoker's throat and smoker's cough, as well as to shortness of breath. Other respiratory effects of smoking include a worsening of allergy and asthma symptoms and an increase in the smoker's susceptibility to colds.

Additional Health, Cosmetic, and Economic Concerns
Smokers are more likely to develop peptic ulcers and to die from them. Smoking reduces fertility in both men and women and is linked to pregnancy complications; men who smoke are twice as likely as nonsmokers to experience impotence. Smoking dulls the senses of taste and smell and

coronary heart disease (CHD) Cardiovascular disease caused by hardening of the arteries that supply oxygen to the heart muscle; also called *coronary artery disease*.

emphysema A disease characterized by a loss of lung tissue elasticity and breakup of the air sacs, impairing the lungs' ability to obtain oxygen and remove carbon dioxide.

chronic bronchitis Recurrent, persistent inflammation of the bronchial tubes.

Terms

A 2000 study revealed that rates of tobacco use among college students are even higher than previously suspected. Earlier surveys looked solely at cigarette smoking; however, this survey of students at over 100 college campuses looked at all forms of tobacco use. When cigarette smoking alone was measured, the percentage of college students who had ever used tobacco was 53%. But when cigar, pipe, and spit tobacco users were also counted, the percentage rose to 61%.

According to the survey, nearly half of all college students used tobacco in the past year—one-third within the past month. Cigarettes were the most common form of tobacco used, followed by cigars. Despite nearly identical smoking rates for men (28.5%) and women (28.4%), *total* tobacco use was higher among men (38%) than women (30%) due to greater use of cigars and spit tobacco among men. More than one-third of college students have smoked a cigar, including more than half of the men and one-quarter of the women; 16% of men and 4% of women report cigar use within the past month. Surprisingly, unlike patterns of use for other tobacco products, cigar use by first- and second-year students exceeds that of juniors and seniors. This may indicate that cigar use is a relatively new phenomenon on college campuses and reflect the growing popularity of cigars among adolescents, who bring their habit with them to college.

Most college students who have used tobacco used more than one product; the most frequent combinations are cigarettes and cigars (20% of tobacco users), cigarettes and pipes (12% of users), and cigarettes, cigars, and spit tobacco (6% of users). Men were much more likely than women to have used more than one kind of tobacco product; 37% of men but only 11% of women had used more than one product in the past month.

Although many students report smoking, most do not smoke in large quantities. Of those who had smoked in the past 30 days, 32% smoke less than 1 cigarette per day, 44% smoke 1 to 10 cigarettes per day, and 13% smoke 1 or more pack per day. Of course, smoking in any quantity has health risks and also lays the groundwork for increased nicotine dependence.

The results of this survey indicate that more needs to be done to highlight the dangers of all forms of tobacco use. Although cigarette use among college students, which increased dramatically between 1993 and 1997, does seem to have stabilized since 1997, use of other forms of tobacco is high and possibly increasing. Although college is a time of experimentation, it can be hoped that fewer students will start using tobacco in any form in years to come.

SOURCE: Rigotti, N. A., J. E. Lee, and H. Wechsler. 2000. U.S. college students' use of tobacco products. *Journal of the American Medical Association* 284(6): 699–705.

increases the risk of hearing loss and blindness. Further research may link tobacco use to still other disorders.

Smoking can cause premature skin wrinkling and baldness, tooth decay and stains, gum disease, discolored fingers, and a persistent tobacco odor in clothes and hair. Smokers have higher rates of motor vehicle crashes, fire-related injuries, and back pain. Smoking is also expensive—about $1000 per year for a pack-a-day habit, in addition to higher insurance premiums and cleaning bills.

Cumulative Effects   The cumulative effects of tobacco use fall into two general categories. The first category is reduced life expectancy. A male who takes up smoking before age 15 and continues to smoke is only half as likely to live to age 75 as a male who never smokes. If he inhales deeply, he risks losing a minute of life for every minute of smoking. Females who have similar smoking habits also have a reduced life expectancy. On average, smokers live 8 years less than nonsmokers.

The second category involves quality of life. A national health survey begun in 1964 shows that smokers spend one-third more time away from their jobs because of illness than nonsmokers. Both men and women smokers show a greater rate of acute and chronic disease than those who have never smoked. Smokers become disabled at younger ages than nonsmokers and have more years of unhealthy life in addition to a shorter life span.

Ww. Other Forms of Tobacco Use

Many smokers have switched from cigarettes to other forms of tobacco, such as cigars, pipes, clove cigarettes, and spit (smokeless) tobacco. However, each of these alternatives is far from safe.

Spit (Smokeless) Tobacco   More than 5 million adults and about 7% of all high school students are current spit tobacco users. Spit tobacco comes in two major forms—snuff and chewing tobacco ("chew"). In snuff, the tobacco leaf is processed into a coarse, moist powder and mixed with flavorings. Users place a "pinch," "dip," or "quid" between the lower lip or cheek and gum and suck on it. In chewing tobacco, the tobacco leaf may be shredded ("leaf"), pressed into bricks or cakes ("plugs"), or dried and twisted into ropelike strands ("twists"). Users place a wad of tobacco in their mouth and then chew or suck it to release the nicotine. All types of smokeless tobacco cause an increase in saliva production, and resulting tobacco juice is spit out or swallowed.

The nicotine in spit tobacco—along with flavorings and additives—is absorbed through the gums and lining of the mouth. Holding an average-size dip in the mouth for 30 minutes delivers about the same amount of nicotine as two or three cigarettes. Because of its nicotine content, spit tobacco is highly addictive. Some users keep it in their mouth even while sleeping.

Although not as dangerous as cigarettes, the use of spit tobacco carries many health risks. Changes can occur in the mouth after only a few weeks of use: Gums and lips become dried and irritated and may bleed. White or red patches may appear inside the mouth; this condition, known as *leukoplakia,* can lead to oral cancer. About 25% of regular spit tobacco users have *gingivitis* (inflammation) and recession of the gums and bone loss around the teeth, especially where the tobacco is usually placed. The senses of taste and smell are usually dulled. In addition, many people find the presence of wads of tobacco in the mouth, stained teeth, bad breath, and behaviors such as frequent spitting to be unpleasant.

One of the most serious effects of spit tobacco is an increased risk of oral cancer—cancers of the lip, tongue, cheek, throat, gums, roof and floor of the mouth, and larynx. Spit tobacco contains at least 28 chemicals known to cause cancer, and long-term snuff use may increase the risk of oral cancer by as much as 50 times. Surgery to treat oral cancer is often disfiguring and may involve removing parts of the face, tongue, cheek, or lip.

Dipping and chewing tobacco produce blood levels of nicotine similar to those in cigarette smokers. High blood levels of nicotine have dangerous effects on the cardiovascular system, including elevation of blood pressure, heart rate, and blood levels of certain fats. Other chemicals in spit tobacco are believed to pose risks to developing fetuses.

Cigars and Pipes After more than two decades of decline, cigar smoking has increased by nearly 50% since 1993. The popularity of cigars is highest among white males age 18–44 with higher than average income and education, but women are also smoking cigars in record numbers. Cigar use is also growing among young people: In the latest government surveys, 15% of high school students reported having smoked at least one cigar in the previous month. An estimated 2% of Americans, mostly males who also smoke cigarettes, are pipe smokers.

Cigars are made from rolled whole tobacco leaves; pipe tobacco is made from shredded leaves and often flavored. Users absorb nicotine through the gums and lining of the mouth. Cigars contain more tobacco than cigarettes and so contain more nicotine and produce more tar when smoked. Large cigars may contain as much tobacco as a whole pack of cigarettes and take 1–2 hours to smoke.

The smoke from cigars contains many of the same chemicals as the smoke from cigarettes, some in much higher quantities. The health risks of cigars depend on the number of cigars smoked and whether or not the

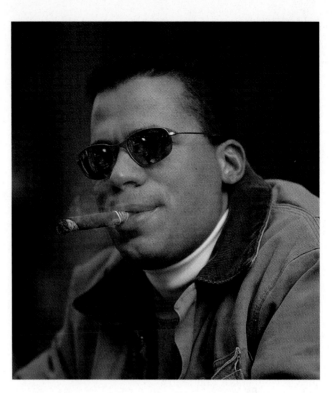

Cigars contain more tobacco than cigarettes and so produce more tar when smoked. Cigar smokers face an increased risk of cancer even if they don't inhale the smoke.

smoker inhales. Because most cigar and pipe users do not inhale, they have a lower risk of cancer and cardiovascular and respiratory diseases than cigarette smokers. However, their risks are substantially higher than those of nonsmokers.

Nicotine addiction is another concern. Most adults who smoke cigars do so only occasionally, and there is little evidence that use of cigars by adults leads to addiction. The recent rise in cigar use among teens has raised concerns, however, because nicotine addiction almost always develops in the teen or young adult years. In June of 2000 the FTC announced an agreement to put warning labels on cigar boxes, 34 years after warning labels first appeared on cigarette packages.

Clove Cigarettes and Bidis Clove cigarettes, also called "kreteks" or "chicartas," are made of tobacco mixed with chopped cloves; they are imported primarily from Indonesia and Pakistan. Clove cigarettes contain almost twice as much tar, nicotine, and carbon monoxide as conventional cigarettes and so have all the same health hazards. Some chemical constituents of cloves may also be dangerous. For example, eugenol, an anesthetic compound found in cloves, may impair the respiratory system's ability to detect and defend against foreign particles. There have been a number of serious respiratory injuries and deaths from the use of clove cigarettes.

Bidis, or "beadies," are small cigarettes imported from India that contain species of tobacco different from those used by U.S. cigarette manufacturers. The tobacco in bidis is hand-rolled in Indian ebony leaves (tendu) and then often flavored; clove, mint, chocolate, and fruit varieties are available. Bidis contain up to four times more nicotine and twice as much tar as U.S. cigarettes.

THE EFFECTS OF SMOKING ON THE NONSMOKER

In a watershed decision in 1993, the U.S. Environmental Protection Agency (EPA) designated environmental tobacco smoke (ETS) a Class A carcinogen—an agent known to cause cancer in humans. In 2000, the Department of Health and Human Services' National Toxicology Program classified ETS as a "known human carcinogen." These designations put ETS in the same category as notorious cancer-causing agents like asbestos. Every year, ETS causes thousands of deaths from lung cancer and heart disease and is responsible for hundreds of thousands of respiratory infections in young children.

Environmental Tobacco Smoke

Environmental tobacco smoke, commonly known as *secondhand smoke,* consists of mainstream smoke and sidestream smoke. Smoke exhaled by smokers is referred to as **mainstream smoke. Sidestream smoke** enters the atmosphere from the burning end of a cigarette, cigar, or pipe. Undiluted sidestream smoke, because it is not filtered through either a cigarette filter or a smoker's lungs, has significantly higher concentrations of the toxic and carcinogenic compounds found in mainstream smoke. For example, compared to mainstream smoke, sidestream smoke has (1) twice as much tar and nicotine; (2) three times as much benzo(a)pyrene, a carcinogen; (3) almost three times as much carbon monoxide, which displaces oxygen from red blood cells and forms *carboxyhemoglobin,* a dangerous compound that seriously limits the body's ability to use oxygen; and (4) three times as much ammonia.

Nearly 85% of the smoke in a room where someone is smoking comes from sidestream smoke. Of course, sidestream smoke is diffused through the air, so nonsmokers don't inhale the same concentrations of toxic chemicals that the smoker does. Still, the concentrations can be considerable. In rooms where people are smoking, levels of carbon monoxide, for instance, can exceed those permitted by Federal Air Quality Standards for outside air.

The secondhand smoke from a cigar can be even more dangerous than that from cigarettes. The EPA has found that the output of carcinogenic particles from a cigar exceeds that of three cigarettes, and cigar smoke contains up to 30 times more carbon monoxide.

ETS Effects Studies show that up to 25% of nonsmokers subjected to ETS develop coughs, 30% develop headaches and nasal discomfort, and 70% suffer from eye irritation. Other symptoms range from breathlessness to sinus problems. People with allergies tend to suffer the most. The odor of tobacco smoke clings to skin and clothes—another unpleasant effect of ETS.

But ETS causes more than just annoyance and discomfort; it causes 3000 lung cancer deaths annually. People who live, work, or socialize among smokers face a 24–50% increase in lung cancer risk. ETS is also responsible for about 60,000 deaths from heart disease each year. Scientists have been able to measure changes that contribute to lung tissue damage and tumor promotion in healthy young test subjects who spend just 3 hours in a smoke-filled room. And nonsmokers can still be affected by the harmful effects of ETS hours after they have left a smoky environment. Carbon monoxide, for example, lingers in the bloodstream 5 hours later.

Infants, Children, and ETS The National Cancer Institute recently estimated that ETS causes up to 2700 SIDS deaths and up to 18,600 cases of low birth weight each year. Children under 5 whose primary caregiver smokes 10 or more cigarettes per day have measurable blood levels of nicotine and tobacco carcinogens. Chemicals in tobacco smoke also show up in breast milk, and breastfeeding may pass more chemicals to the infant of a smoking mother than direct exposure to ETS.

ETS triggers 150,000–300,000 cases of bronchitis, pneumonia, and other respiratory infections in infants and toddlers, resulting in 7500–15,000 hospitalizations. ETS is a risk factor for asthma in children who have not previously displayed symptoms of the disease, and it aggravates the symptoms of the 200,000 to 1 million children who already have asthma. ETS is also linked to reduced lung function and fluid buildup in the middle ear, a contributing factor in middle-ear infections.

Why are infants and children so vulnerable? Because they breathe faster than adults, they inhale more air—and more of the pollutants in the air. Because they also weigh less, they inhale three times more pollutants per unit of body weight than adults do. And because their young lungs are still growing, this intake can impair optimal development. The problem is widespread. The American Academy of Pediatrics estimates that some 9 million American children are exposed to ETS.

Terms

mainstream smoke Smoke that is inhaled by a smoker and then exhaled into the atmosphere.

sidestream smoke Smoke that comes from the burning end of a cigarette, cigar, or pipe.

Everyone knows that smoking shortens life expectancy and increases the risk of cancer, lung disease, and heart disease. But did you know that smoking carries special risks for women? Many of these risks are associated with reproduction and the reproductive organs. Rates of cervical cancer and vulvar cancer, for example, are higher in women who smoke than in women who don't. Smoking diminishes fertility, and for pregnant women, smoking increases the risk of ectopic pregnancy, miscarriage, preterm birth, preeclampsia, and stillbirth.

The combination of smoking and taking oral contraceptives is dangerous; women who smoke and take the pill have a higher risk of potentially fatal blood clots, heart attacks, and strokes than other women. Women smokers are also at increased risk for irregular and painful menstruation, early menopause, and more menopause symptoms.

Smoking increases a woman's chance of developing osteoporosis, a disease in which bones become thinner and more brittle. Older women who smoke are thus more likely to suffer hip fractures from falls. Women who smoke are also at increased risk for thyroid-related diseases and depression.

For the first time in U.S. history, teenage girls are taking up smoking in greater numbers than teenage boys. Female smokers are expected to soon outnumber male smokers in the adult population. We can expect to see a corresponding increase in tobacco-related diseases among women. Already, lung cancer has surpassed breast cancer as the most common cause of cancer death in American women. According to several recent studies, female smokers are more vulnerable than male smokers to lung cancer and bladder cancer. Unless smoking rates decline significantly, we can expect to see more of these life-threatening and debilitating tobacco-related diseases affecting women.

SOURCE: Centers for Disease Control and Prevention. 2001. *Women and Smoking: A Report of the Surgeon General*. Atlanta, Ga.: CDC Office on Smoking and Health.

Avoiding ETS   Given the health risks of exposure to ETS, try these strategies to keep the air around you safe:

- *Speak up tactfully.* Try saying something like, "Would you mind putting your cigarette out or moving to another spot? The smoke is bothering me."

- *Display reminders.* Put up signs asking smokers to refrain in your home, work area, and car.

- *Don't allow smoking in your home or room.* Get rid of ashtrays and ask smokers to light up outside.

- *Open a window.* If you cannot avoid being in a room with a smoker, try to provide some ventilation.

- *Sit in the nonsmoking section in restaurants and other public areas.* Complain to the manager if none exists.

- *Fight for a smoke-free work environment.* Join with your coworkers to either eliminate all smoking indoors or to confine it to certain areas.

- *Discuss quitting strategies.* Social pressure is a major factor in many former smokers' decision to quit. Help the smokers in your life by sharing quitting strategies with them.

Smoking and Pregnancy

Smoking almost doubles a pregnant woman's chance of having a miscarriage, and it significantly increases her risk of ectopic pregnancy. Maternal smoking causes an estimated 4600 infant deaths in the United States each year, primarily due to premature delivery and smoking-related problems with the placenta. Maternal smoking is a major factor in low birth weight, which puts newborns at high risk for infections and other serious problems. If a nonsmoking mother is regularly exposed to ETS, her infant is also at greater risk for low birth weight. Recent studies have also shown that babies whose mothers smoked during pregnancy had higher rates of colic, clubfoot, cleft lip and palate, and impaired lung function.

Babies born to mothers who smoke more than two packs a day perform poorly on developmental tests in the first hours after birth, compared to babies of nonsmoking mothers. Later in life, hyperactivity, short attention span, and lower scores on spelling and reading tests all occur more frequently in children whose mothers smoked during pregnancy than in those born to nonsmoking mothers. Prenatal tobacco exposure has also been associated with behavioral problems in children, including immaturity, emotional instability, physical aggression, and hyperactivity. Males born to smoking mothers have higher rates of adolescent and adult criminal activity, suggesting that maternal smoking may cause brain damage that increases the risk of criminal behavior.

The Cost of Tobacco Use to Society

The health care costs associated with smoking exceed $70 billion per year. If the cost of lost productivity from sickness, disability, and premature death is included, the total is closer to $125 billion. This works out to $5 per pack of cigarettes, far more than the average $0.39 per pack tax collected by states to offset tobacco-related medical costs.

In order to recoup public health care expenditures, 43 state attorneys general filed suit against tobacco companies. In November 1998, an agreement was reached that settled 39 state lawsuits and applied to seven states that never filed suit. (Four states—Florida, Minnesota, Mississippi, and Texas—settled their suits separately for a total of $40 billion.) The 1998 settlement requires the tobacco companies to pay states $206 billion over 25 years; it also limits or bans certain types of advertising, promotions, and lobbying. Many of the provisions of the deal are designed to limit youth exposure and access to tobacco. In exchange, the tobacco industry settles the state lawsuits and is protected from future suits by states, counties, towns, and other public entities. For current information on this settlement and other political and legal activities, call or visit the Web site of one of the tobacco control advocacy groups listed in the For More Information section at the end of the chapter.

WHAT CAN BE DONE?

Every hour, 60 Americans die from preventable smoking-related diseases. Today there are more avenues than ever before for individual and group action against this major public health threat.

Action at Many Levels

Evidence is mounting that smoking restrictions do encourage smokers to quit. In recent years, thousands of local anti-smoking ordinances have been passed by school boards, town councils, and county boards of supervisors to restrict or ban smoking in schools, restaurants, stores, and workplaces. Many private employers, fearing worker's compensation claims based on exposure to workplace smoke, have banned smoking on the job. State legislatures have also passed many tough new anti-tobacco laws. California has one of the most aggressive—and successful—programs, combining taxes on cigarettes, graphic advertisements, and bans on smoking in bars and restaurants. In the past decade, per-capita cigarette consumption fell by 50% in California, lung cancer cases dropped 14%, and heart disease deaths were reduced by more than 30,000.

At the federal level, smoking has been banned on virtually all domestic airplane flights. Many other countries also restrict smoking, and the World Health Organization has taken the lead in international anti-tobacco efforts through sponsorship of World No-Tobacco Day and the promotion of an international tobacco control treaty.

What You Can Do

When a smoker violates a no-smoking designation, complain. If your favorite restaurant or shop doesn't have a nonsmoking policy, ask the manager to adopt one. If you see children buying tobacco, report this illegal activity to the facility manager or the police. Learn more about addiction and tobacco cessation so you can better support the tobacco users you know. Vote for candidates who support anti-tobacco measures; contact local, state, and national representatives to express your views.

Cancel your subscriptions to magazines that carry tobacco advertising; send a letter to the publisher explain-

ing your decision. Voice your opinion about other positive representations of tobacco use. (A recent study found that more than two-thirds of children's animated feature films have featured tobacco or alcohol use with no clear message that such practices were unhealthy.) Volunteer with the American Lung Association, the American Cancer Society, or the American Heart Association.

These are just some of the many ways individuals can help support tobacco prevention and stop-smoking efforts. Nonsmokers not only have the right to breathe clean air, but they also have the right to take action to help solve one of society's most serious public health threats.

> **COMMUNICATE!** Does someone you care about use tobacco or drink too much? Try speaking to that person honestly and offering your support. For example, "I love you very much, and I worry about your smoking. I wish you would quit." Or, "I'm really worried about your drinking, and I hope you won't get mad at me for saying so. You've come back to our room really drunk four times in the last week, and you've been driving yourself home when you're drunk. I really wish you'd talk to a counselor at the health center about your drinking. I'd be happy to go with you, if you want."

Controlling the Tobacco Companies

With their immensely profitable industry shrinking, tobacco companies are concentrating on appealing to narrower and narrower market segments with an ever-increasing array of brands and styles—over 350 in all. As tobacco use has declined among better-educated, wealthier segments of the American population, tobacco companies have redirected their marketing efforts toward minorities, the poor, and young women, populations among whom smoking rates are still high.

With cigarette sales falling in the United States, tobacco companies have also begun focusing on increasing the export of cigarettes, particularly to developing nations. As companies compete for customers in the years ahead, the need to exercise public pressure to keep the powerful tobacco companies in check will persist.

WWW. HOW A TOBACCO USER CAN QUIT

Since 1964, over 50% of all adults who have ever smoked have quit. Giving up tobacco is a long-term, intricate process. Research shows that tobacco users move through predictable stages—from being uninterested in stopping, to thinking about change, to making a concerted effort to stop, to finally maintaining abstinence. But most attempt to quit several times before they finally succeed. Relapse is a normal part of the process.

Table 8-3	Benefits of Quitting Smoking

Within 20 minutes of your last cigarette:
- You stop polluting the air
- Blood pressure drops to normal
- Pulse rate drops to normal
- Temperature of hands and feet increases to normal

8 hours:
- Carbon monoxide level in blood drops to normal
- Oxygen level in blood increases to normal

24 hours:
- Chance of heart attack decreases

48 hours:
- Nerve endings start regrowing
- Ability to smell and taste things is enhanced

2–3 months:
- Circulation improves
- Walking becomes easier
- Lung function increases up to 30%

1–9 months:
- Coughing, sinus congestion, fatigue, and shortness of breath all decrease
- Cilia regrow in lungs, reduce infection

1 year:
- Heart disease death rate is half that of a smoker

5 years:
- Stroke risk drops nearly to the risk for nonsmokers

10 years:
- Lung cancer death rate drops to 50% of that of continuing smokers
- The incidence of other cancers (mouth, throat larynx, esophagus, bladder, kidney, and pancreas) decreases

15 years:
- Risk of lung cancer is about 25% of that of continuing smokers
- Risks of heart disease and stroke are the same as for nonsmokers

SOURCE: American Cancer Society. 2000 *Quitting Smoking* (http://www.cancer.org/tobacco/quitting.html; retrieved July 10, 2000). American Lung Association. 1999. *Benefits of Quitting* (http//www.lungusa.org/tobacco/quit_ben.html; retrieved October 14, 2000).

The Benefits of Quitting

Giving up tobacco provides both immediate and long-term health benefits to men and women of all ages (Table 8-3). The younger people are when they stop smoking, the more pronounced the health improvements. And these improvements gradually but invariably increase as the period of nonsmoking lengthens. It's never too late to quit, though. According to a U.S. Surgeon General's report, people who quit smoking, regardless of age, live longer than people who continue to smoke.

Options for Quitting

Most tobacco users—76% in a recent survey—want to quit, and half of those who want to quit will make an attempt this year. No single method works for everyone, but each does work for some people some of the time. Choosing to quit requires developing a strategy for success. Some people quit "cold turkey," while others taper off more slowly. There are over-the-counter and prescription products that help many people. Behavioral factors that have been shown to increase the chances of a smoker's permanent smoking cessation are support from others and regular exercise. Support can come from friends and family and/or formal group programs sponsored by organizations such as the American Cancer Society, the American Lung Association, and the Seventh-Day Adventist Church or by your college health center or community hospital.

Most smokers in the process of quitting experience both physical and psychological effects of nicotine withdrawal, and exercise can help with both. For many smokers, their tobacco use is associated with certain times and places—following a meal, for example. Resolving to walk after dinner instead of lighting up provides a distraction from cravings and eliminates the cues that trigger a desire to smoke. In addition, many people worry about weight gain associated with quitting. Although most ex-smokers do gain a few pounds, at least temporarily, incorporating exercise into a new tobacco-free routine lays the foundation for healthy weight management. The health risks of adding a few pounds are far outweighed by the risks of continued smoking; it's estimated that a smoker would have to gain 75–100 pounds to equal the health risks of smoking a pack a day.

As with any significant change in health-related behavior, giving up tobacco requires planning, sustained effort, and support. It is an ongoing process, not a one-time event.

Nicotine Replacement Therapy

As the name suggests, nicotine replacement therapy involves supplying the tobacco user with nicotine from a source other than standard tobacco products. This allows a user to overcome the psychological and behavioral aspects of a tobacco habit without having to simultaneously endure the physical symptoms of withdrawal. Although still harmful, nicotine replacement provides a cleaner form of nicotine. It avoids the thousands of poisons and tars that are found in burning tobacco and delivers a lower dose of nicotine than most smokers receive. After a few weeks or months of use, the reforming tobacco user begins to taper off use of the replacement, alleviating withdrawal symptoms.

There are several types of nicotine replacement, each with advantages and disadvantages. None of them are safe to use if the smoker plans to continue using tobacco; nicotine is a powerful stimulant and an overdose can cause serious health complications. Studies have shown that combining nicotine replacement therapy with behavioral counseling can double the number of smokers who quit.

Nicotine patches can be purchased in varying strengths without a prescription. The patches release a controlled and steady supply of nicotine through the skin for 16 or 24 hours, depending on the type selected. Smokers often begin using a full-strength patch and then switch to a weaker one to decrease the nicotine dosage. The most common side effects of the patch are skin irritation and redness, which can often be cleared up by switching to another brand.

Another nonprescription option is *nicotine gum.* When chewed, the gum releases nicotine that is absorbed through the mucous membranes of the mouth. Most users chew one to two pieces per hour. An advantage of the gum versus the patch is that it allows the user to control the nicotine doses, so that the smoker can chew more during a craving. Long-term dependence seems to be a problem for some gum users. Research has shown that 15–20% of gum users who successfully quit smoking continued using the gum for a year or longer, despite the recommended 6-month limit on use.

Nicotine nasal spray and *nicotine inhalers* are available only by prescription. The nasal spray immediately relieves withdrawal symptoms by delivering nicotine to the bloodstream through the nose. The most common side effects are nasal irritation and sinus problems. Inhalers are plastic rods with a nicotine plug. When the smoker puffs on the rod, the plug produces a nicotine vapor that goes to the mouth instead of the lungs. A benefit of the inhaler is that it mimics hand and mouth actions of smoking.

Non-Nicotine Medications

One of the most exciting developments in smoking cessation has been the recent use of bupropion (Zyban), a prescription antidepressant that affects neurotransmitters related to nicotine cravings. In one study of quitting success, 36% of nicotine patch users quit for at least the month, 49% of bupropion users quit, and 58% of users of both the patch and bupropion quit. Another study found that quitters who use bupropion tend to gain less weight than quitters who do not; an especially significant difference was seen among women. Bupropion has also been shown to be successful in helping even the most hardened smokers quit. If bupropion is not effective, there are two other drugs that may be prescribed, clonidine and nortriptyline; however, neither has been approved by the FDA specifically for nicotine dependence.

Each smoking cessation product may be successful for some people, but any attempt to quit must address both the psychological and the physical aspects of nicotine dependence. Plan carefully how you will quit, to maximize your chance of conquering this powerful addiction.

Tips for Today

Alcohol and tobacco cause far more injuries and deaths in the United States than any other drug. To achieve wellness, it's important to avoid tobacco use and ETS exposure and to use alcohol in moderation, if at all. If tobacco or alcohol use is a problem for you or someone you care about, there are many things you can do to improve the situation.

Right now you can

- Ask your roommates or friends if they know that binge drinking can be fatal; if they don't know, give them the facts about it; also share with them the information in this chapter about dealing with an alcohol emergency.

- If you drink, plan ahead for the next party you attend, figuring out how you can limit yourself to one or two drinks.

- If you smoke, think about the next time you'll want a cigarette, such as while taking on the phone this afternoon or relaxing after dinner tonight. Visualize yourself enjoying this activity without a cigarette in your hand. Imagine yourself as a healthier, more robust person. See if you get pleasure or satisfaction from thinking of yourself as a nonsmoker, an ex-smoker, or someone liberated from dependence on cigarettes.

- If you use tobacco, go outside for a short walk or a stretch to limber up. Breathe deeply. Tell a friend you've just decided to quit.

You can look forward to a longer and healthier life if you join the 47 million Americans who have quit using tobacco. The steps for quitting described below are discussed in terms of the most popular tobacco product in the United States—cigarettes—but they can be adapted for all forms of tobacco use.

Gather Information

Collect personal smoking information in a detailed journal about your smoking behavior. Write down the time you smoke each cigarette of the day, the situation you are in, how you feel, and how strong your craving for the cigarette is, plus any other information that seems relevant. Part of the job is to identify patterns of smoking that are connected with routine situations (for example, the coffee break smoke, the after-dinner cigarette, the tension-reduction cigarette). Use this information to discover the behavior patterns involved in your smoking habit.

Make the Decision to Quit

Choose a date in the near future when you expect to be relatively stress-free and can give quitting the energy and attention it will require. Consider making quitting a gift: Choose your birthday as your quit date, for example, or make quitting a Father's Day or Mother's Day present. You might also want to coordinate your quit date with a buddy—a fellow tobacco user who wants to quit or a nonsmoker who wants to give up another bad habit or begin an exercise program. Tell your friends and family when you plan to quit. Ask them to offer encouragement and help hold you to your goal.

Decide what approach to quitting will work best for you. Will you go cold turkey, or will you taper off? Will you use nicotine patches or gum? Will you join a support group? Prepare a contract for quitting, and post it in a prominent place.

Prepare to Quit

Many smokers find that they use cigarettes to help them unwind in tense situations or to relax at other times. If this is true for you, you'll need to find and develop effective substitutes. It takes time to become proficient at relaxation techniques, so begin practicing before your quit date. Refer to the detailed discussion of relaxation techniques in Chapter 2.

Other things you can do to help prepare for quitting include the following:

- Make an appointment to see your physician. Ask about OTC and prescription aids for tobacco cessation and whether one or more might be appropriate for you.

- Make a dentist's appointment to have your teeth cleaned the day after your target quit date.

- Start an easy exercise program, if you're not exercising regularly already.

- Buy some sugarless gum. Stock your kitchen with low-calorie snacks.

- Clean out your car, and air out your house. Send your clothes out for dry cleaning.

- Throw away all your cigarette-related paraphernalia (ashtrays, lighters, etc.).

- The night before your quit day, get rid of all your cigarettes. Have fun with this—get your friends or family to help you tear them up.

- Make your last few days of smoking inconvenient: Smoke only outdoors and when alone. Don't do anything else while you smoke.

Quitting

Your first few days without cigarettes will probably be the most difficult. It's hard to give up such a strongly ingrained habit, but remember that millions of Americans have done it—and you can too. Plan and rehearse the steps you will take when you experience a powerful craving. Avoid or control situations that you know from your journal are powerfully associated with your smoking. If your hands feel empty without a cigarette, try holding or fiddling with a small object such as a paper clip or pencil.

Social support can also be a big help. Arrange with a buddy to help you with your weak moments, and call him or her whenever you feel overwhelmed by an urge to smoke. Tell people you've just quit. You may discover many inspiring former smokers who can encourage you and reassure you that it's possible to quit and lead a happier, healthier life. Find a formal support group to join if you think it will help.

Maintaining Nonsmoking

The lingering smoking urges that remain once you've quit should be carefully tracked and controlled because they can cause relapses if left unattended. Keep track of these urges in your journal to help you deal with them. If certain situations still trigger the urge for a cigarette, change something about the situation to break past associations. If stress or boredom causes strong smoking urges, use a relaxation technique, take a brisk walk, have a stick of gum, or substitute some other activity for smoking.

Don't set yourself up for a relapse. If you allow yourself to get overwhelmed at school or work or to gain weight, it will be easier to convince yourself that now isn't the right time to quit. This *is* the right time. Continue to practice time-management and relaxation techniques. Exercise regularly, eat sensibly, and get enough sleep. These habits will not only ensure your success at remaining tobacco-free, but they will also serve you well in stressful times throughout your life. In fact, former smokers who have quit for at least 3 months report reduced stress levels, probably because quitting smoking lowers overall arousal.

Watch out for patterns of thinking that can make nonsmoking more difficult. Focus on the positive aspects of not smoking, and give yourself lots of praise—you deserve it. Stick with the schedule of rewards you developed for your contract.

Keep track of the emerging benefits that come from having quit. Items that might appear on your list include improved stamina, an increased sense of pride at having kicked a strong addiction, a sharper sense of taste and smell, no more smoker's cough, and so on. Keep track of the money you're saving by not smoking, and spend it on things you really enjoy. And if you do lapse, be gentle with yourself. Lapses are a normal part of quitting. Forgive yourself, and pick up where you left off.

SUMMARY

- After being absorbed into the bloodstream in the stomach and small intestine, alcohol is transported throughout the body. If people drink more alcohol each hour than their body can metabolize, blood alcohol concentration (BAC) increases.

- Alcohol is a CNS depressant. At low doses, it tends to make people feel relaxed. At higher doses, alcohol interferes with motor and mental functioning; at very high doses, alcohol poisoning, coma, and death can occur.

- Alcohol use increases the risk of injury and violence; drinking before driving is particularly dangerous.

- Continued alcohol use has negative effects on the digestive and cardiovascular systems and increases cancer risk and overall mortality.

- Women who drink while pregnant risk giving birth to children with a cluster of birth defects known as fetal alcohol syndrome (FAS).

- Alcohol abuse involves drinking in dangerous situations or drinking to a degree that causes academic, professional, interpersonal, or legal difficulties.

- Alcohol dependence, or alcoholism, is characterized by more extensive problems with alcohol, usually involving tolerance and withdrawal.

- Binge drinking is a common form of alcohol abuse on college campuses that has negative effects on both drinking and nondrinking students.

- Treatment approaches include mutual support groups like AA, job- and school-based programs, inpatient hospital programs, and pharmacological treatments.

- Smoking is the largest preventable cause of ill health and death in the United States. Regular tobacco use causes physical dependence on nicotine, characterized by loss of control, tolerance, and withdrawal.

- Tobacco smoke is made up of several hundred different chemicals, including some that are carcinogenic or poisonous or that damage the respiratory system.

- Nicotine acts on the nervous system as a stimulant or a depressant. It can cause blood pressure and heart rate to increase, straining the heart.

- Smoking causes cardiovascular disease, lung and other cancers, respiratory damage, and many other disorders. Tobacco use leads to lower life expectancy and to a diminished quality of life.

- The use of spit tobacco leads to nicotine addiction and is linked to oral cancers. Cigars, pipes, clove cigarettes, and bidis are not safe alternatives to cigarettes.

- Environmental tobacco smoke (ETS) contains high concentrations of toxic chemicals and can cause headaches, eye and nasal irritation, sinus problems, lung cancer, and heart disease.

- Children whose parents smoke are especially susceptible to respiratory diseases. Smoking during pregnancy increases the risk of miscarriage, stillbirth, congenital abnormalities, premature birth, and low birth weight.

- Giving up smoking is a difficult and long-term process. Although most ex-smokers quit on their own, some smokers benefit from stop-smoking programs, OTC and prescription medications, and support groups.

TAKE ACTION

1. Interview some of your fellow students about their drinking habits. How much do they drink, and how often? Are they more likely to drink on certain days or in certain circumstances? Are there any habits that seem to be common to most students? How do your own drinking habits compare to those of people you interviewed?

2. Plan an alcohol-free party. What would you serve to eat and drink? What would you tell people about the party when you invite them?

3. Interview one or two former tobacco users about their experiences with tobacco and the methods they used to quit. Why did they start smoking or using tobacco, how old were they when they started, and how long did their habit continue? What made them decide to quit? How did they quit? What could a current tobacco user learn from their experience of quitting?

1. *Critical Thinking* Look at advertisements for alcoholic beverages in magazines and on billboards. Analyze several of these ads. What psychological techniques are used to sell the products? What are the hidden messages? Write an essay outlining your opinion of alcohol advertising and marketing. Do you think it's ethical to sell a potentially dangerous substance by appealing to people's desires and vulnerabilities? Do you think liquor manufacturers ought to be held responsible for the damage alcohol inflicts on some people? Explain your reasoning.

2. Write a list of statements or questions you might use to talk with (1) a person you think is developing a drinking problem; (2) a person planning to drive under the influence of alcohol, with and without you in the car; and (3) a person you want to ask about your own behavior when you drink. Consider using statements from your list when an appropriate situation arises.

3. *Critical Thinking* Restrictions on smoking are increasing in our society. Do you think they're fair? Do they infringe on people's rights? Do they go too far or not far enough? Write a brief essay stating your position on smoking restrictions. Be sure to explain your reasoning. What are the most important factors in your decision? Why do you think you have the opinion you do?

FOR MORE INFORMATION

Books

Brigham, J. 1998. *Dying to Quit: Why We Smoke and How We Stop.* Washington, D.C.: National Academy Press. *A discussion of the process and nature of nicotine addiction from both the scientific and personal perspective.*

Dimeff, L. A., et al. 1999. *Brief Alcohol Screening and Interventions for College Students (BASICS). A Harm Reduction Approach.* New York: Guilford Press. *Presents a model designed to help students reduce their alcohol consumption and the risks they face from heavy drinking; includes handouts and assessment forms.*

Jerslid, D. 2001. *Happy Hours: Alcohol in a Woman's Life.* New York: Cliff Street Books. *Provides facts about the effects of drinking on women along with personal stories of recovery.*

Kessler, D. 2001. *A Question of Intent: A Great American Battle with a Deadly Industry.* New York: Public Affairs. *A description of the federal government's attempts to regulate tobacco, written by the former head of the FDA.*

Kinney, J., and G. Leaton. 2000. *Loosening the Grip: A Handbook of Alcohol Information,* 6th ed. St. Louis: Mosby. *A fascinating book about alcohol, including information on physical effects, abuse, alcoholism, and cultural aspects of alcohol use.*

Kleinman, L. 2000. *The Complete Idiot's Guide to Quitting Smoking.* Indianapolis: Macmillan. *A self-help book for smokers who want to quit.*

Parker-Pope, T. 2001. *Cigarettes: Anatomy of an Industry from Seed to Smoke.* New York: New Press. *An entertaining history of cigarettes, with information on the industry and on individual smokers.*

VWW. Organizations, Hotlines, and Web Sites

Al-Anon Family Group Headquarters. Provides information and referrals to local Al-Anon and Alateen groups. The Web site includes a self-quiz to determine if you are affected by someone's drinking.
888-4AL-ANON
http://www.al-anon.alateen.org

Alcoholics Anonymous (AA) World Services. Provides general information on AA, literature on alcoholism, and information about AA meetings and related 12-step organizations.
212-870-3400
http://www.alcoholics-anonymous.org

Alcohol Treatment Referral Hotline. Provides referrals to local intervention and treatment providers.
800-ALCOHOL

American Cancer Society (ACS). Sponsor of the annual Great American Smokeout; provides information on the dangers of tobacco, as well as tools for prevention and cessation for both smokers and users of spit tobacco.
800-ACS-2345
http://www.cancer.org

American Lung Association. Provides information on lung diseases, tobacco control, and environmental health.
800-LUNG-USA; 212-315-8700
http://www.lungusa.org

Bacchus and Gamma Peer Education Network. An association of college- and university-based peer education programs that focus on prevention of alcohol abuse.
http://www.bacchusgamma.org
http://www.habitsmart.com

CDC's Tobacco Information and Prevention Source (TIPS). Provides research results, educational materials, and tips on how to quit smoking; Web site includes special sections for kids and teens.
800-CDC-1311
http://www.cdc.gov/tobacco

Had Enough.Org. Provides information and a self-quiz on binge drinking among college students.
http://www.hadenough.org

Mothers Against Drunk Driving (MADD). Supports efforts to develop solutions to the problems of drunk driving and underage drinking; provides news, information, and brochures about many topics, including a guide for giving a safe party.
http://www.madd.org

National Association for Children of Alcoholics (NACoA). Provides information and support for children of alcoholics.
888-554-COAS; 301-468-0985
http://www.nacoa.net

National Council on Alcoholism and Drug Dependence (NCADD). Provides information on alcoholism and counseling referrals.
212-269-7797; 800-NCA-CALL (24-hour Hope Line)
http://www.ncadd.org

National Institute on Alcohol Abuse and Alcoholism (NIAAA). Provides booklets and other publications on a variety of alcohol-related topics, including fetal alcohol syndrome, alcoholism treatment, and alcohol use and minorities.
301-443-3860
http://www.niaaa.nih.gov

Quitnet. Provides interactive tools and questionnaires, support groups, a library, news on tobacco issues, and quitting programs for both smokers and spit tobacco users.
http://www.quitnet.org

Tobacco BBS. A resource center on tobacco and smoking issues that includes news and information, assistance for smokers who want to quit, and links to related sites.
http://www.tobacco.org

Tobacco Control Resource Center and Tobacco Products Liability Project (TPLP). Provides current information about tobacco-related court cases and legislation.
http://www.tobacco.neu.edu

See also the listings for Chapters 7 and 12.

SELECTED BIBLIOGRAPHY

Centers for Disease Control and Prevention. 2000. Alcohol policy and sexually transmitted disease rates—United States 1981–1995. *Morbidity and Mortality Weekly Report* 49: 346–349.

Centers for Disease Control and Prevention. 2000. Cigarette smoking among adults—United States, 1998. *Morbidity and Mortality Weekly Report* 49(39): 881–884.

Centers for Disease Control and Prevention. 2000. Declines in lung cancer rates—California, 1988–1997. *Morbidity and Mortality Weekly Report* 49(47): 1066–1069.

Centers for Disease Control and Prevention. 2000. Tobacco use among middle and high school students—United States, 1999. *Morbidity and Mortality Weekly Report* 49(03): 49–53.

Centers for Disease Control and Prevention. 2001. *Women and Smoking: A Report of the Surgeon General.* Atlanta, Ga.: CDC Office on Smoking and Health.

Dawson, D. A. 2000. Alcohol consumption, alcohol dependence, and all-cause mortality. *Alcoholism: Clinical and Experimental Research* 24(1): 72–81.

DeHertog, S. A., et al. 2001. Relation between smoking and skin cancer. *Journal of Clinical Oncology* 19(1): 231–238.

Feldman, H. A., et al. 2000. Erectile dysfunction and coronary risk factors: Prospective results from the Massachusetts male aging study. *Preventive Medicine* 30(4): 328–338.

Fichtenberg, C. M., and S. A. Glantz. 2000. Association of the California Tobacco Control Program with declines in cigarette consumption and mortality from heart disease. *New England Journal of Medicine* 343(24): 1772–1777.

Fiore, M. C., et al. 2000. *Treating Tobacco Use and Dependence.* Clinical Practice Guidelines. Rockville, Md.: U.S. Department of Health and Human Services.

Gilliland, F. D., Y. F. Li, and J. M. Peters. 2001. Effects of maternal smoking during pregnancy and environmental tobacco smoke on asthma and wheezing in children. *American Journal of Respiratory and Critical Care Medicine* 163(2): 429–436.

Goldberg, I. J., et al. 2001. Wine and your heart: A science advisory for healthcare professionals from the Nutrition Committee, Council on Epidemiology and Prevention, and Council on Cardiovascular Nursing of the American Heart Association. *Circulation* 103: 472–475.

Green, G. A., et al. 2001. NCAA study of substance use and abuse habits of college student-athletes. *Clinical Journal of Sports Medicine* 11(1): 51–56.

Harris Poll. 2001. *The Power of Tobacco Addiction* (http://www.louisharris.com/harris_poll/index.asp?PID=220; retrieved April 17, 2001.)

Hashim, R., W. M. Thomson, and A. R. Pack. 2001. Smoking in adolescence as a predictor of early loss of periodontal attachment. *Community Dentistry and Oral Epidemiology* 29(2): 130–135.

Hines, L. S., et al. 2001. Genetic variation in alcohol dehydrogenase and the beneficial effect of moderate alcohol consumption on myocardial infarction. *New England Journal of Medicine* 344(8): 549–555.

Imhof, A., et al. 2001. Effect of alcohol consumption on systemic markers of inflammation. *Lancet* 357(9258): 763–767.

Institute of Medicine. 2001. *Clearing the Smoke: Assessing the Science Base for Tobacco Harm Reduction.* Washington, D.C.: National Academy Press.

Jarvis, M. J., et al. 2001. Nicotine yield from machine-smoked cigarettes and nicotine intakes in smokers: Evidence from a representative population survey. *Journal of the National Cancer Institute* 93(2): 134–138.

Lahmann, C., et al. 2001. Matrix metalloproteinase-1 and skin ageing in smokers. *Lancet* 357(9260): 935–936.

Malarcher, A. M., et al. 2001. Alcohol intake, type of beverage, and the risk of cerebral infarction in young women. *Stroke* 32(1): 77–83.

Mannino, D. M., et al. 2001. Health effects related to environmental tobacco smoke exposure in children in the United States. *Archives of Pediatrics and Adolescent Medicine* 155: 36–41.

National Highway Traffic Safety Administration. 2000. *Impaired Driving in the United States* (http://www.nhtsa.dot.gov/people/injury/alcohol/US.htm; retrieved October 12, 2000).

National Institute on Alcohol Abuse and Alcoholism. 2000. *10th Special Report to the U.S. Congress on Alcohol and Health.* Washington, D.C.: U.S. Department of Health and Human Services.

National Toxicology Program. 2000. *Ninth Report on Carcinogens.* Research Triangle Park, N.C.: U.S. Department of Health and Human Services.

Philip, P., et al. 2001. Fatigue, alcohol, and serious road crashes in France: Factorial study of national data. *British Medical Journal* 322(7290): 829–830.

Reynaud, M., et al. 2001. Patients admitted to emergency services for drunkenness: Moderate alcohol users or harmful drinkers? *American Journal of Psychiatry* 158(1): 96–99.

Rigotti, N. A., J. E. Lee, and H. Wechsler. 2000. U.S. college students' use of tobacco products: Results of a national survey. *Journal of the American Medical Association* 284(6): 699–705.

Shaw, M., R. Mitchell, and D. Dorling. 2000. Time for a smoke? One cigarette reduces your life by 11 minutes. *British Medical Journal* 320(7226): 53.

Substance Abuse and Mental Health Services Administration. 2000. *National Household Survey on Drug Abuse, 1999.* Rockville, Md.: Substance Abuse and Mental Health Services Administration.

Wechsler, H. 2000. College binge drinking in the 1990s: A continuing problem. Results of the Harvard School of Public Health 1999 College Alcohol Study. *Journal of American College Health* 48: 199–210.

Wechsler, H., et al. 2001. Drinking levels, alcohol problems, and second-hand effects in substance-free college residences: Results of a national study. *Journal of Studies on Alcohol* 62(1): 23–31.

Weiss, J., et al. 2000. The alcohol hangover. *Annals of Internal Medicine* 132(11): 897–902.

World Health Organization. 2000. *Tobacco Free Initiative: Burden of Disease* (http://tobacco.who.int/en/health/burden.html; retrieved October 14, 2000).

Nutrition Basics

9

LOOKING AHEAD

After reading this chapter, you should be able to

- List the essential nutrients, and describe the functions they perform in the body

- Describe the guidelines that have been developed to help people choose a healthy diet, avoid nutritional deficiencies, and protect themselves from diet-related chronic diseases

- Discuss nutritional guidelines for vegetarians and for special population groups

- Explain how to use food labels and other consumer tools to make informed choices about foods

- Put together a personal nutrition plan based on affordable foods that you enjoy and that will promote wellness, today as well as in the future

In your lifetime, you'll spend about 6 years eating—about 70,000 meals and 60 tons of food. What you choose to eat can have profound effects on your health and well-being. Of particular concern is the connection between lifetime nutritional habits and the risk of major chronic diseases, including heart disease, cancer, stroke, and diabetes. Choosing foods that provide adequate amounts of the nutrients you need, while limiting the substances linked to disease, should be an important part of your daily life. The food choices you make will significantly influence your health—both now and in the future.

This chapter provides the basic principles of **nutrition.** It introduces the six classes of essential nutrients, explaining their roles in the functioning of the body. It also provides different sets of guidelines that you can use to design a healthy diet plan. Finally, it offers practical tools and advice to help you apply the guidelines to your own life. Diet is an area of your life in which you have almost total control. Using your knowledge and understanding of nutrition to create a healthy diet plan is a significant step toward wellness.

NUTRITIONAL REQUIREMENTS: COMPONENTS OF A HEALTHY DIET

When you think about your diet, you probably do so in terms of the foods you like to eat—a turkey sandwich and a glass of milk or a steak and a baked potato. What's important for your health, though, are the nutrients contained in those foods. Your body requires proteins, fats, carbohydrates, vitamins, minerals, and water—about 45

---

nutrition The science of food and how the body uses it in health and disease.

Terms

183

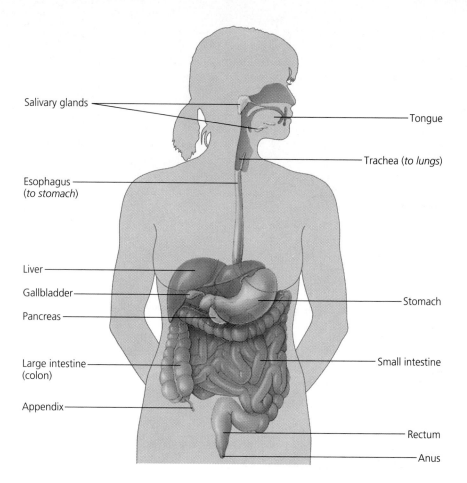

Figure 9-1 The digestive system. Food is partially broken down by being chewed and mixed with saliva in the mouth. As food moves through the digestive tract, it is mixed by muscular contractions and broken down by chemicals. After traveling to the stomach via the esophagus, food is broken down further by stomach acids. Most absorption of nutrients occurs in the small intestine, aided by secretions from the pancreas, gallbladder, and intestinal lining. The large intestine reabsorbs excess water; the remaining solid wastes are collected in the rectum and excreted through the anus.

Salivary glands

Tongue

Trachea (*to lungs*)

Esophagus (*to stomach*)

Liver

Gallbladder

Pancreas

Stomach

Large intestine (colon)

Small intestine

Appendix

Rectum

Anus

essential nutrients. The word *essential* in this context means that you must get these substances from food because your body is unable to manufacture them at all, or at least not fast enough to meet your physiological needs. Your body obtains these nutrients through the process of **digestion,** in which the foods you eat are broken down into compounds your gastrointestinal tract can absorb and your body can use (Figure 9-1).

The energy in foods is expressed as **kilocalories.** One kilocalorie represents the amount of heat it takes to raise the temperature of 1 liter of water 1°C. You need about 2000 kilocalories per day to meet your energy needs. In common usage, people usually refer to kilocalories as *calories,* which is a much smaller energy unit: 1 kilocalorie contains 1000 calories. We'll use the familiar word *calorie* in this chapter to stand for the larger energy unit.

Three classes of nutrients supply energy: protein, carbohydrates, and fats. Fats provide the most energy, at 9 calories per gram; protein and carbohydrates each provide 4 calories per gram. The high caloric content of fat is one reason experts advise against high fat consumption; most of us do not need the extra calories. Alcohol, though it is not an essential nutrient and has no nutritional value, also supplies energy—7 calories per gram.

But just meeting energy needs is not enough; our bodies require adequate amounts of all the essential nutrients to grow and function properly.

Terms

essential nutrients Substances the body must get from foods because it cannot manufacture them at all or fast enough to meet its needs. These nutrients include proteins, fats, carbohydrates, vitamins, minerals, and water.

digestion The process of breaking down foods in the gastrointestinal tract into compounds the body can absorb.

kilocalorie A measure of energy content in food; 1 kilocalorie represents the amount of heat needed to raise the temperature of 1 liter of water 1°C; commonly referred to as *calorie.*

protein An essential nutrient; a compound made of amino acids that contain carbon, hydrogen, oxygen, and nitrogen.

amino acids The building blocks of proteins.

legumes Vegetables such as peas and beans that are high in fiber and are also important sources of protein.

saturated fat A fat with no carbon-carbon double bonds; usually solid at room temperature.

monounsaturated fat A fat with one carbon-carbon double bond; liquid at room temperature.

polyunsaturated fat A fat containing two or more carbon-carbon double bonds; liquid at room temperature.

Proteins—The Basis of Body Structure

Proteins form important parts of the body's main structural components: muscles and bones. Proteins also form important parts of blood, enzymes, some hormones, and cell membranes. As mentioned above, proteins can provide energy for the body (4 calories per gram).

Amino Acids   The building blocks of proteins are called **amino acids.** Twenty common amino acids are found in food; nine of these are essential: histidine, isoleucine, leucine, lysine, methionine, phenylalanine, threonine, tryptophan, and valine. The other 11 amino acids can be produced by the body, given the presence of the needed components supplied by foods.

Complete and Incomplete Proteins   Individual protein sources are considered "complete" if they supply all the essential amino acids in adequate amounts and "incomplete" if they do not. Meat, fish, poultry, eggs, milk, cheese, and soy provide complete proteins. Incomplete proteins, which come from other plant sources such as **legumes** and nuts, are good sources of most essential amino acids, but are usually low in one or two.

Combining two vegetable proteins, such as wheat and peanuts in a peanut butter sandwich, allows each vegetable protein to make up for the amino acids missing in the other protein. The combination yields a complete protein. Your concern with amino acids and complete protein in your diet should focus on what you consume throughout the day, rather than at each meal. Proteins consumed throughout the course of the day can complement each other to form a pool of amino acids the body can draw from to produce the necessary proteins.

Recommended Protein Intake   About two-thirds of the protein in the American diet comes from animal sources; therefore, the American diet is rich in essential amino acids. Most Americans consume more protein than they need each day. Protein consumed beyond what the body needs is synthesized into fat for energy storage or burned for energy requirements. Consuming somewhat above our needs is not harmful, but it can contribute fat to the diet because protein-rich foods are often fat-rich as well. The amount of protein you eat should represent about 10–15% of your total daily calorie intake.

Fats—Essential in Small Amounts

Fats, also known as *lipids,* are the most concentrated source of energy, at 9 calories per gram. The fats stored in your body represent usable energy; they help insulate your body, and they support and cushion your organs. Fats in the diet help your body absorb fat-soluble vitamins, as well as add important flavor and texture to foods. Fats are the major fuel for the body during rest and light

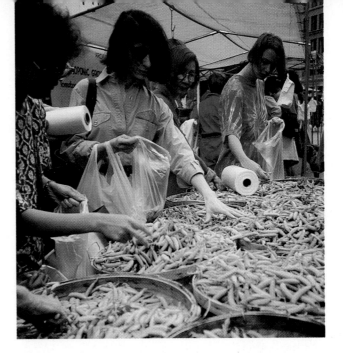

Our bodies require adequate amounts of all essential nutrients—water, proteins, carbohydrates, fats, vitamins, and minerals—in order to grow and function properly. Choosing foods to satisfy these nutritional requirements is an important part of a healthy lifestyle.

activity. Two fats—linoleic acid and alpha-linolenic acid—are essential components of the diet.

Types and Sources of Fats   Most of the fats in food are in the form of triglycerides, which are composed of a glycerol molecule (an alcohol) plus three fatty acids. A fatty acid is made up of a chain of carbon atoms with oxygen attached at one end and hydrogen atoms attached along the length of the chain. Fatty acids differ in the length of their carbon atom chains and in their degree of saturation (the number of hydrogens attached to the chain). If every available bond from each carbon atom in a fatty acid chain is attached to a hydrogen atom, the fatty acid is said to be **saturated.** If not all the available bonds are taken up by hydrogens, the carbon atoms in the chain will form double bonds with each other. Such fatty acids are called unsaturated fats. If there is only one double bond, the fatty acid is called **monounsaturated.** If there are two or more double bonds, the fatty acid is called **polyunsaturated.**

Food fats are often composed of both saturated and unsaturated fatty acids; the dominant type of fatty acid determines the fat's characteristics. Food fats containing large amounts of saturated fatty acids are usually solid at room temperature; they are generally found naturally in animal products. The leading sources of saturated fat in the American diet are red meats (hamburger, steak, roasts), whole milk, cheese, hot dogs, and lunch meats. Food fats containing large amounts of monounsaturated and polyunsaturated fatty acids are usually from plant sources and are liquid at room temperature. Olive, canola, safflower, and peanut oils contain mostly monounsaturated fatty acids. Soybean, corn, and cottonseed oils contain mostly polyunsaturated fatty acids.

There are notable exceptions to these generalizations. When unsaturated vegetable oils undergo the process of **hydrogenation,** a mixture of saturated and unsaturated fatty acids is produced. Hydrogenation turns many of the double bonds in unsaturated fatty acids into single bonds, increasing the degree of saturation and producing a more solid fat from a liquid oil. Hydrogenation also changes some unsaturated fatty acids to **trans fatty acids,** unsaturated fatty acids with an atypical shape that affects their behavior in the body.

Leading sources of trans fats in the American diet are deep-fried fast foods such as french fries and fried chicken; baked and snack foods such as pot pies, cakes, cookies, pastries, doughnuts, and chips; and stick margarine. In general, the more solid a hydrogenated oil is, the more saturated and trans fats it contains; for example, stick margarines typically contain more saturated and trans fats than do tub or squeeze margarines. Small amounts of trans fatty acids are found naturally in meat and milk.

Hydrogenated vegetable oils are not the only plant fats that contain saturated fats. Palm and coconut oils, although derived from plants, are also highly saturated. On the other hand, fish oils, derived from an animal source, are rich in polyunsaturated fats.

Fats and Health   Different types of fats have very different effects on health. Many studies have examined the effects of dietary fat intake on blood **cholesterol** levels and the risk of heart disease. Saturated and trans fatty acids raise blood levels of **low-density lipoprotein**

(LDL), or "bad" cholesterol, thereby increasing a person's risk of heart disease. Unsaturated fatty acids, on the other hand, lower LDL. Monounsaturated fatty acids, such as those found in olive and canola oils, may also increase levels of **high-density lipoproteins (HDL),** or "good" cholesterol, providing even greater benefits for heart health. In large amounts, trans fatty acids may lower HDL. Thus, to reduce the risk of heart disease, it is important to substitute unsaturated fats for saturated and trans fats. (See Chapter 12 for more on cholesterol.)

Most Americans consume more saturated fat than trans fat (11% versus 2–4% of total daily calories). However, health experts are particularly concerned about trans fats because of their double negative effect on heart health—they both raise LDL and lower HDL—and because there is less public awareness of trans fats. The saturated fat content of prepared foods has been listed on nutrition labels since 1994. The FDA has proposed that information on trans fat content also be listed on food labels, but until that change goes into effect, consumers can check for the presence of trans fats by examining the ingredient list of a food: If a food contains "partially hydrogenated oil" or "vegetable shortening," it contains trans fat.

Although saturated and trans fats pose health hazards, other fats are beneficial. Monounsaturated fatty acids, as found in avocados, most nuts, and olive, canola, peanut, and safflower oils, improve cholesterol levels and may help protect against some cancers. **Omega-3 fatty acids,** a form of polyunsaturated fat found primarily in fish, may be even more healthful. Omega-3s are produced when the endmost double bond of a polyunsaturated fat occurs three carbons from the end of the fatty acid chain. Omega-3s have a number of heart-healthy effects, and nutritionists recommend that Americans increase the proportion of omega-3s in their diet by eating fish two or more times a week.

Another form of polyunsaturated fat, omega-6 fatty acid, is produced if the endmost double bond occurs at the sixth carbon atom. Most of the polyunsaturated fats currently consumed by Americans are omega-6s, primarily from corn oil and soybean oil. Foods rich in omega-6s are important because they contain the essential nutrient linoleic acid. However, some nutritionists recommend that people reduce the proportion of omega-6s they consume in favor of omega-3s. To make this adjustment, use canola oil rather than corn oil in cooking, and check for corn, soybean, or cottonseed oil in products such as mayonnaise, margarine, and salad dressing.

In addition to its effects on heart disease risk, dietary fat can affect health in other ways. Diets high in fatty red meat are associated with an increased risk of certain forms of cancer, especially colon cancer. A high-fat diet can also make weight management more difficult. Because fat is a concentrated source of calories (9 calories per gram versus 4 calories per gram for protein and carbohydrate), a high-fat diet is often a high-calorie diet that can lead to weight gain. In addition, there is some evidence that calo-

Terms

hydrogenation A process by which hydrogens are added to unsaturated fats, increasing the degree of saturation and turning liquid oils into solid fats. Hydrogenation produces a mixture of saturated fatty acids and standard and trans forms of unsaturated fatty acids.

trans fatty acid A type of unsaturated fatty acid produced during the process of hydrogenation; trans fats have an atypical shape that affects their chemical activity.

cholesterol A waxy substance found in the blood and cells and needed for cell membranes, vitamin D, and hormone synthesis.

low-density lipoprotein (LDL) Blood fat that transports cholesterol to organs and tissues; excess amounts result in the accumulation of deposits on artery walls.

high-density lipoprotein (HDL) Blood fat that helps transport cholesterol out of the arteries, thereby protecting against heart disease.

omega-3 fatty acids Polyunsaturated fatty acids commonly found in fish oils that are beneficial to cardiovascular health; the endmost double bond occurs three carbons from the end of the fatty acid chain.

Type of Fatty Acid	Found In[a]	Possible Effects on Health
SATURATED *Keep Intake Low*	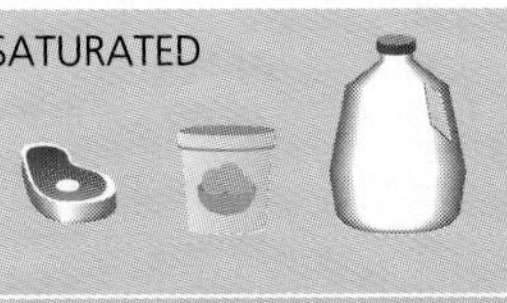 Animal fats (especially fatty meats and poultry fat and skin) Butter, cheese, and other high-fat dairy products Palm and coconut oils	Raises total cholesterol and "bad" (LDL) cholesterol levels Increases risk of heart disease May increase risk of colon and prostate cancers
TRANS 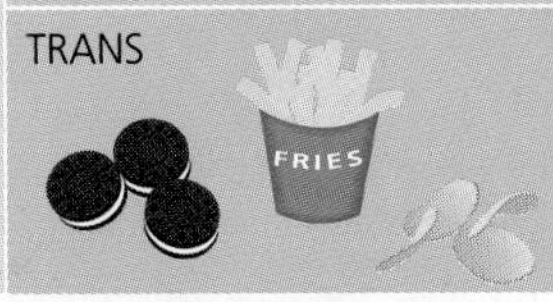	French fries and other deep-fried fast foods Stick margarines, shortening Packaged cookies and crackers Processed snacks and sweets	Raises total cholesterol and "bad" (LDL) cholesterol levels Lowers "good" (HDL) cholesterol levels May increase risk of heart disease and breast cancer
MONOUNSATURATED *Choose Moderate Amounts*	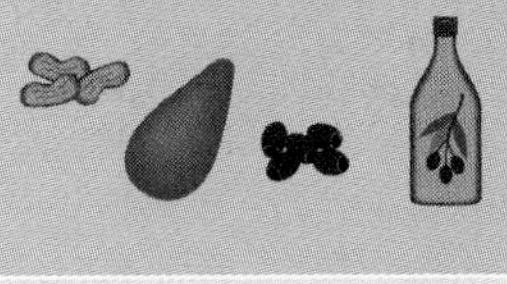 Olive, canola, and safflower oils Avocados, olives Peanut butter (without added fat) Many nuts, including almonds, cashews, pecans, pistachios	Lowers total cholesterol and "bad" (LDL) cholesterol levels May reduce blood pressure and lower triglyceride levels (a risk factor for CVD) May reduce risk of heart disease, stroke, and some cancers
POLYUNSATURATED (two groups)[b]		
Omega-3 fatty acids 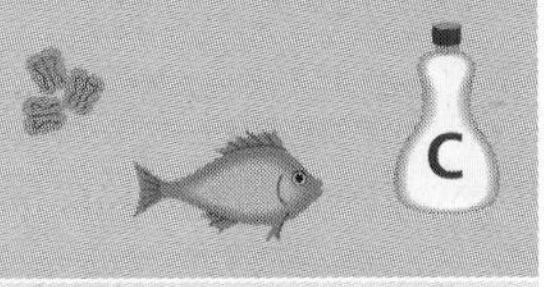	Fatty fish, including salmon, white albacore tuna, mackerel, anchovies, and sardines Lesser amounts in walnut, flaxseed, canola, and soybean oils; tofu; walnuts; flaxseeds; and dark-green, leafy vegetables	Reduces blood clotting and inflammation and inhibits abnormal heart rhythms Lowers triglyceride levels (a risk factor for CVD) May lower blood pressure in some people May reduce risk of fatal heart attack, stroke and some cancers
Omega-6 fatty acids 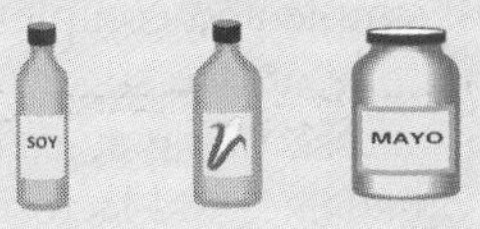	Corn, soybean, and cottonseed oils (often used in margarine, mayonnaise, and salad dressing)	Lowers total cholesterol and "bad" (LDL) cholesterol levels May lower "good" (HDL) cholesterol levels May reduce risk of heart disease May slightly increase risk of cancer if omega-6 intake is high and omega-3 intake is low

[a] Food fats contain a combination of types of fatty acids in various proportions; for example, canola oil is composed mainly of monounsaturated fatty acids (62%) but also contains polyunsaturated (32%) and saturated (6%) fatty acids. Food fats are categorized here according to their predominant fatty acid.

[b] The essential fatty acids are polyunsaturated: Linoleic acid is an omega-6 fatty acid and alpha-linolenic acid is an omega-3 fatty acid.

Figure 9-2 Types of fatty acids and their possible effects on health. The health effects of dietary fats are still being investigated. In general, nutritionists recommend that we consume a diet moderate in fat overall and that we substitute unsaturated fats for saturated and trans fats. Monounsaturated fats and omega-3 polyunsaturated fats may be particularly good choices for promoting health. Eating lots of fat of any type can provide excess calories because all types of fats are rich sources of energy (9 calories per gram).

ries from fat are more easily converted to body fat than calories from protein or carbohydrate.

Although more research is needed on the precise effects of different types and amounts of fat on overall health, a great deal of evidence points to the fact that most people benefit from lowering their overall fat intake to recommended levels and substituting unsaturated fats for saturated and trans fats. The types of fatty acids and their effects on health are summarized in Figure 9-2.

Recommended Fat Intake You need only about 1 tablespoon (15 grams) of vegetable oil per day incorporated into your diet to supply the essential fats. The average American diet supplies considerably more than this amount; in fact, fats make up about 33% of our total calorie intake. (This is the equivalent of about 75 grams, or 5 tablespoons, of fat per day for someone who consumes 2000 calories.) Health experts recommend that most Americans reduce their total fat intake to 30% or less of total calories, with less than 10% coming from saturated fat. A 2001 report by the National Cholesterol Education Program (NCEP) suggests total fat intake of 25–35%, with less than 7% coming from saturated fat, up to 10% from polyunsaturated fat, and up to 20% from monounsaturated fat. The NCEP diet also recommends that trans fat intake be kept low and that total calorie intake allow for the maintenance of a healthy weight.

Table 9-1

Table 9-1 Recommended Daily Intake for Fat, Protein, and Carbohydrate

	Energy/Gram	Percent of Total Calories	Recommended Daily Nutrient Intake Goal or Limit		
			Calories and Grams for Three Levels of Energy Intake		
			1600 Calories	2200 Calories	2800 Calories
Fat	9 calories/gram	30% or less	480 calories = 53 grams	660 calories = 73 grams	840 calories = 93 grams
Saturated fat	*9 calories/gram*	*less than 10%*	*160 calories = 18 grams*	*220 calories = 24 grams*	*280 calories = 31 grams*
Protein	4 calories/gram	15%	240 calories = 60 grams	330 calories = 83 grams	420 calories = 105 grams
Carbohydrate	4 calories/gram	55%	880 calories = 220 grams	1210 calories = 303 grams	1540 calories = 385 grams
Added sugars	*4 calories/gram*		*6 teaspoons = 24 grams*	*12 teaspoons = 48 grams*	*18 teaspoons = 72 grams*

The number of calories and grams of fat that correspond to the 30% (total fat) and 10% (saturated fat) limits are shown in Table 9-1 for diets consisting of 1600, 2200, and 2800 calories per day. To determine how close you are to meeting these intake goals for fat, keep a running total over the course of the day. For prepared foods, food labels list the number of grams of fat, protein, and carbohydrate; the breakdown for popular fast-food items can be found in the Appendix. Nutrition information is also available in many grocery stores, published in inexpensive nutrition guides, and online (see For More Information at the end of the chapter). In reducing fat intake to recommended levels, the emphasis should be on lowering saturated and trans fats. You can still eat high-fat foods, but it makes good sense to limit the size of your portions and to balance your intake with low-fat foods.

COMMUNICATE! Fast-food restaurants are convenient, fast, and inexpensive—but feature many high-fat, high-sodium options. The next time your friends or family want to go get a burger, try persuading them to make a different choice. Engage both their minds and their emotions by pointing out the facts about fat and salt and appealing to their desire to be fit and active. End with specific suggestions, such as going to a salad bar or an ethnic restaurant or cooking a meal together at home.

Carbohydrates—An Ideal Source of Energy

Carbohydrates are needed in the diet primarily to supply energy for body cells. Some cells, such as those found in the brain and other parts of the nervous system and in blood,

use only carbohydrates for fuel. During high-intensity exercise, muscles also use primarily carbohydrates for fuel.

Simple and Complex Carbohydrates Carbohydrates are classified into two groups: simple and complex. Simple carbohydrates contain only one or two sugar units in each molecule; they include sucrose (table sugar), fructose (fruit sugar), maltose (malt sugar), and lactose (milk sugar). Simple carbohydrates provide sweetness in foods and are found naturally in fruits and milk and are added to soft drinks, fruit drinks, candy, and desserts.

Complex carbohydrates consist of chains of many sugar molecules; they include starches and most types of dietary fiber. Starches are found in a variety of plants, especially grains (wheat, rye, rice, oats, barley, millet), legumes (dry beans, peas, and lentils), and tubers (potatoes and yams). Most other vegetables contain a mixture of starches and simple carbohydrates. Dietary fiber is found in grains, fruits, and vegetables.

During digestion in the mouth and small intestine, your body breaks down starches and double sugars into single sugar molecules, such as **glucose,** for absorption. Once glucose is in the bloodstream, the pancreas releases the hormone insulin, which allows cells to take up glucose and use it for energy. The liver and muscles also take up glucose to provide carbohydrate storage in the form of glycogen. Some people have problems controlling blood glucose levels, a disorder called diabetes mellitus.

Refined Carbohydrates Versus Whole Grains Complex carbohydrates can be further divided between refined, or processed, carbohydrates and unrefined carbohydrates, or whole grains. Before they are processed, all grains are **whole grains,** consisting of an inner layer of

What Are Whole Grains?

The first step in increasing your intake of whole grains is to correctly identify them. The following are whole grains:

whole wheat	whole-grain corn
whole rye	popcorn
whole oats	brown rice
oatmeal	barley

More unusual choices include bulgur (cracked wheat), millet, kasha (roasted buckwheat kernels), quinoa, wheat and rye berries, amaranth, graham flour, whole-grain kamut, whole-grain spelt, and whole-grain triticale.

Wheat flour, unbleached flour, enriched flour, and degerminated corn meal are not whole grains. Wheat germ and wheat bran are also not whole grains, but they are the constituents of wheat typically left out when wheat is processed and so are healthier choices than regular wheat flour, which typically contains just the endosperm.

Reading Food Packages to Find Whole Grains

To find packaged foods rich in whole grains, read the list of ingredients and check for special health claims related to whole grains. The *first* item on the list of ingredients should be one of the whole grains listed above. In addition, the FDA allows manufacturers to include special health claims for foods that contain 51% or more whole-grain ingredients. Such products may contain a statement such as the following on their packaging: "Rich in whole grain," "Made with 100% whole grain," or "Diets rich in whole-grain foods may help reduce the risk of heart disease and certain cancers." However, many whole-grain products will not carry such claims.

Incorporating Whole Grains into Your Daily Diet

- *Bread:* Look for sandwich breads, bagels, English muffins, buns, and pita breads with a whole grain listed as the first ingredient.
- *Breakfast cereals:* Check the ingredient list for whole grains. Whole-grain choices include oatmeal, muesli, shredded wheat, and some types of raisin bran, bran flakes, wheat flakes, toasted oats, and granola.
- *Rice:* Choose brown rice or rice blends that include brown rice.
- *Pasta:* Look for whole-wheat, whole-grain kamut, or whole-grain spelt pasta.
- *Tortillas:* Choose whole-wheat or whole-corn tortillas.
- *Crackers and snacks:* Some varieties of crackers are made from whole grains, including some flatbreads or crispbreads, woven wheat crackers, and rye crackers. Other whole-grain snack possibilities include popcorn, popcorn cakes, brown rice cakes, whole-corn tortilla chips, and whole-wheat fig cookies. Be sure to check food labels for fat content, as many popular snacks are also high in fat.
- *Mixed-grain dishes:* Combine whole grains with other foods to create healthy mixed dishes such as tabouli; soups made with hulled barley or wheat berries; and pilafs, casseroles, and salads made with brown rice, whole-wheat couscous, kasha, millet, wheat bulgur, and quinoa.

If your grocery store doesn't carry all of these items, try your local health food store.

germ, a middle layer called the endosperm, and an outer layer of bran. During processing, the germ and bran are often removed, leaving just the starchy endosperm. The refinement of whole grains transforms whole-wheat flour to white flour, brown rice to white rice, and so on.

Refined carbohydrates usually retain all the calories of their unrefined counterparts, but they tend to be much lower in fiber, vitamins, minerals, and other beneficial compounds. Unrefined carbohydrates tend to take longer to chew and digest than refined ones. This slower digestive pace tends to make people feel full sooner and for a longer period, lessening the chance that they will overeat. A slower rise in blood glucose levels following consumption of complex carbohydrates may help in the management of diabetes. Whole grains are also high in dietary fiber and so have all the benefits of fiber. Consumption of whole grains has been linked to reduced risk for heart disease, diabetes, high blood pressure, stroke, and certain forms of cancer. For all these reasons, whole grains are recommended over those that have been refined.

Recommended Carbohydrate Intake   On average, Americans consume over 250 grams of carbohydrate per day, well above the minimum of 50–100 grams of essential carbohydrate required by the body. However, health experts recommend that most Americans increase their consumption of carbohydrates to 55–60% of total daily calories, or about 275–300 grams of carbohydrate for someone consuming 2000 calories per day. The focus should be on consuming a variety of foods rich in complex carbohydrates, especially whole grains.

carbohydrate An essential nutrient; sugars, starches, and dietary fiber are all carbohydrates.

glucose A simple sugar that is the body's basic fuel.

whole grain The entire edible portion of a grain such as wheat, rice, or oats, including the germ, endosperm, and bran. During milling or processing, parts of the grain are removed, often leaving just the endosperm.

Terms

Experts also recommend that Americans alter the proportion of simple and complex carbohydrates in the diet, lowering simple carbohydrate intake from about 25% to about 10–15% of total daily calories. To accomplish this change, reduce your intake of foods like soft drinks, candy, sweet desserts, and sweetened fruit drinks, which are high in simple sugars but low in other nutrients. The bulk of the simple carbohydrates in your diet should come from fruits, which are rich in vitamins and minerals, and milk, which is high in protein and calcium.

Dietary Fiber—A Closer Look

Dietary fiber consists of carbohydrate plant substances that are difficult or impossible for humans to digest. Instead, fiber passes through the intestinal tract and provides bulk for feces in the large intestine, which in turn facilitates elimination. In the large intestine, some types of fiber are broken down by bacteria into acids and gases, which explains why consuming too much fiber can lead to intestinal gas.

Types of Dietary Fiber Nutritionists classify fibers as soluble or insoluble. **Soluble fiber** slows the body's absorption of glucose and binds cholesterol-containing compounds in the intestine, lowering blood cholesterol levels and reducing the risk of cardiovascular disease. **Insoluble fiber** binds water, making the feces bulkier and softer so they pass more quickly and easily through the large intestine.

Both kinds of fiber contribute to disease risk reduction and management. A diet high in soluble fiber can help people manage diabetes and high blood cholesterol levels. A diet high in insoluble fiber can help prevent a variety of health problems, including constipation, hemorrhoids, and **diverticulitis.** Some studies have linked high-fiber diets with a reduced risks of colon and rectal cancer; more recent evidence suggests that other characteristics of diets rich in fruits, vegetables, and whole grains may be responsible for this reduction in risk.

Sources of Dietary Fiber All plant foods contain some dietary fiber. Fruits, legumes, oats (especially oat bran), barley, and psyllium (found in some cereals and laxatives) are particularly rich in soluble fiber. Wheat (especially wheat bran), cereals, grains, and vegetables are all good sources of insoluble fiber. However, the processing of packaged foods can remove fiber, so it's important to depend on fresh fruits and vegetables and foods made from whole grains as sources of dietary fiber.

Recommended Intake of Dietary Fiber Most Americans consume about 16 grams of dietary fiber a day, whereas the recommended daily amount is 20–35 grams of fiber. Fiber should come from foods, not supplements, which should only be used under medical supervision. To increase the amount of fiber in your diet, try the following:

- Choose whole-grain foods instead of those made from processed grains. Select a breakfast cereal with 5 or more grams of fiber per serving.
- Eat whole, unpeeled fruits rather than drinking fruit juice. Top cereals, yogurt, and desserts with berries, unpeeled apple slices, or other fruit.
- Include legumes in soups and salads. Combine raw vegetables with pasta, rice, or beans in salads.
- Substitute bean dip for cheese-based or sour cream-based dips or spreads. Use raw vegetables rather than chips for dipping.

Vitamins—Organic Micronutrients

Vitamins are organic (carbon-containing) substances required in very small amounts to regulate various processes within living cells (Table 9-2). Humans need 13 vitamins. Four are fat-soluble (A, D, E, and K), and nine are water-soluble (C, and the eight B-complex vitamins: thiamin, riboflavin, niacin, vitamin B-6, folate, vitamin B-12, biotin, and pantothenic acid).

Functions of Vitamins Many vitamins help chemical reactions take place. They provide no energy to the body directly but help unleash the energy stored in carbohydrates, proteins, and fats. Vitamins are critical in the production of red blood cells and the maintenance of the nervous, skeletal, and immune systems. Some vitamins act as **antioxidants,** which help preserve healthy cells in the body. Key vitamin antioxidants include vitamin E, vitamin C, and the vitamin A precursor beta-carotene.

Sources of Vitamins The human body does not manufacture most of the vitamins it requires and must obtain them from foods. Vitamins are abundant in fruits, vegetables, and grains. In addition, many processed foods, such

| Table 9-2 | | Facts About Vitamins | | |

Vitamin	Important Dietary Sources	Major Functions	Signs of Prolonged Deficiency	Toxic Effects of Megadoses
Fat-Soluble				
Vitamin A	Liver, milk, butter, cheese, and fortified margarine; carrots, spinach, and other orange and deep-green vegetables and fruits	Maintenance of vision, skin, linings of the nose, mouth, digestive and urinary tracts, immune function	Night blindness; dry, scaling skin; increased susceptibility to infection; loss of appetite; anemia; kidney stones	Headache, vomiting and diarrhea, vertigo, double vision, bone abnormalities, liver damage, miscarriage and birth defects
Vitamin D	Fortified milk and margarine, fish liver oils, butter, egg yolks (sunlight on skin also produces vitamin D)	Development and maintenance of bones and teeth, promotion of calcium absorption	Rickets (bone deformities) in children; bone softening, loss, and fractures in adults	Kidney damage, calcium deposits in soft tissues, depression, death
Vitamin E	Vegetable oils, whole grains, nuts and seeds, green leafy vegetables, asparagus, peaches	Protection and maintenance of cellular membranes	Red blood cell breakage and anemia, weakness, neurological problems, muscle cramps	Relatively nontoxic, but may cause excess bleeding or formation of blood clots
Vitamin K	Green leafy vegetables; smaller amounts widespread in other foods	Production of factors essential for blood clotting	Hemorrhaging	Anemia, jaundice
Water-Soluble				
Vitamin C	Peppers, broccoli, spinach, brussels sprouts, citrus fruits, strawberries, tomatoes, potatoes, cabbage, other fruits and vegetables	Maintenance and repair of connective tissue, bones, teeth, and cartilage; promotion of healing; aid in iron absorption	Scurvy, anemia, reduced resistance to infection, loosened teeth, joint pain, poor wound healing, hair loss, poor iron absorption	Urinary stones in some people, acid stomach from ingesting supplements in pill form, nausea, diarrhea, headache, fatigue
Thiamin	Whole-grain and enriched breads and cereals, organ meats, lean pork, nuts, legumes	Conversion of carbohydrates into usable forms of energy, maintenance of appetite and nervous system function	Beriberi (symptoms include muscle wasting, mental confusion, anorexia, enlarged heart, nerve changes)	None reported
Riboflavin	Dairy products, enriched breads and cereals, lean meats, poultry, fish, green vegetables	Energy metabolism; maintenance of skin, mucous membranes, and nervous system structures	Cracks at corners of mouth, sore throat, skin rash, hypersensitivity to light, purple tongue	None reported
Niacin	Eggs, poultry, fish, milk, whole grains, nuts, enriched breads and cereals, meats, legumes	Conversion of carbohydrates, fats, and protein into usable forms of energy	Pellagra (symptoms include diarrhea, dermatitis, inflammation of mucous membranes, dementia)	Flushing of the skin, nausea, vomiting, diarrhea, liver dysfunction, glucose intolerance
Vitamin B-6	Eggs, poultry, fish, whole grains, nuts, soybeans, liver, kidney, pork	Protein and neurotransmitter metabolism; red blood cell synthesis	Anemia, convulsions, cracks at corners of mouth, dermatitis, nausea, confusion	Neurological abnormalities and damage
Folate	Green leafy vegetables, yeast, oranges, whole grains, legumes, liver	Amino acid metabolism, synthesis of RNA and DNA, new cell synthesis	Anemia, weakness, fatigue, irritability, shortness of breath, swollen tongue	Masking of vitamin B-12 deficiency
Vitamin B-12	Eggs, milk, meats, other animal foods	Synthesis of blood cells; other metabolic reactions	Anemia, fatigue, nervous system damage, sore tongue	None reported
Biotin	Cereals, yeast, egg yolks, soy flour, liver, widespread in foods	Metabolism of fats, carbohydrates, and proteins	Rash, nausea, vomiting, weight loss, depression, fatigue, hair loss	None reported
Pantothenic acid	Animal foods, whole grains, broccoli, legumes; widespread in foods	Metabolism of fats, carbohydrates, and proteins	Fatigue, numbness and tingling of hands and feet, gastrointestinal disturbances	None reported

SOURCES: Food and Nutrition Board, National Academy of Sciences, 2000. *Dietary Reference Intakes for Vitamin C, Vitamin E, Selenium, and Carotenoids.* Washington, D.C.: National Academy Press. Food and Nutrition Board; National Academy of Sciences. 1998. *Dietary Reference Intakes for Thiamin, Riboflavin, Niacin, Vitamin B₆, Folate, Vitamin B₁₂, Pantothenic Acid, and Choline.* Washington, D.C.: National Academy Press. National Research Council. 1989. *Recommended Dietary Allowances,* 10th ed. Washington, D.C.: National Academy Press. Shils, M.E., et al., eds. 1998 *Modern Nutrition in Health and Disease,* 9th ed. Baltimore; Williams & Wilkins.

as flour and breakfast cereals contain added vitamins. A few vitamins are made in certain parts of the body: The skin makes vitamin D when it is exposed to sunlight, and intestinal bacteria make vitamin K.

Vitamin Deficiencies and Excesses If your diet lacks sufficient amounts of a particular vitamin, characteristic symptoms of deficiency develop (see Table 9-2.) For example, vitamin A deficiency can cause blindness and vitamin B-6 deficiency can cause seizures. Vitamin deficiency diseases are most often seen in developing countries; they are relatively rare in the United States because vitamins are readily available from our food supply. However, intakes below recommended levels can have adverse effects on health even if they are not low enough to cause a deficiency disease. For example, low intake of folate and vitamins B-6 and B-12 has been linked to increased heart disease risk.

Extra vitamins in the diet can be harmful, especially when taken as supplements. High doses of vitamin A are toxic and increase the risk of birth defects, for example. Even when vitamins are not taken in excess, relying on supplements can be a problem. There are many substances in foods other than vitamins and minerals, and some of these compounds may have important health effects. Later in the chapter we will discuss when a vitamin supplement is advisable. For now, keep in mind that it's best to obtain most of your vitamins from foods rather than supplements.

Minerals—Inorganic Micronutrients

Minerals are inorganic (non–carbon-containing) elements you need in relatively small amounts to help regulate body functions, aid in the growth and maintenance of body tissues, and help release energy (Table 9-3). There are about 17 essential minerals. The major minerals, those that the body needs in amounts exceeding 100 milligrams, include calcium, phosphorus, magnesium, sodium, potassium, and chloride. The essential trace minerals, those that

you need in minute amounts, include copper, fluoride, iodide, iron, selenium, and zinc.

Characteristic symptoms develop if an essential mineral is consumed in a quantity too small or too large for good health. The minerals most commonly lacking in the American diet are iron, calcium, zinc, and magnesium. Focus on good food choices for these. Lean meats are rich in iron and zinc, while low-fat or fat-free dairy products are excellent choices for calcium. Plant foods such as whole grains and leafy vegetables are good sources of magnesium. Iron-deficiency **anemia** is a problem in many age groups, and researchers fear poor calcium intakes are sowing the seeds for future **osteoporosis,** especially in women.

Water—Vital But Often Ignored

Water is the major component in both foods and the human body: You are composed of about 60% water. Your need for other nutrients, in terms of weight, is much less than your need for water. You can live up to 50 days without food, but only a few days without water.

Water is distributed all over the body, among lean and other tissues and in blood and other body fluids. Water is used in the digestion and absorption of food and is the medium in which most of the chemical reactions take place within the body. Some water-based fluids like blood transport substances around the body, while other fluids serve as lubricants or cushions. Water also helps regulate body temperature.

Water is contained in almost all foods, particularly in liquids, fruits, and vegetables. The foods and fluids you consume provide 80–90% of your daily water intake; the remainder is generated through metabolism. You lose water each day in urine, feces, and sweat and through evaporation from your lungs. To maintain a balance between water consumed and water lost, you need to take in about 1 milliliter of water for each calorie you burn—about 2 liters, or 8 cups, of fluid per day—more if you live in a hot climate or engage in vigorous exercise.

Other Substances in Food

Many substances in food are not essential nutrients but may influence health.

Antioxidants When the body uses oxygen or breaks down certain fats or proteins as a normal part of metabolism, it gives rise to substances called **free radicals.** Environmental factors like cigarette smoke, exhaust fumes, radiation, excessive sunlight, certain drugs, and stress can increase free radical production. A free radical is a chemically unstable molecule that will react with fats, proteins, and DNA, damaging cell membranes and mutating genes. Because of this, free radicals have been implicated in aging, cancer, cardiovascular disease, and other degenerative diseases like arthritis.

Terms

minerals Inorganic compounds needed in relatively small amounts for regulation, growth, and maintenance of body tissues and functions.

anemia A deficiency in the oxygen-carrying material in the red blood cells.

osteoporosis A condition in which the bones become extremely thin and brittle and break easily.

free radical An electron-seeking compound that can react with fats, proteins, and DNA, damaging cell membranes and mutating genes in its search for electrons; produced through chemical reactions in the body and by exposure to environmental factors such as sunlight and tobacco smoke.

phytochemical A naturally occurring substance found in plant foods that may help prevent and treat chronic diseases like cancer and heart disease; *phyto* means plant.

| Table 9-3 | Facts About Selected Minerals |

Mineral	Important Dietary Sources	Major Functions	Signs of Prolonged Deficiency	Toxic Effects of Megadoses
Calcium	Milk and milk products, tofu, fortified orange juice and bread, green leafy vegetables, bones in fish	Maintenance of bones and teeth, control of nerve impulses and muscle contraction	Stunted growth in children, bone mineral loss in adults urinary stone	Constipation, calcium deposits in soft tissues, inhibition of mineral absorption
Fluoride	Fluoride-containing drinking water, tea, marine fish eaten with bones	Maintenance of tooth and bone structure	Higher frequency of tooth decay	Increased bone density, mottling of teeth, impaired kidney function
Iodine	Iodized salt, seafood	Essential part of thyroid hormones, regulation of body metabolism	Goiter (enlarged thyroid), cretinism (birth defect)	Depression of thyroid activity, hyperthyroidism in susceptible people
Iron	Meat, legumes, eggs, enriched flour, dark-green vegetables, dried fruit, liver	Component of hemoglobin, myoglobin, and enzymes	Iron-deficiency anemia, weakness, impaired immune function, gastrointestinal distress	Liver and kidney damage, joint pains, sterility, disruption of cardiac function, death
Magnesium	Widespread in foods and water (except soft water); especially found in grains, legumes, nuts, seeds, green vegetables	Transmission of nerve impulses, energy transfer, activation of many enzymes	Neurological disturbances, cardiovascular problems, kidney disorders, nausea, growth failure in children	Nausea, vomiting, diarrhea, central nervous system depression, coma; death in people with impaired kidney function
Phosphorus	Present in nearly all foods, especially milk, cereal, legumes, meat, poultry, fish	Bone growth and maintenance, energy transfer in cells	Impaired growth, weakness, kidney disorders, cardiorespiratory and nervous system dysfunction	Drop in blood calcium levels, calcium deposits in soft tissues, bone loss
Potassium	Meats, milk, fruits, vegetables, grains, legumes	Nerve function and body water balance	Muscular weakness, nausea, drowsiness, paralysis, confusion, disruption of cardiac rhythm	Cardiac arrest
Selenium	Seafood, meat, eggs, whole grains	Protection of cells from oxidative damage, immune response	Muscle pain and weakness, heart disorders	Hair and nail loss, nausea and vomiting, weakness, irritability
Sodium	Salt, soy sauce, salted foods, tomato juice	Body water balance, acid-base balance, nerve function	Muscle weakness, loss of appetite, nausea, vomiting; deficiency is rarely seen	Edema, hypertension in sensitive people
Zinc	Whole grains, meat, eggs, liver, seafood (especially oysters)	Synthesis of proteins, RNA, and DNA; wound healing; immune response; ability to taste	Growth failure, loss of appetite, impaired taste acuity, skin rash, impaired immune function, poor wound healing	Vomiting, impaired immune function, decline in blood HDL levels, impaired copper absorption

SOURCES: Food and Nutrition Board, National Academy of Sciences. 2001. *Dietary Reference Intakes for Vitamin A, Vitamin K, Arsenic, Boron, Chromium, Copper, Iodine, Iron, Manganese, Molybdenum, Nickel, Silicon, Vanadium, and Zinc.* Washington, D. C.: National Academy Press. Food and Nutrition Board, National Academy of Sciences, 2000. *Dietary Reference Intakes for Vitamin C, Vitamin E, Selenium, and the Carotenoids.* Washington, D.C.: National Academy Press. Food and Nutrition Board, National Academy of Sciences, 1997. *Dietary Reference Intakes for Calcium, Phosphorus, Magnesium, Vitamin D, and Fluoride,* Washington, D.C.: National Academy Press. Shils, M. E., et al., eds. 1998. *Modern Nutrition in Health and Disease,* 9th ed. Baltimore: Williams & Wilkins.

Antioxidants found in foods can help protect the body from damage by free radicals in several ways. Some dietary antioxidants prevent or reduce the formation of free radicals; others remove free radicals from the body by reacting with them directly by donating electrons. Antioxidants can also repair some types of free radical damage after it occurs. Some antioxidants, such as vitamin C, vitamin E, and selenium, are also essential nutrients; others, such as carotenoids, found in yellow, orange, and deep-green vegetables, are not. Many fruits and vegetables are rich in antioxidants.

Phytochemicals Antioxidants are a particular type of **phytochemical,** a substance found in plant foods that may help prevent chronic disease. Researchers have just begun to identify and study all the different compounds found in foods, and many preliminary findings are promising (see Chapter 12). For example, certain substances

Osteoporosis is a condition in which bones become dangerously thin and fragile over time. It currently afflicts over 28 million Americans, 80% of them women, and results in over 1.5 million bone fractures each year. Most bone mass is built by age 18, and after bone density peaks between the ages of 25 and 35, bone mass is slowly lost over time. To prevent osteoporosis, the best strategy is to build as much bone as possible during your young years and then do everything you can to maintain it as you age. Up to 50% of bone loss is determined by controllable lifestyle factors, especially diet and exercise habits. Key nutrients include the following:

Calcium   Consuming an adequate amount of calcium is important throughout life to build and maintain bone mass. Milk, yogurt, and calcium-fortified orange juice, bread, and cereals are all good sources.

Vitamin D   Vitamin D is necessary for bones to absorb calcium; a daily intake of 400–800 IU is recommended by the National Osteoporosis Foundation. Vitamin D can be obtained from foods and is manufactured by the skin when exposed to sunlight. Candidates for vitamin D supplements include people who don't eat many foods rich in vitamin D; those who don't expose their face, arms, and hands to the sun (without sun-

screen) for 5–15 minutes a few times each week; and people who live north of an imaginary line roughly between Boston and the Oregon–California border (the sun is weaker in northern latitudes).

Vitamin K   Vitamin K promotes the synthesis of proteins that help keep bones strong. Broccoli and leafy-green vegetables are rich in vitamin K.

Other Nutrients   Other nutrients that may play an important role in bone health include vitamin C, magnesium, potassium, manganese, zinc, copper, and boron. On the flip side, there are several dietary substances that may have a *negative* effect on bone health, especially if consumed in excess: alcohol, protein, sodium, caffeine, retinol (a form of vitamin A), and soda. For healthy bones, it is important to be moderate in your intake of these compounds.

Finally, it is important to combine a healthy diet with regular exercise. Weight-bearing aerobic activities, if performed regularly, help build and maintain bone mass throughout life. Strength training improves bone density, muscle mass, strength, and balance, protecting against both bone loss and falls, a major cause of fractures.

---

found in soy foods may help lower cholesterol levels. Sulforaphane, a compound isolated from broccoli and other **cruciferous vegetables,** may render some carcinogenic compounds harmless. Allyl sulfides, a group of chemicals found in garlic and onions, appear to boost the activity of cancer-fighting immune cells.

If you want to increase your intake of phytochemicals, eat a variety of fruits, vegetables, and grains rather than relying on supplements. Like many vitamins and minerals, isolated phytochemicals may be harmful if taken in high doses. In addition, it is likely that their health benefits are the result of chemical substances working in combination.

NUTRITIONAL GUIDELINES:
PLANNING YOUR DIET

Various tools have been created by scientific and government groups to help people design healthy diets. The **Dietary Reference Intakes (DRIs)** are standards for nutrient intake designed to prevent nutritional deficiencies and reduce the risk of chronic disease. The **Food Guide Pyramid** translates these nutrient recommendations into a balanced food-group plan that includes all essential nutrients. To provide further guidance, **Dietary Guidelines for Americans** have been established to address the prevention of diet-related chronic diseases.

Dietary Reference Intakes (DRIs)

How much vitamin C, iron, calcium, and other nutrients do you need to stay healthy? The Food and Nutrition Board of the National Academy of Sciences establishes dietary standards, or recommended intake levels, for Americans of all ages. The current set of standards, called Dietary Reference Intakes (DRIs), is relatively new, having been introduced in 1997. An earlier set of standards, called the **Recommended Dietary Allowances (RDAs),** focused on preventing nutritional deficiency diseases such as anemia; the RDAs were established in 1941 and updated periodically, most recently in 1989. The newer DRIs have a broader focus because recent research has looked not just at the prevention of nutrient deficiencies but also at the role of nutrients in promoting optimal health and preventing chronic diseases such as cancer, osteoporosis, and heart disease.

The DRIs include standards for both recommended intakes and maximum safe intakes. The recommended intake of each nutrient is expressed as either a *Recommended Dietary Allowance (RDA)* or *Adequate Intake (AI)*. An AI is set when there is not enough information available to set an RDA value; regardless of the type of standard used, however, the DRI represents the best available estimate of intake for optimal health. The *Tolerable Upper Intake Level (UL)* sets the maximum daily intake by a healthy person that is unlikely to cause health problems. (However, there

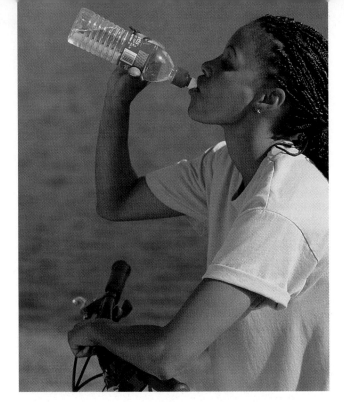

Often overlooked but absolutely crucial to life, water is an essential part of the diet. You need to drink about 8 cups of fluid per day—more if you live in a hot climate or exercise vigorously.

is no established benefit from consuming nutrients at levels above the RDA or AI.)

The DRIs are being issued in stages, and, by early 2001, they had been set for most vitamins and minerals. The DRIs established to date can be found in the Nutrition Resources section at the end of the chapter (pp. 212–215); there you can also find an abridged version of the 1989 RDAs, which includes recommended intakes for nutrients for which DRIs have not yet been set. (For more on updates and additions to the DRIs, visit the Web site of the Food and Nutrition Board; see For More Information at the end of the chapter.)

Should You Take Supplements? The aim of the DRIs is to guide you in meeting your nutritional needs primarily with food, rather than with vitamin and mineral supplements. This goal is important because recommendations have not yet been set for some essential nutrients. Many supplements contain only nutrients with established recommendations, so using them to meet nutrient needs can leave you deficient in other nutrients. Supplements also lack potentially beneficial phytochemicals that are found only in whole foods. Nutrition scientists generally agree that most Americans can obtain most of the vitamins and minerals they need by consuming a varied, nutritionally balanced diet.

The question of whether or not to take supplements is a serious one. Some vitamins and minerals are dangerous when ingested in excess, as shown in Tables 9-2 and 9-3. Large doses of particular nutrients can also cause health problems by affecting the absorption of other vitamins and minerals. For all these reasons, you should think carefully about whether or not to take supplements; consider consulting a physician or registered dietitian.

In setting the DRIs, the Food and Nutrition Board recommended supplements of particular nutrients for the following groups:

- Women who are capable of becoming pregnant should take 400 μg per day of folic acid (the synthetic form of the vitamin folate) from fortified foods and/or supplements in addition to folate from a varied diet. Research indicates that this level of folate intake will reduce the risk of neural tube defects, which occur early in pregnancy. Since 1998, enriched breads, flours, corn meals, rice, noodles, and other grain products have been fortified with small amounts of folic acid. Folate is found naturally in leafy green vegetables, legumes, oranges and orange juice, and strawberries.

- People over age 50 should consume foods fortified with vitamin B-12, B-12 supplements, or a combination of the two in order to meet the majority of the DRI of 2.4 mg of B-12 daily. Up to 30% of people over 50 may have problems absorbing protein-bound B-12 in foods. Vitamin B-12 in supplements and fortified foods is more readily absorbed and can help prevent a deficiency.

Terms

cruciferous vegetables Vegetables of the cabbage family, including cabbage, broccoli, brussels sprouts, kale, and cauliflower; the flower petals of these plants form the shape of a cross, hence the name.

Dietary Reference Intakes (DRIs) An umbrella term for four types of nutrient standards: Adequate Intake (AI), Estimated Average Requirement (EAR), and Recommended Dietary Allowance (RDA) set levels of intake considered adequate to prevent nutrient deficiencies and reduce the risk of chronic disease; Tolerable Upper Intake Level (UL) sets the maximum daily intake that is unlikely to cause health problems.

Food Guide Pyramid A food-group plan that provides practical advice to ensure a balanced intake of the essential nutrients.

Dietary Guidelines for Americans General principles of good nutrition intended to help prevent certain diet-related diseases.

Recommended Dietary Allowances (RDAs) Amounts of certain nutrients considered adequate to prevent deficiencies in most healthy people; will eventually be replaced by the Dietary Reference Intakes (DRIs).

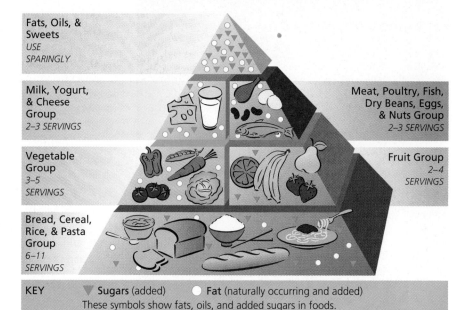

Figure 9-3 The Food Guide Pyramid: a guide to daily food choices. The Pyramid is an outline of what to eat each day—not a rigid prescription, but a general guide that lets you choose a healthful diet that's right for you. It calls for eating a variety of foods to get the nutrients you need and at the same time the right amount of calories to maintain a healthy weight. The Pyramid also focuses on fat because many Americans eat too much fat, especially saturated fat.

SOURCE: U.S. Department of Agriculture, Center for Nutrition Policy and Promotion. 1996. *The Food Guide Pyramid*. Home and Garden Bulletin No. 252.

Fats, Oils, & Sweets *USE SPARINGLY*

Milk, Yogurt, & Cheese Group 2–3 SERVINGS

Meat, Poultry, Fish, Dry Beans, Eggs, & Nuts Group 2–3 SERVINGS

Vegetable Group 3–5 SERVINGS

Fruit Group 2–4 SERVINGS

Bread, Cereal, Rice, & Pasta Group 6–11 SERVINGS

KEY ▼ Sugars (added) ○ Fat (naturally occurring and added) These symbols show fats, oils, and added sugars in foods.

Because of the oxidative stress caused by smoking, the Food and Nutrition Board also recommends that smokers consume 35 mg *more* vitamin C per day than the DRI intake level set for their age and sex (for adults, recommended daily vitamin C intakes for nonsmokers are 90 mg for men and 75 mg for women). However, supplements are not usually needed because this extra vitamin C can easily be obtained from foods. For example, one cup of orange juice has about 100 mg of vitamin C.

Supplements may also be recommended in other cases. Women with heavy menstrual flows may need extra iron to compensate for monthly loss. Some vegetarians may need supplemental calcium, iron, zinc, and vitamin B-12, depending on their food choices. Newborns need a single dose of vitamin K, which must be administered under the direction of a physician. People who consume few calories, who have certain diseases, or who take certain medications may need specific vitamin and mineral supplements; such supplement decisions must be made by a physician because some vitamins and minerals counteract the actions of certain medications.

In deciding whether to take a vitamin and mineral supplement, consider whether you already regularly consume a fortified breakfast cereal. Many breakfast cereals contain almost as many nutrients as a vitamin pill! If you do decide to take a supplement, choose a balanced formulation that contains 50–100% of the Daily Value for

vitamins and minerals. Avoid supplements containing large doses of particular nutrients.

Daily Values Because the DRIs are too cumbersome to use as a basis for food labels, the Food and Drug Administration developed another set of dietary standards, the **Daily Values.** The Daily Values are based on several different sets of guidelines and represent appropriate intake levels for a 2000-calorie diet. The percent Daily Value shown on a food label shows how well that food contributes to your recommended daily intake. Food labels are described in more detail later in the chapter.

The Food Guide Pyramid

The Food Guide Pyramid is a food-group plan developed by the U.S. Department of Agriculture that gives a recommended number of servings for five different major food groups (Figure 9-3). A range of servings is given for each group: The smaller number is for people who consume about 1600 calories a day, such as many sedentary women; the large number for those who consume about 2800 calories a day, such as active men. The fundamental principles of the Food Guide Pyramid are moderation, variety, and balance—a theme echoed throughout this chapter.

It is important to choose a variety of foods within each group because different foods have different combinations of nutrients: for example, within the vegetable group potatoes are high in vitamin C, while spinach is a rich source of vitamin A. Foods also vary in their amount of calories and nutrients, and people who do not need many calories should focus on nutrient-dense foods within each group (foods that are high in nutrients rela-

Terms **Daily Values** A simplified version of the RDAs used on food labels; also included are values for nutrients with no RDA per se.

Studies have shown that most people underestimate the size of their food portions, in many cases by as much as 50%. If you need to retrain your eye, try using measuring cups and spoons and an inexpensive kitchen scale when you eat at home. For quick estimates, use the following equivalents:

- 1 teaspoon of margarine = the tip of your thumb
- 1 ounce of cheese = your thumb, four dice stacked together, or an ice cube
- 3 ounces of chicken or meat = a deck of cards or an audio-cassette tape
- ½ cup of rice or cooked vegetables = an ice cream scoop or one-third of a soda can

- 2 tablespoons of peanut butter = a ping pong ball or large marshmallow
- 1 cup of pasta = a small fist or a tennis ball
- 1 medium potato = a computer mouse
- 1–2 ounce muffin or roll = plum or large egg
- 1-ounce bagel = hockey puck or yo-yo
- 1 medium fruit (apple or orange) = baseball
- ¼ cup nuts = golf ball
- Small cookie or cracker = poker chip

tive to the number of calories they contain). For example, whole-grain bread is more nutrient-dense than white bread, and 100% orange juice is more nutrient-dense than an orange-flavored drink. Many foods you eat contain servings from more than one food group.

Bread, Cereals, Rice, and Pasta (6–11 Servings)
Foods from this group are usually low in fat and rich in complex carbohydrates, dietary fiber (if grains are unrefined), and many vitamins and minerals, including thiamin, riboflavin, iron, niacin, folate, and zinc. Although 6–11 servings may seem like a large amount of food, many people eat several servings at a time. A single serving is the equivalent of the following:

- 1 slice of bread or half of a hamburger bun, English muffin, or bagel
- 1 small roll, biscuit, or muffin
- 1 ounce of ready-to-eat cereal
- ½ cup cooked cereal, rice, or pasta
- 5–6 small or 2–3 large crackers

For maximum nutrition, choose whole-grain breads, high-fiber cereals, whole-wheat pasta, and brown rice.

Vegetables (3–5 Servings)   Vegetables are low in fat and rich in carbohydrates, dietary fiber, vitamin A, vitamin C, folate, magnesium, and other nutrients. A serving of vegetables is equivalent to the following:

- 1 cup raw leafy vegetables
- ½ cup raw or cooked vegetables
- ¾ cup vegetable juice
- ½ cup tomato sauce
- ½ cup cooked dry beans

Good choices from this group include dark-green leafy vegetables such as spinach, chard, and collards; deep-orange and red vegetables such as carrots, winter squash, red bell peppers, and tomatoes; broccoli, cauliflower, and other cruciferous vegetables; peas; green beans; potatoes; and corn. Dry beans (legumes) such as pinto, navy, kidney, and black beans can be counted as servings of vegetables or as alternatives to meat.

Fruits (2–4 Servings)   Like vegetables, fruits are rich in carbohydrates, dietary fiber, and many vitamins, especially vitamin C. The serving sizes used in the Pyramid are as follows:

- 1 medium (apple, banana, peach, orange, pear) or 2 small (apricot, plum) whole fruit(s)
- 1 melon wedge
- ½ cup berries, cherries, or grapes
- ½ grapefruit
- ¼ cup dried fruit
- ½ cup chopped, cooked, canned, or frozen fruit
- ¾ cup fruit juice (100% juice)

Good choices from this group are citrus fruits and juices, melons, pears, apples, bananas, and berries. Choose whole fruits often—they are higher in fiber and ofen lower in calories than fruit juices. Fruit *juices* typically contain more nutrients than fruit *drinks*. For canned fruits, choose those packed in fruit juice or water rather than in syrup.

Milk, Yogurt, and Cheese (2–3 Servings)   Foods from this group are high in protein, carbohydrate, calcium, riboflavin, and vitamin D. To limit the fat in your diet, it is best to choose servings of low-fat or nonfat items from this group:

- 1 cup milk or yogurt
- 1½ ounces cheese
- 2 ounces processed cheese

Cottage cheese is lower in calcium than most other cheeses, and 1 cup of cottage cheese counts as only half a serving for this food group. Ice cream is also lower in calcium than many other dairy products (½ cup is equivalent to ⅓ serving); in addition, it is high in sugar and fat.

Meat, Poultry, Fish, Dry Beans, Eggs, and Nuts (2–3 Servings) This group of foods provides protein, niacin, iron, vitamin B-6, zinc, and thiamin; the animal foods in the group also provide vitamin B-12. The Pyramid recommends 2–3 servings each day of foods from this group. The total amount of these servings should be the equivalent of 5–7 ounces of cooked lean meat, poultry, or fish per day. Many people misjudge what makes up a single serving for this food group:

- 2–3 ounces cooked lean meat, poultry, or fish (an average hamburger or a medium chicken breast half is about 3 ounces; 4 thin slices of bologna, 6 slices of hard salami, or ½ cup of drained canned tuna counts as about 2 ounces)

- The following portions of nonmeat foods are equivalent to 1 ounce of lean meat: ½ cup cooked dry beans (if not counted as a vegetable), 1 egg, 2 tablespoons peanut butter, ⅓ cup nuts, ¼ cup seeds, and ½ cup tofu

One egg at breakfast, a cup of pinto beans at lunch, and a hamburger at dinner would add up to the equivalent of 6 ounces of lean meat for the day. To limit your intake of fat and saturated fat, choose lean cuts of meat and skinless poultry, and watch your serving sizes carefully. Choose at least one serving of plant proteins, such as black beans, lentils, or tofu, every day.

Fats, Oils, and Sweets The tip of the Pyramid includes fats, oils, and sweets—foods such as salad dressings, oils, butter, margarine, gravy, mayonnaise, soft drinks, candy, jellies and jams, syrups and sweet desserts. Foods from the tip of the Pyramid provide calories but few nutrients; they should not replace foods from the other groups. The total amount of fats, oils, and sweets you consume should be determined by your overall energy needs.

The colored triangles and circles in the Pyramid appear in all the other food groups to remind you that food choices in those groups can also be high in fats and added sugars (see Figure 9-3). ("Added sugars" are sugars added to foods in processing or at the table, not the sugars found naturally in fruits and milk.) Overconsumption of fat and added sugars leaves fewer calories available for healthier food choices from the five major food groups. General strategies for controlling intake of fat and added sugars include choosing lower-fat foods within each food group, eating fewer foods that are high in sugar and fat and low

in other nutrients, and limiting the amount of fats and sugars added to foods during cooking or at the table.

COMMUNICATE! Maintaining a healthy diet when eating out may involve making special requests. Many people request that certain items be left off their selections (for example, "I'd like that without the cheese," "I'd like the salad dressing on the side"), ask for substitutions ("Could I have a baked potato instead of the fries?"), request information about menu items ("Do you know if the crab cakes are made with mayonnaise?"), or ask for different preparations ("May I have the halibut broiled instead of fried?"). The next time you're eating out, make sure you're getting the healthiest meal you can. If you feel awkward making such requests, ask your dining partners for their support.

Dietary Guidelines for Americans

To provide further guidance for choosing a healthy diet, the U.S. Department of Agriculture (USDA) and the U.S. Department of Health and Human Services (DHHS) have issued Dietary Guidelines for Americans, most recently in 2000. These guidelines are intended for healthy children ages 2 years and older and adults of all ages. Following these guidelines promotes health and reduces risk for chronic diseases, including heart disease, cancer, diabetes, stroke, and obesity. Ten guidelines are provided, organized under three messages, the "ABCs for Health":

Aim for fitness.

Build a healthy base.

Choose sensibly.

What follows is a brief summary of the guidelines.

Aim for Fitness The two guidelines in this category emphasize that a lifestyle combining sensible eating with regular physical activity promotes long-term health and fitness and enables people to enjoy life and feel their best.

AIM FOR A HEALTHY WEIGHT Evaluate your body weight in terms of body mass index (BMI), a measure of relative body weight that also takes height into account. (See Chapter 11 for instructions on how to determine your BMI.) If your current weight is healthy, aim to avoid weight gain. If you are overweight, first aim to prevent further weight gain, and then lose weight to improve your health. Plan to lose weight gradually—about 10% of your weight over about 6 months—through a combination of sensible eating, physical activity, and behavior change.

BE PHYSICALLY ACTIVE EVERY DAY Become active if you are inactive, and maintain or increase physical activity if you are already active. Aim to accumulate at least 30 minutes (adults) or 60 minutes (children) of moderate physical activity on most days, preferably every day. Moderate physical activity is any activity that requires about as much energy as walking 2 miles in 30 minutes. You can do the activity all at once or spread it out over two to three periods during the day. If you already get 30 minutes of physical activity daily, you can gain even more health benefits by increasing the intensity or duration of your activity. Aerobic activities and activities for strength and flexibility are especially beneficial. (See Chapter 10 for advice on increasing daily physical activity and creating a complete exercise program.)

Build a Healthy Base The four guidelines in this category provide a foundation for healthy eating.

LET THE PYRAMID GUIDE YOUR FOOD CHOICES To ensure that you get all the nutrients you need, choose the recommended number of daily servings from each of the five major food groups shown in the Food Guide Pyramid. Healthy eating patterns start with plant foods, represented in the three groups at the base of the Pyramid: grains, vegetables, and fruits. Plan your meals around a variety of foods from these groups, keeping a close eye on serving sizes. Everyone, especially adolescent girls and women, should take special care to meet their recommended intakes for calcium, iron, and folic acid.

CHOOSE A VARIETY OF GRAINS DAILY, ESPECIALLY WHOLE GRAINS Grains such as wheat, oats, corn, and rice are rich in complex carbohydrates and tend to be low in fat; whole grains provide more fiber and nutrients than refined grains. Make grains the foundation of your diet— eat six or more servings daily. If your calorie needs are low, eat only six servings of a sensible size. Include several servings of whole grains daily, choosing a variety of grains, such as whole wheat, brown rice, oats, and whole corn. Prepare or choose grain products with little added saturated fat and sugar.

EAT A VARIETY OF FRUITS AND VEGETABLES DAILY Different fruits and vegetables are rich in different nutrients, so it's important to choose a variety. For example, carrots, dark-green leafy vegetables, and cantaloupe are excellent sources of carotenoids; citrus fruits, potatoes, and broccoli are rich in vitamin C; spinach, legumes, and orange juice are high in folate; and bananas, winter squash, and dried fruits are good sources of potassium. Fresh fruits and vegetables, especially when eaten with the peel, are also good sources of dietary fiber. Eat at least two servings of fruit and three servings of vegetables daily.

KEEP FOOD SAFE TO EAT Safe foods are those that pose little risk from harmful bacteria, viruses, parasites, or chemical contaminants. It is especially important to be careful with perishable foods such as eggs, meats, poultry, fish, shellfish, milk products, and fresh fruits and vegetables. If food has been left out for too long or refrigerated for too long, it may not be safe to eat even if it looks and

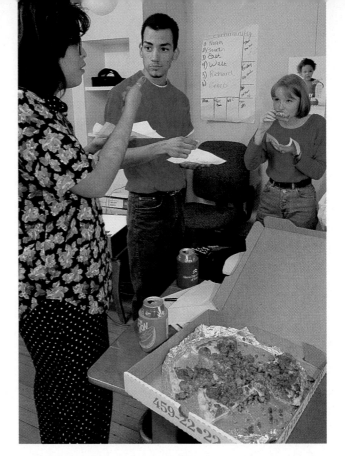

Eating on the run is a common—but not always healthy—habit among college students. After a lunch of pizza and soda, these students should complete their day's diet with a low-fat, nutrient-rich dinner.

smells fine. The CDC estimates that 76 million illnesses, 325,000 hospitalizations, and 5,200 deaths occur each year in the United States due to foodborne illness.

Choose Sensibly The four guidelines in this category help you make food choices that promote health and reduce the risk of certain chronic diseases.

CHOOSE A DIET LOW IN SATURATED FAT AND CHOLESTEROL AND MODERATE IN TOTAL FAT A diet low in saturated fat (less than 10% of daily calories) and cholesterol (less than 300 milligrams per day) helps keep blood cholesterol levels low and reduces the risk of cardiovascular disease. Moderate fat intake (no more than 30% of total calories) also helps with weight control. To control your intake of saturated and total fat, choose lean meat, fish, and poultry and dry beans as protein sources; use nonfat or low-fat dairy products; and limit your consumption of high-fat foods. Choose vegetable oils rather than solid fats like those in meat, butter, and margarine.

Cholesterol is found only in animal foods. To limit your cholesterol intake, follow the Pyramid recommendations for consumption of animal foods, and pay particular attention to serving sizes. In addition, limit your intake of foods that are particularly high in cholesterol, including

- Don't buy food in containers that leak, bulge, or are severely dented. Refrigerated foods should be cold, and frozen foods should be solid.

- Refrigerate perishable items as soon as possible after purchase. Use or freeze fresh meats within 3–5 days and fresh poultry, fish, and ground meat within 1–2 days.

- Store raw meat, poultry, fish, and shellfish in containers in the refrigerator so that the juices don't drip onto other foods. Keep these items away from other foods, surfaces, utensils, or serving dishes to prevent cross-contamination.

- Thaw frozen food in the refrigerator or in the microwave oven, not on the kitchen counter. Cook foods immediately after thawing.

- Thoroughly wash your hands with warm soapy water for 20 seconds before and after handling food, especially raw meat, fish, shellfish, poultry, or eggs.

- Make sure counters, cutting boards, dishes, utensils, and other equipment are thoroughly cleaned before and after use using hot soapy water. Wash dishcloths and kitchen towels frequently.

- If possible, use separate cutting boards for meat, poultry, and seafood and for foods that will be eaten raw, such as fruits and vegetables. Replace cutting boards once they become worn or develop hard-to-clean grooves.

- Thoroughly rinse and scrub fruits and vegetables with a brush, if possible, or peel off the skin.

- Cook foods thoroughly, especially beef, poultry, fish, pork, and eggs. Use a food thermometer to ensure that foods are cooked to a safe temperature. If using a microwave, turn or stir the food to make sure it is heated evenly throughout.

When eating out, order hamburger cooked "well-done" and make sure foods are served piping not.

- Refrigerate foods within 2 hours of purchase or preparation, and within 1 hour if the air temperature is above 90°F. Refrigerate foods at or below 40°F and freeze at or below 0°F. Use refrigerated leftovers within 3–4 days.

- Don't eat raw animal products, including raw eggs in homemade hollandaise sauce or eggnog. Use only pasteurized milk and juice, and look for pasteurized eggs, which are now available in some states.

- Cook eggs until they're firm, and fully cook foods containing eggs. Store eggs in the coldest part of the refrigerator, not in the door, and use them within 3–5 weeks.

- Avoid raw sprouts. Even sprouts grown under clean conditions in the home can be risky. Cook sprouts before eating them.

- According to the USDA, "When in doubt, throw it out." Even if a food looks and smells fine, it may not be safe. If you aren't sure that a food has been prepared, served, and stored safely, don't eat it.

The effects of foodborne illness are usually not serious, although some groups, such as children, pregnant women, and the elderly, are more at risk for severe complications. If you experience symptoms of foodborne illness—diarrhea, vomiting, fever, and weakness—drink plenty of clear fluids to prevent dehydration, and rest to speed recovery. A fever higher than 102°F, blood in the stool, or dehydration deserves a physician's evaluation, especially if the symptoms persist for more than 2–3 days. If you experience neurological symptoms such as double vision, paralysis, or dizziness, consult a physician immediately.

---

egg yolks, dairy fats, and liver and other organ meats. Food labels provide the fat, saturated fat, and cholesterol content of foods.

CHOOSE BEVERAGES AND FOODS TO MODERATE YOUR INTAKE OF SUGARS   Sugar doesn't cause hyperactivity, but it does promote tooth decay. In addition, many foods high in sugar are relatively high in calories but low in other nutrients. The Pyramid recommends no more than about 6 teaspoons (24 g) of added sugars a day if you eat 1600 calories, 12 teaspoons (48 g) at 2200 calories, or 18 teaspoons (72 g) at 2800 calories. Most Americans consume much more than this—one can of regular soda, the leading source of added sugars in the American diet, supplies about 10 teaspoons of sugar. To reduce sugar consumption, cut back on soft drinks, candies, sweet desserts (cakes, cookies, pies), fruit drinks, and other foods high in added sugars. Try drinking water rather than sweetened drinks, and don't let sodas and other sweets crowd out more nutritious foods, such as low-fat milk.

CHOOSE AND PREPARE FOODS WITH LESS SALT   Many people can reduce their chance of developing high blood pressure by consuming less salt. It is recommended that you limit sodium intake to no more than 2400 mg per day, the equivalent of about 1 teaspoon of salt. Salt is found mainly in processed and prepared foods and may also be added during cooking or at the table. To lower your intake of salt, choose fresh or plain frozen meat, poultry, seafood, and vegetables most often; they are lower in salt than more processed forms. Check and compare the sodium content in processed foods; add less salt during cooking and at the table; and limit your use of high-sodium condiments like soy sauce, ketchup, mustard, pickles, and olives. Use lemon juice, herbs, and spices instead of salt to enhance the flavor of foods.

IF YOU DRINK ALCOHOLIC BEVERAGES, DO SO IN MODERATION   Alcoholic beverages supply calories but few nutrients; excess alcohol alters judgement and can lead to dependency and other serious health problems (see

Your overall goal is to limit total fat intake to no more than 30% of total calories. Within that limit, favor unsaturated fats from vegetable oils, nuts, and fish over saturated and trans fats from animal products and foods made with hydrogenated vegetable oils or shortening. Limit saturated fat to less than 10% of total calories.

- Be moderate in your consumption of foods high in fat, including fast food, commercially prepared baked goods and desserts, deep fried foods, meat, poultry, nuts and seeds, and regular dairy products.

- When you do eat high-fat foods, limit your portion sizes, and balance your intake with foods low in fat.

- Choose lean cuts of meat, and trim any visible fat from meat before and after cooking. Remove skin from poultry before or after cooking.

- Drink fat-free or low-fat milk instead of whole milk, and use lower-fat varieties in puddings, soups, and baked products. Substitute plain low-fat yogurt, blender-whipped low-fat cottage cheese, or buttermilk in recipes that call for sour cream.

- To reduce saturated and trans fat, use vegetable oil instead of butter or margarine. Use tub or squeeze margarine instead of stick margarine. Look for margarines that are free of trans fats.

- Season vegetables, seafood, and meats with herbs and spices rather than with creamy sauces, butter, or margarine.

- Try lemon juice on salad, or use a yogurt-based salad dressing instead of mayonnaise or sour cream dressings.

- Steam, boil, bake, or microwave vegetables, or stir-fry them in a small amount of vegetable oil.

- Roast, bake, or broil meat, poultry, or fish so that fat drains away as the food cooks.

- Use a nonstick pan for cooking so that added fat will be unnecessary; use a vegetable spray for frying.

- Chill broths from meat or poultry until the fat becomes solid. Spoon off the fat before using the broth.

- Substitute egg whites for whole eggs when baking; limit the number of egg yolks when scrambling eggs.

- Choose fruits as desserts most often.

- Eat a low-fat vegetarian main dish at least once a week.

Chapter 8). Drinking in moderation is defined as no more than one drink a day for women and no more than two drinks a day for men. People who should not drink at all include individuals who cannot restrict their drinking to moderate levels, women who are or may become pregnant, individuals who plan to drive or operate machinery, and individuals taking medications that can interact with alcohol. If you choose to drink alcoholic beverages, do so sensibly, moderately, and with meals; never drink in situations where it may put you or others at risk.

The Vegetarian Alternative

Some people choose a diet with one essential difference from the diets we've already described—foods of animal origin (meat, poultry, fish, eggs, milk) are eliminated or restricted. Many do so for health reasons; vegetarian diets tend to be lower in saturated fat, cholesterol, and animal protein and higher in complex carbohydrates, dietary fiber, folate, vitamins C and E, carotenoids, and phytochemicals. Some people adopt a vegetarian diet out of concern for the environment, for financial considerations, or for reasons related to ethics or religion.

Types of Vegetarian Diets   There are various vegetarian styles; the wider the variety of the diet eaten, the easier it is to meet nutritional needs. **Vegans** eat only plant foods. **Lacto-vegetarians** eat plant foods and dairy products. **Lacto-ovo-vegetarians** eat plant foods, dairy products, and eggs. According to recent polls, about 5 million American adults never eat meat, poultry, or fish and fall into one of these three groups. Others can be categorized as **partial, semivegetarians,** or **pescovegetarians;** these individuals eat plant foods, dairy products, eggs, and usually a small selection of poultry, fish, and other seafood.

A Food Pyramid for Vegetarians   Several organizations have adapted the USDA Food Guide Pyramid for vegetarian diets; the version shown in Figure 9-4 was created by the American Dietetic Association. At its base are the same three plant-based food groups found on the USDA Pyramid. The basic dairy group is also the same in this vegetarian pyramid; however, vegans and other vege-

---

vegan A vegetarian who eats no animal products at all.

lacto-vegetarian A vegetarian who includes milk and cheese products in the diet.

lacto-ovo-vegetarian A vegetarian who eats no meat, poultry, or fish, but does eat eggs and milk products.

partial, semivegetarian, or **pescovegetarian** A vegetarian who includes eggs, dairy products, and small amounts of poultry and seafood in the diet.

Terms

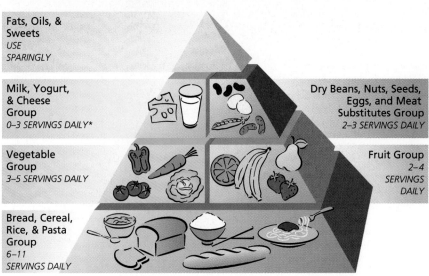

Figure 9-4 Food Guide Pyramid for vegetarian meal planning. A healthy vegetarian diet includes a variety of foods, including whole grains, vegetables, fruits, legumes, nuts, seeds, and, if desired, dairy products and eggs. SOURCE: American Dietetic Association, 1997. Vegetarian diets—Position of ADA. *Journal of the American Dietetic Association* 97: 1317–1321.

Fats, Oils, & Sweets
USE SPARINGLY

Milk, Yogurt, & Cheese Group
*0–3 SERVINGS DAILY**

Dry Beans, Nuts, Seeds, Eggs, and Meat Substitutes Group
2–3 SERVINGS DAILY

Vegetable Group
3–5 SERVINGS DAILY

Fruit Group
2–4 SERVINGS DAILY

Bread, Cereal, Rice, & Pasta Group
6–11 SERVINGS DAILY

*Vegetarians who choose not to use milk, yogurt, or cheese need to select other food sources rich in calcium.

tarians who do not consume any dairy products must find other rich sources of calcium. The Dry Beans, Nuts, Seeds, Eggs, and Meat Substitutes group includes such foods as soy milk, legumes, eggs or egg whites, nuts, seeds, tofu (soybean curd), tempeh (a cultured soy product), and peanut butter. Daily consumption of a variety of plant foods in amounts that meet total energy needs can provide all needed nutrients, although special care (and supplements) may be needed to obtain adequate amounts of vitamin B-12, vitamin D, calcium, iron, and zinc.

Dietary Challenges for Women and Men

The Food Guide Pyramid and Dietary Guidelines for Americans provide a basis that everyone can use to create a healthy diet. However, women and men face special dietary challenges.

Women Women tend to be smaller and weigh less than men, meaning they have lower energy needs and therefore consume fewer calories. Because of this, women have more difficulty getting adequate amounts of all essential nutrients and need to focus on nutrient-dense foods. Low calcium intake may be linked to the development of osteoporosis in later life. Nonfat and low-fat dairy products and fortified cereal, bread, and orange juice are good choices. Iron is also a concern: Menstruating women have higher iron requirements than other groups, and a lack of iron in the diet can lead to iron-deficiency anemia. Lean red meat, green leafy vegetables, and fortified breakfast cereals are good sources of iron. As discussed earlier, all women capable of becoming pregnant should consume adequate folic acid from fortified foods and/or supplements.

Men Men are seldom thought of as having nutritional deficiencies because they generally have high-calorie diets. However, many men have a diet that does not follow the Food Guide Pyramid but that includes more red meat and fewer fruits, vegetables, and grains than recommended. This dietary pattern is linked to heart disease and some types of cancer. A high intake of calories can lead to weight gain in the long term if a man's activity level decreases as he ages. Men should use the Pyramid as a basis for their overall diet and focus on increasing their consumption of fruits, vegetables, and grains to obtain vitamins, minerals, fiber, and phytochemicals.

COMMUNICATE! Fast-food restaurants spend millions of advertising dollars to get you to eat their food. What appeals do you find most memorable and difficult to resist? What subtle messages do the ads send? The next time you see a TV ad for a fast-food restaurant, examine it carefully. What are the verbal and visual messages of the ad and what do they convey? Who do you think is being targeted by the ad? What does the ad suggest about people who eat at the restaurant—in terms of lifestyle or personality characteristics?

WW. A PERSONAL PLAN: MAKING INFORMED CHOICES ABOUT FOOD

Now that you understand the basis of good nutrition and a healthy diet, you can put together a diet that works for you. Focus on the likely causes of any health problems in your life, and make specific dietary changes to address them. You may also have some specific areas of concern, such as interpreting food labels and dietary supplement

General Guidelines

- Eat slowly, and enjoy your food. Set aside a separate time to eat, and don't eat while you study.

- Eat a colorful, varied diet. The more colorful your diet is, the more varied and rich in fruits and vegetables it will be. Many Americans eat few fruits and vegetables, despite the fact that these foods are typically inexpensive, delicious, rich in nutrients, and low in fat and calories.

- Eat breakfast. You'll have more energy in the morning and be less likely to grab an unhealthy snack later on.

- Choose healthy snacks—fruits, vegetables, grains, and cereals—as often as you can.

- Combine physical activity with healthy eating. You'll feel better and have a much lower risk of many chronic diseases. Even a little exercise is better than none.

Eating in the Dining Hall

- Choose a meal plan that includes breakfast, and don't skip it.

- Accept that dining hall food is not going to be as good as home cooking. Find dishes that you like and that are nutritious. Pay attention to portion sizes.

- If menus are posted or distributed, decide what you want to eat before you get in line, and stick to your choices. Consider what you plan to do and eat for the rest of the day before making your choices.

- Ask for large servings of vegetables and small servings of meat and other high-fat main dishes. Build your meals around grains and vegetables.

- Try whole grains like brown rice, whole-wheat bread, and whole-grain cereals.

- Choose leaner poultry, fish, or bean dishes rather than high-fat meats and fried entrees.

- Ask that gravies and sauces to be served on the side; limit your intake.

- Choose broth-based or vegetable soups rather than cream soups.

- At the salad bar, load up on leafy greens, beans, and fresh vegetables. Avoid mayonnaise-coated salads, bacon, croutons, and high-fat dressings. Put dressing on the side, and dip your fork into it rather than pouring it over the salad.

- Drink nonfat milk, water, mineral water, or 100% fruit juice rather than heavily sweetened fruit drinks, whole milk, soft drinks, or beer.

- Choose fruit for dessert rather than pastries, cookies, or cakes.

Eating in Fast-Food Restaurants

- Most fast-food chains can provide a brochure with a nutritional breakdown of the foods on the menu. Ask for it. (See also the information in the Appendix.)

- Order small single burgers with no cheese instead of double burgers with many toppings. If possible, ask for them broiled instead of fried.

- Ask for items to be prepared without mayonnaise, tartar sauce, sour cream, or other high-fat sauces. Ketchup, mustard, and fat-free mayonnaise or sour cream are better choices and are available at many fast-food restaurants.

- Choose whole-grain buns or bread for burgers and sandwiches.

- Choose chicken items made from chicken breast, not processed chicken.

- Order vegetable pizzas.

- If you order french fries or onion rings, get the smallest size, and/or share them with a friend.

Eating on the Run

Are you chronically short of time? The following healthy and filling items can be packed for a quick snack or meal: fresh or dried fruit, fruit juices, raw fresh vegetables like carrots, plain bagels, bread sticks, whole-wheat fig bars, low-fat cheese sticks or cubes, low-fat crackers or granola bars, nonfat or low-fat yogurt, snack-size cereal boxes, pretzels, rice or corn cakes, plain popcorn, soup (if you have access to a microwave), or water.

---

labels, avoiding foodborne illnesses, and understanding food allergies. We turn to these and other topics next.

Reading Food Labels

Consumers can get help in applying the principles of the Food Guide Pyramid and the Dietary Guidelines for Americans from food labels. Since 1994, all processed foods regulated by either the FDA or the USDA have included standardized nutrition information on their labels. Every food label shows serving sizes and the amount of fat, saturated fat, cholesterol, sodium, total carbohydrate, dietary fiber, sugars, and protein in each serving. To make intelligent choices about food, learn to read and understand food labels.

Reading Dietary Supplement Labels

Dietary supplements include vitamins, minerals, amino acids, herbs, glandular extracts, enzymes, and other compounds. Although dietary supplements are often thought to be safe and "natural," they do contain powerful, bioactive chemicals that have the potential for harm. About one-quarter of all pharmaceutical drugs are derived from

Food labels are designed to help consumers make food choices based on the nutrients that are most important to good health. In addition to listing nutrient content by weight, the label puts the information in the context of a daily diet of 2000 calories that includes no more than 65 grams of fat (approximately 30% of total calories). For example, if a serving of a particular product has 13 grams of fat, the label will show that the serving represents 20% of the daily fat allowance. If your daily diet contains fewer or more than 2000 calories, you need to adjust these calculations accordingly (see Table 9-1).

Food labels contain uniform serving sizes. This means that if you look at different brands of salad dressing, for example, you can compare calories and fat content based on the serving amount. Regulations also require that foods meet strict definitions if their packaging includes the terms "light," "lowfat," or "high-fiber" (see below). Health claims such as "good source of dietary fiber" or "low in saturated fat" on packages are signals that those products can wisely be included in your diet. Overall, the food label is an important tool to help you choose a diet that conforms to the Food Guide Pyramid and the Dietary Guidelines.

Selected Nutrient Claims and What They Mean

Healthy A food that is low in fat, low in saturated fat, has no more than 360–480 mg of sodium and 60 mg of cholesterol, *and* provides 10% or more of the Daily Value for vitamin A, vitamin C, protein, calcium, iron, or dietary fiber.

Light or lite One-third fewer calories or 50% less fat than a similar product.

Reduced or fewer At least 25% less of a nutrient than a similar product; can be applied to fat ("reduced fat"), saturated fat, cholesterol, sodium, and calories.

Extra or added 10% or more of the Daily Value per serving when compared to a similar product.

Good source 10–19% of the Daily Value for a particular nutrient.

High, rich in, or excellent source of 20% or more of the Daily Value for a particular nutrient.

Low calorie 40 calories or less per serving.

High fiber 5 g or more of fiber per serving.

Good source of fiber 2.5–4.9 g of fiber per serving.

Fat-free Less than 0.5 g of fat per serving.

Lowfat 3 g of fat or less per serving.

Saturated fat-free Less than 0.5 g of saturated fat and 0.5 g of trans fatty acids per serving.

Low saturated fat 1 g or less of saturated fat per serving and no more than 15% of total calories.

Cholesterol free Less than 2 mg of cholesterol and 2 g or less of saturated fat per serving.

Low cholesterol 20 mg or less of cholesterol and 2 g or less of saturated fat per serving.

Low sodium 140 mg or less of sodium per serving.

Very low sodium 35 mg or less of sodium per serving.

Lean Cooked seafood, meat, or poultry with less than 10 g of fat, 4.5 g or less of saturated fat, and less than 95 mg of cholesterol per serving.

Extra lean Cooked seafood, meat, or poultry with less than 5 g of fat, 2 g of saturated fat, and 95 mg of cholesterol per serving.

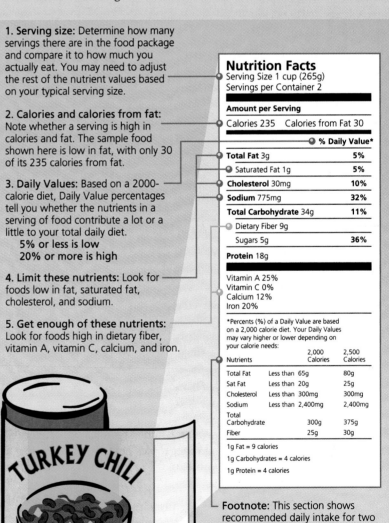

1. Serving size: Determine how many servings there are in the food package and compare it to how much you actually eat. You may need to adjust the rest of the nutrient values based on your typical serving size.

2. Calories and calories from fat: Note whether a serving is high in calories and fat. The sample food shown here is low in fat, with only 30 of its 235 calories from fat.

3. Daily Values: Based on a 2000-calorie diet, Daily Value percentages tell you whether the nutrients in a serving of food contribute a lot or a little to your total daily diet.
   5% or less is low
   20% or more is high

4. Limit these nutrients: Look for foods low in fat, saturated fat, cholesterol, and sodium.

5. Get enough of these nutrients: Look for foods high in dietary fiber, vitamin A, vitamin C, calcium, and iron.

Nutrition Facts
Serving Size 1 cup (265g)
Servings per Container 2

Amount per Serving

Calories 235   Calories from Fat 30

	% Daily Value*
Total Fat 3g	**5%**
Saturated Fat 1g	**5%**
Cholesterol 30mg	**10%**
Sodium 775mg	**32%**
Total Carbohydrate 34g	**11%**
Dietary Fiber 9g	
Sugars 5g	**36%**
Protein 18g	

Vitamin A 25%
Vitamin C 0%
Calcium 12%
Iron 20%

*Percents (%) of a Daily Value are based on a 2,000 calorie diet. Your Daily Values may vary higher or lower depending on your calorie needs:

Nutrients		2,000 Calories	2,500 Calories
Total Fat	Less than	65g	80g
Sat Fat	Less than	20g	25g
Cholesterol	Less than	300mg	300mg
Sodium	Less than	2,400mg	2,400mg
Total Carbohydrate		300g	375g
Fiber		25g	30g

1g Fat = 9 calories

1g Carbohydrates = 4 calories

1g Protein = 4 calories

Footnote: This section shows recommended daily intake for two levels of calorie consumption and values for dietary calculations; it's the same on all labels.

botanical sources, and even essential vitamins and minerals can have toxic effects if consumed in excess.

In the United States, supplements are not legally considered drugs and are not regulated the way drugs are. Before they are approved by the FDA and put on the market, drugs undergo clinical studies to determine safety, effectiveness, side effects and risks, possible interactions with other substances, and appropriate dosages. The FDA does not authorize or test dietary supplements, and supplements are not required to demonstrate either safety or effectiveness prior to marketing. Although dosage guidelines exist for some of the compounds in dietary supplements, dosages for many are not well established.

Although in many ingredients in dietary supplements have been used for centuries in Eastern or European herbal medicine, some have been found to be dangerous to interact with prescription or over-the-counter drugs in dangerous ways. Garlic supplements, for example, can cause bleeding if taken with anticoagulant ("blood thinning") medications. Even products that are generally considered safe can have side effects—St. John's wort, for example, increases the skin's sensitivity to sunlight and may decrease the effectiveness of drugs used to treat HIV infection, oral contraceptives, and other medications.

There are also key differences between how drugs and supplements are manufactured. FDA-approved medications are standardized for potency, and quality control and proof of purity are required. Dietary supplement manufacture is not so closely regulated, and there is no guarantee that a product even contains a given ingredient, let alone in the appropriate amount. The potency of herbal supplements tends to vary widely due to differences in growing and harvesting conditions, preparation methods, and storage. In addition, herbs can be contaminated or misidentified at any stage from harvest to packaging.

With increased consumer knowledge and demand, it is likely that both the research base and the manufacturing standards for dietary supplements will improve. In an effort to provide consumers with more reliable and consistent information about supplements, standard labels similar to those found on foods are required for dietary supplements.

Finally, it is important to remember that dietary supplements are no substitute for a healthy diet. Supplements do not provide all the known—or yet-to-be-discovered—benefits of whole foods. Supplements should also not be used as a replacement for medical treatment for serious illnesses.

Organic Foods

Some people who are concerned about pesticides and other environmental contaminants choose to buy foods that are **organic.** In December 2000, the USDA enacted a new, national standard for organic foods to replace the older system of local, state, and private standards. To be certified as organic, foods must meet strict production,

processing, handling, and labeling criteria. Organic crops must meet limits on pesticide residues; for meat, milk, eggs, and other animal products to be certified organic, animals must be given organic feed and access to the outdoors and may not be given antibiotics or growth hormones. The use of genetic engineering, ionizing radiation, and sewage sludge are prohibited. Products can be labeled "100% organic" if they contain all organic ingredients and "organic" if they contain at least 95% organic ingredients; all such products may carry the new USDA organic seal. A product with at least 70% organic ingredients can be labeled "made with organic ingredients" but cannot use the USDA seal.

Foods that are organic are not chemical-free, however, They may be contaminated with pesticides used on neighboring lands or on foods transported in the same train or truck. However, they do tend to have lower levels of pesticide residues than conventionally grown crops. There are strict pesticide limits for all foods—organic and conventional—and the debate about the potential health effects of long-term exposure to small amounts of pesticide residues is ongoing.

Additives in Food

Today, some 2800 substances are intentionally added to foods for one or more of the following reasons: (1) to maintain or improve nutritional quality, (2) to maintain freshness, (3) to help in processing or preparation, or (4) to alter taste or appearance. Additives make up less than 1% of our food. The most widely used are sugar, salt, and corn syrup; these three, plus citric acid, baking soda, vegetable colors, mustard, and pepper, account for 98% by weight of all food additives used in the United States.

Some additives, such as sulfites and monosodium glutamate (MSG), may be of concern for certain people, because either they are consumed in large quantities or they cause some type of reaction. To protect yourself, eat a variety of foods in moderation. If you have a sensitivity to an additive, check food labels when you shop, and ask questions when you eat out.

Food Irradiation

Food irradiation is the treatment of foods with gamma rays, X rays, or high-voltage electrons to kill potentially

---

organic A designation applied to foods grown and produced according to strict guidelines limiting the use of pesticides, nonorganic ingredients, hormones, antibiotics, genetic engineering, irradiation, and other practices.

food irradiation The treatment of foods with gamma rays, X rays, or high-voltage electrons to kill potentially harmful pathogens and increase shelf life.

Terms

Since 1999, specific types of information have been required on the labels of dietary supplements. In addition to basic information about the product, labels include a "Supplement Facts" panel, modeled after the "Nutrition Facts" panel used on food labels (see the figure). Under the Dietary supplement Health and Education Act (DSHEA) and food labeling laws, supplement labels can make three types of health-related claims.

- *Nutrient-content claims,* such as "high in calcium," "excellent source of vitamin C," or "high potency." The claims "high in" and "excellent source of" mean the same as they do on food labels. A "high potency" single-ingredient supplement must contain 100% of its Daily Value; a "high potency" multi-ingredient product must contain 100% or more of the Daily Value of at least two-thirds of the nutrients present for which Daily Values have been established.

- *Disease claims,* if they have been authorized by the FDA or another authoritative scientific body. The association between adequate calcium intake and lower risk of osteoporosis is an example of an approved disease claim.

- *Structure-function claims,* such as "antioxidants maintain cellular integrity" or "this product enhances energy levels." Because these claims are not reviewed by the FDA, they must carry a disclaimer (see the sample label).

Tips for Choosing and Using Dietary Supplements

- Check with your physician before taking a supplement. Many are not meant for children, elderly people, women who are pregnant or breastfeeding, people with chronic illnesses, or people taking prescription or OTC medications.

- Choose brands made by nationally known food and drug manufacturers or "house brands" from large retail chains.

Due to their size and visibility, such sources are likely to have higher manufacturing standards.

- Look for the *USP* or *NF* designation, indicating that the product meets some minimum safety and purity standard developed by the U.S. Pharmacopeia. (The U.S. Pharmacopeia develops standards for purity and potency for pharmaceutical drugs and has also set standards for vitamins, minerals, and some herbal products.) The designation *NNFA* indicates that the manufacturer has met the National Nutritional Foods Association standards for quality control and cleanliness. Other, smaller association and labs, including ConsumerLab.Com, also test and rate dietary supplements.

- Follow the cautions, instructions for use, and dosage given on the label.

- If you experience side effects, discontinue use of the product and contact your physician. Report any serious reactions to the FDA's MedWatch monitoring program (800-FDA-1088; http://www.fda.gov/medwatch).

For More Information About Dietary Supplements

ConsumerLab.Com: http://www.consumerlab.com

Food and Drug Administration: http:// vm.cfsan.fda.gov/~dms/supplmnt.html

National Institutes of Health, Office of Dietary Supplements: http://dietary-supplements.info.nih.gov

National Nutritional Foods Association: http:// www.nnfa.org

U.S. Department of Agriculture: http:// www.nal.usda.gov/fnic/etext/000015.html

U.S. Pharmacopeia: http:// www.usp.org/dietary

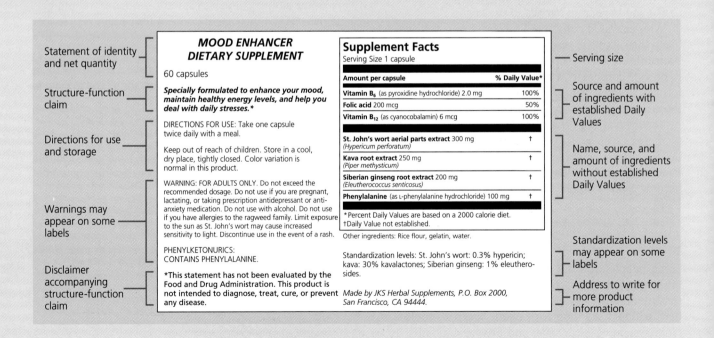

Genetic modification of foods, also frequently referred to as genetic engineering or biotechnology, has become a scientific, economic, and political issue around the world. Genetic engineering involves altering the characteristics of a plant, animal, or microorganism by adding, rearranging, or replacing genes in its DNA; the result is a **genetically modified (GM) organism.** New DNA may come from related species or organisms or from entirely different types of organisms. A number of genetically engineered products are already widely used, including insulin to treat diabetes and the enzyme chymosin to produce cheese. Over half of the current U.S. soybean crop has been genetically modified to be resistant to an herbicide used to kill weeds, and nearly a quarter of the U.S. corn crop carries genes for herbicide resistance or to produce a protein lethal to a destructive type of caterpillar. Products made with GM organisms include juice, soda, nuts, tuna, frozen pizza, spaghetti sauce, canola oil, chips, salad dressing, and soup.

The potential benefits of GM foods cited by supporters include improved yields overall and in difficult growing conditions, increased disease resistance, improved nutritional content, lower prices, and less use of pesticides. For example, scientists have used genetic engineering to develop a new type of rice that is rich in beta-carotene. Introducing this plant in developing countries could reduce the incidence of vitamin A deficiency, a major worldwide health problem that causes a million deaths and over 300,000 cases of blindness among children each year. GM food supporters argue that all crops are genetically modified, either by traditional plant breeding or by newer biotechnology methods. Genetic engineering techniques are more effective than traditional breeding methods because the process is much quicker and more precise.

Critics of biotechnology argue that unexpected effects may occur. Gene manipulation could elevate levels of naturally oc-

curring toxins and allergens or could permanently change the gene pool and reduce biodiversity. Critics also fear that transfer of genes could result in pesticide-resistant insects, herbicide-resistant weeds, and antibiotic-resistant bacteria. In 2000, a form of GM corn approved for use only in animal feed was found to have co-mingled with other varieties of corn and to have been used in human foods; this mistake sparked fears of allergic reactions and led to recalls. Opposition to GM foods is particularly strong in Europe, where many countries are demanding GM-free imports. In many developing nations that face food shortages, responses to genetically engineered crops have tended to be more positive.

Another major concern has been labeling. Under current rules, the FDA requires special labeling only when a food's composition is changed significantly or when a known allergen is introduced. For example, soybeans that contain a gene from a peanut would have to be labeled because peanuts are a common allergen. Surveys indicate that most Americans don't have strong views about the safety of GM foods, but the majority want to know if their foods contain GM ingredients. (Foods labeled as organic do not include GM ingredients.)

In April 2000, the National Academy of Sciences released a report stating that there is no proof that GM food on the market is unsafe but that regulatory changes are needed. The report called for better assessment of potential allergens in GM crops, more research into the spread of pest-resistant genes, and better coordination of regulatory agencies. The FDA is reconsidering how it reviews GM foods, and it may begin requiring new GM foods to undergo a mandatory (rather than the current voluntary) federal safety review. Further testing may help sort out the health and safety issues surrounding GM foods, while increased regulation, labeling, and consumer education may lead to more widespread acceptance of biotechnology.

harmful pathogens, including bacteria, parasites, insects, and fungi that cause foodborne illness. It also reduces spoilage and extends shelf life. Even though irradiation has been generally endorsed by agencies such as the World Health Organization, the Centers for Disease Control and Prevention, and the American Medical Association, few irradiated foods are currently on the market due to consumer resistance and skepticism. Studies haven't conclusively identified any harmful effects of food irradiation, and researchers have found that when consumers are given information about the process of irradiation and the benefits of irradiated foods, most want to purchase them. All primary irradiated foods (meat, vegetables, and so on) are labeled with the flowerlike radura symbol. It is important to remember that although irradiation kills most pathogens, proper handling of irradiated foods is still critical to prevent foodborne illness.

Food Allergies and Food Intolerances

For some people, consuming a particular food causes symptoms such as itchiness, swollen lips, or abdominal pain. Adverse reactions like these may be due either to a food allergy or to a food intolerance, and symptoms may range from annoying to life-threatening.

Food Allergies   A true **food allergy** is a reaction of the body's immune system to a food or food ingredient. This

genetically modified (GM) organism A plant, animal, or microorganism in which genes have been added, rearranged, or replaced through genetic engineering.

food allergy An adverse reaction to a food or food ingredient in which the immune system perceives a particular substance (allergen) as foreign and acts to destroy it.

Terms

immune reaction can occur within minutes of ingesting the food, resulting in symptoms that affect the skin (hives), gastrointestinal tract (cramps or diarrhea), respiratory tract (asthma), or mouth (swelling of the lips or tongue). The most severe response is a systemic reaction called anaphylaxis, which involves a potentially life-threatening drop in blood pressure.

Food allergies affect only about 2% of the adult population and about 4–6% of infants. Although numerous food allergens have been identified, just a few foods account for more than 90% of the food allergies in the United States: cow's milk, eggs, peanuts, tree nuts (walnuts, cashews, and so on), soy, wheat, fish, and shellfish. Individuals with food allergies, especially those prone to anaphylaxis, must diligently avoid trigger foods.

Food Intolerances   Many people who believe they have food allergies may actually suffer from a much more common source of adverse food reactions, a **food intolerance.** In the case of a food intolerance, the problem usually lies with metabolism rather than with the immune system. Lactose intolerance, for example, occurs in people who are deficient in the enzyme lactase, which is needed to digest milk sugar (lactose). A more serious condition is intolerance of gluten, a protein component of some grains; in affected individuals, consumption of gluten damages the lining of the small intestine. Many people with food intolerances can consume small amounts of the food that affects them, and through trial and error, they can adjust their intake of the trigger food to an appropriate level.

If you suspect that you have a food allergy or intolerance, a good first step is to keep a food diary. Note everything you eat or drink, any symptoms you develop, and how long after eating the symptoms appear. Then make an appointment with your physician to go over your diary and determine if any additional tests are needed.

Tips for Today

Eating is one of life's great pleasures. There are many ways to satisfy your nutrient needs, so you can create a healthy diet that takes into account your personal preferences and favorite foods. If your current eating habits are not as healthy as they could be, you can choose equally delicious foods that offer both short-term and long-term health benefits. Opportunities to improve your diet present themselves every day, and small changes add up.

Terms   **food intolerance** An adverse reaction to a food or food ingredient that doesn't involve the immune system; intolerances are often due to a problem with metabolism.

Right now you can

- Substitute a healthy snack—an apple, a banana, or popcorn—for a bag of chips or cookies.
- Drink a glass of water, and put a bottle of water in your backpack for tomorrow.
- For your next serving of grains, choose a whole-grain food—for example, whole-wheat bread, whole-grain pasta, or brown rice.
- Plan to make healthy selections when you go to dinner, such as a baked potato instead of french fries or salmon instead of steak.

SUMMARY

- To function at its best, the human body requires about 45 essential nutrients in specific proportions. People get the nutrients needed to fuel their bodies and maintain tissues and organ systems from foods.
- Proteins, made up of amino acids, form muscles and bones and help make up blood, enzymes, hormones, and cell membranes.
- Fats, a concentrated source of energy, also help insulate the body and cushion the organs. Dietary fat intake should be limited to 30% of total daily calories. Unsaturated fats should be favored over saturated and trans fats.
- Carbohydrates supply energy to the brain and other parts of the nervous system as well as to red blood cells. The body needs 50–100 grams of carbohydrates a day, but much more is recommended.
- Dietary fiber includes plant substances that are difficult or impossible for humans to digest. Insoluble fiber holds water and increases bulk in the stool. Soluble fiber binds cholesterol-containing compounds in the intestine and slows glucose absorption.
- The 13 vitamins needed in the diet are organic substances that promote specific chemical and cell processes within living tissue. Deficiencies or excesses can cause serious illnesses and even death.
- The approximately 17 minerals needed in the diet are inorganic substances that regulate body functions, aid in the growth and maintenance of body tissues, and help in the release of energy from foods.
- Water is used to digest and absorb food, transport substances around the body, lubricate joints and organs, and regulate body temperature.
- Dietary Reference Intakes (DRIs) are recommended intakes for essential nutrients that meet the needs of healthy people.

After reading this chapter and completing the dietary assessment in Wellness Worksheet 9 in the Study Guide, you can probably identify several changes you could make to improve your diet. Here, we focus on choosing healthy beverages to increase intake of nutrients and decrease intake of empty calories from added sugars and fat. However, this model of dietary change can be applied to any modification you'd like to make to your diet.

Gather Data and Establish a Baseline

Begin by tracking your beverage consumption in your health journal. Write down the types and amounts of beverages you drink, including water. Also note where you were at the time and whether you obtained the beverage on site or brought it with you. At the same time, investigate your options. Find out what other beverages you can easily obtain over the course of your daily routine. For example, what drinks are available in the dining hall where you eat lunch or at the student union where you often grab snacks? How many drinking fountains do you walk by over the course of the day? This information will help you put together a successful plan for change.

Analyze Your Data and Set Goals

Evaluate your beverage consumption by dividing your typical daily consumption between healthy and less healthy choices. Use the following guide as a basis, and add other beverages to the lists as needed.

Choose less often:

- Regular soda
- Sweetened bottled iced tea
- Fruit beverages made with little fruit juice (usually labeled fruit drinks, punches, beverages, blends, or ades)
- Whole milk

Choose more often:

- Water—plain, mineral, and sparkling
- Low-fat or nonfat milk
- Fruit juice (100% juice)
- Unsweetened herbal tea

How many beverages do you consume daily from each category? What would be a healthy and realistic goal for change? For example, if your beverage consumption is currently evenly divided between the "choose more often" and "choose less often"

categories (four from each list), you might set a final goal for your behavior change program of increasing your healthy choices by two (six from the "more often" list and two from the "less often" list).

Develop a Plan for Change

Once you've set your goal, you need to develop strategies that will help you choose healthy beverages more often. Consider the following possibilities:

- Keep healthy beverages on hand; if you live in a student dorm, rent a small refrigerator or keep juice, nonfat milk, and other healthy choices in the dorm's kitchen refrigerator.
- Plan ahead, and put a bottle of water or 100% juice in your backpack every day.
- Check food labels on beverages for serving sizes, calories, and nutrients; comparison shop to find the healthiest choices, and watch your serving sizes. Use this information to make your "choose more often" list longer and more specific.
- If you eat out frequently, examine all the beverages available at the places you typically eat your meals. You'll probably find that healthy choices are available; if not, bring along your own drink or find somewhere else to eat.
- For a snack, try water and a piece of fruit rather than a heavily sweetened beverage.
- Create healthy beverages that appeal to you; for example, try adding slices of citrus fruit to water or mixing 100% fruit juice with sparkling water.

You may also need to make some changes in your routine to decrease the likelihood that you'll make unhealthy choices. For example, you might discover from your health journal that you always buy a soda after class when you pass a particular vending machine. If this is the case, try another route that allows you to avoid the machine. And try to guard against impulse buying by carrying water or a healthy snack with you every day.

To complete your plan, try some of the other behavior change strategies described in Chapter 1: Develop and sign a contract, set up a system of rewards, involve other people in your program, and develop strategies for challenging situations. Once your plan is complete, take action. Keep track of your progress in your health journal by continuing to monitor and evaluate your beverage consumption.

- The Food Guide Pyramid contains six food groups; choosing foods from each group every day helps ensure the appropriate amounts of necessary nutrients.
- The Dietary Guidelines for Americans address the prevention of diet-related diseases; they advise us to aim for a healthy weight through diet and physical activity; build a healthy base for our diets by follow-

ing the Pyramid, choosing a variety of plant foods, and handling foods safely; and make sensible food choices that consider intake of fat, sugar, salt, and alcohol.

- Other dietary issues of concern include food and supplement labels, organic foods, food irradiation, and food allergies and intolerances.

1. Read the list of ingredients on three or four canned or packaged foods that you enjoy eating. If any ingredients are unfamiliar to you, find out what they are and why they have been used. A nutrition textbook from the library may be a helpful resource.

2. Investigate the nutritional and dietary guidelines that are used to prepare the food served in your school. Are they consistent with what you've learned in this chapter? If not, try to find out more about the guidelines that have been used and why they were chosen.

3. Prepare a flavorful low-fat vegetarian and/or ethnic meal. (Use the suggestions in the chapter, and check your local library for appropriate cookbooks.) How do the foods included in the meal and the preparation methods differ from what you're used to?

JOURNAL ENTRY

1. In your health journal, keep track of everything you eat and drink for 3–4 days. Calculate the average number of servings from each food group you consume each day. Then see how well your average daily intake meets the guidelines in the Food Guide Pyramid.

2. Put together three sample daily menus that follow the Food Guide Pyramid. Keep the dietary guidelines in mind as you make your food selections from each group. Also, be sure to base your menus on foods you enjoy eating.

3. *Critical Thinking* Analyze patterns of food advertising on television by recording the number and types of ads that appear each hour. If possible, compare the number and types of products advertised during an hour of cartoons or other children's programs, an hour of daytime programs, and an hour of prime-time programs. What patterns do you see? What types of information do the ads present? Are they geared toward different segments of the population? Do they encourage healthy eating?

FOR MORE INFORMATION

Books

American Dietetic Association. 1999. *The Essential Guide to Nutrition and the Foods We Eat: Everything You Need to Know about the Foods You Eat.* New York: HarperCollins. *An excellent review of current nutrition information and issues.*

Insel, P., R. E. Turner, and D. Ross. 2001. *Nutrition.* Sudbury, Mass.: Jones and Bartlett. *A comprehensive review of major concepts in nutrition.*

Selkowitz, A. 2000. *The College Student's Guide to Eating Well on Campus.* Bethesda, Md.: Tulip Hill Press. *Provides practical advice for students, including how to make healthy choices when eating in a dorm or restaurant and how to stock a first pantry.*

Wolfe, F. A. 2000. *The Complete Idiot's Guide to Being a Vegetarian,* 2nd ed. Indianapolis: Macmillan. *Provides information on the health benefits of vegetarian diets and how to plan healthy meals; advice is given for vegetarian diets for special population groups, including children.*

Newsletters

Environmental Nutrition (800-829-5384)

Nutrition Action Health Letter (202-332-9110; http://www.cspinet.org)

Tufts University Health & Nutrition Letter (800-274-7581; http://www.healthletter.tufts.edu)

Organizations, Hotlines, and Web Sites

American Dietetic Association. Provides a wide variety of nutrition-related educational materials.
    800-366-1655
    http://www.eatright.org

American Heart Association. Delicious Decisions. Provides basic information about nutrition, tips for shopping and eating out, and heart-healthy recipes.
    http://www.deliciousdecisions.org

Ask the Dietitian. Questions and answers on many topics relating to nutrition.
    http://www.dietitian.com

CyberDiet. Provides a variety of resources, including a profile that calculates calorie and nutrient needs and a database that provides nutrition information in food label format.
    http://www.CyberDiet.com

FDA Center for Food Safety and Applied Nutrition. Offers information about topics such as food labeling, food additives, dietary supplements, and foodborne illness.
    http://vm.cfsan.fda.gov

Food Safety Hotlines. Provide information on safe purchase, handling, cooking, and storage of food.
    888-SAFEFOOD (FDA)
    800-535-4555 (USDA)

Gateways to Government Nutrition Information. Provide access to government resources relating to nutrition and food safety.

http://www.nutrition.gov

http://www.foodsafety.gov

National Academies' Food and Nutrition Board. Provides information about the Dietary Reference Intakes and related guidelines.

http://www4.nationalacadamies.org/IOM/IOMHome.nsf/Pages/Food+and+Nutrition+Board

National Cancer Institute: *5-A-Day.* Provides tips and recipes to help consumers increase their intake of fruits and vegetables.

http://5aday.nci.nih.gov

Tufts University Nutrition Navigator. Provides descriptions and ratings for many nutrition-related Web pages.

http://navigator.tufts.edu

USDA Center for Nutrition Policy and Promotion. Includes information on the Dietary Guidelines and the Food Guide Pyramid; also provides the Healthy Eating Index, an individualized online assessment of overall dietary quality.

http://www.usda.gov/cnpp

USDA Food and Nutrition Information Center. Provides a variety of materials and extensive links relating to the Dietary Guidelines, food labels, the Food Guide Pyramid, and many other topics.

http://www.nal.usda.gov/fnic

Other USDA Web sites and programs of interest include the *Animal and Plant Health Inspection Service,* which provides information on biotechnology (http://www.aphis.usda.gov/biotechnology); the *Food Safety and Inspection Service,* which provides consumer resources on food safety and irradiation (http://www.fsis.usda.gov); and the *Agricultural Marketing Service,* which provides information on food standards, including the National Organic Program. *Vegetarian Resource Group.* Information and links for vegetarians and people interested in learning more about vegetarian diets.

http://www.diet.vrg.org

You can also obtain recipes at many Web sites; the following are a few of the large, searchable recipe sites:

Nutrition Analysis Tool, University of Illinois, Urbana/Champaign.

http://www.ag.uiuc.edu/~food-lab/nat

USDA Nutrient Data Laboratory

http://www.nal.usda.gov/fnic/foodcomp

See also the resources listed in the dietary supplements box on p. 206 and in the For More Information sections in Chapters 10–12.

SELECTED BIBLIOGRAPHY

American Heart Association Nutrition Committee. 2000. AHA Dietary Guidelines: Revision 2000. *Circulation* 102: 2296–2311.

Bock, S. A., A. Munoz-Furlong, and H. A. Sampson. 2001. Fatalities due to anaphylactic reactions to foods. *Journal of Allergy and Clinical Immunology* 107(1): 191–193.

Booth, S. L., et al. 2000. Dietary vitamin K intakes are associated with hip fractures but not with bone mineral density in elderly men and women. *American Journal of Clinical Nutrition* 71: 1201–1208.

Centers for Disease Control and Prevention. 2001. Diagnosis and management of foodborne illnesses. *MMWR Recommendations and Reports* 50(RR-2).

Food and Drug Administration, Center for Drug Evaluation and Research. 2000. *FDA Public Health Advisory: Risk of Drug Interactions with St. John's Wort and Indinavir and Other Drugs* (http://www.fda.gov/cder/drug/advisory/stjwort.htm; retrieved May 31, 2000).

Food and Drug Administration, Center for Food Safety and Applied Nutrition. 2000. *Guidance on How to Understand and Use the Nutrition Facts Panel on Food Labels* (http://vm.cfsan.fda.gov/~dms/foodlab.html; retrieved July 14, 2000).

Food and Nutrition Board. National Academy of Sciences. 2001. *Dietary Reference Intakes for Vitamin A, Vitamin K, Arsenic, Boron, Chromium, Copper, Iodine, Iron, Manganese, Molybdenum, Nickel, Silicon, Vanadium, and Zinc.* Washington, D.C.: National Academy Press.

French, S. A., et al. 2001. Pricing and promotion effects on low-fat vending snack purchases. *American Journal of Public Health* 91: 112–117.

Fung, T. T., et al. 2001. Association between dietary patterns and plasma biomarkers of obesity and cardiovascular disease risk. *American Journal of Clinical Nutrition* 73: 61–67.

Henkel, J. 2000. Soy: Health claims for soy protein, questions about other compounds. *FDA Consumer,* May/June.

IFT Expert Report on Biotechnology and Foods: Introduction. 2000. *Food Technology* 54(8): 124–136.

Insel, P., R. E. Turner, and D. Ross. 2001. *Nutrition.* Sudbury, Mass.: Jones and Bartlett.

Iso, H., et al. 2001. Intake of fish and omega-3 fatty acids and risk of stroke in women. *Journal of the American Medical Association* 285(3): 304–312.

Jacobs, D. R., H. E. Meyer, and K. Solvoll. 2001. Reduced mortality among whole grain bread eaters in men and women in the Norwegian County Study. *European Journal of Clinical Nutrition* 55(2): 137–143.

Kant, A. K. 2000. Consumption of energy-dense, nutrient-poor foods by adult Americans: Nutritional and health implications. *American Journal of Clinical Nutrition* 72(4): 929–936.

Liu, S., et al. 2000. Whole grain consumption and risk of ischemic stroke in women. *Journal of the American Medical Association* 284(12): 1534–1540.

National Research Council. 2000. *Genetically Modified Pest-Protected Plants: Science and Regulation.* Washington, D.C.: National Academy Press.

Oomen, C. M., et al. 2001. Association between trans fatty acid intake and 10-year risk of coronary heart disease in the Zutphen Elderly Study: A prospective population-based study. *Lancet* 357(9258): 746–751.

Patterson, R. E., et al. 2001. Is there a consumer backlash against the diet and health message? *Journal of the American Dietetic Association* 101(1): 37–41.

Pew Initiative on Food and Biotechnology. 2001. *Public Sentiment About Genetically Modified Food* (http://pewagbiotech.org/research; retrieved April 18, 2001).

Thompson, L. 2000. Are bioengineered foods safe? *FDA Consumer,* January/February.

U.S. Department of Agriculture, Agricultural Marketing Service. 2000. *Organic Foods: Labeling and Marketing Information* (http://www.ams.usda.gov/nop/facts/labeling; retrieved January 8, 2001).

U.S. Department of Agriculture, Food Safety and Inspection Service. 2000. *Irradiation of Raw Meat and Poultry: Questions and Answers* (http://www.fsis.usda.gov/OA/pubs/qa_irrad.htm; retrieved October 23, 2000).

U.S. Department of Agriculture, National Agricultural Statistics Service. 2000. *Acreage, June 2000* (http://usda.mannlib.cornell.edu/reports/nassr/field/pcp-bba/acrg0600.txt; retrieved October 24, 2000).

U.S. Department of Agriculture and U.S. Department of Health and Human Services. 2000. *Nutrition and Your Health: Dietary Guidelines for Americans,* 5th ed. Home and Garden Bulletin No. 232.

Wyshak, G. 2000. Teenaged girls, carbonated beverage consumption, and bone fracture. *Archives of Pediatric and Adolescent Medicine* 154: 610–613.

Table 1   Dietary Reference Intakes (DRIs): Recommended Levels for Individual Intake

Life Stage	Group	Calcium (mg/day)	Phosphorus (mg/day)	Magnesium (mg/day)	Vitamin D (µg/day)[a,b]	Fluoride (mg/day)	Thiamin (mg/day)	Riboflavin (mg/day)	Niacin (mg/day)[c]	Vitamin B-6 (mg/day)	Folate (µg/day)[d]	Vitamin B-12 (µg/day)	Pantothenic Acid (mg/day)	Biotin (µg/day)
Infants	0–5 months	210	100	30	5	0.01	0.2	0.3	2	0.1	65	0.4	1.7	5
	6–11 months	270	275	75	5	0.5	0.3	0.4	3	0.3	80	0.5	1.8	6
Children	1–3 years	500	460	80	5	0.7	0.5	0.5	6	0.5	150	0.9	2	8
	4–8 years	800	500	130	5	1	0.6	0.6	8	0.6	200	1.2	3	12
Males	9–13 years	1300	1250	240	5	2	0.9	0.9	12	1.0	300	1.8	4	20
	14–18 years	1300	1250	410	5	3	1.2	1.3	16	1.3	400	2.4	5	25
	19–30 years	1000	700	400	5	4	1.2	1.3	16	1.3	400	2.4	5	30
	31–50 years	1000	700	420	5	4	1.2	1.3	16	1.3	400	2.4	5	30
	51–70 years	1200	700	420	10	4	1.2	1.3	16	1.7	400	2.4[e]	5	30
	>70 years	1200	700	420	15	4	1.2	1.3	16	1.7	400	2.4[e]	5	30
Females	9–13 years	1300	1250	240	5	2	0.9	0.9	12	1.0	300	1.8	4	20
	14–18 years	1300	1250	360	5	3	1.0	1.0	14	1.2	400[f]	2.4	5	25
	19–30 years	1000	700	310	5	3	1.1	1.1	14	1.3	400[f]	2.4	5	30
	31–50 years	1000	700	320	5	3	1.1	1.1	14	1.3	400[f]	2.4	5	30
	51–70 years	1200	700	320	10	3	1.1	1.1	14	1.5	400	2.4[e]	5	30
	>70 years	1200	700	320	15	3	1.1	1.1	14	1.5	400	2.4[e]	5	30
Pregnancy	≤18 years	1300	1250	400	5	3	1.4	1.4	18	1.9	600[g]	2.6	6	30
	19–30 years	1000	700	350	5	3	1.4	1.4	18	1.9	600[g]	2.6	6	30
	31–50 years	1000	700	360	5	3	1.4	1.4	18	1.9	600[g]	2.6	6	30
Lactation	≤18 years	1300	1250	360	5	3	1.5	1.6	17	2.0	500	2.8	7	35
	19–30 years	1000	700	310	5	3	1.5	1.6	17	2.0	500	2.8	7	35
	31–50 years	1000	700	320	5	3	1.5	1.6	17	2.0	500	2.8	7	35

NOTE: This table includes Dietary Reference Intakes for those nutrients for which DRIs had been set through June 2001. The table includes values for the type of DRI standard—Adequate Intake (AI) or Recommended Dietary Allowance (RDA)—that has been established for that particular nutrient and life stage. RDAs are shown in **bold type.**

[a]As cholecalciferol. 1 µg cholecalciferol = 40 IU vitamin D.

[b]In the absence of adequate exposure to sunlight.

[c]As niacin equivalents. 1 mg of niacin = 60 mg of tryptophan.

[d]As dietary folate equivalents (DFE). 1 DFE = 1 µg food folate = 0.6 µg of folic acid (from fortified food or supplement) consumed with food = 0.5 µg of synthetic (supplemental) folic acid taken on an empty stomach.

[e]Because 10–30% of older people may malabsorb food-bound B-12, it is advisable for those older than 50 years to meet their RDA mainly by consuming foods fortified with B-12 or a B-12-containing supplement.

[f]In view of evidence linking folate intake with neural tube defects in the fetus, it is recommended that all women capable of becoming pregnant consume 400 µg of synthetic folic acid from fortified food and/or supplements in addition to intake of food folate from a varied diet.

[g]It is assumed that women will continue consuming 400 µg of folic acid until their pregnancy is confirmed and they enter prenatal care, which ordinarily occurs after the end of the periconceptional period—the critical time for formation of the neural tube.

Table 1 Dietary Reference Intakes (DRIs): Recommended Levels for Individual Intake (Continued)

Life Stage	Group	Choline (mg/day)[h]	Vitamin C (mg/day)	Vitamin E (mg/day)[i]	Selenium (μg/day)	Vitamin A (μg/day)[j]	Vitamin K (μg/day)	Chromium (μg/day)	Copper (μg/day)	Iodine (μg/day)	Iron (mg/day)[k]	Manganese (mg/day)	Molybdenum (μg/day)	Zinc (mg/day)[l]
Infants	0–5 months	125	40	4	15	400	2.0	0.2	200	110	0.27	0.003	2	2
	6–11 months	150	50	6	20	500	2.5	5.5	220	130	11	0.6	3	3
Children	1–3 years	200	15	6	20	300	30	11	340	90	7	1.2	17	3
	4–8 years	250	25	7	30	400	55	15	440	90	10	1.5	22	5
Males	9–13 years	375	45	11	40	600	60	25	700	120	8	1.9	34	8
	14–18 years	550	75[m]	15	55	900	75	35	890	150	11	2.2	43	11
	19–30 years	550	90[m]	15	55	900	120	35	900	150	8	2.3	45	11
	31–50 years	550	90[m]	15	55	900	120	35	900	150	8	2.3	45	11
	51–70 years	550	90[m]	15	55	900	120	30	900	150	8	2.3	45	11
	>70 years	550	90[m]	15	55	900	120	30	900	150	8	2.3	45	11
Females	9–13 years	375	45	11	40	600	60	21	700	120	8	1.6	34	8
	14–18 years	400	65[m]	15	55	700	75	24	890	150	15	1.6	43	9
	19–30 years	425	75[m]	15	55	700	90	25	900	150	18	1.8	45	8
	31–50 years	425	75[m]	15	55	700	90	25	900	150	18	1.8	45	8
	51–70 years	425	75[m]	15	55	700	90	20	900	150	8	1.8	45	8
	>70 years	425	75[m]	15	55	700	90	20	900	150	8	1.8	45	8
Pregnancy	≤18 years	450	80	15	60	750	75	29	1000	220	27	2.0	50	13
	19–30 years	450	85	15	60	770	90	30	1000	220	27	2.0	50	11
	31–50 years	450	85	15	60	770	90	30	1000	220	27	2.0	50	11
Lactation	≤18 years	550	115	19	70	1200	75	44	1300	290	10	2.6	50	14
	19–30 years	550	120	19	70	1300	90	45	1300	290	9	2.6	50	12
	31–50 years	550	120	19	70	1300	90	45	1300	290	9	2.6	50	12

[h]Although AIs have been set for choline, there are few data to assess whether a dietary supply of choline is needed at all stages of the life cycle, and it may be that the choline requirement can be met by endogenous synthesis at some of these stages.

[i]As α-Tocopherol.

[j]As retinol activity equivalents (RAE): 1 RAE = 1 μg retinol = 12 μg β-carotene = 24 μg of other provitamin A carotenoids. Preformed vitamin A (retinol) is abundant in animal-derived foods; provitamin A carotenoids are abundant in some dark-yellow, orange, red, and deep-green fruits and vegetables.

[k]Because the absorption of iron from plant foods is low compared to that from animal foods, the RDA for strict vegetarians is approximately 1.8 times higher than the values established for omnivores (14 mg/day for adult male vegetarians; 33 mg/day for premenopausal female vegetarians). Oral contraceptives (OCs) reduce menstrual blood losses, so women taking them need less daily iron; the RDA for premenopausal women taking OCs is 10.9 mg/day. For more on iron requirements for other special situations, refer to *Dietary Reference Intakes for Vitamin A, Vitamin K, Arsenic, Boron, Chromium, Copper, Iodine, Iron, Manganese, Molybdenum, Nickel, Silicon, Vanadium, and Zinc.*

[l]Vegetarians may need up to 50% more zinc because a chemical in plants (phytate) hinders zinc absorption in the body.

SOURCES: Food and Nutrition Board, National Academy of Sciences. 2000. *Dietary Reference Intakes for Vitamin C, Vitamin E, Selenium, and Carotenoids.* Washington, D.C.: National Academy Press. Food and Nutrition Board, National Academy of Sciences. 2001. *Dietary Reference Intakes for Vitamin A, Vitamin K, Arsenic, Boron, Chromium, Copper, Iodine, Iron, Manganese, Molybdenum, Nickel, Silicon, Vanadium, and Zinc.* Washington, D.C.: National Academy Press. Reprinted with permission from National Academy of Sciences. Copyright © 1998 by the National Academy of Sciences.

Table 2	Tolerable Nutrient Upper Intake Levels for Adults

Nutrient	Upper Intake Level
Calcium	2,500 mg/day
Phosphorus	4,000 mg/day
Magnesium (nonfood sources)	350 mg/day
Vitamin D	50 µg/day
Fluoride	10 mg/day
Niacin	35 mg/day
Vitamin B-6	100 mg/day
Folate	1,000 µg/day
Choline	3,500 mg/day
Vitamin C	2,000 mg/day
Vitamin E	1,000 mg/day
Selenium	400 µg/day
Vitamin A	3,000 µg/day
Boron	20 mg/day
Copper	10,000 µg/day
Iodine	1,100 µg/day
Iron	45 mg/day
Manganese	11 mg/day
Molybdenum	2,000 µg/day
Nickel	1.0 mg/day
Vanadium	1.8 mg/day
Zinc	40 mg/day

This table includes the adult Tolerable Upper Intake Level (UL) standard of the Dietary Reference Intakes (DRIs). For some nutrients, there is insufficient data on which to develop a UL. This does not mean that there is no potential for adverse effects from high intake, and when data about adverse effects are limited, extra caution may be warranted. In healthy individuals, there is no established benefit from nutrient intakes above the RDA or AI.

SOURCES: Food and Nutrition Board, National Academy of Sciences. 1997. *Dietary Reference Intakes for Calcium, Phosphorus, Magnesium, Vitamin D, and Fluoride.* Washington, D.C.: National Academy Press. Food and Nutrition Board, National Academy of Sciences. 1998. *Dietary Reference Intakes for Thiamin, Riboflavin, Niacin, Vitamin B6, Folate, Vitamin B12, Pantothenic Acid, Biotin, and Choline.* Washington, D.C.: National Academy Press. Food and Nutrition Board, National Academy of Sciences. 2000. *Dietary Reference Intakes for Vitamin C, Vitamin E, Selenium, and Carotenoids.* Washington, D.C.: National Academy Press. Food and Nutrition Board, National Academy of Sciences. 2001. *Dietary Reference Intakes for Vitamin A, Vitamin K, Arsenic, Boron, Chromium, Copper, Iodine, Iron, Manganese, Molybdenum, Nickel, Silicon, Vanadium, and Zinc.* Washington, D.C.: National Academy Press. Copyright © 1998 by the National Academy of Sciences. Reprinted with permission from National Academy Press, Washington, D.C.

Table 3	Recommended Dietary Allowances, Revised 1989[a,b] (Abridged)

Category	Age (Years) or Condition	Protein (g/kg)[c]
Infants	0.0–0.5	2.2
	0.5–1.0	1.6
Children	1–3	1.2
	4–6	1.1
	7–10	1.0
Males	11–14	1.0
	15–18	0.9
	19–24	0.8
	25–50	0.8
	51+	0.8
Females	11–14	1.0
	15–18	0.8
	19–24	0.8
	25–50	0.8
	51+	0.8
Pregnant		+10g
Lactating	1st 6 Months	+15g
	2nd 6 Months	+12g

[a]This table includes RDAs for those nutrients for which DRIs had not yet been established as of June 2001. The allowances, expressed as average daily intakes over time, are intended to provide for individual variations among most normal people as they live in the United States under usual environmental stresses. Diet should be based on a variety of common foods in order to provide other nutrients for which human requirements have been less well defined.
[b]Estimated Minimum Requirements of healthy adults: 500 mg sodium; 750 mg chloride; 2000 mg potassium. (For information on other age groups, see *Recommended Dietary Allowances,* 10th ed.)
[c]The RDA for protein is expressed as grams of protein per kilogram of body weight. To calculate the RDA, multiply body weight in kilograms (1 kilogram = 2.2 pounds) by the appropriate number from the protein column. For example, a 19-year-old male who weighs 165 pounds would calculate his protein RDA as follows: 165 lb ÷ 2.2 kg/lb = 75 kg × 0.8 g/kg (from table) = 60 g protein per day. For pregnant or lactating women, calculate RDA based on age and then add the appropriate number of additional grams listed in the table.

SOURCE: Reprinted with permission from *Recommended Dietary Allowances:* 10th Edition. Copyright © 1989 by the National Academy of Sciences. Courtesy of the National Academy Press, Washington, D.C.

		Calorie Level		
		1600	2200	2800
Breakfast	Cantaloupe	¼ medium	¼ medium	¼ medium
	Whole-wheat pancakes	2	2	3
	Blueberry sauce	¼ cup	¼ cup	6 tablespoons
	Margarine		1 teaspoon	2 teaspoons
	Turkey patty		1½ ounces	1½ ounces
	Milk	skim, 1 cup	skim, 1 cup	2%, 1 cup
Lunch	Chili-stuffed baked potato	¾ cup chili, 1 potato	¾ cup chili, 1 potato	¾ cup chili, 1 potato
	Low-fat, low-sodium cheddar cheese		3 tablespoons	3 tablespoons
	Spinach-orange salad	1 cup	1 cup	1 cup
	Wheat crackers	6	6	6
	Grapes			12
	Fig bars			2
	Milk		skim, 1 cup	2%, 1 cup
Dinner	Apricot-glazed chicken	1 breast half	1 breast half	1 breast half
	Rice-pasta pilaf	¾ cup	¾ cup	¾ cup
	Steamed zucchini			½ cup
	Tossed salad	1 cup	1 cup	1 cup
	Reduced-calorie Italian dressing	1 tablespoon	1 tablespoon	
	Regular Italian dressing			1 tablespoon
	Hard roll(s)	1 small	2 small	2 small
	Margarine		2 teaspoons	2 teaspoons
	Vanilla ice milk	½ cup	½ cup	½ cup
Snacks	Fig bar	1		
	Skim milk	¾ cup		
	Apple		½ medium	½ medium
	Soft pretzel		1 large	1 large
	Lemonade			1 cup
	2% fat milk			1 cup
Number of Servings	Bread group	6	9	11
	Vegetable group	4¼	4¼	5¼
	Fruit group	2⅓	2¾	4
	Milk group	2	2⅔	3⅔
	Meat group (ounces)	5½	7	7
Nutrient Data	Calories	1,665	2,199	2,859
	Fat*, grams (percent calories)	38 (20%)	59 (24%)	87 (27%)
	Saturated fat*, grams (percent calories)	11 (6%)	17 (7%)	27 (8%)
	Cholesterol, mg	183	236	309
	Sodium, mg	1861	3138	3508
	Dietary fiber, g	23	25	31

*Values have been rounded to the nearest whole number.

SOURCE: Shaw, A., et al. 1997. *Using the Food Guide Pyramid: A Resource for Health Educators.* Washington, D.C.: U.S. Department of Agriculture.

Exercise for Health and Fitness

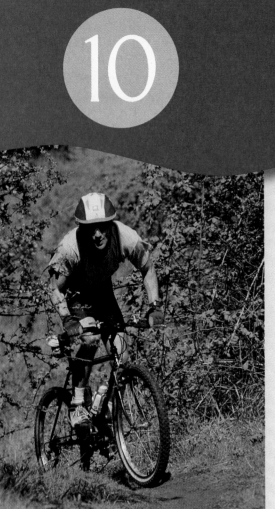

LOOKING AHEAD

After reading this chapter, you should be able to

- Define physical fitness and list the health-related components of fitness
- Explain the wellness benefits of physical activity and exercise
- Describe how to develop each of the health-related components of fitness
- Discuss how to choose appropriate exercise equipment, how to eat and drink for exercise, how to assess fitness, and how to prevent and manage injuries
- Put together a personalized exercise program that you enjoy and that will enable you to achieve your fitness goals

Your body is a wonderful moving machine. Your bones, joints, and ligaments provide a support system for movement; your muscles perform the motions of work and play; your heart and lungs nourish your cells as you move through your daily life. But your body is made to work best when it is physically active. It readily adapts to practically any level of activity and exercise: The more you ask of your body—your muscles, bones, heart, lungs —the stronger and more fit it becomes. The opposite is also true. Left unchallenged, bones lose their density, joints stiffen, muscles become weak, and cellular energy systems begin to degenerate. To be truly healthy, human beings must be active.

The benefits of physical activity are both physical and mental, immediate and far-reaching. Being physically fit makes it easier to do everyday tasks, such as lifting; it provides reserve strength for emergencies; and it helps people to look and feel good. Over the long term, physically fit individuals are less likely to develop heart disease, cancer, high blood pressure, diabetes, and many other de-

generative diseases. Their cardiorespiratory systems tend to resemble those of people 10 or more years younger than themselves. As they get older, they may be able to avoid weight gain, muscle and bone loss, fatigue, memory loss, and other problems associated with aging. With a healthy heart, strong muscles, a lean body, and a repertoire of physical skills they can call on for recreation and enjoyment, fit people can maintain their physical and mental well-being throughout their entire lives.

Unfortunately, modern life for most Americans provides few built-in occasions for vigorous activity. Technological advances have made our lives increasingly sedentary. According to *Healthy People 2010,* levels of physical activity remain low for all populations of Americans. In 1996, the U.S. Surgeon General published *Physical Activity and Health,* a report designed to reverse these trends and get Americans moving. The report's conclusions include the following:

- People of all ages, both male and female, benefit from regular physical activity.

- People can obtain significant health benefits by including a moderate amount of physical activity on most, if not all, days of the week.
- Additional health benefits can be gained through greater amounts of physical activity. People who can maintain a regular regimen of more vigorous or longer-duration activity are likely to obtain even greater benefits.
- Physical activity reduces the risk of premature mortality, improves psychological health, and is important for the health of muscle, bones, and joints.

Are you one of the 60% of Americans who are not regularly active? Or one of the 25% who are not active at all? This chapter will give you the basic information you need to put together a physical fitness program that will add fun and joy to your life and provide the foundation for a lifetime of fitness.

WHAT IS PHYSICAL FITNESS?

Physical fitness is a set of physical attributes that allows the body to respond or adapt to the demands and stress of physical effort—that is, to perform moderate-to-vigorous levels of physical activity without becoming overly tired. Physical fitness has many components, some related to general health and others related to particular sports or activities. The five components of fitness most important for health are cardiorespiratory endurance, muscular strength, muscular endurance, flexibility, and body composition (proportion of fat to fat-free mass).

Cardiorespiratory Endurance

Cardiorespiratory endurance is the ability to perform prolonged, large-muscle, dynamic exercise at moderate-to-high levels of intensity. When levels of cardiorespiratory fitness are low, the heart has to work very hard during normal daily activities and may not be able to work hard enough to sustain high-intensity physical activity in an emergency. As cardiorespiratory fitness improves, the heart begins to function more efficiently. It doesn't have to work as hard at rest or during low levels of exercise. The heart pumps more blood per heartbeat, resting heart rate slows down, blood volume increases, blood supply to the tissues improves, and resting blood pressure decreases. A healthy heart can better withstand the strains of everyday life, the stress of occasional emergencies, and the wear and tear of time.

Cardiorespiratory endurance is considered a critically important component of health-related fitness because the functioning of the heart and lungs is so essential to overall wellness. A person simply cannot live very long or very well without a healthy heart. Low levels of cardiorespiratory fitness are linked with heart disease, the leading

cause of death among Americans. Cardiorespiratory endurance is developed by activities that involve continuous rhythmic movements of large-muscle groups like those in the legs—for example, walking, cycling, and aerobic dance.

Muscular Strength

Muscular strength is the amount of force a muscle can produce with a single maximum effort. Strong, powerful muscles are important for the smooth and easy performance of everyday activities, such as climbing stairs, as well as for emergency situations. They help keep the skeleton in proper alignment, preventing back and leg pain and providing the support necessary for good posture. Muscular strength has obvious importance in recreational activities. Strong people can hit a tennis ball harder, kick a soccer ball farther, and are able to ride a bicycle uphill more easily.

Muscle tissue is an important element of overall body composition. Greater muscle mass makes possible a higher rate of metabolism and faster energy use, which help to maintain a healthy body weight. Strength training has also been shown to benefit cardiovascular health. Muscular strength can be developed by training with weights or by using the weight of the body for resistance during calisthenic exercises such as push-ups and sit-ups.

Muscular Endurance

Muscular endurance is the ability to sustain a given level of muscle tension—that is, to hold a muscle contraction for a long period of time, or to contract a muscle over and over again. Muscular endurance is important for good posture and for injury prevention. It helps people cope with the physical demands of everyday life and enhances performance in sports and work. Like muscular strength, muscular endurance is developed by stressing the muscles with a greater load (weight) than they are used to. The degree to which strength or endurance develops depends on the type and amount of stress that is applied.

physical fitness A set of physical attributes that allows the body to respond or adapt to the demands and stress of physical effort.

cardiorespiratory endurance The ability of the body to perform prolonged, large-muscle, dynamic exercise at moderate-to-high levels of intensity.

muscular strength The amount of force a muscle can produce with a single maximum effort.

muscular endurance The ability of a muscle or group of muscles to remain contracted or to contract repeatedly for a long period of time.

Terms

Flexibility

Flexibility is the ability to move the joints through their full range of motion. Although range of motion is not a significant factor in everyday activities for most people, inactivity causes the joints to become stiffer with age. Stiffness often causes older people to assume unnatural body postures, and it can lead to back, shoulder, or neck pain. The majority of Americans experience low-back pain at some time in their lives. Stretching exercises can help ensure a normal range of motion.

Body Composition

Body composition refers to the proportion of fat and fat-free mass (muscle, bone, and water) in the body. Healthy body composition involves a high proportion of fat-free mass and an acceptably low level of body fat. A person with excessive body fat is more likely to experience a variety of health problems, including heart disease, high blood pressure, stroke, joint problems, diabetes, gallbladder disease, cancer, and back pain. The best way to lose fat is through a lifestyle that includes a sensible diet and exercise. The best way to add muscle mass is through resistance training such as weight training.

COMMUNICATE! Do you want to exercise more but find you just can't fit it into your day? Listen carefully to what you're telling yourself, perhaps by writing down your "self-talk" about exercise for a few days. Are you rationalizing, making excuses, or procrastinating? For example, "I'm too busy with my classes this semester to fit exercise into my schedule," or "Right now I want to spend all my free time with my new girlfriend/boyfriend," or "I'll try to start running once the weather gets warmer." Can you think of ways to counter these statements and change your exercise habits? For example, "I see a lot of other busy people who are exercising, and I can probably do it too"; "I could ask my girlfriend/boyfriend to go for a hike in the hills with me"; "I can use the exercise equipment at the gym until the weather warms up." Remember that when you rationalize and make excuses, the only one who loses is you.

THE BENEFITS OF EXERCISE

As mentioned above, the greater the demands made on the body, the more fit it becomes. Over time, immediate,

short-term adjustments translate into long-term changes and improvements (Figure 10-1). For example, when breathing and heart rate increase during exercise, the heart gradually develops the ability to pump more blood with each beat. Then, during exercise, it doesn't have to beat as fast to meet the body's demand for oxygen.

Exercise is one of the most important things you can do to improve your level of wellness. Regular exercise increases energy levels, improves emotional and psychological well-being, boosts the immune system, and prevents many kinds of diseases. At any age, people who exercise are less likely to die from all causes than their sedentary peers.

Improved Cardiorespiratory Functioning

During exercise, the cardiorespiratory system (heart, lungs, and circulatory system) must work harder to meet the body's increased demand for oxygen. Regular endurance exercise improves the functioning of the heart and the ability of the cardiorespiratory system to carry oxygen to body tissues.

More Efficient Metabolism

Endurance exercise improves metabolism, the process by which food is converted to energy and tissue is built. A physically fit person is better able to generate energy, to use carbohydrates and fats for energy, and to regulate hormones. Physical training may also protect the body's cells from damage from free radicals, which are produced during normal metabolism (see Chapter 9).

Improved Body Composition

Exercise can improve body composition in several ways. Endurance exercise significantly increases daily calorie expenditure; it can also slightly raise *metabolic rate,* the rate at which the body burns calories, for several hours after an exercise session. Strength training increases muscle mass, thereby tipping the body composition ratio toward fat-free mass and away from fat. It can also help with losing fat because metabolic rate is directly proportional to fat-free mass: The more muscle mass, the higher the metabolic rate.

Disease Prevention and Management

Regular physical activity lowers your risk of many chronic, disabling diseases. It can also help people with those diseases improve their health.

Cardiovascular Disease A sedentary lifestyle is one of the six major risk factors for **cardiovascular disease (CVD)** (see Chapter 12). People who are sedentary have CVD death rates significantly higher than those of fit individuals. There is a dose-response relationship between exercise and CVD: The benefit of physical activity occurs at moderate levels of activity and increases with increas-

---

Terms

flexibility The range of motion in a joint or group of joints; flexibility is related to muscle length.

body composition The proportion of fat and fat-free mass (muscle, bone, and water) in the body.

cardiovascular disease (CVD) A collective term for diseases of the heart and blood vessels.

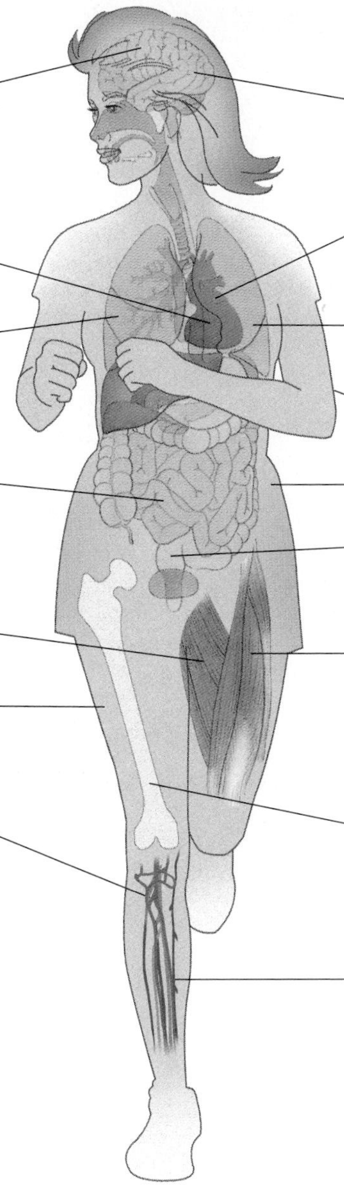

Increased levels of neurotransmitters; constant or slightly increased blood flow to the brain.

Increased heart rate and stroke volume (amount of blood pumped per beat).

Increased pulmonary ventilation (amount of air breathed into the body per minute). More air is taken into the lungs with each breath and breathing rate increases.

Reduced blood flow to the stomach, intestines, liver, and kidneys, resulting in less activity in the digestive tract and less urine output.

Increased energy production in muscles.

Increased blood flow to the skin and increased sweating to help maintain a safe body temperature.

Increased systolic blood pressure; increased blood flow and oxygen transport to working skeletal muscles and the heart; increased oxygen consumption.

Improved self-image, cognitive functioning, and ability to manage stress; decreased depression, anxiety, and risk for stroke.

Increased heart size and resting stroke volume; lower resting heart rate. Risk of heart disease and heart attack significantly reduced.

Improved ability to extract oxygen from air during exercise. Reduced risk of colds and upper respiratory tract infections.

Increased sweat rate and earlier onset of sweating, helping to cool the body.

Decreased body fat.

Reduced risk of colon cancer and certain other forms of cancer.

Muscle cell changes that allow for greater energy production and power output during exercise. Insulin sensitivity remains constant or improves, helping to prevent Type 2 diabetes. Muscle mass may also increase somewhat.

Increased density and breaking strength of bones, ligaments, and tendons; reduced risk for low-back pain, injuries, and osteoporosis; improved range of motion in joints.

Increased blood volume and capillary density; higher levels of high-density lipoproteins (HDL) and lower levels of triglycerides; lower resting blood pressure and reduced platelet stickiness (a factor in coronary heart disease).

Figure 10-1 Immediate and long-term effects of regular exercise. When exercise is performed regularly, short-term changes in the body develop into more permanent adaptations; these long-term effects include improved ability to exercise, reduced risk of many chronic diseases, improved psychological and emotional well-being, and increased life expectancy.

ing levels of activity. Endurance exercise and strength training improve blood fat levels by increasing levels of high-density lipoproteins and decreasing levels of low-density lipoproteins and triglycerides. Endurance exercise and strength training reduce high blood pressure and lower the risk of coronary heart disease and stroke.

Cancer Some studies have shown a relationship between increased physical activity and a reduction in a person's risk of all types of cancer, but these findings are not conclusive. There is strong evidence that exercise reduces the risk of colon cancer, and promising data that it reduces the risk of cancer of the breast and reproductive organs in women and prostate cancer in men.

Osteoporosis A special benefit of exercise, especially for women, is protection against osteoporosis. Weight-bearing exercise, which includes almost everything except swimming, helps build bone during the teens and twenties. People with denser bones can better endure the bone loss that occurs with aging. Strength training can increase bone density throughout life.

If you've ever gone for a long, brisk walk after a hard day's work, you know how refreshing exercise can be. Exercise can improve mood, stimulate creativity, clarify thinking, relieve anxiety, and provide an outlet for anger or aggression. But why does exercise make you feel good? Does it simply take your mind off your problems? Or does it cause a physical reaction that affects your mental state?

Current research indicates that exercise triggers many physical changes in the body that can alter mood. Scientists are now trying to explain how and why exercise affects the mind. One theory has to do with the physical structure of the brain. The area of the brain responsible for the movement of muscles is near the area responsible for thought and emotion. As muscles work vigorously, the resulting stimulation in the muscle center of the brain may also stimulate the thought and emotion center, producing improvements in mood and cognitive functions.

Other researchers suggest that exercise stimulates the release of **endorphins,** chemicals in the brain that can suppress fatigue, decrease pain, and produce euphoria. The "runner's high" often experienced after running several miles may be due to an increased production of endorphins.

A third area of research focuses on changes in brain activity during and after exercise. One change is an increase in alpha brain wave activity. Alpha waves indicate a highly relaxed state; meditation also induces alpha wave activity. A second change is an alteration in the levels of **neurotransmitters,** brain chemicals that increase alertness and reduce stress. Higher levels of

neurotransmitters such as serotonin may explain how exercise improves mild to moderate cases of depression. Researchers have found that exercise can be as effective as psychotherapy in treating depression, and even more effective when used in conjunction with other therapies. In addition to boosting neurotransmitter activity, exercise provides a distraction from stressful stimuli, enhances self-esteem, and may provide opportunity for positive social interactions. Regular exercise also improves body image.

Although most people don't associate exercise with mental skills, physical activity has been shown to have positive effects on cognitive functioning in both the short term and the long term. Exercise improves alertness and memory and can help you perform cognitive tasks at your peak level. Exercise may also help boost creativity. In a study of college students, those who ran regularly or took aerobic dance classes scored significantly higher on standard psychological tests of creativity than sedentary students. Over the long term, exercise can slow and possibly even reverse certain age-related declines in cognitive performance, including slowed reaction time and loss of short-term memory and nonverbal reasoning skills.

The message from this research is that exercise is a critical factor in developing *all* the dimensions of wellness, not just physical health. Even moderate exercise like walking briskly a few times per week can significantly improve your well-being. A lifetime of physical activity can leave you with a healthier body and a sharper, happier, more creative mind.

Diabetes   Recent studies have shown that exercise prevents the development of Type 2 diabetes, the most common form. Exercise burns excess sugar and makes cells more sensitive to insulin. Exercise also helps keep body fat at healthy levels. (Obesity is a key risk factor for Type 2 diabetes.)

Improved Psychological and Emotional Wellness

People who are physically active experience many social, psychological, and emotional benefits. They experience less stress and are buffered against the dangerous physical effects of stress. They are less likely to experience anxiety and depression. Exercise offers an arena for harmonious interaction with other people, as well as opportunities to strive and excel.

Improved Immune Function

Exercise can have either positive or negative effects on the immune system, the physiological processes that protect us from disease. Moderate endurance exercise boosts immune function, while excessive training depresses it. Physically fit people get fewer colds and upper respiratory tract infections than people who are not fit.

Prevention of Injuries and Low-Back Pain

Increased muscle strength protects against injury because it helps people maintain good posture and appropriate body mechanics when carrying out everyday activities like walking, lifting, and carrying. Strong muscles in the abdomen, hips, low back, and legs support the back in proper alignment and help prevent low-back pain.

Improved Wellness over the Life Span

Although people differ in the maximum levels of fitness they can achieve through exercise, the wellness benefits of exercise are available to everyone. All the benefits of exercise continue to accrue but gain new importance as the resilience of youth begins to wane. Simply stated, exercising can help you live a longer and healthier life.

Terms   **endorphins** Brain chemicals that seem to be involved in modulating pain and producing euphoria.

neurotransmitters Brain chemicals that transmit nerve impulses.

Physical fitness and athletic achievement are not limited to the able-bodied. People with disabilities can also attain high levels of fitness and performance, as shown by the elite athletes who compete in the Paralympics. The premier event for athletes with disabilities, the Paralympics are held in the same year and city as the Olympics. The athletes who participate include people with cerebral palsy, people with visual impairments, paraplegics, quadriplegics, and others. They compete in wheelchair races and wheelchair basketball, tandem cycling, in which a blind cyclist pedals with a sighted athlete, and other events. The performance of these skilled athletes makes it clear that people with disabilities can be active, healthy, and extraordinarily fit.

Currently, some 50 million Americans are estimated to have significant disabilities. Some disabilities are the result of injury, such as spinal cord injuries sustained in car crashes. Other disabilities result from illness, such as the blindness that may occur as a complication of diabetes or the joint stiffness that accompanies arthritis. And some disabilities are present at birth, as in the case of congenital limb deformities or cerebral palsy.

Exercise and physical activity are as important for people with disabilities as for able-bodied individuals—if not *more* important. Being active helps prevent secondary conditions that may result from prolonged inactivity, such as circulatory or muscular problems. It provides an emotional boost that helps support a positive attitude as well as opportunities to make new friends, increase self-confidence, and gain a sense of accomplishment. Currently, about 12% of people with disabilities engage in regular moderate activity.

Some health clubs offer activities and events geared for people of all ages and types of disabilities. They may have modified aerobics classes, special weight training machines, classes involving mild exercise in warm water, and other activities adapted for people with disabilities. Popular sports and recreational activities include adapted horseback riding, golf, swimming, and skiing. Competitive sports are also available—for example, there are wheelchair versions of billiards, tennis, hockey, and basketball, as well as sports for people with hearing, visual, or mental impairments. For those who prefer to get their exercise at home, special videos are available geared to individuals who use wheelchairs or who have arthritis, hearing impairments, or many other disabilities.

If you have a disability and want to be more active, check with your physician about what's appropriate for you. Call your local community center, YMCA/YWCA, independent living center, or health club to locate potential facilities; look for a club or facility with experienced personnel and appropriate adaptive equipment. For specialized videos, check with hospitals and health associations that are geared to specific disabilities, such as the Arthritis Foundation. Remember that no matter what your level of ability or disability, it's possible to make physical activity an integral part of your life.

SOURCES: U.S. Department of Health and Human Services. 2000. *Healthy People 2010*, 2nd ed. Washington, D.C.: DHHS. National Center on Physical Activity and Disability. 2000. *White Paper: Spinal Cord Injury and Fitness*. Chicago: National Center on Physical Activity and Disability. U.S. Department of Health and Human Services. 1996. *Physical Activity and Health: A Report of the Surgeon General*. Atlanta: DHHS.

DESIGNING YOUR EXERCISE PROGRAM

The best exercise program has two primary characteristics: It promotes your health and it's fun to do. Exercise does not have to be a chore. On the contrary, it can provide some of the most pleasurable moments of your day, once you make it a habit.

Physical Activity and Exercise for Health and Fitness

Physical activity can be defined as any body movement carried out by skeletal muscles and requiring energy—standing up, walking down the hall, carrying a child, and so on. The term *exercise* is usually used to refer to a subset of physical activity—planned, structured, repetitive movement of the body designed specifically to improve or maintain physical fitness. To develop fitness, a person must perform a sufficient amount of physical activity to stress the body and cause long-term physiological changes.

Lifestyle Physical Activity for Health Promotion The Surgeon General's report recommends that all Americans include a moderate amount of physical activity on most, preferably all, days of the week. The report suggests a goal of expending 150 calories per day, or about 1000 calories per week, in physical activity. Because energy expenditure is a function of both intensity and duration of activity, the same amount of benefit can be obtained in longer sessions of moderate-intensity activities as in shorter sessions of more strenuous activities. Thus, 15 minutes of running is equivalent to 30 minutes of brisk walking; both activities use about 150 calories of energy. Other moderate activities include playing volleyball for 45 minutes, gardening for 30–45 minutes, wheeling oneself in a wheelchair for 30–40 minutes, bicycling 5 miles in 30 minutes, jumping rope for 15 minutes, and stairwalking for 15 minutes. In addition to recommending moderate-intensity physical activity, the Surgeon General's report recommends that people perform resistance training (exercising against an opposing force such as a weight) at least twice a week to build and maintain strength.

By increasing lifestyle physical activity, people can expect to significantly improve their health and well-being. Such a program may not necessarily increase physical fitness, however.

"Too little time" is a common excuse for not being physically active. Learning to manage your time successfully is crucial if you are to maintain a wellness lifestyle. You can begin by keeping a record of how you are currently spending your time; in your health journal, use a grid broken into blocks of 15, 20, or 30 minutes to track your daily activities. Then analyze your record: List each type of activity and the total time you engaged in it on a given day—for example, sleeping, 7 hours; eating, 1.5 hours; studying, 3 hours; and so on. Next, prioritize your activities according to how important they are to you, from essential to somewhat important to not important at all.

Based on the priorities you set, make changes in your daily schedule by subtracting time from some activities in order to make time for physical activity. Look particularly carefully at your leisure time activities and your methods of transportation; these are areas where it is easy to build in physical activity. Make changes using a system of tradeoffs. For example, you may decide to watch television for 10 minutes less in the morning in order to change your 5-minute drive to class into a 15-minute walk.

The following are just a few ways to become more active:

- Take the stairs instead of the elevator or escalator.
- Walk to the mailbox, bank, or library whenever possible.
- Park your car a mile or even just a few blocks from your destination, and walk briskly.
- Do at least one chore every day that requires physical activity: wash the windows or your car, clean your room or house, mow the lawn, rake the leaves.
- Take study or work breaks to avoid sitting for more than 30 minutes at a time. Get up and walk around the library, your office, or your home; go up and down a flight of stairs.
- Stretch when you stand in line or watch TV.
- When you take public transportation, get off one stop early and walk to your destination.
- Go dancing instead of to a movie.
- Walk to visit a neighbor or friend rather than calling him or her on the phone. Go for a walk while you chat.
- Put your remote controls in storage; when you want to change TV or radio stations, get up and do it by hand.

Exercise Programs to Develop Physical Fitness   The Surgeon General's report concluded that people can obtain even greater health benefits by increasing the duration and intensity of activity. Thus a person who engages in a structured, formal exercise program designed to measurably improve physical fitness will obtain even greater improvements in quality of life and greater reductions in disease and mortality risk.

How Much Physical Activity Is Enough?   Some experts feel that people get most of the health benefits of a formal exercise program simply by becoming more active over the course of the day. Others feel that the lifestyle approach sets too low an activity goal and that people should exercise long and intensely enough to improve physical fitness. More research is needed to resolve this debate, but there is probably truth in both of these positions. Regular physical activity, regardless of intensity, makes you healthier and can help protect you from many chronic diseases, but you obtain even more benefits when you are physically fit.

Where does this leave you? Most experts agree that some physical activity is better than none, but that more—as long as it does not result in injury—is probably better than some. A physical activity pyramid to guide you in meeting these goals for physical activity is shown in Figure 10-2. If you are sedentary, start at the bottom of the pyramid and gradually increase the amount of moderate-intensity physical activity in your daily life. You don't have to exercise vigorously, but you should experience a moderate increase in your heart and breathing rates. For even greater benefits, move up to the next two levels of the pyramid, which illustrate parts of a formal exercise program. The American College of Sports Medicine has established guidelines for creating an exercise program that includes **cardiorespiratory endurance (aerobic) exercise**, strength training, and flexibility training (Table 10-1). Such a program will develop all the health-related components of physical fitness. For a summary of the health and fitness benefits of different levels of physical activity, refer to Figure 10-3.

Medical Clearance

Previously inactive men over 40 and women over 50 should get a medical examination before beginning an exercise program. Diabetes, asthma, heart disease, and extreme obesity are conditions that may call for a modified program. If you have risk factors for heart disease, you should have a physical checkup, including an **electrocardiogram (ECG or EKG)**, before beginning an exercise program. This checkup will help ensure that your program will be a benefit to your health, rather than a potential hazard.

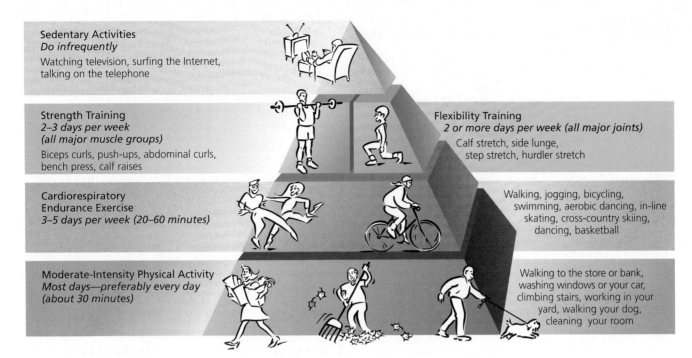

Sedentary Activities
Do infrequently
Watching television, surfing the Internet, talking on the telephone

Strength Training
2–3 days per week (all major muscle groups)
Biceps curls, push-ups, abdominal curls, bench press, calf raises

Flexibility Training
2 or more days per week (all major joints)
Calf stretch, side lunge, step stretch, hurdler stretch

Cardiorespiratory Endurance Exercise
3–5 days per week (20–60 minutes)

Walking, jogging, bicycling, swimming, aerobic dancing, in-line skating, cross-country skiing, dancing, basketball

Moderate-Intensity Physical Activity
Most days—preferably every day (about 30 minutes)

Walking to the store or bank, washing windows or your car, climbing stairs, working in your yard, walking your dog, cleaning your room

Figure 10-2   Physical activity pyramid.   Similar to the Food Guide Pyramid, this physical activity pyramid is designed to help people become more active. If you are currently sedentary, begin at the bottom of the pyramid and gradually increase the amount of moderate-intensity physical activity in your life. If you are already moderately active, begin a formal exercise program that includes cardiorespiratory endurance exercise, flexibility training, and strength training to help you develop all the health-related components of fitness.

Cardiorespiratory Endurance Exercises

Exercises that condition your heart and lungs should have a central role in your fitness program. The best exercises for developing cardiorespiratory endurance are those that stress a large portion of the body's muscle mass for a prolonged period of time. These include walking, jogging, running, swimming, bicycling, and aerobic dancing. Many popular sports and recreational activities such as racquetball, tennis, basketball, and soccer are also good if the skill level and intensity of the game are sufficient to provide a vigorous workout.

Frequency   The optimal workout schedule for endurance training is 3–5 days per week. Beginners should start with 3 and work up to 5 days. Training more than 5 days a week may lead to injury; and while you do get health benefits from exercising very vigorously only 1–2 days per week, you risk injury because your body never adapts fully to regular exercise training.

Intensity   Intensity is the crucial factor in attaining a significant training effect—that is, in increasing the body's cardiorespiratory capacity. A primary purpose of endurance training is to increase **maximal oxygen consumption (MOC)**. MOC represents the maximum ability of the cells to use oxygen and is considered the best measure of cardiorespiratory capacity. Intensity of training is the crucial factor in improving MOC.

One of the easiest ways to determine exactly how intensely you should work involves measuring your heart rate. It is not necessary or desirable to exercise at your maximum heart rate—the fastest heart rate possible before exhaustion sets in—in order to improve your cardiorespiratory capacity. Beneficial effects occur at lower heart rates with a much lower risk of injury. **Target heart rate** is the rate at which you should exercise to obtain cardiorespiratory benefits.

cardiorespiratory endurance (aerobic) exercise Rhythmical, large-muscle exercise for a prolonged period of time; partially dependent on the ability of the cardiovascular system to deliver oxygen to tissues.

electrocardiogram (ECG or EKG) A recording of the changes in electrical activity of the heart.

maximal oxygen consumption (MOC) The body's maximum ability to transport and use oxygen.

target heart rate The heart rate at which exercise yields cardiorespiratory benefits.

Terms

Table 10-1   Exercise Recommendations for Healthy Adults

Exercise to Develop and Maintain Cardiorespiratory Endurance and Body Composition

Mode of activity	Any activity that uses large-muscle groups, can be maintained continuously, and is rhythmical and aerobic in nature; for example, walking-hiking, running-jogging, cycling-bicycling, cross-country skiing, aerobic dance, and other forms of group exercise, rope skipping, rowing, stairclimbing, swimming, skating, and endurance game activities.
Frequency of training	3–5 days per week.
Intensity of training	55/65–90% of maximum heart rate or 40/50–85% of maximum oxygen uptake reserve. The lower intensity values (55–64% of maximum heart rate and 40–49% of maximum oxygen uptake reserve) are most applicable to individuals who are quite unfit. For average individuals, intensities of 70–85% of maximum heart rate are appropriate; see p. 226 for instructions for determining target heart rate.
Duration of training	20–60 total minutes of continuous or intermittent (in sessions lasting 10 or more minutes) aerobic activity. Duration is dependent on the intensity of activity; thus, lower-intensity activity should be conducted over a longer period of time (30 minutes or more). Lower-to-moderate-intensity activity of longer duration is recommended for the nonathletic adult.

Exercise to Develop and Maintain Muscular Strength and Endurance, Flexibility, and Body Composition

Resistance training	One set of 8–10 exercises that condition the major muscle groups should be performed 2–3 days per week. Most people should complete 8–12 repetitions of each exercise; for older and more frail people (approximately 50–60 years of age and above), 10–15 repetitions with a lighter weight may be more appropriate. Multiple-set regimens may provide greater benefits if time allows.
Flexibility training	Stretches for the major muscle groups should be performed a minimum of 2–3 days per week; at least four repetitions, held for 10–30 seconds, should be completed.

SOURCES: American College of Sports Medicine. 1998. ACSM position stand. The recommended quantity and quality of exercise for developing and maintaining cardiorespiratory and muscular fitness and flexibility in healthy adults. *Medicine and Science in Sports and Exercise* 30(6): 975–991.

Duration   A total duration of 20–60 minutes is recommended; exercise can take place in a single session or in multiple bouts lasting 10 or more minutes. The total duration of exercise depends on its intensity. To improve cardiorespiratory endurance during a low- to moderate-intensity activity such as walking or slow swimming, you should exercise for 45–60 minutes. For high-intensity exercise performed at the top of your target heart rate zone, a duration of 20 minutes is sufficient. It is usually best to start off with less-vigorous activities and only gradually increase intensity.

The Warm-Up and Cool-Down   It is always important to warm up before you exercise and to cool down afterward. Warming up enhances your performance and decreases your chances of injury. A warm-up session should include low-intensity movements similar to those in the activity that will follow. Examples of low-intensity movements are hitting forehands and backhands before a tennis game and running a 12-minute mile before progressing to an 8-minute one. Some experts also recommend warm-up stretching exercises for flexibility after the general warm-up and before intense activity.

Cooling down after exercise is important to restore the body's circulation to its normal resting condition. When you are at rest, a relatively small percentage of your total blood volume is directed to muscles, but during exercise, as much as 85% of the heart's output is directed to them. During recovery from exercise, it is important to continue exercising at a low level to provide a smooth transition to the resting state.

 Developing Muscular Strength and Endurance

Any program designed to promote health should include exercises that develop muscular strength and endurance.

Types of Strength Training Exercises   Muscular strength and endurance can be developed in many ways, from weight training to calisthenics. Common exercises such

Terms

resistance exercise Exercise that forces muscles to contract against increased resistance; also called *strength training*.

isometric exercise The application of force without movement; also called *static exercise*.

isotonic exercise The application of force with movement.

	Lifestyle physical activity	Moderate exercise program	Vigorous exercise program
Description	Moderate physical activity—an amount of activity that uses about 150 calories per day	Cardiorespiratory endurance exercise (20–60 minutes, 3–5 days per week); strength training and stretching exercises (2–3 days per week)	Cardiorespiratory endurance exercise (20–60 minutes, 3–5 days per week); interval training; strength training (3–4 days per week); and stretching exercises (3–5 days per week)
Sample activities or program	*One of the following:* • Walking to and from work, 15 minutes each way • Cycling to and from class, 10 minutes each way • Raking leaves for 30 minutes • Dancing (fast) for 30 minutes • Playing basketball for 20 minutes	• Jogging for 30 minutes, 3 days per week • Weight training, 1 set of 8 exercises, 2 days per week • Stretching exercises, 3 days per week	• Running for 45 minutes, 3 days per week • Intervals: running 400 m at high effort 4 sets, 2 days per week • Weight training, 3 sets of 10 exercises, 3 days per week • Stretching exercises, 5 days per week
Health and fitness benefits	Better blood cholesterol levels, reduced body fat, better control of blood pressure, improved metabolic health, and enhanced glucose metabolism; improved quality of life; reduced risk of some chronic diseases	All the benefits of lifestyle physical activity, plus improved physical fitness (increased cardiorespiratory endurance, muscular strength and endurance, and flexibility) and even greater improvements in health and quality of life and reductions in chronic disease risk	All the benefits of lifestyle physical activity and a moderate exercise program, with greater increases in fitness and somewhat greater reductions in chronic disease risk Participating in a vigorous exercise program may increase risk of injury and overtraining

Figure 10-3   Health and fitness benefits of different amounts of physical activity and exercise.

as sit-ups, push-ups, pull-ups, and wall-sitting (leaning against a wall in a seated position and supporting yourself with your leg muscles) maintain the muscular strength of most people if they practice them several times a week. To condition and tone your whole body, choose exercises that work the major muscles of the shoulders, chest, back, arms, abdomen, and legs.

To increase strength, you must do **resistance exercise**—exercises in which your muscles must exert force against a significant amount of resistance. Resistance can be provided by weights, exercise machines, or your own body weight. **Isometric exercises** involve applying force without movement, such as when you contract your abdominal muscles. For maximum strength gains, hold an isometric contraction for 6 seconds; do 5–10 repetitions. Don't hold your breath—that can restrict blood flow to your heart and brain. Within a few weeks, you will notice the effect of this exercise. Isometrics are particularly useful when recovering from an injury.

Isotonic exercises involve applying force with movement, as, for example, in weight training exercises such as the bench press. These are the most popular type of exercises for increasing muscle strength and seem to be most valuable for developing strength that can be transferred to other forms of physical activity. They include exercises using barbells, dumbbells, weight machines, and the body's own weight, as in push-ups or sit-ups.

Choosing Equipment   Weight machines are preferred by many people because they are safe, convenient, and easy to use. You just set the resistance (usually by placing a pin in the weight stack), sit down at the machine, and start working. Machines make it easy to isolate and work specific muscles. Free weights require more care, balance, and coordination to use, but they strengthen your body in ways that are more adaptable to real life. For free weights, you need to use a spotter, someone who stands by to assist in case you lose control over a weight.

Choosing Exercises   A complete weight training program works all the major muscle groups: neck, upper back, shoulders, arms, chest, abdomen, lower back, thighs, buttocks, and calves. Different exercises work different muscles, so it usually takes about 8–10 exercises to get a complete workout for general fitness—for example, bench presses to develop the chest, shoulders,

Your target heart rate is the rate at which you should exercise to experience cardiorespiratory benefits. Your target heart rate is based on your maximum heart rate, which can be estimated from your age. (If you are a serious athlete or face possible cardiovascular risks from exercise, you may want to have your maximum heart rate determined more accurately through a treadmill test in a physician's office, hospital, or sports medicine laboratory.) Your target heart rate is actually a range; the lower value corresponds to moderate-intensity exercise, while the higher value is associated with high-intensity activities. Target heart rates are shown in the accompanying table.

You can monitor the intensity of your workouts by measuring your pulse either at your wrist or at one of your carotid arteries, located on either side of your Adam's apple. Your pulse rate drops rapidly after exercise, so begin counting immediately after you have finished exercising. You will obtain the most accurate results by counting beats for 15 seconds and then multiplying by 4 to get your heart rate in beats per minute (bpm). The 15-second counts corresponding to each target heart rate range are also shown in the table at the right.

Age (years)	Target Heart Rate Range (bpm)*	15-Second Count (beats)*
20–24	127–182	32–46
25–29	124–176	31–44
30–34	121–171	30–43
35–39	118–167	30–42
40–44	114–162	29–41
45–49	111–158	28–40
50–54	108–153	27–38
55–59	105–149	26–37
60–64	101–144	25–36
65+	97–140	24–35

*Target heart rates lower than those shown here are appropriate for individuals who are quite unfit. Ranges are based on the following formula. Target heart rate = 0.65 to 0.90 of maximum heart rate, assuming maximum heart rate = 220 − age.

and upper arms; pull-ups to work the biceps and upper back; squats to develop the legs and buttocks; toe raises to work the calves; and so on. (A complete sample weight training program for general fitness can be found on the *Core Concepts Interactive* CD-ROM that accompanies the text.)

Intensity and Duration   The amount of weight (resistance) you lift in weight training exercises is equivalent to intensity in cardiorespiratory endurance training; the number of repetitions of each exercise is equivalent to duration. In order to improve fitness, you must do enough repetitions of each exercise to temporarily fatigue your muscles. The number of repetitions needed to cause fatigue depends on the amount of resistance: the heavier the weight, the fewer repetitions to reach fatigue. In general, a heavy weight and a low number of repetitions (1–5) build strength, while a light weight and a high number of repetitions (20–25) build endurance. For a general fitness program to build both strength and endurance, try to do 8–12 repetitions of each exercise; a few exercises, such as abdominal crunches and calf raises, may require more.

Begin with a weight that you can lift fairly easily, and do 8–12 repetitions of each exercise. As you progress, add weight when you can do more than 12 repetitions of an exercise. For developing strength and endurance for general fitness, a single set (group) of each exercise is sufficient, provided you use enough resistance (weight) to fatigue your muscles. Doing more than 1 set of each exercise may increase strength development, and most serious weight trainers do at least 3 sets of each exercise. If you do

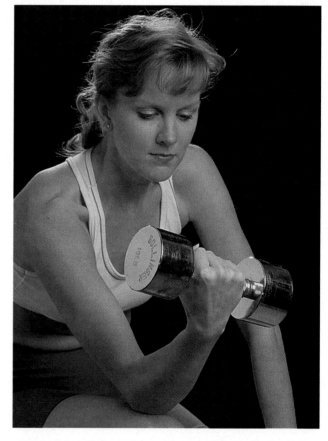

Building muscular strength is an important component of a fitness program. Weight training is just one way to increase strength, improve muscle tone, and enhance the overall appearance of the body.

The 2000 Olympic Games in Sydney made headlines not just for athletic achievements but also for the number of athletes testing positive for performance-enhancing drugs. Some athletes were banned from competition before or during the games, while others had medals taken away after they failed postcompetition drug tests. The Olympic Movement Anti-Doping Code calls for the elimination of the use of performance-enhancing drugs in sports in order to both ensure respect for sports ethics and protect the health of athletes.

Drugs intended to enhance athletic performance are used not only by elite Olympic athletes but also by active individuals of all fitness levels. Two to 3% of high school and college students report having used steroids, and over-the-counter dietary supplements are much more popular. Many such substances are ineffective and expensive, and many are also dangerous. For example, supplements marketed to bodybuilders containing gamma butyrolactone or butanediol, CNS depressants related to the illegal drug gamma hydroxybutyrate (GHB), may cause vomiting, seizures, coma, and potentially fatal withdrawal reactions (see Chapter 7). A few of the most widely used compounds are described below.

Anabolic Steroids   These synthetic derivatives of testosterone are taken to increase strength, power, speed, endurance, muscle size, and aggressiveness. **Anabolic steroids** have dangerous side effects, including disruption of the body's hormone system, liver disease, acne, breast development and testicular shrinkage in males, masculinization in women and children, and increased risk of heart disease and cancer. Steroid use is also associated with an increased risk of drug abuse and HIV infection.

Adrenal Androgens   This group of drugs, which includes dehydroepiandrosterone (DHEA) and androstenedione, are typically taken to stimulate muscle growth and aid in weight control. The few studies of these agents done on humans show that they are of very little value in improving athletic performance, and they have side effects similar to those of anabolic steroids, especially when taken in high doses.

Erythropoietin (EPO)   A naturally occurring hormone that boosts the concentration of red blood cells, EPO is typically used by endurance athletes to improve their performance. EPO can cause blood clots and death.

Creatine Monohydrate   Use of creatine supplements may improve performance in short-term, high-intensity, repetitive exercise; however, in 2000, a panel of ACSM experts concluded that there is no evidence that creatine supplements increase the aerobic power of muscles. They may increase water retention in muscles, giving the feeling of increased muscularity without an actual increase in muscle size. The long-term effects of creatine use, especially among young people, are not well established.

Protein, Amino Acid, and Polypeptide Supplements   Little research supports the use of such supplements, even in athletes on extremely heavy training regimens. The protein requirements of athletes are not much higher than those of sedentary individuals, and most people take in more than enough protein in their diets. By substituting supplements for food sources of protein, people may risk deficiencies in other key nutrients typically found in such foods, including iron and B vitamins.

Chromium Picolinate   Sold over the counter, chromium picolinate is a more easily digested form of the trace mineral chromium. Although often marketed as a means to build muscle and reduce fat, most studies have found no positive effects. Long-term use of high dosages may have serious health consequences.

---

perform more than 1 set of an exercise, rest long enough between sets to allow your muscles to recover. Be sure to warm up before every weight training session and cool down afterward.

Frequency   For general fitness, the American College of Sports Medicine recommends a frequency of 2–3 days per week. Allow your muscles a day of rest between workouts to avoid soreness and injury. If you enjoy weight training and would like to train more often, try working different muscle groups on alternate days.

Gender Differences in Muscle Size and Strength   Men are generally stronger than women because they typically have larger bodies overall and larger muscles. But when the amount of muscle tissue is taken into account, men are only 1–2% stronger than women in the upper body and about equal to women in the lower body. (Men have a larger proportion of muscle tissue in the upper body, so it's easier for them to build upper-body strength than it is

for women.) This disparity is probably due in large part to androgens, naturally occurring male hormones that promote the growth of muscle tissue. Androgen levels are about 6–10 times higher in men than in women.

However, both men and women can increase strength through resistance training. Men tend to build larger, stronger muscles. Women tend to lose inches and increase strength without developing excessively bulky muscles. (Because of their lower levels of androgens, women do not develop large muscles from moderate strength training.)

A Caution About Supplements   No nutritional supplement or drug will change a weak, untrained person into a strong, fit person. Those changes require regular training

---

anabolic steroids Synthetic male hormones used to increase muscle size and strength.   Terms

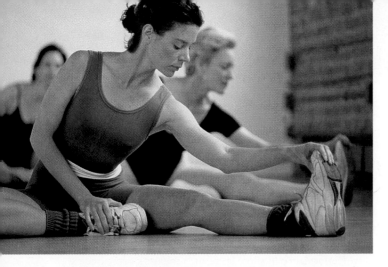

When performed regularly, stretching exercises help maintain or improve the range of motion in joints. For each exercise, stretch to the point of tightness in the muscle and hold the position for 10–30 seconds.

that stresses the body and causes physiological adaptations. Supplements or drugs that promise quick, large gains in strength usually don't work and are often either dangerous or expensive, or both. The long-term effects of many supplements have not been studied. Use your critical thinking skills to evaluate claims made about supplements, and stay with the proven method of a steady, progressive fitness program to build strength.

Flexibility Exercises

Flexibility, or stretching, exercises are important for maintaining the normal range of motion in the major joints of the body. Some exercises, such as running, can actually decrease flexibility because they require only a partial range of motion. Like a good weight training program, a good stretching program includes exercises for all the major muscle groups and joints of the body: neck, shoulders, back, hips, thighs, hamstrings, and calves. (See the sample stretching program on *Core Concepts Interactive*.)

Proper Stretching Technique   Stretching should be performed statically. "Bouncing" (known as ballistic stretching) is dangerous and counterproductive. Stretching can be either active or passive. In active stretching, a muscle is stretched by a contraction of opposing muscles. In passive stretching, an outside force or resistance provided by yourself, a partner, gravity, or a weight helps your joints move through their range of motion. You can achieve a greater range of motion and a more intense stretch using passive stretching, but there is a greater risk of injury. The safest and most convenient technique may be active static stretching with a passive assist. For example, you might do a seated stretch of your calf muscles both by contracting the muscles on the top of your shin and by grabbing your feet and pulling them toward you.

Intensity and Duration   For each exercise, stretch to the point of tightness in the muscle, and hold the position for 10–30 seconds. Rest for 30–60 seconds, and then repeat, trying to stretch a bit farther. Relax and breathe easily as you stretch. You should feel a pleasant, mild stretch as you let the muscles relax; stretching should not be painful. Do at least 4 repetitions of each exercise. A complete flexibility workout usually takes about 20–30 minutes.

Increase your intensity gradually over time. Improved flexibility takes many months to develop. There are large individual differences in joint flexibility. Don't feel you have to compete with others during stretching workouts.

Frequency   Do stretching exercises a minimum of 2–3 days per week. You may develop more flexibility if you do them after exercise, during your cool-down, because your muscles are warmer then and can be stretched farther.

Training in Specific Skills

The final component in your fitness program is learning the skills required for the sports or activities in which you choose to participate. The first step in learning a new skill is getting help. Sports like tennis, golf, sailing, and skiing require mastery of basic movements and techniques, so instruction from a qualified teacher can save you hours of frustration and increase your enjoyment of the sport. Skill is also important in conditioning activities such as jogging, swimming, and cycling. Even if you learned a sport as a child, additional instruction now can help you refine your technique.

COMMUNICATE!   Our choice of fitness activities is influenced by many factors, including the messages communicated to us by the media and through other cultural channels. We get messages about the activities considered appropriate for our age, gender, socioeconomic status, level of ability, and so on. For example, what image comes to mind when you think of golf, basketball, salsa dancing, ballet, ice hockey, boxing, weight lifting? Are your images stereotypes? Where do you think you got them, and how valid are they? If there is an activity you'd like to try but haven't because of media influences, try critically analyzing those influences and revising your thinking.

WW. Putting It All Together

Now that you know the basic components of a fitness program, you can put them all together in a program that works for you. Remember to include the following:

- *Cardiorespiratory endurance exercise:* Do at least 20 minutes of aerobic exercise at your target heart rate three to five times a week.

- *Muscular strength and endurance:* Work the major muscle groups (1 or more sets of 8–10 exercises) two to three times a week.
- *Flexibility exercise:* Do stretches at least two or three times a week.
- *Skill training:* Incorporate some or all of your aerobic or strengthening exercise into an enjoyable sport or physical activity.

GETTING STARTED AND STAYING ON TRACK

Once you have a program that fulfills your basic fitness needs and suits your personal tastes, adhering to a few basic principles will help you improve at the fastest rate, have more fun, and minimize the risk of injury.

Selecting Instructors, Equipment, and Facilities

One of the best places to get help and advice about exercise is a class, where an expert instructor can help you learn the basics of training and answer your questions. A qualified personal trainer can also get you started on an exercise program or a new form of training. Make sure that your instructor or trainer has proper qualifications, such as a college degree in exercise physiology or physical education and certification by the American College of Sports Medicine (ACSM), American Council on Exercise (ACE), or another professional organization.

When you are selecting equipment, try to purchase the best you can afford. Good equipment will enhance your enjoyment and decrease your risk of injury. Appropriate safety equipment, such as pads and helmets for in-line skating, is particularly important.

Before you buy a new piece of equipment, investigate it. Is it worth the money? Does it produce the results its proponents claim for it? Is it safe? Does it fit properly, and is it in good working order? Does it provide a genuine workout? Will you really use it regularly? Ask the experts (coaches, physical educators, and sports instructors) for their opinion. Better yet, educate yourself. Every sport, from running to volleyball, has its own magazine. A little effort to educate yourself will be well rewarded.

If you are thinking of joining a health club or fitness center, be sure to choose one that has the right programs and equipment available at the times you will use them. Ask for a free trial workout, 1-day pass, or an inexpensive 1- to 2-week trial membership before committing to a long-term contract. Be wary of promotional gimmicks and high-pressure sales tactics. Also make sure the facility is certified; look for the displayed names American College of Sports Medicine (ACSM), American Council on Exercise (ACE), or Aerobics and Fitness Association of America (AFAA). These trade associations have established standards to help protect consumer health, safety, and rights.

Eating and Drinking for Exercise

Most people do not need to change their eating habits when they begin a fitness program. In almost every case, a well-balanced diet contains all the energy and nutrients needed to sustain an exercise program. A balanced diet is also the key to improving your body composition when you begin to exercise more. One of the promises of a fitness program is a decrease in body fat and an increase in muscular body mass. The best way to control body fat is to follow a diet containing adequate but not excessive calories and to be physically active.

One of the most important principles to follow when exercising is to drink enough water. Sweating during exercise depletes the body's water supply and can lead to dehydration if fluids are not replaced. Serious dehydration can cause reduced blood volume, accelerated heart rate, elevated body temperature, muscle cramps, heat stroke, and other problems. Drinking water before and during exercise is important to prevent dehydration and enhance athletic performance.

Thirst alone is not a good indication of how much you need to drink, because thirst is quickly depressed by drinking even small amounts of water. As a rule of thumb, try to drink about 8 ounces of water (more in hot weather) for every 30 minutes of heavy exercise. Bring a water bottle with you when you exercise so you can replace your fluids while they're being depleted. For workouts lasting less than 60–90 minutes, cool water is an appropriate fluid replacement; for longer workouts or for exercise in especially hot and humid conditions, a commercial sports beverage that contains carbohydrates may be beneficial.

Managing Your Fitness Program

How can you tell when you're in shape? When do you stop improving and start maintaining? How can you stay motivated? If your program is going to become an integral part of your life, these are very important questions.

Consistency: The Key to Physical Improvement   It is important to be able to recognize when you have achieved the level of fitness that is appropriate for you. Your body gets into shape by adapting to increasing levels of physical stress. If you don't push yourself by increasing the intensity of your workout, no change will occur in your body. But if you subject your body to overly severe stress, it will break down and become distressed, or injured. Your body needs time to adapt to increasingly higher levels of stress. If you feel extremely sore and tired the day after exercising, then you have worked too hard.

Consistency is the key to getting into shape without injury. The best way to ensure consistency is to keep a training journal in which you record the details of your workouts: how far you ran, how much weight you lifted, how

Footwear is perhaps the most important item of equipment for almost any activity. Shoes protect and support your feet and improve your traction. When you jump or run, you place as much as six times more force on your feet than when you stand still. Shoes can help cushion against the stress that this additional force places on your lower legs, thereby preventing injuries. Some athletic shoes are also designed to help prevent ankle rollover, another common source of injury.

When choosing athletic shoes, first consider the activity you've chosen for your exercise program. Shoes appropriate for different activities have very different characteristics. For example, running shoes typically have highly cushioned midsoles, rubber outsoles with elevated heels, and a great deal of flexibility in the forefoot. The heels of walking shoes tend to be lower, less padded, and more beveled than those designed for running. For aerobic dance, shoes must be flexible in the forefoot and have straight, nonflared heels to allow for safe and easy lateral movements. Court shoes also provide substantial support for lateral movements; they typically have outsoles made from white rubber that will not damage court surfaces.

Also consider the location and intensity of your workouts. If you plan to walk or run on trails, you should choose shoes with water-resistant, highly durable uppers and more outsole traction. If you work out intensely or have a relatively high body weight, you'll need thick, firm midsoles to avoid bottoming-out the cushioning system of your shoes.

Foot type is another important consideration. If your feet tend to roll inward excessively, you may need shoes with additional stability features on the inner side of the shoe to counteract this movement. If your feet tend to roll outward excessively, you may need highly flexible and cushioned shoes that promote foot motion. For aerobic dancers with feet that tend to roll inward or outward, mid-cut to high-cut shoes may be more appropriate than low-cut aerobic shoes or cross-trainers (shoes designed to be worn for several different activities). Compared with men, women have narrower feet overall and narrower heels relative to the forefoot. Most women will get a better fit if they choose shoes that are specifically designed for women's feet rather than those that are downsized versions of men's shoes.

For successful shoe shopping, keep the following strategies in mind:

- Shop at an athletic shoe or specialty store that has personnel trained to fit athletic shoes and a large selection of styles and sizes.

- Shop late in the day or, ideally, following a workout. Your foot size increases over the course of the day and as a result of exercise.

- Wear socks like those you plan to wear during exercise. If you have an old pair of athletic shoes, bring them with you. The wear pattern on your old shoes can help you select a pair with extra support or cushioning in the places you need it the most.

- Ask for help. Trained salespeople know which shoes are designed for your foot type and your level of activity. They can also help fit your shoes properly.

- Don't insist on buying shoes in what you consider to be your typical shoe size. Sizes vary from shoe to shoe. In addition, foot sizes change over time, and many people have one foot that is larger or wider than the other. Try several sizes in several widths, if necessary. Don't buy shoes that are too small.

- Try on both shoes, and wear them around for 10 or more minutes. Try walking on a noncarpeted surface. Approximate the movements of your activity: walk, jog, run, jump, and so on.

- Check the fit and style carefully:

    Is the toe box roomy enough? Your toes will spread out when your foot hits the ground or you push off. There should be at least one thumb's width of space from the longest toe to the end of the toe box.

    Do the shoes have enough cushioning? Do your feet feel supported when you bounce up and down? Try bouncing on your toes and on your heels.

    Do your heels fit snugly into the shoe? Do they stay put when you walk, or do they rise up?

    Are the arches of your feet right on top of the shoes' arch supports?

    Do the shoes feel stable when you twist and turn on the balls of your feet? Try twisting from side to side while standing on one foot.

    Do you feel any pressure points?

- If the shoes are not comfortable in the store, don't buy them. Don't expect athletic shoes to stretch over time in order to fit your feet properly.

---

many laps you swam, and so on. This record will help you evaluate your progress and plan your workout sessions intelligently. Don't increase your exercise volume by more than 5–10% per week.

Assessing Your Fitness   When are you "in shape"? It depends. One person may be out of shape running a mile in 5 minutes; another may be in shape running a mile in 12 minutes. As mentioned earlier, your ultimate level of fitness depends on your goals, your program, and your natural ability. The important thing is to set goals that make sense for you.

If you are interested in finding out exactly how fit you are before you begin a program, the best approach is to get an assessment from a modern sports medicine laboratory. Such laboratories can be found in university physical

Injury	Symptoms	Treatment
Blister	Accumulation of fluid in one spot under the skin	Don't pop or drain it unless it interferes too much with your daily activities. If it does pop, clean the area with antiseptic and cover with a bandage. Do not remove the skin covering the blister.
Bruise	Pain, swelling, and discoloration (contusion)	R-I-C-E: rest, ice, compression, elevation.
Joint sprain	Pain, tenderness, swelling, discoloration, and loss of function	R-I-C-E; apply heat after 36–48 hours if swelling has disappeared. Stretch and strengthen the affected area.
Muscle cramp	Painful, spasmodic muscle contractions	Gently stretch for 15–30 seconds at a time, and/or massage the cramped area. Drink fluids.
Muscle soreness or stiffness	Pain and tenderness in the affected muscle	Stretch the affected muscle gently; exercise at a low intensity; apply heat.
Muscle strain	Pain, tenderness, swelling, and loss of strength in the affected muscle	R-I-C-E; apply heat after 36–48 hours if swelling has disappeared. Stretch and strengthen affected area.
Shin splints	Pain and tenderness on the front of the lower leg; sometimes also pain in the calf	Rest; apply ice to the affected area several times a day; wrap with tape for support. Stretch and strengthen muscles in the lower legs. Purchase good-quality footwear, and run on soft surfaces.
Side stitch	Pain on the side of the abdomen	Decrease the intensity of your workout, or stop altogether; bend over in the direction of the stitch.

SOURCE: Fahey, T. D., P. M. Insel, and W. T. Roth. 2001. *Fit and Well: Core Concepts and Labs in Physical Fitness and Wellness*, 4th ed. Mountain View, Calif.: Mayfield.

education departments and medical centers. Here you will receive an accurate profile of your capacity to exercise. Typically, your endurance will be measured on a treadmill or bicycle, your body fat will be estimated, and your strength and flexibility will be tested. This evaluation will reveal whether your physical condition is consistent with good health, and the staff members at the laboratory can suggest an exercise program that will be appropriate for your level of fitness.

Preventing and Managing Athletic Injuries   It is important to learn how to deal with injuries so they don't derail your fitness program (Table 10-2). Some injuries require medical attention. Consult a physician for head and eye injuries, possible ligament injuries, broken bones, and internal disorders such as chest pain, fainting, and intolerance to heat. Also seek medical attention for apparently minor injuries that do not get better within a reasonable amount of time.

For minor cuts and scrapes, stop the bleeding and clean the wound with soap and water. Treat soft tissue injuries (muscles and joints) with the R-I-C-E principle:

Rest: Stop using the injured area as soon as you experience pain, and avoid any activity that causes pain.

Ice: Apply ice to the injured area to reduce swelling and alleviate pain. Apply ice immediately for 10–20 minutes, and repeat every few hours until the swelling disappears. Let the injured part return to normal temperature between icings, and do not apply ice to one area for more than 20 minutes (10 minutes if you are using a cold gel pack).

Compression: Wrap the injured area with an elastic or compression bandage between icings. If the area starts throbbing or begins to change color, the bandage may be wrapped too tightly. Do not sleep with the wrap on.

Elevation: Raise the injured area above heart level to decrease the blood supply and reduce swelling.

After about 36–48 hours, apply heat if the swelling has completely disappeared to help relieve pain, relax muscles, and reduce stiffness. Immerse the affected area in warm water or apply warm compresses, a hot water bottle, or a heating pad.

To prevent injuries in the future, follow a few basic guidelines:

1. Stay in condition; haphazard exercise programs invite injury.

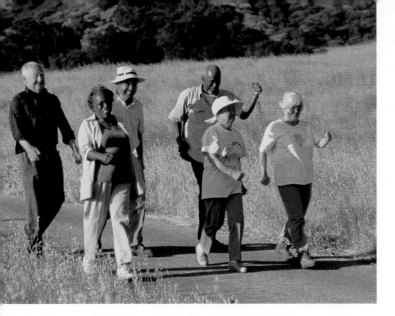

It makes sense to choose activities that will add enjoyment to your life for years to come. In this group of older people, we can see the rewards of a lifetime of fitness and smart exercise habits.

2. Warm up thoroughly before exercise.

3. Use proper body mechanics when lifting objects or executing sports skills.

4. Don't exercise when you're ill or overtrained (experiencing extreme fatigue due to overexercising).

5. Use the proper equipment.

6. Don't return to your normal exercise program until athletic injuries have healed.

Staying with Your Program Once you have attained your desired level of fitness, you can maintain it by exercising regularly at a consistent intensity, three to five times a week. In general, if you exercise at the same intensity over a long period, your fitness will level out and can be maintained easily.

What if you run out of steam? Although good health is an important *reason* to exercise, it's a poor *motivator* for consistent adherence to an exercise program. It's a good idea to have a meaningful goal, anything from fitting into the same-size jeans you used to wear to successfully skiing down a new slope; just make sure your goals are realistic. Signing a contract, exercising with a friend, and giving yourself frequent rewards are additional strategies.

Varying your program is another key strategy. Some people alternate two or more activities—swimming and jogging, for example—to improve a particular component of fitness. The practice, called **cross-training**, can help prevent boredom and overuse injuries. Explore many exercise options, and try new activities, especially ones that you will

Terms   **cross-training** Participating in two or more activities to develop a particular component of fitness.

be able to do for the rest of your life. Every step you take will bring you closer to your ultimate goal—fitness and wellness that last a lifetime.

Tips for Today

Physical activity and exercise offer benefits in nearly every area of wellness, helping you generate energy, manage stress, control your weight, improve your mood, and, of course, become physically stronger and healthier. Building a program of regular exercise into your life is well worth the effort, even if it seems complicated or difficult at first. Even a low-to-moderate level of activity provides valuable health benefits. The important thing is to get moving.

Right now you can

- Get up and stretch.

- Go outside and take a brisk walk.

- Look at your calendar for the rest of the week and write in some physical activity—such as walking, running, biking, skating, swimming, hiking, or playing Frisbee—on as many days as you can; schedule the activity for a specific time, and stick to it.

- If you don't yet use the gym or fitness facility on your campus, go there now and begin planning how to use it.

- Call a friend and invite him or her to start a regular exercise program with you.

SUMMARY

- The five components of physical fitness most important to health are cardiorespiratory endurance, muscular strength, muscular endurance, flexibility, and body composition.

- Exercise improves the functioning of the heart and the ability of the cardiorespiratory system to carry oxygen to the body's tissues. It also increases the efficiency of the body's metabolism and improves body composition.

- Exercise lowers the risk of cardiovascular disease, cancer, osteoporosis, and diabetes. It improves immune function and psychological health and helps prevent injuries and low-back pain.

- Everyone should accumulate at least 30 minutes per day of moderate endurance-type physical activity. Additional health and fitness benefits can be achieved through longer or more vigorous activity.

- Cardiorespiratory endurance exercises stress a large portion of the body's muscle mass. Endurance exercise should be performed 3–5 days per week for a total of 20–60 minutes per day. Intensity can be evaluated by measuring the heart rate.

Although most people recognize the importance of incorporating exercise into their lives, many find it difficult to do. No single strategy will work for everyone, but the general steps outlined here should help you create an exercise program that fits your goals, preferences, and lifestyle. A carefully designed contract and program plan can help you convert your vague wishes into a detailed plan of action.

Step 1: Set Goals

Setting specific goals to accomplish by exercising is an important first step in a successful fitness program because it establishes the direction you want to take. Your goals might be specifically related to health, such as lowering your blood pressure and risk of heart disease, or they might relate to other aspects of your life, such as improving your tennis game or the fit of your clothes. If you can decide why you're starting to exercise, it can help you keep going.

Think carefully about your reasons for incorporating exercise into your life, and then fill in the goals portion of the fitness contract in Wellness Worksheet 10 (see the Study Guide).

Step 2: Select Activities

As discussed in the chapter, the success of your fitness program depends on the consistency of your involvement. Select activities that encourage your commitment: The right program will be its own incentive to continue; poor activity choices create obstacles and can turn exercise into a chore.

When choosing activities for your fitness program, consider the following:

- Is this activity fun? Will it hold my interest over time?

- Will this activity help me reach the goals I have set?

- Will my current fitness and skill level enable me to participate fully in this activity?

- Can I easily fit this activity into my daily schedule? Are there any special requirements (facilities, partners, equipment, etc.) that I must plan for?

- Can I afford any special costs required for equipment or facilities?

- (If you have special exercise needs due to a particular health problem.) Does this activity conform to my special health needs? Will it enhance my ability to cope with my specific health problem?

Using the guidelines listed above, select a number of sports and activities. Fill in the program plan portion of the fitness contract.

Step 3: Make a Commitment

Complete your fitness contract by signing it and having it witnessed and signed by someone who can help make you accountable for your progress. By completing a written contract, you will make a firm commitment and will be more likely to follow through until you meet your goals.

Step 4: Begin and Maintain Your Program

Start out slowly to allow your body time to adjust. Be realistic and patient—meeting your goals will take time. The following guidelines may help you start and stick with your program:

- Set aside regular periods for exercise. Choose times that fit in best with your schedule, and stick to them. Allow an adequate amount of time for warm-up, cool-down, and a shower.

- Take advantage of any opportunity for exercise that presents itself (for example, walk to class).

- Do what you can to avoid boredom. Do stretching exercises or jumping jacks to music, or watch the evening news while riding your stationary bicycle.

- Exercise with a group that shares your goals and general level of competence.

- Vary the program. Change your activities periodically. Alter your route or distance if biking or jogging. Change racquetball partners, or find a new volleyball court.

Step 5: Record and Assess Your Progress

Keeping a record that notes the daily results of your program will help remind you of your ongoing commitment to your program and give you a sense of accomplishment. Create daily and weekly program logs that you can use to track your progress. Record the activity type, frequency, and duration. Keep your log handy, and fill it in immediately after each exercise session. Post it in a visible place to remind you of your activity schedule and provide incentive for improvement.

SOURCE: Adapted from Kusinitz, I., and M. Fine. 1995. *Your Guide to Getting Fit,* 3rd ed. Mountain View, Calif.: Mayfield.

- Warming up before exercising and cooling down afterward improve your performance and decrease your chances of injury.

- Exercises that develop muscular strength and endurance involve exerting force against a significant resistance. A strength training program for general fitness typically involves 1 set of 8–12 repetitions of 8–10 exercises, 2–3 days per week.

- A good flexibility program includes exercises for all the major muscle groups and joints of the body. A

series of active, static stretches should be done 2 or more days per week; each stretch should be held for 10–30 seconds and repeated at least 4 times.

- A well-balanced diet contains all the energy and nutrients needed to sustain a fitness program; remember to drink enough fluids.

- Rest, ice, compression, and elevation (R-I-C-E) are the appropriate treatments for many injuries.

1. Go to your school's physical education office and ask for a listing of all the exercise and fitness facilities available on your campus. Visit the facilities, and investigate the activities that are done there. If there are activities you'd like to try, consider doing so.

2. Investigate the fitness clubs in your community. How do they compare with each other? How do they measure up in terms of the guidelines provided in this chapter?

WW. JOURNAL ENTRY

1. In your health journal, list the positive behaviors and attitudes that help you avoid a sedentary lifestyle and stay fit. How can you strengthen these behaviors and attitudes? Then list the negative behaviors and attitudes that block a physically active lifestyle. Which ones can you change? How can you change them?

2. Habit helps us conserve energy as we go through our daily lives, but it also blinds us to areas we could change. Make a list of ten ways you can incorporate more physical activity into your life by changing a habit, such

as walking instead of riding the bus, taking the stairs in a certain building instead of the elevator, and so on.

3. *Critical Thinking* Study the ads for fitness products and clubs on television, in popular magazines, and in your local newspaper. What markets are they targeting? How do they try to appeal to their audience? What other messages are they sending? Write a short essay describing your findings.

FOR MORE INFORMATION

Books

Anderson, B., and J. Anderson. 2000. *Stretching,* 20th anniv. ed. Bolinas, Calif.: Shelter Publications. *Updated edition of a classic, with more than 200 stretches for 60 sports and activities.*

Fahey, T. 2000. *Basic Weight Training for Men and Women,* 4th ed. Mountain View, Calif.: Mayfield. *A practical guide to developing training programs tailored to individual needs.*

Fahey, T., P. Insel, and W. Roth. 2001. *Fit and Well: Core Concepts and Labs in Physical Fitness and Wellness,* 4th ed. Mountain View, Calif.: Mayfield. *A comprehensive guide to developing a complete fitness program.*

Nieman, D. C. 1999. *Exercise Testing and Prescription. A Health-Related Approach,* 4th ed. Mountain View, Calif.: Mayfield. *A comprehensive discussion of the effects of exercise and exercise testing and prescription.*

U.S. Department of Health and Human Services. 1996. *Physical Activity and Health: A Report of the Surgeon General.* Atlanta: Department of Health and Human Services. (Also available online: http://www.cdc.gov/nccdphp/sgr/sgr.htm.) *Provides a summary of the evidence for the benefits of physical activity as well as recommendations for activity and exercise.*

WW. Organizations, Hotlines, and Web Sites

American College of Sports Medicine. Provides brochures, publications, and audio- and videotapes on the positive effects of exercise.
317-637-9200
http://www.acsm.org

American Council on Exercise. Promotes exercise and fitness for all Americans; the Web site features fact sheets on many consumer

topics, including choosing shoes, cross-training, steroids, and getting started on an exercise program.
800-529-8227
http://www.acefitness.org

American Heart Association: Just Move. Provides practical advice for people of all fitness levels plus an online fitness diary.
http://www.justmove.org

Canada's Physical Activity Guide. Offers many suggestions for increasing physical activity; also includes the Physical Activity Readiness Questionnaire (PAR-Q) to assess safety of exercise.
http://www.hc-sc.gc.c2/hppb/paguide

Disabled Sports USA. Provides sport and recreation services to people with physical or mobility disorders.
http://www.dsusa.org

Exercise: A Guide from the National Institute on Aging and the National Aeronautics and Space Administration. Provides practical advice on fitness for seniors; includes animated instructions for specific weight training and flexibility exercises.
http://weboflife.arc.nasa.gov/exerciseandaging/index.html

Georgia State University: Exercise and Physical Fitness Page. Provides information about the benefits of exercise and how to get started on a fitness program.
http://www.gsu.edu/~wwwfit

National Institute on Drug Abuse: Anabolic Steroid Abuse. Provides information and links about the dangers of anabolic steroids.
http://www.steroidabuse.org

Shape Up America! Fitness Center. Includes fitness assessments, information on the benefits of exercise, tips for overcoming barriers, and tracking forms.
http://shapeup.org/fitness

Strong Women. Provides practical fitness advice for women, including sample programs and training tips.

http://www.strongwomen.com

Workout.Com. A commercial site that includes a wide variety of illustrated exercises and fitness programs.

http://www.workout.com

Information on many specific sports, activities, and fitness issues is available on the Web; use the following sites that provide many links or use a search engine to locate appropriate sites.

Fitness Find

http://www.fitnessfind.com

Fitness Link

http://www.fitnesslink.com

Fitness Partner Connection Jumpsite

http://www.primusweb.com/fitnesspartner

NetSweat: The Internet's Fitness Resource

http://www.sickbay.com/netsweat

Yahoo! Recreation and Sports

http://dir.yahoo.com/recreation/sports

See also the listings for Chapters 9, 11, and 12.

SELECTED BIBLIOGRAPHY

Andersen, L. B., et al. 2000. All-cause mortality associated with physical activity during leisure time, work, sports, and cycling to work. *Archives of Internal Medicine* 160(11): 1621–1628.

Babyak, M., et al. 2000. Exercise treatment for major depression: Maintenance of therapeutic benefit at 10 months. *Psychosomatic Medicine* 62(5): 633–638.

Boutelle, K. N., et al. 2000. Associations between exercise and health behaviors in a community sample of working adults. *Preventive Medicine* 30(3): 217–224.

Brooks, G. A., et al. 2000. *Exercise Physiology: Human Bioenergetics and Its Applications,* 3rd ed. Mountain View, Calif.: Mayfield.

Centers for Disease Control and Prevention. 2000. Compliance with physical activity recommendations by walking for exercise. *Morbidity and Mortality Weekly Report* 49(25): 560–565.

Centers for Disease Control and Prevention. 2001. Physical activity trends—United States, 1990–1998. *Morbidity and Mortality Weekly Report* 50(9): 166–169.

Centers for Disease Control and Prevention. 2001. Prevalence of disabilities and associated health conditions among adults—United States, 1999. *Morbidity and Mortality Weekly Report* 50(7): 120–125.

Daley, M. J., and W. L. Spinks. 2000. Exercise, mobility and aging. *Sports Medicine* 29(1): 1–12.

Fahey, T., P. Insel, and W. Roth. 2001. *Fit and Well: Core Concepts and Labs in Physical Fitness and Wellness,* 4th ed. Mountain View, Calif.: Mayfield.

Galloway, M. T., and P. Jolk. 2000. Aging successfully: The importance of physical activity in maintaining health and function. *Journal of the American Academy of Orthopaedic Surgeons* 8(1): 37–44.

Geffken, D. F., et al. 2001. Association between physical activity and markers of inflammation in a healthy elderly population. *American Journal of Epidemiology* 153(3): 242–250.

Hu, F. B., et al. 2000. Physical activity and risk of stroke in women. *Journal of the American Medical Association* 283(22): 2961–2967.

Jakes, R. W., et al. 2001. Patterns of physical activity and ultrasound attenuation by heel bone among Norfolk cohort of European Prospective Investigation of Cancer (EPIC Norfolk). *British Medical Journal* 322: 140.

Kriketos, A. D., et al. 2000. Effects of aerobic fitness on fat oxidation and body fatness. *Medicine and Science in Sports and Exercise* 32(4): 805–811.

Lakka, T. A., et al. 2001. Cardiorespiratory fitness and the progression of carotid atherosclerosis in middle-aged men. *Annals of Internal Medicine* 134(1): 12–20.

Laukkanen, J. A., et al. 2001. Cardiovascular fitness as a predictor of mortality in men. *Archives of Internal Medicine* 161(6): 825–831.

Lee, I. M., and R. S. Paffenbarger. 2000. Associations of light, moderate, and vigorous intensity physical activity with longevity. The Harvard Alumni Health Study. *American Journal of Epidemiology* 151(3): 293–299.

McAuley, E., et al. 2000. Physical activity, self-esteem, and self-efficacy relationships in older adults: A randomized controlled trial. *Annals of Behavioral Medicine* 22(2): 131–139.

National Institute on Drug Abuse. 2001. *Steroids (Anabolic-Androgenic)* (http://www.drugabuse.gov/Infofax/steroids.html; retrieved April 16, 2001).

Paluska, S. A., and T. L. Schwenk. 2000. Physical activity and mental health: Current concepts. *Sports Medicine* 29(3): 167–180.

Pollock, M. L., et al. 2000. AHA Science Advisory. Resistance exercise in individuals with and without cardiovascular disease: Benefits, rationale, safety, and prescription. *Circulation* 101(7): 828–833.

Sader, M. A., et al. 2001. Androgenic anabolic steroids and arterial structure and function in male bodybuilders. *Journal of the American College of Cardiology* 37(1): 224–230.

Salmon, P. 2001. Effects of physical exercise on anxiety, depression, and sensitivity to stress. *Clinical Psychology Review* 21(1): 33–61.

Stampfer, M. J., et al. 2000. Primary prevention of coronary heart disease in women through diet and lifestyle. *New England Journal of Medicine* 343(1): 16–22.

Tanji, J. L. 2000. The benefits of exercise for women. *Clinics in Sports Medicine* 19(2): 175–185, vii.

University of Florida News. 2001. *Study: Sports Participation Has Mental Perks for All* (http://www.napa.ufl.edu/2001news/bodyimag.htm; retrieved April 19, 2001).

Wallace, L. S., et al. 2000. Characteristics of exercise behavior among college students: Application of social cognitive theory to predicting stage of change. *Preventive Medicine* 31(5): 494–505.

Weight Management

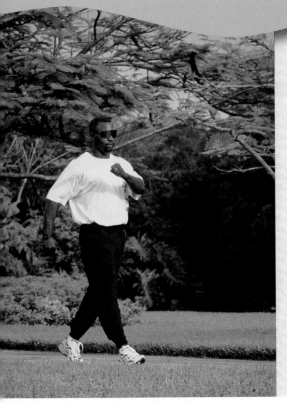

LOOKING AHEAD

After reading this chapter, you should be able to

- Discuss different methods for assessing body weight and body composition

- Explain the health risks associated with overweight and obesity

- Explain factors that may contribute to a weight problem, including genetic, physiological, lifestyle, and psychosocial factors

- Describe lifestyle factors that contribute to weight gain and loss, including the role of diet, exercise, and emotional factors

- Identify and describe the symptoms of eating disorders and the health risks associated with them

- Design a personal plan for successfully managing body weight

Achieving and maintaining a healthy body weight is a serious public health challenge in the United States and a source of distress for many Americans. Under standards developed by the National Institutes of Health, about 60% of American adults are overweight, including more than 20% who are obese (Table 11-1). And while millions struggle to lose weight, others fall into dangerous eating patterns such as binge eating or self-starvation.

Although not completely understood, managing body weight is not a mysterious process. The "secret" is balancing calories consumed with calories expended in daily activities—in other words, eating a moderate diet and exercising regularly. This chapter takes a closer look at weight management through lifestyle and suggests specific strategies for reaching and maintaining a healthy weight.

BASIC CONCEPTS OF WEIGHT MANAGEMENT

How many times have you or one of your friends said, "I'm too fat. I need to lose weight"? If you are like most people, you are concerned about what you weigh. But how do you decide if your weight is healthy? How heavy is too heavy, and how thin is too thin?

Body Composition

The human body can be divided into fat-free mass and body fat. Fat-free mass is composed of all the body's nonfat tissues: bone, water, muscle, connective tissue, organ tissues, and teeth. Body fat includes both essential and nonessential body fat. **Essential fat** includes lipids incorporated in the nerves and organs. These fat deposits, crucial for normal

Terms

essential fat The fat in the body necessary for normal body functioning.

nonessential (storage) fat Extra fat or fat reserves stored in the body.

percent body fat The percentage of total body weight that is composed of fat.

Overweight and obesity are epidemic in the United States. More than half of all adults are overweight and nearly a quarter are obese. The rate of obesity has nearly doubled since 1960, and it continues to rise. If current rates of weight gain continue, *all* American adults will be overweight by 2030. The health problems associated with overweight have also increased, including a 33% rise in the rate of diabetes in just the past decade. It's estimated that inactivity and overweight account for more than 300,000 premature deaths annually in the United States, second only to tobacco-related deaths.

At the same time that Americans are getting fatter, more and more of them are becoming unhappy with their bodies. In recent surveys, more than half of Americans have stated that they are dissatisfied with their weight, and only about 10% report being completely satisfied with their bodies. Dissatisfaction with body weight and shape is at the core of eating disorders, including anorexia, bulimia, and binge eating. Rising levels of overweight accompanied by increased body dissatisfaction have led to an increase in dieting. In surveys, about 30% of adult males and 55% of adult females report having tried to lose weight within the past year; the rate of dieting among adolescent girls and female college students is even higher.

Healthy People 2010 sets the goal of decreasing the number of people who are obese to no more than 15% of adults and 5% of children and adolescents. Despite widespread dieting, however, the trend has definitely been away from this goal, and many Americans appear to be losing the battle to manage their weight. At the root of the problem is energy balance: Americans currently consume about 160 more calories per day than they did 20 years ago, and they engage in less physical activity. Some of the factors that help explain this shift include the following:

- More meals eaten outside the home
- Increased portion sizes
- Increased consumption of soft drinks, fast food, and convenience foods
- More time spent in sedentary activities
- Greater numbers of labor-saving devices
- Fewer daily gym classes for children and adolescents
- Fewer short trips on foot and more by automobile

Public health officials have called for the development of a comprehensive national plan to address the obesity epidemic, one that targets both behavior and environment. Goals include preventing weight gain in adults who are at a healthy weight or who are overweight, promoting weight loss for the obese, and increasing physical activity for Americans of all ages. Proposed strategies include government subsidies for fruits and vegetables and a "sin tax" on high-calorie foods, with the proceeds going to create bike paths, parks, and other facilities that promote physical activity. As officials debate different solutions, there are many actions that individuals can take. At the 2000 National Nutrition Summit, Secretary of Health and Human Services Donna Shalala stressed the importance of good nutrition and exercise and challenged everyone to turn off the television and get off the couch.

---

body functioning, make up about 3% of total body weight in men and 12% in women. The larger percentage in women is due to fat deposits in the breasts, uterus, and other sites specific to females. **Nonessential (storage) fat** exists primarily within fat cells, or *adipose tissue,* often located just below the skin and around major organs. The amount of storage fat varies from person to person based on many factors, including gender, age, heredity, metabolism, diet, and activity level. When we talk about wanting to "lose weight," most of us are referring to storage fat.

What is most important for health is not total weight but rather the proportion of the body's total weight that is fat—the **percent body fat.** For example, two women may both be 5 feet, 5 inches tall and weigh 130 pounds. But one woman, an endurance runner, may have only 15% of her body weight as fat, while the second, sedentary, woman could have 32% body fat. While 130 pounds is not considered "overweight" for women of this height by most standards, the second woman may be overfat. Since most people use the word "overweight" to describe the condition of having too much body fat, we will use it in this chapter, although "overfat" is actually a more accurate term.

VITAL STATISTICS

Table 11-1	The Prevalence of Obesity: Populations of Special Concern		

Group	Estimated Prevalence of Obesity*	Healthy People 2010 Target
Children (age 6–11)	11%	5%
Adolescents (age 12–19)	10	5
Adults (age 20–74)	23	15
Men	20	15
Women	25	15
Low-income people	29	15
People with disabilities	30	15
Black women	38	15
Mexican American women	35	15

*Children and adolescents are classified as obese if they have a BMI at or above the appropriate 95th percentile for body mass index (BMI); adults are classified as obese if they have a BMI of 30 or above.

SOURCE: U.S. Department of Health and Human Services. 2000. *Healthy People 2010,* 2nd ed. Washington, D.C.: DHHS.

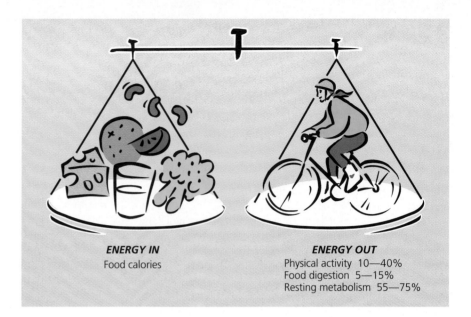

Figure 11-1 The energy balance equation. In order to maintain your current weight, you must burn up as many calories as you take in as food each day.

ENERGY IN
Food calories

ENERGY OUT
Physical activity 10—40%
Food digestion 5—15%
Resting metabolism 55—75%

Energy Balance

The key to keeping a healthy ratio of fat to fat-free mass is maintaining an energy balance (Figure 11-1). You take in energy (calories) from the food you eat. Your body uses energy (calories) to maintain vital body functions (resting metabolism), to digest food, and to fuel physical activity. When energy in equals energy out, you maintain your current weight. To change your weight and body composition, you must tip the energy balance equation in a particular direction. If you take in more calories daily than your body burns, the excess calories will be stored as fat, and you will gain weight over time. If you eat fewer calories than you burn each day, you will lose some of that storage fat and probably lose weight.

The two parts of the energy balance equation over which you have the most control are the energy you take in as food and the energy you burn during physical activity. To lose weight and body fat, you can increase the amount of energy you burn by increasing your level of physical activity and/or decrease the amount of energy you take in by consuming fewer calories.

Terms

overweight Body weight that falls above the range associated with minimum mortality.

obesity The condition of having an excess of nonessential body fat; having a body mass index of 30 or greater or having a percent body fat greater than 24% for men and 31% for women.

body mass index (BMI) A measure of relative body weight that takes height into account and is highly correlated with more direct measures of body fat; calculated by dividing total body weight (in kilograms) by the square of height (in meters).

Evaluating Body Weight and Body Composition

Overweight is usually defined as total body weight above the recommended range for good health (as determined by large-scale population surveys). **Obesity** is defined as a more serious degree of overweight. Many methods are available for measuring and evaluating body weight and percent body fat.

Height-Weight Charts In the past, many people relied on height-weight charts to evaluate their body weight. Based on insurance company statistics, these list a range of "ideal" or "recommended" body weights associated with the lowest mortality for people of a particular sex, age, and height. Although easy to use, height-weight charts can be highly inaccurate for some people, and they provide only an indirect measure of body fatness.

Body Mass Index Although also based on the concept that a person's weight should be proportional to height, **body mass index (BMI)** is a more accurate assessment method than height-weight charts. BMI is defined as body weight (in kilograms) divided by the square of height (in meters); you can determine your BMI by referring to Figure 11-2. Under standards issued by the National Institutes of Health, a BMI between 18.5 and 24.9 is considered healthy; a person with a BMI of 25 or above is classified as overweight; and a person with a BMI of 30 or above is classified as obese. A person with a BMI below 18.5 is classified as underweight, although low BMI values may be healthy in some cases if they are not the result of smoking, an eating disorder, or an underlying disease; a BMI value of 17.5 or less is sometimes used as a diagnostic criterion for anorexia nervosa.

	<18.5 Underweight		18.5–24.9 Normal						25–29.9 Overweight					30–34.9 Obesity (Class I)					35–39.9 Obesity (Class II)					≥40 Extreme obesity
BMI	17	18	19	20	21	22	23	24	25	26	27	28	29	30	31	32	33	34	35	36	37	38	39	40
Height											Body Weight (pounds)													
4' 10"	81	86	91	96	101	105	110	115	120	124	129	134	139	144	148	153	158	163	168	172	177	182	187	192
4' 11"	84	89	94	99	104	109	114	119	124	129	134	139	144	149	154	159	163	168	173	178	183	188	193	198
5'	87	92	97	102	108	113	118	123	128	133	138	143	149	154	159	164	169	174	179	184	190	195	200	205
5' 1"	90	95	101	106	111	117	122	127	132	138	143	148	154	159	164	169	175	180	185	191	196	201	207	212
5' 2"	93	98	104	109	115	120	126	131	137	142	148	153	159	164	170	175	181	186	191	197	202	208	213	219
5' 3"	96	102	107	113	119	124	130	136	141	147	153	158	164	169	175	181	186	192	198	203	209	215	220	226
5' 4"	99	105	111	117	122	128	134	140	146	152	157	163	169	175	181	187	192	198	204	210	216	222	227	233
5' 5"	102	108	114	120	126	132	138	144	150	156	162	168	174	180	186	192	198	204	210	216	222	229	235	241
5' 6"	105	112	118	124	130	136	143	149	155	161	167	174	180	186	192	198	205	211	217	223	229	236	242	248
5' 7"	109	115	121	128	134	141	147	153	160	166	173	179	185	192	198	204	211	217	224	230	236	243	249	256
5' 8"	112	118	125	132	138	145	151	158	165	171	178	184	191	197	204	211	217	224	230	237	244	250	257	263
5' 9"	115	122	129	136	142	149	156	163	169	176	183	190	197	203	210	217	224	230	237	244	251	258	264	271
5' 10"	119	126	133	139	146	153	160	167	174	181	188	195	202	209	216	223	230	237	244	251	258	265	272	279
5' 11"	122	129	136	143	151	158	165	172	179	187	194	201	208	215	222	230	237	244	251	258	265	273	280	287
6'	125	133	140	148	155	162	170	177	184	192	199	207	214	221	229	236	243	251	258	266	273	280	288	295
6' 1"	129	137	144	152	159	167	174	182	190	197	205	212	220	228	235	243	250	258	265	273	281	288	296	303
6' 2"	132	140	148	156	164	171	179	187	195	203	210	218	226	234	242	249	257	265	273	281	288	296	304	312
6' 3"	136	144	152	160	168	176	184	192	200	208	216	224	232	240	248	256	264	272	280	288	296	304	312	320
6' 4"	140	148	156	164	173	181	189	197	206	214	222	230	238	247	255	263	271	280	288	296	304	312	321	329

Figure 11-2 Body mass index (BMI). To determine your BMI, find your height in the left column. Move across the appropriate row until you find the weight closest to your own. The number at the top of the column is the BMI at that height and weight.   SOURCE: Ratings from National Heart, Lung, and Blood Institute. 1998. *Clinical Guidelines on the Identification, Evaluation, and Treatment of Overweight and Obesity in Adults: The Evidence Report.* Bethesda, Md.: National Institutes of Health.

Body Composition Analysis   The most accurate and direct way to evaluate body composition is to determine percent body fat; a variety of methods are available. Refer to Table 11-2 for body composition ratings based on percent body fat.

• Hydrostatic (underwater) weighing. One of the most accurate techniques is hydrostatic weighing, in which a person is submerged and weighed under water. Muscle has a higher density and fat a lower density than water, so people with more fat tend to float and weigh less under water, while lean people tend to sink and weigh relatively more under water.

• Skinfold measurements. The skinfold thickness technique measures the thickness of fat under the skin. A technician grasps a fold of skin at a predetermined location and measures it using an instrument called a caliper. Measurements are taken at several sites and plugged into formulas that predict body fat percentages.

• Electrical impedance analysis. In this method, electrodes are attached to the body and a harmless electrical current is transmitted from electrode to electrode. A computer can calculate fat percentages from current measurements.

Table 11-2	Percent Body Fat Standards for Men and Women	
	Men	Women
At risk[a]	≤5%	≤8%
Below average	6–14	9–22
Average	15	23
Above average	16–24	24–31
At risk[b]	≥25	≥32

[a]At risk for diseases and disorders associated with malnutrition
[b]At risk for diseases associated with obesity

Note: These percentages represent approximate standards for body composition; percent body fat associated with good health varies, depending on health status and risk factors for disease. For example, a man with high blood pressure and high cholesterol levels might want to reduce his percentage of body fat, even if it is average for the general population.

SOURCE: Heyward, V. H. 1998. *Advanced Fitness Assessment and Exercise Prescription.* Champaign, Ill.: Human Kinetics.

Excess Body Fat and Wellness

The amount of fat in the body—and its location—can have profound effects on health.

Symptoms of diabetes:

• Frequent urination

• Extreme thirst and hunger

• Unexplained weight loss

• Extreme fatigue

• Blurred vision

• Frequent infections

• Slow wound healing

• Tingling or numbness inhands and feet

• Dry, itchy skin

Note: In the early stages, diabetes often has no symptoms.

Esophagus

Stomach

Pancreas

Small intestine

Normal:
Insulin binds to receptors on the surface of a cell and signals special transporters in the cell to transport glucose inside.

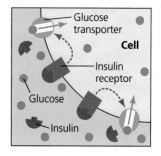

Glucose transporter

Cell

Insulin receptor

Glucose

Insulin

Type 1 diabetes:
The pancreas produces little or no insulin. Thus, no signal is sent instructing the cell to transport glucose, and glucose builds up in the bloodstream.

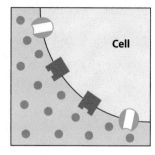

Cell

Type 2 diabetes:
The pancreas produces too little insulin and/or the body's cells are resistant to it. Some insulin binds to receptors on the cell's surface, but the signal to transport glucose is blocked. Glucose builds up in the bloodstream.

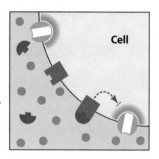

Cell

Figure 11-3 Diabetes mellitus. During digestion, carbohydrates are broken down in the small intestine into glucose, a simple sugar that enters the bloodstream. The presence of glucose signals the pancreas to release insulin, a hormone that helps cells take up glucose; once inside a cell, glucose can be converted to energy. In diabetes, this process is disrupted, resulting in a buildup of glucose in the bloodstream.

The Health Risks of Excess Body Fat Obese people have an overall mortality rate almost twice that of non-obese people. Obesity is associated with unhealthy cholesterol and triglyceride levels, impaired heart function, and death from cardiovascular disease. Other health risks associated with obesity include hypertension, many kinds of cancer, impaired immune function, gallbladder and kidney diseases, skin problems, sleep disorders, arthritis, and other bone and joint disorders.

Of particular note is the strong association between excess body fat and diabetes mellitus, a disease that causes a disruption of normal metabolism. The pancreas, a long, thin organ located behind the stomach, normally secretes the hormone insulin, which stimulates cells to take up glucose to produce energy (Figure 11-3). In a person with diabetes, this process is disrupted, causing a buildup of glucose in the bloodstream. Over the long term, diabetes is associated with kidney failure; nerve damage; circula-tion problems; retinal damage and blindness; and increased rates of heart attack, stroke, and hypertension.

The risks from obesity increase with its severity, and they are much more likely to occur in people who are more than twice their desirable body weight. The National Institutes of Health recommends weight loss for people whose BMI places them in the obese category and for those who are overweight *and* have two or more major risk factors for disease such as tobacco use and high blood pressure. If your BMI is 25 or above, consult a physician for help in determining a healthy BMI for you.

Obesity can affect psychological as well as physical wellness. Being perceived as fat can be a source of ridicule, ostracism, and sometimes discrimination from others; it can contribute to psychological problems such as depression, anxiety, and low self-esteem. For some, the stigma associated with obesity can give rise to a negative body image, body dissatisfaction, and eating disorders.

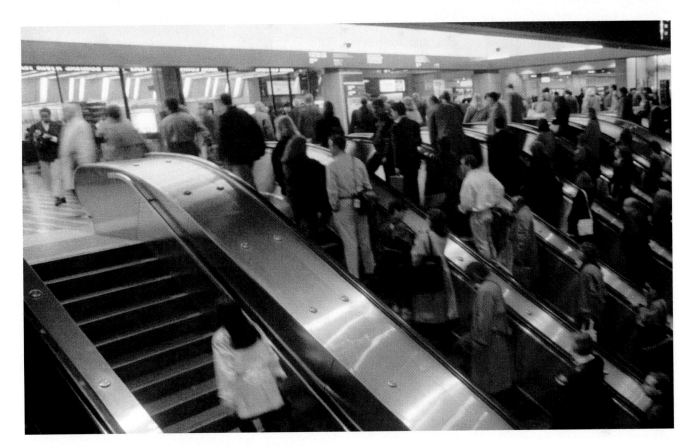

The typical American lifestyle does not lead naturally to healthy weight management. Labor-saving technology helps reinforce our sedentary habits.

maintain vital body functions, including respiration, heart rate, body temperature, and blood pressure, while the body is at rest. As shown in Figure 11-1, RMR accounts for 55–75% of daily energy expenditure. The energy required to digest food accounts for an additional 5–15% of daily energy expenditure. The remaining 10–40% is expended during physical activity.

Both heredity and behavior affect metabolic rate. Men, who have a higher proportion of muscle mass than women, have a higher RMR (muscle tissue is more metabolically active than fat). Also, some individuals inherit a higher or lower RMR than others. A higher RMR means that a person burns more calories while at rest and can therefore take in more calories without gaining weight.

Weight loss or gain also affects metabolic rate. When a person loses weight, both RMR and the energy required to perform physical tasks decrease. The reverse occurs when weight is gained. Exercise has a positive effect on metabolism. When people exercise, they slightly increase their RMR—the number of calories their bodies burn at rest. They also increase their muscle mass, which is associated with a higher metabolic rate. The exercise itself also burns calories, raising total energy expenditure. The higher the energy expenditure, the more the person can eat without gaining weight.

Lifestyle Factors

While genes and metabolism may increase risk for excess body fat, they are not sufficient to explain the increasingly high rate of obesity seen in the United States. The gene pool has not changed dramatically in the past 40 years, during which time the rate of obesity among Americans has doubled. Clearly, other factors are at work—particularly lifestyle factors such as increased energy intake and decreased physical activity.

Eating Americans have access to an abundance of highly palatable and calorie-dense foods, and many have eating habits that contribute to weight gain. Most overweight adults will admit to eating more than they should

female athlete triad A condition consisting of three interrelated disorders: abnormal eating patterns (and excessive exercising) followed by lack of menstrual periods (amenorrhea) and decreased bone density (premature osteoporosis).

amenorrhea The absence of menstruation.

resting metabolic rate (RMR) The energy required to maintain vital body functions, including respiration, heart rate, body temperature, and blood pressure, while the body is at rest.

Terms

of high-fat, high-sugar, high-calorie foods. Americans eat out more frequently now than in the past, and we rely more heavily on fast food and packaged convenience foods. Restaurant and convenience food portion sizes tend to be very large, and the foods themselves are more likely to be high in fat, sugar, and calories and low in nutrients. Studies have consistently found that people underestimate portion sizes by as much as 25%.

Physical Activity   Activity levels among Americans are declining, beginning in childhood and continuing throughout the life cycle. Most adults drive to work, sit all day, and then relax in front of the TV at night. During leisure time, both children and adults surf the Internet, play video games, or watch TV rather than bike, participate in sports, or just do yardwork or chores around the house. On average, Americans exercise 15 minutes per day and watch 150 minutes of TV. Modern conveniences such as remote controls, elevators, and power mowers have also reduced daily physical activity.

Psychosocial Factors

Many people have learned to use food as a means of coping with stress and negative emotions. Eating can provide a powerful distraction from difficult feelings—loneliness, anger, boredom, anxiety, shame, sadness, inadequacy. It can be used to combat low moods, low energy levels, and low self-esteem. When food and eating become the primary means of regulating emotions, binge eating or other disturbed eating patterns can develop.

Obesity is strongly associated with socioeconomic status. The prevalence of obesity goes down as income level goes up. More women are obese at lower income levels than men, but men are somewhat more obese at higher levels. These differences may reflect the greater sensitivity and concern for a slim physical appearance among upper-income women, as well as greater access to information about nutrition and to low-fat and low-calorie foods. It may also reflect the greater acceptance of obesity among certain ethnic groups, as well as different cultural values related to food choices.

In some families and cultures, food is used as a symbol of love and caring. It is an integral part of social gatherings and celebrations. In such cases, it may be difficult to change established eating patterns because they are linked to cultural and family values.

COMMUNICATE!   When food is intertwined with cultural and social meanings, such as at a company picnic, a wedding banquet, or a holiday party, we often feel pressured to eat more than we need or even want. If you have such an event on your calendar, think ahead about how you can make healthy choices without breaking social norms. For example, instead of accepting seconds and thirds at Thanksgiving dinner, you could say simply, "Everything tastes wonderful, but I'm full!" If you're pressed, try saying, "Maybe I could take a piece of pie home with me for tomorrow."

ADOPTING A HEALTHY LIFESTYLE FOR SUCCESSFUL WEIGHT MANAGEMENT

Permanent weight loss is not something you start and stop. You need to adopt healthy behaviors that you can maintain throughout your life.

Diet and Eating Habits

In contrast to "dieting," which involves some form of food restriction, "diet" refers to your daily food choices. Everyone has a diet, but not everyone is dieting. You need to develop a diet that you enjoy and that enables you to maintain a healthy body composition. Use the Food Guide Pyramid as the basis for planning a healthy diet (see Chapter 9). For weight management, you may need to pay special attention to total calories, portion sizes, energy density, fat and sugar intake, and eating habits.

Total Calories   The Food Guide Pyramid suggests the following approximate daily energy intakes:

- 1600 calories: Many sedentary women and some older adults
- 2200 calories: Most children, teenage girls, active women, and many sedentary men
- 2800 calories: Teenage boys, many active men, and some very active women

However, energy balance may be a more important consideration for weight management than total calories consumed (see Figure 11-1). To maintain your current weight, the total number of calories you eat must equal the number you burn. To lose weight, you must decrease your calorie intake and/or increase the number of calories you burn; to gain weight, the reverse is true. The best approach for weight loss is combining an increase in physical activity with moderate calorie restriction. Don't go on a "crash diet." You need to adopt a level of food intake that provides all the essential nutrients and that you can live with over the long term.

Portion Sizes   Overconsumption of total calories is closely tied to portion sizes. Most of us significantly underestimate the amount of food we eat. Limiting portion sizes to those recommended in the Food Guide Pyramid is critical for maintaining good health. To counteract portion distortion, weigh and measure your food at home for a few days every now and then. In addition, check the serving sizes listed on packaged foods. For many people, concentrating on portion sizes is also a much easier

For successful weight management, some people find it helpful to limit their intake of foods high in fat and simple sugars. Foods made with fat and sugar substitutes are often promoted for weight loss. However, whether fat and sugar substitutes help you achieve and maintain a healthy weight depends on your lifestyle—your overall eating and activity habits. When evaluating foods containing fat and sugar substitutes, consider these issues:

• *Is the food lower in calories or just lower in fat?* Reduced-fat foods often contain extra sugar to improve the taste and texture lost when fat is removed, so such foods may be as high or even higher in total calories than their fattier counterparts. Limiting fat intake is an important goal for weight management, but so is controlling total calories.

• *Are you choosing foods with fat and/or sugar substitutes* instead of *foods you typically eat or* in addition to *foods you typically eat?* If you consume low-fat, no-sugar-added ice cream instead of regular ice cream, you may save calories. But if you add such ice cream to your daily diet simply because it is lower in fat and sugar, your overall calorie consumption—and your weight—may increase.

• *How many foods containing fat and sugar substitutes do you consume each day?* Although the FDA has given at least provisional approval to all the fat and sugar substitutes currently available, health concerns about some of these products linger. For example, the fat substitute Olestra, marketed under the trade name Olean, reduces the absorption of fat-soluble nutrients and certain antioxidants and causes gastrointestinal distress in some people. One way to limit any potential adverse effects is to read labels and monitor how much of each product you consume. Remember that fat and sugar substitutes are found in a wide variety of products.

• *Is an even healthier choice available?* Many of the foods containing fat and sugar substitutes are low-nutrient snack foods. Although substituting a lower-fat or lower-sugar version of the same food may be beneficial, fruits, vegetables, and whole grains are healthier snack choices.

method of monitoring and managing total food intake than counting calories.

Energy (Calorie) Density   To cut back on calories and still feel full, favor foods with a low energy density—that is, those that are relatively heavy but have few calories. For example, for the same 100 calories, you could consume 21 baby carrots or 4 pretzel twists; you are more likely to feel full after eating the serving of carrots because it weighs 10 times that of the serving of pretzels (10 ounces versus 1 ounce). Fresh fruits and vegetables, with their high water and fiber content, are low in energy density, as are whole-grain foods. Meat, ice cream, potato chips, croissants, crackers, and low-fat cakes and cookies are examples of foods high in energy density. Strategies for lowering the energy density of your diet include the following:

• Eat fruit with breakfast and for dessert.
• Add extra vegetables to sandwiches, casseroles, stir-fry dishes, pizza, pasta dishes, and fajitas.
• Start meals with a bowl of broth-based soup; include a green salad or fruit salad.
• Snack on fresh fruits and vegetables rather than crackers, chips, or other energy-dense snack foods.
• Limit serving sizes of energy-dense foods such as butter, mayonnaise, cheese, chocolate, fatty meats, croissants, and snack foods that are fried or high in added sugars (including reduced-fat products).

Fat Calories   Although some fat is needed in the diet to provide essential nutrients, you should avoid overeating fatty foods. There is some evidence that fat calories are more easily converted to body fat than calories from protein or carbohydrate. Limiting fat in the diet can also help you limit your total calories. As described in Chapter 9, fat should supply no more than 30% of your average total daily calories, which translates into no more than 66 grams of fat in a 2000-calorie diet each day. Foods rich in fat include oils, margarine, butter, cream, and lard, which are almost pure fat; meat and processed foods, which contain a great deal of "hidden" fat; and nuts, seeds, and avocados, which are plant sources of fats. Moving toward a diet strong in complex carbohydrates and fresh fruits and vegetables, and away from a reliance on meat and processed foods, is an effective approach to reducing fat consumption. Watch out for processed foods labeled "fat-free" or "reduced fat," as they may be high in calories.

Complex Carbohydrates   It has long been the fashion among dieters to cut back on bread, pasta, and potatoes to control weight. But complex carbohydrates from these sources, as well as from vegetables, legumes, and whole grains, are precisely the nutrients that can help you achieve and maintain a healthy body weight. Foods high in complex carbohydrates help provide a feeling of satiety, or fullness, that can keep you from overeating. Carbohydrates should make up 55–65% of total daily calories for most people.

Simple Sugars and Refined Carbohydrates   Foods high in added sugar provide calories but few nutrients. Choose fresh fruits and whole grains instead of foods high in added sugars and refined carbohydrates. Avoid

If you gaze into the mirror and wish you could change the way your body looks, consider getting some exercise—not to reshape your contours but to firm up your body image and enhance your self-esteem. In a recent study, 82 adults completed a 12-week aerobic exercise program and had 12 months of follow-up. Compared with the control group, these participants improved their fitness and also benefited psychologically in tests of mood, anxiety, and self-concept. These same physical and psychological benefits were still significant at the 1-year follow-up.

One reason for the findings may be that people who exercise regularly often gain a sense of mastery and competence that enhances their self-esteem and body image. In addition, exercise contributes to a more toned look, which many adults prefer. Research suggests that physically active people are more comfortable with their bodies and their image than sedentary people are. In one workplace study, 60 employees were asked to complete a 36-session stretching program whose main purpose was to prevent muscle strains at work. At the end of the program,

besides the significant increase by all participants in measurements of flexibility, their perceptions of their bodies improved and so did their overall sense of self-worth.

Similar results were obtained in a Norwegian study, in which 219 middle-aged people at risk for heart disease were randomly assigned to one of four groups: diet, diet plus exercise, exercise, and no intervention. The greater the participation of individuals in the exercise component of the program, the higher were their scores in perceived competence/self-esteem and coping.

SOURCES: DiLorenzo, T. M., et al. 1999. Long-term effects of aerobic exercise on psychological outcomes. *Preventive Medicine* 28(1): 75–85. Sorensen, M., et al. 1999. The effect of exercise and diet on mental health and quality of life in middle-aged individuals with elevated risk factors for cardiovascular disease. *Journal of Sports Science* 17(5): 369–377. Moore, T. M. 1998. A workplace stretching program. *AAOHN Journal* 46(12): 563–568.

or minimize consumption of sugary soft drinks and fruit drinks, which are often high in calories.

Protein   The typical American consumes more than an adequate amount of protein, and protein not needed by the body for growth and tissue repair will be stored as fat. Foods high in protein are often also high in fat. Stick to the recommended protein intake of 10–15% of total daily calories.

Eating Habits   Equally important to weight management is eating small, frequent meals—three or more a day plus snacks—on a dependable, regular schedule. Skipping meals leads to excessive hunger, feelings of deprivation, and increased vulnerability to binge eating or snacking on high-calorie, high-fat, or sugary foods. A regular pattern of eating, along with some personal "decision rules" governing food choices, is a way of thinking about a healthy, low-fat diet. Decision rules governing breakfast might be these, for example: Choose a sugar-free, high-fiber cereal with nonfat milk most of the time; once in a while (no more than once a week), have a hard-boiled egg; save pancakes and waffles for special occasions. Making the healthier choice more often than not is the essence of moderation.

Physical Activity and Exercise

Physical activity and exercise burn calories and keep the metabolism geared to using food for energy instead of storing it as fat. Making significant cuts in food intake in order to lose weight is a difficult strategy to maintain; increasing your physical activity is a much better approach.

The first step in becoming more active is to incorporate more physical activity into your daily life. Accumulate 30 minutes or more of moderate-intensity physical activity—walking, gardening, housework, and so on—on most, or preferably all, days of the week. In the long term, even a small increase in activity level can help maintain your current weight or help you lose a modest amount of weight. In fact, research suggests that fidgeting—stretching, squirming, standing up, and so on—may help prevent weight gain in some people. If you are overweight and want to lose weight, a greater amount of physical activity can help. Researchers have found that people who lose weight and don't regain it typically burn about 2800 calories per week in physical activity—the equivalent of about 1 hour of brisk walking per day.

Once you become more active every day, consider beginning a formal exercise program that includes cardiorespiratory endurance exercise, resistance training, and stretching exercises. Moderate cardiorespiratory endurance exercise, sustained for 45 minutes to 1 hour, can help trim body fat permanently. Strength training helps increase fat-free mass, which results in more calorie burning even outside of exercise periods. The message about exercise is that regular exercise, maintained throughout life, makes weight management easier and improves quality of life.

Thinking and Emotions

The way you think about yourself and your world influences and is influenced by how you feel and how you act. Certain kinds of thinking produce negative emotions, which can undermine a healthy lifestyle. Research on people who have a weight problem indicates that low self-esteem and the negative emotions that accompany it are significant problems. This often results in part from mentally comparing the actual self to an internally held picture of the "ideal self." The greater the discrepancy, the larger the impact on self-esteem and the more likely the presence of negative emotions.

Often our internalized "ideal self" is the result of having adopted perfectionistic goals and beliefs about how we and others "should" be. Examples of such beliefs are "If I don't do things perfectly, I'm a failure" and "It's terrible if I'm not thin." These irrational beliefs may cause stress and emotional disturbance. The remedy is to challenge such beliefs and replace them with more realistic ones. (See Chapter 3 for tips on developing realistic self-talk.) A healthy lifestyle is supported by having realistic beliefs and goals and by engaging in positive self-talk and problem-solving efforts.

Coping Strategies

Adequate and appropriate coping strategies for dealing with the stresses and challenges of life are another lifestyle factor in weight management. One strategy that some people adopt for coping is eating. Food may be used to alleviate loneliness or as entertainment or a pickup for fatigue. Eating provides distraction from difficult problems and is a means of punishing the self or others for real or imagined transgressions.

People with a healthy lifestyle have more effective ways to get their needs met. Having learned to communicate assertively and to manage interpersonal conflict effectively, they don't shrink from problems or overreact. The person with a healthy lifestyle knows how to create and maintain relationships with others and has a solid network of friends and loved ones. Food is used appropriately—to fuel life's activities and gain personal satisfaction, not to manage stress.

APPROACHES TO OVERCOMING A WEIGHT PROBLEM

What should you do if you are overweight? There are several options available to you.

Doing It Yourself

Research indicates that people are far more successful than was previously thought at losing weight and keeping it off. One study found that about 64% of the subjects achieved long-term success without joining a formal program or getting special help. Other researchers investigated the characteristics that distinguished those who lost at least 20% of their body weight and maintained this loss for 2 years or more. Although some had used diet alone to lose weight, some had used exercise alone, and others had used a combination of diet and exercise, virtually all maintained their success by making exercise a permanent part of their lifestyle. They kept tabs on their weight and habits; they learned to develop their own diet, exercise, and maintenance plans, and they became more involved in and excited by activities other than eating—such as careers, projects, and special interests. Long-term success depends on maintaining the lifestyle changes that helped you lose the weight in the first place.

If you need to lose weight, focus on adopting the healthy lifestyle described throughout this book. The "right" weight for you will naturally evolve, and you won't have to diet. However, if you must diet, do so in combination with exercise, and avoid very-low-calorie diets. Don't try to lose more than 0.5–2 pounds per week. Realize that most low-calorie diets cause a rapid loss of body water at first. When this phase passes, weight loss declines. As a result, dieters are often misled into believing that their efforts are not working. They then give up, not realizing that smaller losses later in the diet are actually better than the initial big losses, because later loss is mostly fat loss, whereas initial loss was primarily fluid.

For more tips on losing weight on your own, refer to the Behavior Change Strategy at the end of the chapter.

Diet Books

Many people who try to lose weight by themselves fall prey to one or more of the dozens of diet books on the market. Although a very few of these do contain useful advice and tips for motivation, most make empty promises. Some guidelines for evaluating and choosing a diet book are as follows:

1. Reject books that advocate an unbalanced way of eating. These include books advocating high-carbohydrate-only diets or low-carbohydrate, high-protein diets. Also reject books promoting a single food, such as cabbage or grapefruit.

2. Reject books that claim to be based on a "scientific breakthrough" or to have the "secret" to success.

3. Reject books that use gimmicks, like matching eating to blood type, hyping insulin resistance as the single cause of obesity, combining foods in special ways to achieve weight loss, or purporting that a weight problem is due to food allergies or sensitivities, yeast infections, or hormone imbalances.

4. Reject books that promise quick weight loss or that limit the selection of foods.

5. Accept books that advocate a balanced approach to diet plus exercise and sound nutrition advice.

A recent crop of popular books has advocated diets high in protein, low in carbohydrate, and relatively high in fat. The American College of Sports Medicine, the

Food Choices

- Follow the recommendations in the Food Guide Pyramid for eating a moderate, varied diet.

- Check food labels for serving sizes, calories, and nutrient levels. Favor foods with a low energy density and a high nutrient density.

- Watch for hidden calories. Reduced-fat foods often have as many calories as their full-fat versions. Condiments like butter, margarine, mayonnaise, and salad dressings provide about 100 calories per tablespoon; added sugars such as jams, jellies, and syrup are also packed with calories.

- Drink fewer calories. Many Americans consume high-calorie beverages such as soda, fruit drinks, sports drinks, alcohol, and specialty coffees and teas.

- For problem foods, try eating small amounts under controlled conditions. Go out for a scoop of ice cream, for example, rather than buying half a gallon for your freezer.

Planning and Serving

- Keep a log of what you eat. Before you begin your program, your log will provide a realistic picture of your current diet. Once you start your program, a log will keep you focused on your food choices and portion sizes.

- Eat three meals a day, including breakfast. Replace impulse snacking with planned, healthy snacks. Keep low-calorie snacks on hand to combat the "munchies": baby carrots, popcorn, and fresh fruits and vegetables are good choices.

- When shopping for food, make a list and stick to it. Don't shop when you're hungry. Avoid aisles that contain problem foods.

- Use measuring cups and spoons and a food scale to become more familiar with appropriate portion sizes.

- Serve meals on small plates and in small bowls to help you eat smaller portions without feeling deprived.

- Eat only in specifically designated spots. Remove food from other areas of your house or apartment.

- When you eat, just eat—don't do anything else, such as read or watch TV.

- Eat more slowly. Take small bites and chew food thoroughly. Pay attention to every bite, and enjoy your food. Between bites, try putting your fork or spoon down and taking sips of water or another beverage.

- When you're done eating, remove your plate. Cue yourself that the meal is over—drink a glass of water, suck on a mint, chew gum, or brush your teeth.

Special Occasions

- When you eat out, choose a restaurant where you can make healthy food choices. Ask the server not to put bread on the table before the meal, and request that sauces and salad dressings be served on the side. If portion sizes are large, take half your food home for a meal later in the week.

- If you cook a large meal for friends, send leftovers home with your guests.

- If you're eating at a friend's, eat a little and leave the rest. Don't eat to be polite; if someone offers you food you don't want, thank the person and decline firmly: "No thank you, I've had enough" or "It's delicious, but I'm full."

- Take care during the winter holidays. Research indicates that people gain less than they think during the winter holidays (about a pound) but that the weight isn't lost during the rest of the year, leading to slow, steady weight gain.

Physical Activity and Stress Management

- Increase your level of daily physical activity.

- Begin a formal exercise program that includes endurance exercise, strength training, and stretching.

- Develop techniques for handling stress—go for a walk or use a relaxation technique. Practice positive self-talk.

- Develop strategies for coping with non-hunger cues to eat, such as boredom, sleepiness, or anxiety. Try calling a friend, taking a shower, or reading a magazine.

- Tell family members and friends that you're making lifestyle changes, and ask them to be supportive.

American Dietetic Association, the Cooper Institute for Aerobics Research, and the Women's Sports Foundation released a joint statement saying that such diets are not a good weight-loss strategy, will not improve athletic performance, and can be harmful in some cases. The only reason such plans help some people lose weight is that the diets they advocate provide so few calories; but as with all such plans, they are difficult to maintain over any period of time. Low-carbohydrate diets may also be high in unhealthy saturated fats, and they often limit or elimi-

nate foods such as grains, fruits, and vegetables that are rich in nutrients and fiber.

Dietary Supplements and Diet Aids

The number of dietary supplements and other weight loss aids on the market has also increased in recent years. Promoted in advertisements, magazines, direct mail campaigns, infomercials, and Web sites, these products typically promise a quick and easy path to weight loss. Most

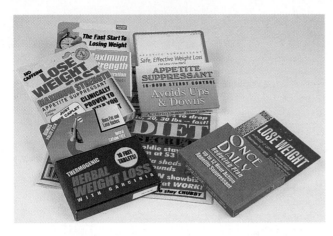

There are many plans and supplements promoted for weight loss, but few have any research supporting their effectiveness for long-term weight management. Developing lifelong healthy eating and exercise habits is the best approach for achieving and maintaining a healthy body composition.

of these products are marketed as dietary supplements and so are subject to fewer regulations than over-the-counter medications. If you are considering one of these products, use your critical thinking skills.

WWW. Weight-Loss Programs

Weight-loss programs come in a variety of types, including noncommercial support organizations, commercial programs, Web sites, and clinical programs.

Noncommercial Weight-Loss Programs Noncommercial programs such as TOPS (Take Off Pounds Sensibly) and Overeaters Anonymous (OA) mainly provide group support. They do not advocate any particular diet, but they do recommend seeking professional advice for creating an individualized diet and exercise plan. These types of programs are generally free. Your physician or a registered dietitian can also provide information and support for weight loss.

Commercial Weight-Loss Programs Commercial programs such as Weight Watchers, Jenny Craig, Diet Workshop, and Richard Simmons Slimmons typically provide group support, nutrition education, physical activity recommendations, and behavior modification advice. Some also make available packaged foods to assist in following dietary advice. Many commercial programs voluntarily belong to the Partnership for Healthy Weight Management established by the Federal Trade Commission in 1999. By doing so, they agree to provide clients with information on staff training and education, the risks associated with each program or product, the costs of the program, and the expected outcomes of the program, including rates of success. A responsible and safe weight-loss program should have the following features:

1. The recommended diet should be safe and balanced, include all the food groups, and meet the DRIs for all nutrients. Physical activity and exercise should be strongly encouraged.

2. The program should promote slow, steady weight loss averaging about $^{1}\!/_{2}$–2 pounds per week.

3. If a participant plans to lose more than 20 pounds, has any health problems, or is taking medication on a regular basis, physician evaluation and monitoring should be recommended. The staff of the program should include qualified counselors and health professionals.

4. The program should include plans for weight maintenance after the weight-loss phase is over.

5. The program should provide information on all fees and costs, including those of supplements and prepackaged foods, as well as data on risks and expected outcomes of participating in the program.

A plan for maintenance is especially important because studies indicate that only 10–15% of program participants maintain their weight loss—the rest gain back all or more than they had lost. One study of participants found that regular exercise was the best predictor of maintaining weight loss, whereas frequent television viewing was the best predictor of weight gain. This reinforces the idea that successful weight management requires long-term lifestyle changes.

Online Weight-Loss Programs A recent addition to the weight-loss program scene is the Internet-based program. Most such Web sites include a cross between self-help and group support through chat rooms, bulletin boards, and e-newsletters. Many sites offer online self-assessment for diet and physical activity habits as well as a meal plan; some provide access to a staff professional for individualized help. The criteria used to evaluate commercial programs can also be applied to Internet-based programs. In addition, check whether a program offers member-to-member support and access to staff professionals.

Clinical Weight-Loss Programs Medically supervised clinical programs are usually located in a hospital or other medical setting. Designed to help those who are severely obese, these programs typically involve a closely monitored very-low-calorie diet. The cost of a clinical program is usually high, but insurance will often cover part of the fee.

Prescription Drugs

The medications most often prescribed for weight loss are appetite suppressants that reduce feelings of hunger or increase feelings of fullness. Appetite suppressants usually work by increasing levels of catecholamine or serotonin, two brain chemicals that affect mood and appetite. All prescription weight-loss drugs have potential side effects.

Many over-the-counter (OTC) products are promoted for appetite control and fat loss, but few have evidence supporting their effectiveness. In addition, use of OTC products doesn't help in the adoption of lifestyle behaviors that can help people achieve and maintain a healthy weight over the long term.

Formula Drinks and Food Bars

Canned diet drinks, powders used to make shakes, and diet food bars and snacks are designed to achieve weight loss by substituting for some or all of a person's daily food intake. However, most people find it difficult to use these products for long periods as a substitute for more satisfying "real" food, and serious health problems may result if they are used as the sole source of nutrition for extended periods of time. Use of such products can result in rapid weight loss for those who can stick with them, but such weight loss is accompanied by loss of muscle mass, and the weight is typically regained.

Herbs and Herbal Products

Although many people believe that because herbs are "natural" they are safe, it is important to remember that herbs contain biologically active compounds that can be dangerous, especially if taken in large doses. As described in Chapter 9, herbs are marketed as dietary supplements, so there is little information about effectiveness, proper dosage, drug interactions, and side effects. In addition, labels may not accurately reflect the ingredients and dosages present, and safe manufacturing practices are not guaranteed. For example, the substitution of a toxic herb for another compound during the manufacture of a Chinese herbal weight-loss preparation caused more than 100 cases of kidney damage and cancer among users in Europe.

Ephedra, also known as ma huang or desert herb, is a popular herb found in weight-loss aids. Its active ingredient, ephedrine, is structurally similar to amphetamine. As a stimulant, ephedra may suppress appetite and increase body temperature and basal metabolic rate, causing calories to be burned at a faster rate. However, few studies have been done to identify safe and effective uses of ephedra, and long-term use is not recommended. In addition, many products containing ephedra also contain other stimulants—caffeine or herbal products that contain caffeine such as guarana seeds or kola nuts. There have been many reports of adverse effects from use of ephedra, including elevated blood pressure, panic attacks, seizures, insomnia,

headache, and nausea; it may also increase the risk of heart attack or stroke in some people, particularly if combined with another stimulant. The FDA is considering new regulations for ephedra, including dosage guidelines and warnings.

Herbal "dieter's teas" often contain a variety of strong botanical laxatives and diuretics such as senna, aloe, buckthorn, rhubarb root, cascara, and castor oil. If used in excess, these can cause extreme diarrhea, nausea, vomiting, dehydration, fainting, and electrolyte imbalances that can lead to heart rhythm problems. If used regularly, the colon may become dependent on the laxative effect, resulting in chronic constipation. Any weight loss that occurs is due to fluid loss, not fat loss.

Other Dietary Supplements and Diet Aids

Supplements containing specific amino acids and proteins are also marketed for weight loss. Promoters claim that amino acids may ward off cravings and the impulse to binge-eat; however, there is little research to support these claims. In addition, even if such products do affect appetite, they may not be very helpful in weight management. Hunger is often not the reason that people consume high-calorie foods or overeat. The use of so-called "fat burners" or "fat inhibitors" such as carnitine, hydroxycitrate, chromium, or pyruvate is also not currently supported by research findings.

Fiber is another common ingredient in OTC diet aids. Manufacturers claim that fiber can swell in the stomach and control appetite by making people feel full. However, dietary fiber acts as a bulking agent in the large intestine, not in the stomach. The FDA has found no data to warrant classifying any type of fiber as an aid in weight control. In addition, most diet aids contain a mere 1–3 grams of fiber, which do not contribute much toward the recommended daily intake of 20–35 grams.

Until 2000, the synthetic compound phenylpropanolamine (PPA) was a common ingredient in OTC diet pills. Like ephedra, PPA acts as a mild stimulant and appetite suppressant. Although originally approved for short-term use, reports of increased risk for stroke led the FDA in 2000 to ask manufacturers to stop marketing products containing PPA.

The bottom line on nonprescription diet aids is *caveat emptor*—let the buyer beware. There is no quick and easy way to lose weight. The most effective approach is to develop healthy diet and exercise habits and make them a permanent part of your lifestyle.

Those that affect catecholamine levels, including phentermine (Ionamin), diethylpropion (Tenuate), and mazindol (Sanorex), may cause sleeplessness, nervousness, and euphoria. Sibutramine (Meridia) acts on both the serotonin and catecholamine systems; it may trigger increases in blood pressure and heart rate.

A newer medication for obesity is orlistat (Xenical), which lowers calorie consumption by blocking fat absorption in the intestines; it prevents about 30% of the fat

in food from being digested. Similar to the fat substitute olestra, orlistat reduces the absorption of fat-soluble vitamins and antioxidants. Side effects include diarrhea, cramping, and other gastrointestinal problems if users do not follow a low-fat diet.

Studies have generally found that appetite suppressants produce modest weight loss—about 5–22 pounds above the loss expected with nondrug obesity treatments. Unfortunately, many people regain the weight they've lost

Body Image and Gender

Women are much more likely than men to be dissatisfied with their bodies, often wanting to lose weight. In one study, only 30% of eighth-grade girls reported being content with their bodies, while 70% of their male classmates expressed satisfaction with their looks. Girls and women are much more likely than boys and men to diet, develop eating disorders, and be obese.

One reason that girls and women are dissatisfied with their bodies is that they are influenced by the media—particularly advertisements and women's fashion magazines. Most teen girls report that the media influence their idea of the perfect body and their decision to diet. In a study of adult women, viewing pictures of thin models in magazines had an immediate negative effect on their mood. Clearly, media images affect women's self-image and self-esteem. For American women of all ages, success is still too often equated with how we look rather than who we are.

It is important to note that the image of the "perfect" woman presented in the media is often unrealistic and even unhealthy. In a review of BMI data for Miss America pageant winners since 1922, researchers noted a significant decline in BMI over time, with an increasing number of recent winners having BMIs in the "underweight" category. The average fashion model is 4–7 inches taller and 20 pounds lighter than the average American woman.

Our culture may be promoting an unattainable masculine ideal as well. Researchers studying male action figures such as GI Joe from the past 40 years noted that they have become increasingly muscular. A recent Batman action figure, if projected onto a man of average height, would result in someone with a 30-inch waist, 57-inch chest, and 27-inch biceps.

Body Image and Ethnicity

The thin, toned look as a feminine ideal is just a fashion, one that is not shared by all cultures. Although some groups espouse thinness as an "ideal" body type, others do not. In many traditional African societies, for example, full-figured women's bodies are seen as symbols of health, prosperity, and fertility. African American teenage girls have a much more positive body image than white girls; in one survey, two-thirds of them defined beauty as "the right attitude," whereas white girls were more preoccupied with weight and body shape. Nevertheless, recent evidence indicates that African American women are as likely to engage in disordered eating behavior, especially binge eating and vomiting, as their Latina, American Indian, and white counterparts. This finding underscores the complex nature of eating disorders and body image.

Avoiding Body Image Problems

To minimize your risk of developing a body image problem, keep the following strategies in mind:

- Focus on healthy habits and good physical health. Eat a moderate, balanced diet, and choose physical activities you enjoy. Avoid chronic or repetitive dieting.

- Focus on good psychological health and put concerns about physical appearance in perspective. Your worth as a human being is not dependent on how you look.

- Find things to appreciate in yourself besides an idealized body image. Men and women whose self-esteem is based primarily on standards of physical attractiveness can find it difficult to age gracefully. Those who can learn to value other aspects of themselves are more accepting of the physical changes that occur naturally with age.

- See the beauty and fitness industries for what they are. Realize that one of their goals is to prompt dissatisfaction with yourself so that you will buy their products.

if they stop taking the drugs. Since most weight-loss medications are approved for only short-term use, regaining weight is a serious problem.

Side effects and risks are other concerns. In 1997, the FDA removed from the market two prescription weight-loss drugs, fenfluramine (Pondimin) and dexfenfluramine (Redux), after their use was linked to potentially life-threatening heart valve problems. (Fenfluramine was used most often in combination with phentermine, an off-label combination referred to as "fen/phen.") It appears that people who took these drugs over a long period or at high dosages are at greatest risk for problems, but the FDA recommends that anyone who has taken either of these drugs be examined by a physician.

Prescription weight-loss drugs are not for people who want to lose a few pounds to wear a smaller size of jeans. The latest federal guidelines advise people to try lifestyle modification for at least 6 months before trying drug therapy. Prescription drugs are recommended—in conjunction with lifestyle changes—only in certain cases: for people who have been unable to lose weight with non-drug options and who have a BMI over 30 (or over 27 if two or more additional risk factors such as diabetes and high blood pressure are present).

Acceptance and Change

Most Americans, young and old, are unhappy with some aspect of their appearance and often their weight. The "can-do" attitude of Americans, together with the belief that there is a solution to this dissatisfaction, leads to even more problems with body image, as well as to dieting, disordered eating, and the desire for cosmetic surgery to "fix" perceived defects.

In fact, there are limits to the changes that can be made to body weight and body shape, both of which are influenced by heredity. The changes that can and should be made are lifestyle changes—engaging in regular physical activity, obtaining adequate nutrition, and maintaining healthy eating habits. With these changes, the body weight and shape that develop will be natural and appropriate for an individual's particular genetic makeup.

Knowing when the limits to healthy change have been reached—and learning to accept those limits—is crucial for overall wellness. Obesity is a serious health risk, but weight management needs to take place in a positive and realistic atmosphere. For an obese person, losing as few as 10 pounds can reduce blood pressure and improve mood. The hazards of excessive dieting and overconcern about body weight need to be countered by a change in attitude about what constitutes the perfect body and a reasonable body weight. A body weight goal must take into account a person's weight history, social circumstances, metabolic profile, and psychological well-being.

WWW. EATING DISORDERS

Problems with body weight and weight control are not limited to excessive body fat. A growing number of people experience **eating disorders,** characterized by severe disturbances in eating patterns and eating-related behaviors. The major eating disorders are anorexia nervosa, bulimia nervosa, and binge-eating disorder. **Anorexia nervosa** is characterized by a refusal to maintain a minimally normal body weight. **Bulimia nervosa** is characterized by repeated episodes of binge eating followed by compensatory behaviors such as self-induced vomiting, the misuse of laxatives or diuretics, fasting, or excessive exercise. **Binge-eating disorder** is characterized by binge eating without regular use of compensatory behaviors.

Terms

eating disorder A serious disturbance in eating patterns or eating-related behavior, characterized by a negative body image and concerns about body weight or body fat.

anorexia nervosa An eating disorder characterized by a refusal to maintain body weight at a minimally healthy level and an intense fear of gaining weight or becoming fat; self-starvation.

bulimia nervosa An eating disorder characterized by recurrent episodes of binge eating and purging: overeating and then using compensatory behaviors such as vomiting, laxatives, and excessive exercise to prevent weight gain.

binge-eating disorder An eating disorder characterized by binge eating and a lack of control over eating behavior in general.

purging The use of vomiting, laxatives, excessive exercise, restrictive dieting, enemas, diuretics, or diet pills to compensate for food that has been eaten and that the person fears will produce weight gain.

At any given time, 0.5–2.0% of Americans suffer from anorexia and 1.0–3.0% have bulimia. Binge-eating disorder may affect 2.0–5.0% of all adults and 8.0% of those who are obese. An even greater number of Americans exhibit disordered eating behavior but do not fully meet the criteria of one of the recognized eating disorders. Anorexia and bulimia affect far more women than men.

Anorexia Nervosa

A person suffering from anorexia nervosa does not eat enough food to maintain a reasonable body weight. Anorexia affects 1–3 million Americans, 95% of them female. Although it can occur later, anorexia typically develops between the ages of 12 and 18.

Characteristics of Anorexia Nervosa People suffering from anorexia have an intense fear of gaining weight or becoming fat. Their body image is distorted, so that even when emaciated, they think they are fat. (Distorted body image is also a hallmark of *muscle dysmorphia,* a disorder experienced by some body builders in which they see themselves as small and out of shape despite being very muscular.) People with anorexia may engage in compulsive behaviors or rituals that help keep them from eating, though some may also binge and purge. They commonly use vigorous and prolonged physical activity to reduce body weight as well. Although they may express a great interest in food, even taking over the cooking responsibilities for the rest of the family, their own diet becomes more and more extreme. People with anorexia often hide or hoard food without eating it.

Anorexic people are typically introverted, emotionally reserved, and socially insecure. They are often "model children" who rarely complain and are anxious to please others and win their approval. Although school performance is typically above average, they are often critical of themselves and not satisfied with their accomplishments. For people with anorexia nervosa, their entire sense of self-esteem may be tied up in their evaluation of their body shape and weight.

Health Risks of Anorexia Nervosa Because of extreme weight loss, females with anorexia often stop menstruating, become intolerant of cold, and develop low blood pressure and heart rate. They develop dry skin that is often covered by fine body hair like that of an infant. Their hands and feet may swell and take on a blue color.

Anorexia nervosa has been linked to a variety of medical complications, including disorders of the cardiovascular, gastrointestinal, and endocrine systems. Death can occur from heart failure caused by electrolyte imbalances. As many as 16% of patients with anorexia nervosa die of complications related to the disorder. Depression is also a serious risk, and about half the fatalities relating to anorexia are suicides.

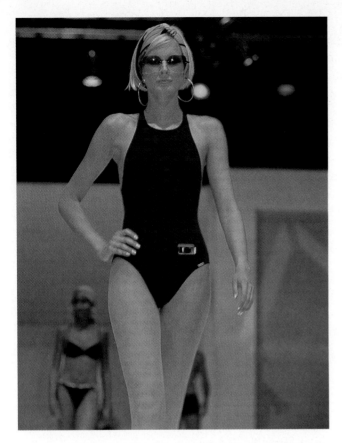

The image of the "ideal" female body promoted by the fashion and fitness industries doesn't reflect the wide range of body shapes and sizes that are associated with good health. An overconcern with body image can contribute to low self-esteem and the development of eating disorders.

Bulimia Nervosa

A person suffering from bulimia nervosa engages in recurrent episodes of binge eating followed by **purging**. Bulimia is often difficult to recognize because sufferers conceal their eating habits and usually maintain a normal weight, although they may experience weight fluctuations of 10–15 pounds. Although bulimia usually begins in adolescence or young adulthood, it has recently begun to emerge at increasingly younger (11–12 years) and older (40–60 years) ages.

Characteristics of Bulimia Nervosa   During a binge, a bulimic person may rapidly consume anywhere from 1,000 to 60,000 calories. This is followed by an attempt to get rid of the food by **purging,** usually by vomiting or using laxatives or diuretics. During a binge, bulimics feel as though they have lost control and cannot stop or limit how much they eat. Some binge and purge only occasionally, while others do so many times every day.

In public, people suffering from bulimia may appear to eat normally, but they are rarely comfortable around food. Binges usually occur in secret and can become nightmarish—ravaging the kitchen for food, going from one grocery store to another to buy food, or even stealing food. During the binge, all feelings are blocked out, and food acts as an anesthetic. Afterward, they feel physically drained and emotionally spent. They usually feel deeply ashamed and disgusted with both themselves and their behavior and terrified that they will gain weight.

Major life changes such as leaving for college, getting married, having a baby, or losing a job can trigger a binge-purge cycle. At such times, stress is high and the person may have no good outlet for emotional conflict or tension. As with anorexia, bulimia sufferers are often insecure and depend on others for approval and self-esteem. They may hide difficult emotions such as anger and disappointment from themselves and others. Binge eating and purging becomes a way of dealing with feelings.

Health Risks of Bulimia Nervosa   The binge-purge cycle of bulimia places a tremendous strain on the body. Contact with vomited stomach acids erodes tooth enamel. Repeated vomiting or the use of laxatives, in combination with deficient calorie intake, can damage the liver and kidneys and cause cardiac arrhythmia. Chronic hoarseness and esophageal tearing with bleeding may also result from vomiting. More rarely, binge eating can lead to rupture of the stomach. Although many bulimic women maintain normal weight, even small amounts of weight loss to a lower-than-normal weight can cause menstrual problems. And although less often associated with suicide, than anorexia, bulimia is associated with increased depression, excessive preoccupation with food and body image, and sometimes disturbances in cognitive functioning.

Binge-Eating Disorder

Binge-eating disorder is characterized by uncontrollable eating, usually followed by feelings of guilt and shame with weight gain. Common eating patterns are eating more rapidly than normal, eating until uncomfortably full, eating when not hungry, and preferring to eat alone. Binge eaters may eat large amounts of food throughout the day, with no planned mealtimes. Binge eaters are almost always obese, so they face all the health risks associated with obesity. In addition, binge eaters may have higher rates of depression and anxiety.

Compulsive overeaters rarely eat because of hunger. Instead, food is used as a means of coping with stress, conflict, and other difficult emotions or to provide solace and entertainment. People who do not have the resources to deal effectively with stress may be more vulnerable to binge-eating disorder. Inappropriate overeating often begins during childhood. In some families, eating may be used as an activity to fill otherwise empty time. Parents may reward children with food for good behavior or withhold food as a means of punishment, thereby creating distorted feelings about the use of food.

- Educate yourself about eating disorders and their risks and about treatment resources in your community.

- Write down specific ways the person's eating problem is affecting you or others in the household. Call a house meeting to talk about how others are affected by the problem and how to take action.

- Consider consulting a professional about the best way to approach the situation. Obtain information about how and where your friend can get help. Attend a local support group.

- Arrange to speak privately with the person, along with other friends or family members. Let one person lead the group and do most of the talking. Discuss specific incidents and the consequences of disordered eating.

- If you are going to speak with your friend, write down ahead of time what your concerns are and what you would like to say. Expect that the person you are concerned about will deny there is a problem, minimize it, or become angry with you. Remain calm and nonjudgmental, and continue to express your concern.

- Avoid giving simplistic advice about eating habits. Gently encourage your friend to eat properly.

- Take time to listen to your friend, and express your support and understanding. Encourage honest communication. Emphasize your friend's good characteristics, and compliment all her or his successes.

- Help maintain the person's sense of dignity by encouraging personal responsibility and decision making. Be patient and realistic; recovery is a long process. Continue to love and support your friend.

- If the situation is an emergency—if the person has fainted or attempted suicide, for example—take immediate action. Call 9-1-1 for help.

- If you feel very upset about the situation, seek professional help. Remember, you are not to blame for another person's eating disorder.

Treating Eating Disorders

The treatment of eating disorders must address both problematic eating behaviors and the misuse of food to manage stress and emotions. Anorexia nervosa treatment first involves averting a medical crisis by restoring adequate body weight; then the psychological aspects of the disorder can be addressed. The treatment of bulimia nervosa or binge-eating disorder involves first stabilizing the eating patterns and then identifying and changing the patterns of thinking that lead to disordered eating and improving coping skills. Concurrent problems, such as depression or anxiety, must also be addressed. In 1996, the antidepressant Prozac became the first medication approved by the FDA for the treatment of bulimia.

Treatment usually involves a combination of psychotherapy and medical management. The therapy may be carried out individually or with the entire family. A support or self-help group can be a useful adjunct to such treatment. Depending on the severity of the disorder, treatment may last from a few months to several years.

Today's Challenge

Eating disorders can be seen as the logical extension of the concern with weight that pervades American society. Although most people don't succumb to irrational or distorted ideas about their bodies, many do become obsessed with dieting. The challenge facing Americans today is achieving a healthy body weight without excessive dieting—by adopting and maintaining sensible eating habits, an active lifestyle, realistic and positive attitudes and emotions, and creative ways of handling stress.

Tips for Today

Maintaining a healthy weight means balancing calories in with calories out. Many forces and factors in contemporary society work against a healthy balance, so it's imperative that individuals take active control of managing their weight. Many approaches work, but the simplest formula is moderate food intake coupled with regular exercise.

Right now you can

- Drink a glass of water instead of a soda.

- Throw away any high-calorie, low-nutrient snack foods in your kitchen and start a list of fruits and vegetables you can buy as snacks instead.

- Put a sign on your refrigerator reminding you of your weight-management goals.

- Go outside and walk, jog, or bike for 15 minutes.

- Review the information on portion sizes in Chapter 9 and consider whether the portions you usually take at meals are larger than they need to be.

SUMMARY

- Body composition is the relative amounts of fat-free mass and fat in the body. *Overweight* and *obesity* refer to body weight or the percentage of body fat that exceeds what is associated with good health.

- The key to weight management is maintaining a balance of calories in (food) and calories out (resting metabolism, food digestion, and physical activity).

The behavior management plan described in Chapter 1 provides an excellent framework for a weight-management program. Following are some suggestions about specific ways you can adapt that general plan to controlling your weight.

Motivation and Commitment

Make sure you are motivated and committed before you begin. Failure at weight loss is a frustrating experience that can make it more difficult to lose weight in the future. Think about the reasons you want to lose weight. Self-focused reasons, such as to feel good about yourself or to have a greater sense of well-being, are often associated with success. Trying to lose weight for others or out of concern for how others view you is a poor foundation for a weight-loss program. Make a list of your reasons for wanting to lose weight, and post it in a prominent place.

Setting Goals

Choose a reasonable weight you think you would like to reach over the long term, and be willing to renegotiate it as you get further along. Break your long-term weight and behavioral goals into a series of short-term goals. Develop a new way of behaving by designing small, manageable steps that will get you to where you want to go.

Creating a Negative Energy Balance

When your weight is constant, you are burning approximately the same number of calories as you are taking in. To tip the energy balance toward weight loss, you must either consume fewer calories or burn more calories through physical activity, or both. One pound of body fat represents 3500 calories. To lose weight at the recommended rate of 0.5–2.0 pounds per week, you must create a negative energy balance of 1750–7000 calories per week or 250–1000 calories per day. To generate your negative energy balance, it's usually best to begin by increasing your activity level rather than decreasing your calorie consumption.

Physical Activity

Consider how you can increase your energy output simply by increasing routine physical activity, such as walking or taking the stairs. If you are not already involved in a regular exercise routine aimed at increasing endurance and building or maintaining muscle mass, seek help from someone who is competent to help you plan and start an appropriate exercise routine. If you are already doing regular physical exercise, evaluate your program according to the guidelines in Chapter 10.

Don't try to use exercise to "spot reduce." Leg lifts, for example, contribute to fat loss only to the extent that they burn calories; they don't burn fat just from your legs. You can make parts of your body appear more fit by exercising them, but the only way you can reduce fat in any specific part of your body is to create an overall negative energy balance.

Diet and Eating Habits

If you can't generate a large enough negative energy balance solely by increasing physical activity, you may want to supplement exercise with modest cuts in your calorie intake. Don't think of this as "going on a diet"; your goal is to make small changes in your diet that you can maintain for a lifetime. Focus on cutting your fat intake and on eating a variety of nutritious foods in moderation. Don't try skipping meals, fasting, or going on a very-low-calorie diet or a diet that is unbalanced.

Making changes in eating habits is another important strategy for weight management. If your program centers on a conscious restriction of certain food items, you're likely to spend all your time thinking about the forbidden foods. Focus on *how* to eat rather than *what* to eat. Refer to the box "Strategies for Successful Weight Management" for suggestions.

Self-Monitoring

Keep a record of your weight and behavior change progress. Try keeping a record of everything you eat. Write down what you plan to eat, in what quantity, *before* you eat. You'll find that just having to record something that is "not OK" to eat is likely to stop you from eating it. If you also note what seems to be triggering your urges to eat (for example, you feel bored, someone offered you something), you'll become more aware of your weak spots and be better able to take corrective action. Also, keep track of your daily activities and your formal exercise program so you can monitor increases in physical activity.

Putting Your Plan into Action

- Examine the environmental cues that trigger poor eating and exercise habits, and devise strategies for dealing with them. For example, you may need to remove "problem" foods from your house temporarily or put a sign on the refrigerator reminding you to go for a walk instead of having a snack. Anticipate problem situations, and plan ways to handle them more effectively.

- Create new environmental cues that will support your new healthy behaviors. Put your walking shoes by the front door. Move fruits and vegetables to the front of the refrigerator.

- Get others to help. Talk to friends and family members about what they can do to support your efforts. Find a buddy to join you in your exercise program.

- Give yourself lots of praise and rewards. Think about your accomplishments and achievements and congratulate yourself. Plan special nonfood treats for yourself, such as a walk or a movie. Reward yourself often and for anything that counts toward success.

- If you do slip, tell yourself to get back on track immediately, and don't waste time on self-criticism. Think positively instead of getting into a cycle of guilt and self-blame. Don't demand too much of yourself.

- Don't get discouraged. Be aware that although weight loss is bound to slow down after the first loss of body fluid, the weight loss at this slower rate is more permanent than earlier, more dramatic losses.

- Remember that weight management is a lifelong project. You need to adopt reasonable goals and strategies that you can maintain over the long term.

- Standards for assessing body weight and body composition include body mass index (BMI) and percent body fat.

- Too much or too little body fat is linked to health problems; the distribution of body fat can also be a significant risk factor.

- An inaccurate or negative body image is common and can lead to psychological distress.

- Factors involved in the regulation of body weight and body fat include heredity and metabolic rate.

- Nutritional guidelines for weight management include consuming a moderate number of calories; limiting portion sizes, energy density, and the intake of fat, simple sugars, refined carbohydrates, and protein to recommended levels; increasing the intake of complex carbohydrates; and developing an eating schedule and decision rules for food choices.

- Activity guidelines for weight management emphasize daily physical activity and regular sessions of endurance exercise and strength training.

- Weight management requires developing positive, realistic self-talk and self-esteem and a repertoire of appropriate techniques for handling stress and other emotional and physical challenges.

- People can be successful at long-term weight loss on their own, usually through diet and exercise.

- Diet books, OTC diet aids and supplements, and formal weight-loss programs should be assessed for safety and efficacy.

- Anorexia nervosa is characterized by self-starvation, distorted body image, and an intense fear of gaining weight. Bulimia nervosa is characterized by recurrent episodes of uncontrolled binge eating and frequent purging. Binge-eating disorder involves binge eating without regular use of compensatory purging.

TAKE ACTION

1. Find out what percentage of your body weight is fat by taking one of the tests described in this chapter at your campus health clinic, sports medicine clinic, or health club. If you have too high or too low a proportion of body fat, consider taking steps to change it.

2. Interview some people who have successfully lost weight and kept it off. What were their strategies and techniques? Do you think their approach would work for others?

WW JOURNAL ENTRY

1. Monitor your diet for a week to see exactly how much fat and sugar you consume. If these amounts are excessive, make a list of specific steps you can take to reduce them.

2. Make a list of at least five things you could do each day to become more physically active—for example, riding your bike to class instead of driving or taking the stairs instead of the elevator. For each, describe the lifestyle adjustments you'd need to make—for example, leaving for class 10 minutes earlier to allow time to ride your bike rather than drive.

3. *Critical Thinking* Evaluate some of the weight-loss resources in your community. First, investigate a commercial weight-management program that operates in your community. Write an evaluation of it in terms of the criteria listed in the chapter. How does the program measure up? Next, look at the frozen diet dinners in your supermarket, such as Weight Watchers, Lean Cuisine, and Healthy Choice. How do they compare in terms of calories, fat content, and nutritional value?

FOR MORE INFORMATION

Books

Hensrud, D. D., ed. 2000. *Mayo Clinic on Healthy Weight.* New York: Kensington. *Presents basic information on determining and achieving a healthy body weight.*

Levenkorn, S. 2000. *Anatomy of Anorexia.* New York: Norton. *An up-to-date reference on the symptoms, diagnosis, and treatment of anorexia for patients, families, friends, and therapists.*

Milchovich, S. K., and B. Dunn-Long. 1999. *Diabetes Mellitus: A Practical Handbook,* 7th ed. Palo Alto, Calif.: Bull. *A user-friendly guide to diabetes.*

Nash, J. D. 1999. *Binge No More: Your Guide to Overcoming Disordered Eating.* Oakland, Calif.: New Harbinger. *Provides information and techniques for overcoming binge eating in the context of all types of disordered eating.*

Pope, H. G., K. A. Phillips, and R. Olivardia. 2000. *Adonis Complex: The Secret Crisis of Male Body Obsession.* New York: Free Press. *Provides a historical review of the changing fashions in male body type and information about male problems with body image.*

Rolls, B. J., and R. A. Barnett. 2001. *Volumetrics: Feel Full on Fewer Calories.* New York: HarperCollins. *Presents a research-based weight-management plan centering on the concept of energy density.*

WW. Organizations and Web Sites

American Diabetes Association. Provides information, a free newsletter, and referrals to local support groups; the Web site includes and online diabetes risk assessment.

800-342-2383; http://www.diabetes.org

Cyberdiet. Provides a variety of assessment and planning tools and practical tips for eating a healthy diet and being physically active.

http://www.cyberdiet.com

National Heart, Lung, and Blood Institute (NHLBI): Aim for a Healthy Weight. Provides information and tips on diet and physical activity, as well as a BMI calculator.

http://www.nhlbi.nih.gov/health/public/heart/obesity/lose_wt

National Institute of Diabetes and Digestive and Kidney Diseases (NIDDK). Health Information: Weight Loss and Control. Provides information and referrals for problems related to obesity, weight control, and nutritional disorders.

877-946-4627

http://www.niddk.nih.gov/health/nutrit/nutrit.htm

Partnership for Healthy Weight Management. Provides information on evaluating weight-loss programs and advertising claims.

http://www.consumer.gov/weightloss

Phys: Weight Loss. A commercial site with resources for self-assessment, goal setting, dietary planning, and exercise; also includes the "diet debunker," which reviews popular diet books.

http://www.phys.com/loseweight

Shape Up America! Provides materials about safe dietary and physical fitness strategies for successful weight management, including an online BMI calculator.

http://shapeup.org

Thrive Online/Weight Control. Information and tools for weight management, including a BMI calculator, a weight-loss readiness quiz, and suggestions for diet and exercise.

http://www.thriveonline.com/weight

There are also many resources for people concerned about eating disorders.

American Anorexia/Bulimia Association
http://www.aabainc.org

Anorexia Nervosa and Related Eating Disorders (ANRED)
http://www.anred.com

Eating Disorders Awareness and Prevention (EDAP)
800-931-2237; http://www.edap.org

National Association of Anorexia Nervosa and Associated Disorders (ANAD)
847-831-3438 (referral line); http://www.anad.org

Something Fishy Website on Eating Disorders
http://www.something-fishy.org

See also the listings in Chapter 9 and 10.

SELECTED BIBLIOGRAPHY

Cohane, G. H., and H. G. Pope. 2001. Body image in boys: A review of the literature. *International Journal of Eating Disorders* 29(4): 373–379.

Crespo, C. J., et al. 2001. Television watching, energy intake, and obesity in US children. *Archives of Pediatric and Adolescent Medicine* 155(3): 360–365.

Food and Drug Administration. 2001. FDA issues public health advisory on phenylpropanolamine in drug products. *FDA Consumer,* January/February.

Guide to rating the weight-loss Websites. 2000. *Tufts University Health and Nutrition Letter,* July Special Supplement.

Haller, C. A., and N. L. Benowitz. 2000. Adverse cardiovascular and central nervous system events associated with dietary supplements containing ephedra alkaloids. *New England Journal of Medicine* 343(25): 1833–1838.

Hu, F. B., et al. 2001. Physical activity and risk for cardiovascular events in diabetic women. *Annals of Internal Medicine* 134: 96–106.

Jick, H. 2000. Heart valve disorders and appetite-suppressant drugs. *Journal of the American Medical Association* 283(13): 1738–1740.

Kernan, W. N., et al. 2000. Phenylpropanolamine and the risk of hemorrhagic stroke. *New England Journal of Medicine* 343(25): 1826–1832.

Khan, L. K., et al. 2001. Use of prescription weight loss pills among U.S. adults in 1996–1998. *Annals of Internal Medicine* 134(4): 282–286.

Leit, R. A., H. G. Pope, and J. J. Gray. 2001. Cultural expectations of muscularity in men: The evolution of playgirl centerfolds. *International Journal of Eating Disorders* 29(1): 90–93.

Liebman, B. 2000. Ten tips for staying lean. *Nutrition Action Healthletter* 26(6): 3–7.

Litt, A. S. 2000. *The College Student's Guide to Eating Well on Campus.* Bethesda, Md.: Tulip Hill Press.

Lotufo, P. A., et al 2001. Diabetes and all-cause and coronary heart disease mortality among U.S. male physicians. *Archives of Internal Medicine* 161: 242–247.

Mokdad, A. H., et al. 2000. The continuing epidemic of obesity in the United States. *Journal of the American Medical Association* 284(13): 1650–1651.

Mokdad, A. H., et al. 2000. Diabetes trends in the U.S.: 1990–1998. *Diabetes Care* 23(9): 1278–1283.

National Center for Health Statistics. 2000. *Prevalence of Overweight and Obesity Among Adults: United States, 1999* (http://www.cdc.gov/nchs/products/pubs/pubd/hestats/obese/obse99.htm; retrieved December 15, 2000).

National Institute of Diabetes and Digestive and Kidney Disorders. 2001. *Prescription Medications for the Treatment of Obesity* (http://www.niddk.nih.gov/health/nutrit/pubs/presmeds.htm; retrieved April 19, 2001).

Pope, H. G., et al. 1999. Evolving ideals of male body image as seen through action toys. *International Journal of Eating Disorders* 26(1): 65–72.

Rubinstein, S., and B. Caballero. 2000. Is Miss America an undernourished role model? *Journal of the American Medical Association* 283(12): 1569.

Seidell, J. C., et al. 2001. Report from a Centers for Disease Control and Prevention workshop on use of adult anthropometry for public health and primary health care. *American Journal of Clinical Nutrition* 73(1): 123–126.

Shalala, D. E. 2000. *Good Nutrition and Public Health: Remarks at the National Nutrition Summit, May 30, 2000* (http://www.hhs.gov/news/speeches/000530.html; retrieved November 3, 2000).

Stevens, V. J., et al. 2001. Long-term weight loss and changes in blood pressure. *Annals of Internal Medicine* 134: 1–11.

Tate, D. F., R. R. Wing, and R. A. Winett. 2001. Using Internet technology to deliver a behavioral weight loss program. *Journal of the American Medical Association* 285(9): 1172–1777.

Wagner, E. H., et al. 2001. Effect of improved glycemic control on health care costs and utilization. *Journal of the American Medical Association* 285(2): 182–189.

Yanovski, J. A., et al. 2000. A prospective study of holiday weight gain. *New England Journal of Medicine* 342(12): 861–867.

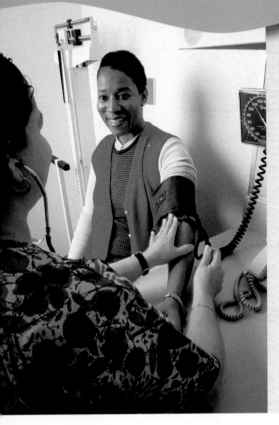

12

Cardiovascular Disease and Cancer

LOOKING AHEAD

After reading this chapter, you should be able to

- List the major components of the cardiovascular system and describe how blood is pumped and circulated throughout the body

- Describe the controllable and uncontrollable risk factors associated with cardiovascular disease

- Discuss the major forms of cardiovascular disease and how they develop

- Explain what cancer is and how it spreads

- List and describe common cancers—their risk factors, signs and symptoms, treatments, and approaches to prevention

- Discuss some of the causes of cancer and how they can be avoided or minimized, and describe how cancer can be detected, diagnosed, and treated

- List specific actions you can take to lower your risk of developing cardiovascular disease and cancer

Cardiovascular disease (CVD) is the leading cause of death in the United States, accounting for nearly half of all deaths. Cancer is the second leading cause, accounting for about a quarter of all deaths. Although genetics and the physical environment play roles, CVD and cancer are primarily lifestyle diseases. This chapter describes the forms and causes of these two killers and provides information about how to reduce your risk of succumbing to them.

THE CARDIOVASCULAR SYSTEM

The cardiovascular system consists of the heart and blood vessels (veins, arteries, and capillaries); together, they pump and circulate blood throughout the body. A person weighing 150 pounds has about 5 quarts of blood, which is circulated about once every minute.

The heart is a four-chambered, fist-size muscle located just beneath the ribs under the left breast (Figure 12-1). Its role is to pump oxygen-poor blood to the lungs and oxygenated (oxygen-rich) blood to the rest of the body. Blood actually travels through two separate circulatory systems: The right side of the heart pumps blood to and from the lungs in what is called *pulmonary circulation,* and the left side pumps blood through the rest of the body in *systemic circulation.*

Used, oxygen-poor blood enters the right upper chamber, or **atrium,** of the heart through the **vena cava,** the largest vein in the body (Figure 12-2). Valves prevent the blood from flowing the wrong way. As the right atrium fills, it contracts and pumps blood into the right lower chamber, or **ventricle,** which, when it contracts, pumps blood through the pulmonary artery into the lungs. There, blood picks up oxygen and discards carbon dioxide. Cleaned, oxygenated blood then flows through the

Blood vessels are classified by size and function. **Veins** carry blood to the heart; **arteries** carry blood away from the heart. Veins have thin walls, but arteries have thick elastic walls that enable them to expand and relax with the volume of the blood being pumped through them. After leaving the heart, the aorta branches into smaller and smaller vessels. Two vital arteries, called the coronary arteries, branch off the aorta to carry blood back to the heart tissues themselves.

The smallest arteries branch still further into **capillaries,** tiny vessels only one cell thick that deliver oxygen and nutrient-rich blood to the tissues and receive oxygen-poor, waste-carrying blood. From the capillaries, this blood empties into small veins and then into larger veins that return it to the heart. From there the cycle is repeated.

RISK FACTORS FOR CARDIOVASCULAR DISEASE

Researchers have identified a variety of factors associated with an increased risk of developing CVD. They are grouped into two categories: major risk factors and contributing risk factors. Some major risk factors, such as use of tobacco, are linked to controllable aspects of lifestyle and can therefore be changed. Others, such as age, sex, and heredity, are beyond an individual's control.

Major Risk Factors That Can Be Changed

The American Heart Association (AHA) has identified six major risk factors for CVD that can be changed: tobacco use, high blood pressure, unhealthy blood cholesterol levels, physical inactivity, obesity, and diabetes.

Tobacco Use About 1 in 5 deaths from CVD is attributable to smoking. People who smoke a pack of cigarettes a day have twice the risk of heart attack that nonsmokers have; smoking two or more packs a day triples the risk. And when smokers do have heart attacks, they are two to

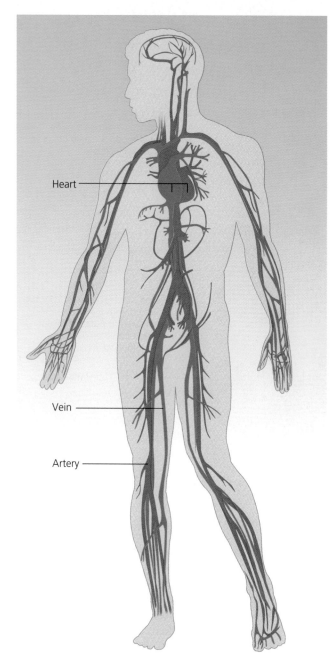

Figure 12-1 The cardiovascular system.

pulmonary veins into the left atrium. As this chamber fills, it contracts and pumps blood into the powerful left ventricle, which pumps it through the **aorta,** the body's largest artery, to be fed into the rest of the body's blood vessels. The period of the heart's contraction is called *systole;* the period of relaxation is called *diastole*.

The heartbeat—the split-second sequence of contractions of the heart's four chambers—is controlled by electrical impulses. These signals originate in a bundle of specialized cells in the right atrium called the pacemaker. Unless the pace is speeded up or slowed down by the brain in response to such stimuli as danger or exhaustion, the heart produces electrical impulses at a steady rate.

Terms

cardiovascular disease (CVD) The collective term for various forms of diseases of the heart and blood vessels.

atria The two upper chambers of the heart in which blood collects before passing to the ventricles; also called *auricles*.

vena cava The large vein through which blood is returned to the right atrium of the heart.

ventricles The two lower chambers of the heart from which blood flows through arteries to the lungs and other parts of the body.

aorta The large artery that receives blood from the left ventricle and distributes it to the body.

veins Vessels that carry blood to the heart.

arteries Vessels that carry blood away from the heart.

capillaries Very small blood vessels that distribute blood to all parts of the body.

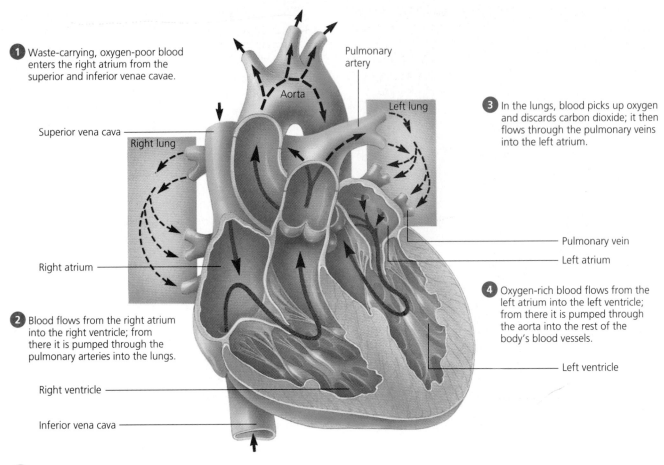

1 Waste-carrying, oxygen-poor blood enters the right atrium from the superior and inferior venae cavae.

Pulmonary artery

3 In the lungs, blood picks up oxygen and discards carbon dioxide; it then flows through the pulmonary veins into the left atrium.

Aorta

Left lung

Superior vena cava

Right lung

Pulmonary vein

Left atrium

Right atrium

4 Oxygen-rich blood flows from the left atrium into the left ventricle; from there it is pumped through the aorta into the rest of the body's blood vessels.

2 Blood flows from the right atrium into the right ventricle; from there it is pumped through the pulmonary arteries into the lungs.

Left ventricle

Right ventricle

Inferior vena cava

Figure 12-2   Circulation in the heart.

four times more likely than nonsmokers to die from them. Women who smoke heavily and use oral contraceptives are up to 32 times more likely to have a heart attack and up to 20 times more likely to have a stroke than women who don't smoke and take the pill.

Smoking harms the cardiovascular system and raises risk for CVD in several ways. Nicotine, a central nervous system stimulant, increases blood pressure and heart rate; the carbon monoxide in cigarette smoke displaces oxygen in the blood, reducing the amount of oxygen available to the heart and other parts of the body. Smoking damages the linings of arteries, and it contributes to unhealthy blood fat levels by reducing levels of high-density lipoproteins (HDL), "good cholesterol," and raising levels of triglycerides and low-density lipoproteins (LDL), "bad cholesterol." It causes the **platelets** in blood to become sticky and cluster, promoting clotting. Smoking also permanently accelerates the rate at which fatty deposits are laid down in arteries.

You don't have to smoke to be affected. The risk of death from coronary heart disease increases up to 30% among those exposed to environmental tobacco smoke (ETS) at home or at work. Researchers estimate that 62,000 nonsmokers die from CVD each year as a result of exposure to ETS.

High Blood Pressure   High blood pressure, or **hypertension,** is a risk factor for many forms of CVD but is also considered a disease itself. High blood pressure occurs when too much force or pressure is exerted against the walls of the arteries. If your blood pressure is high, your heart has to work harder to push the blood forward. Over time, a strained heart weakens and tends to enlarge, which weakens it further. Increased blood pressure also scars and hardens arteries, making them less elastic. Heart attacks, strokes, **atherosclerosis,** and kidney failure can result.

Hypertension usually has no early warning signs, so it's important to have your blood pressure tested at least once every two years (more often if you have CVD risk factors). If yours is consistently high, your physician can help you lower it through diet, weight management, exercise, and, if necessary, medication. (High blood pressure and atherosclerosis are discussed later in the chapter.)

High Levels of Cholesterol   Cholesterol is a fatty, wax-like substance that circulates through the bloodstream and is an important component of cell membranes, sex hormones, vitamin D, the fluid that coats the lungs, and the protective sheaths around nerves. Adequate cholesterol is essential for the proper functioning of the body. However, excess cholesterol can clog arteries and increase the risk of cardiovascular disease. Our bodies obtain cholesterol in two ways: from the liver, which manufactures it, and from the foods we eat. Cholesterol levels vary depending on diet, age, sex, heredity, and other factors.

GOOD VERSUS BAD CHOLESTEROL   Cholesterol is carried in the blood in protein-lipid packages called lipoproteins. Lipoproteins can be thought of as shuttles that transport cholesterol to and from the liver through the circulatory system. **Low-density lipoproteins (LDLs)** shuttle cholesterol from the liver to the organs and tissues that require it. LDL is known as "bad" cholesterol because if there is more than the body can use, the excess is deposited in the blood vessels. If coronary arteries are blocked, the result may be a heart attack; if an artery carrying blood to the brain is blocked, a stroke may occur. **High-density lipoproteins (HDLs)**, or "good" cholesterol, shuttle unused cholesterol back to the liver for recycling. By removing cholesterol from blood vessels, HDL helps protect against atherosclerosis.

RECOMMENDED BLOOD CHOLESTEROL LEVELS   The National Cholesterol Education Program (NCEP) recommends cholesterol testing at least once every 5 years for all adults, beginning at age 20. The recommended test is a lipoprotein profile that measures total cholesterol, LDL cholesterol, HDL cholesterol, and triglycerides (another blood fat). General cholesterol and triglyceride guidelines are given in Table 12-1. In general, high LDL levels and low HDL levels are associated with a high risk for CVD; low levels of LDL and high levels of HDL are associated with lower risk. HDL is important because a high HDL level seems to offer protection from CVD even in cases where total cholesterol is high.

As shown in Table 12-1, LDL levels below 100 mg/dl (milligrams per deciliter) and total cholesterol levels below 200 mg/dl are desirable. An estimated 100 million American adults—over half the population—have total cholesterol levels of 200 mg/dl or higher. The CVD risk associated with elevated cholesterol levels also depends on other factors. For example, an above optimal level of LDL would be of more concern for an individual who also smoked and had high blood pressure than for an individual without these additional CVD risk factors.

IMPROVING CHOLESTEROL LEVELS   Important dietary changes that lower LDL levels include substituting unsaturated for saturated and trans fats and increasing soluble fiber intake. Decreasing your intake of saturated and trans fats is particularly important because they promote the production and excretion of cholesterol by the liver. Exercising regularly and eating more fruits, vegetables, and whole grains also help. You can raise your HDL levels by exercising regularly, losing weight if you are overweight,

Table 12-1	Cholesterol Guidelines
LDL cholesterol (mg/dl)	
Less than 100	Optimal
100–129	Near optimal/above optimal
130–159	Borderline high
160–189	High
190 or more	Very high
Total cholesterol (mg/dl)	
Less than 200	Desirable
200–239	Borderline high
240 or more	High
HDL cholesterol (mg/dl)	
Less than 40	Low
60 or more	High
Triglycerides (mg/dl)	
Less than 150	Normal
150–199	Borderline high
200–499	High
500 or more	Very high

SOURCES: Expert Panel on Detection, Evaluation, and Treatment of High Blood Cholesterol in Adults. 2001. Executive Summary of the Third Report of the National Cholesterol Education Program (NCEP) Expert Panel on Detection, Evaluation, and Treatment of High Blood Cholesterol in Adults (Adult Treatment Panel III). *Journal of the American Medical Association* 285(19).

quitting smoking, and altering the amount and type of fat you consume.

Physical Inactivity   An estimated 35–50 million Americans are so sedentary that they are at high risk for developing CVD. Exercise is thought to be the closest

platelets Microscopic disk-shaped cell fragments in the blood that disintegrate on contact with foreign objects and release chemicals that are necessary for the formation of blood clots.

hypertension Sustained abnormally high blood pressure.

atherosclerosis A form of CVD in which the inner layers of artery walls are made thick and irregular by plaque deposits; arteries become narrow and blood supply is reduced.

low-density lipoproteins (LDL) Blood fat that transports cholesterol from the liver to organs and tissues; excess is deposited on artery walls, where it can eventually block the flow of blood to the heart and brain; "bad" cholesterol.

high-density lipoprotein (HDL) Blood fat that helps transport cholesterol out of the arteries and thus protects against heart diseases; "good" cholesterol.

Terms

thing we have to a "magic bullet" against heart disease. It lowers CVD risk by helping decrease blood pressure, increase HDL levels, maintain desirable weight, and prevent or control diabetes. A minimum of 30 minutes per day of moderate physical activity is recommended; more intense or longer-duration exercise has even greater health benefits (see Chapter 10).

Obesity   A person whose body weight is more than 30% above the recommended level is at higher risk for heart disease and stroke, even if no other risk factors are present. Excess weight increases the strain on the heart by contributing to high blood pressure and high cholesterol. It can also lead to diabetes, another CVD risk factor. As discussed in Chapter 11, distribution of body fat is also significant: Fat that collects in the torso is more dangerous than fat that collects around the hips. A sensible diet and regular exercise are the best ways to achieve and maintain a healthy body weight. For someone who is overweight, even modest weight reduction can reduce CVD risk.

Diabetes   As described in Chapter 11, diabetes is a disorder characterized by elevated blood glucose levels due to either insufficient supply or insufficient action of insulin. People with diabetes are at increased risk for CVD, partly because elevated blood glucose levels can damage the lining of arteries, making them more vulnerable to atherosclerosis; diabetics also often have other risk factors, including hypertension, obesity, and unhealthy cholesterol levels. Even people whose diabetes is under control face an increased risk of CVD, therefore, careful control of other risk factors is critical for people with diabetes.

Contributing Risk Factors That Can Be Changed

Other factors that can be changed also contribute to CVD risk, including triglyceride levels and psychological and social factors.

High Triglyceride Levels   Like cholesterol, triglycerides are blood fats that are obtained from food and manufactured by the body. High triglyceride levels are a reliable predictor of heart disease, especially if associated with other risk factors, such as low HDL levels, obesity, and diabetes. Factors contributing to elevated triglyceride levels include excess body fat, physical inactivity, cigarette smoking, excess alcohol intake, very high carbohydrate diets, and certain diseases and medications.

A full lipid profile should include testing and evaluation of triglyceride levels (see Table 15-1). For people with borderline high triglyceride levels, increased physical activity and weight reduction can help bring levels down into the healthy range; for people with high triglycerides, drug therapy may be recommended. Being moderate in the use of alcohol and quitting smoking are also important.

Psychological and Social Factors   Many of the psychological and social factors that influence other areas of wellness are also important risk factors for CVD.

• *Stress.* Excessive stress can strain the heart and blood vessels over time and contribute to CVD. A full-blown stress response causes blood pressure to rise; blood platelets become more likely to cluster, possibly enhancing the formation of artery-clogging clots. Stress can also trigger abnormal heart rhythms (arrhythmias), with potentially fatal consequences.

• *Chronic hostility and anger.* Certain traits in the hard-driving "Type A" personality—hostility, cynicism, and anger—are associated with increased risk of heart disease. Men prone to anger have two to three times the heart attack risk of calmer men.

• *Suppressing psychological distress.* Suppressing anger and other negative emotions may also be hazardous. People who hide psychological distress appear to have higher rates of heart disease than people who experience similar distress but share it with others. People with so-called Type D personalities tend to be pessimistic, negative, and unhappy and to suppress these feelings.

• *Depression and anxiety.* Both mild and severe depression are linked to an increased risk of CVD, and there is a strong association between anxiety disorders and an increased risk of death from heart disease, particularly sudden death from heart attack.

• *Social isolation.* People with little social support are at higher risk for dying from CVD than people with close ties to others. A strong social support network is a major antidote to stress. Friends and family members can also promote and support a healthy lifestyle.

• *Low socioeconomic status.* Low socioeconomic status and low educational attainment also increase risk for CVD. These associations are probably due to a variety of factors, including lifestyle and access to health care.

COMMUNICATE!   Does someone in your family have any major risk factors for cardiovascular disease that can be changed, such as smoking or physical inactivity? If so, practice how you might talk to the person about altering his or her behavior to reduce risk. Be prepared for some resistance; you may have to have more than one conversation about your concern. You might begin by saying, for instance, "Dad, I'm worried about what smoking might be doing to your heart. Can we talk about that for a minute?"

Major Risk Factors That Can't Be Changed

A number of major risk factors for CVD cannot be changed: heredity, aging, being male, and ethnicity.

Current research suggests that people with a quick temper, a persistently hostile outlook, and a cynical, mistrusting attitude toward life are more likely to develop heart disease than those with a calmer, more trusting attitude. People who are angry frequently, intensely, and for long periods experience the stress response—and its accompanying boosts in heart rate, blood pressure, and stress hormone levels—much more often than more relaxed individuals. Over the long term, these effects may damage arteries and promote CVD.

Are you too hostile? To help answer that question, Duke University researcher Redford Williams, M.D., has devised a short self-test. It's not a scientific evaluation, but it does offer a rough measure of hostility. Are the following statements true or false for you?

1. I often get annoyed at checkout cashiers or the people in front of me when I'm waiting in line.

2. I usually keep an eye on the people I work or live with to make sure they do what they should.

3. I often wonder how homeless people can have so little respect for themselves.

4. I believe that most people will take advantage of you if you let them.

5. The habits of friends or family members often annoy me.

6. When I'm stuck in traffic, I often start breathing faster and my heart pounds.

7. When I'm annoyed with people, I really want to let them know it.

8. If someone does me wrong, I want to get even.

9. I'd like to have the last word in any argument.

10. At least once a week, I have the urge to yell at or even hit someone.

According to Williams, five or more "true" statements suggest that you're excessively hostile and should consider taking steps to mellow out.

To manage your anger, begin by monitoring your angry responses and looking for triggers—people or situations that typically make you angry. Familiarize yourself with the patterns of thinking that lead to angry or hostile feelings, and then try to head them off before they develop into full-blown anger. If you feel your anger starting to build, try reasoning with yourself by asking the following questions:

1. *Is this really important enough to get angry about?* For example, is having to wait an extra 5 minutes for a late bus so important that you should stew about it for the entire 15-minute ride?

2. *Am I really justified in getting angry?* Is the person in front of you really driving slowly, or are you trying to speed?

3. *Is getting angry going to make a real and positive difference in this situation?* Will yelling and slamming the door really help your friend find the concert tickets he misplaced?

If you answer "yes" to all three questions, then calm but assertive communication may be an appropriate response. If your anger isn't reasonable, try distracting yourself or removing yourself from the situation. Exercise, humor, social support, and other stress-management techniques can also help (see Chapter 3 for additional anger-management tips). Your heart—and the people around you—will benefit from your calmer, more positive outlook.

SOURCES: Take it to heart: "Chill out." 2000. *Mind/Body/Health Newsletter* 9(2): 1–2. Anger and heart-disease risk. 2000. *Harvard Heart Letter,* July. QUIZ SOURCE: Is hostility hurting your heart? 1998. *Consumer Reports on Health,* August.

Heredity   The tendency to develop CVD seems to be inherited. High cholesterol levels, hypertension, abnormal blood-clotting problems, diabetes, and obesity are other CVD risk factors that have genetic links. People who inherit a tendency for CVD are not destined to develop it, but they may, have to work harder than other people to prevent CVD.

Aging   The risk of heart attack increases dramatically after age 65. About 70% of all heart attack victims are age 65 or older, and more than four out of five who suffer fatal heart attacks are over 65. For people over 55, the incidence of stroke more than doubles in each successive decade. However, many people in their thirties and forties, especially men, have heart attacks.

Being Male   Although CVD is the leading killer of both men and women in the United States, men face a greater risk of heart attack than women, especially earlier in life. Until age 55, men also have a greater risk of hypertension than women. The incidence of stroke is about 19% higher for males than females. Estrogen production, which is highest during the childbearing years, may offer premenopausal women some protection against CVD.

Ethnicity   Death rates from heart disease vary among ethnic groups in the United States, with African Americans having much higher rates of hypertension, heart disease, and stroke than other groups. Puerto Rican Americans, Cuban Americans, and Mexican Americans

CVD is the leading cause of death for all Americans, but significant differences exist between men and women and between white Americans and African Americans in the incidence, diagnosis, and treatment of this deadly disease.

CVD has been thought of as a "man's disease," but it actually kills more women than men. Polls indicate that women vastly underestimate their risk of dying of a heart attack and overestimate their risk of dying of breast cancer. In reality, nearly 1 in 2 women dies of CVD, while 1 in 23 dies of breast cancer. For women, CVD typically does not develop until after age 50, because of the protective effects of estrogen prior to menopause. Estrogen improves cholesterol levels in the blood by increasing HDL levels and decreasing LDL levels. Some women choose hormone replacement therapy (HRT) after menopause to keep estrogen levels high, although HRT may provide little benefit for women who already have heart disease.

When women do have heart attacks, they are more likely than men to die within a year. One reason is that since they develop heart disease at older ages, they are more likely to have other health problems that complicate treatment. Women also have smaller hearts and arteries than men, possibly making diagnosis and surgery more difficult. Another reason is that medical personnel appear to evaluate and treat women less aggressively than men. Physicians may not immediately recognize the symptoms women describe (women are more likely than men to have a heart attack without chest pain), and they may be more willing to dismiss the health problems of an older woman than those of a man in the "prime of life." Until greater awareness and better diagnostic techniques are in place, women must be persistent in seeking accurate diagnosis and effective treatment.

African Americans also have a different experience of CVD than do white men. The CVD death rate is about 25% higher in black men and 33% higher in black women than in whites. Blacks tend to develop hypertension at an earlier age than whites, and their average blood pressures are much higher. As a result, the stroke rate among blacks is 1.5 times greater than that among whites.

Possible genetic and biological factors in this CVD profile include heightened sensitivities to salt and a physiologically different response to stress, which can lead to high blood pressure and a greater tendency to develop diabetes, another CVD risk factor. Low income is another factor and is associated with reduced access to adequate health care, insurance, and information about prevention. Discrimination may also play a role, both by increasing stress and by affecting treatment by physicians and hospitals.

Although these factors are important, recent evidence favors lifestyle explanations for the higher CVD rate among African Americans. For example, black New Yorkers born in the South have a much higher CVD risk than those born in the Northeast. (Researchers speculate that some lifestyle risk factors for CVD, including smoking and a high-fat diet, may be more common in the South.) People with low incomes, who are disproportionately black, tend to smoke more, use more salt, and exercise less than those with higher incomes. In addition, half of black women and one-third of black men are overweight.

The general preventive strategies recommended for all Americans may be particularly critical for African Americans. In addition, researchers have identified several dietary factors that may be of special importance for blacks. Studies have found that diets high in potassium and calcium improve blood pressure in African Americans. Fruits, vegetables, grains, and nuts are rich in potassium; dairy products are high in calcium.

---

are also more likely to suffer from high blood pressure and angina (a warning sign of heart disease) than non-Hispanic white Americans. These differences may be due in part to differences in education, income, and other socioeconomic factors. Asian Americans historically have had far lower rates of CVD than white Americans. However, cholesterol levels among Asian Americans appear to be rising, presumably because of the adoption of a high-fat American diet.

Possible Risk Factors Currently Being Studied

In recent years, a number of other possible risk factors for cardiovascular disease have been identified.

Elevated blood levels of homocysteine, an amino acid that may damage the lining of blood vessels, are associated with an increased risk of CVD. Men generally have higher homocysteine levels than women, as do individuals with diets low in folic acid, vitamin B-12, and vitamin B-6. Most people can lower homocysteine levels easily by adopting a healthy diet rich in fruits, vegetables, and grains and by taking supplements if needed.

High levels of a specific type of LDL called lipoprotein(a), or Lp(a), have been identified as a possible risk factor for coronary heart disease (CHD), especially when associated with high LDL or low HDL levels. Lp(a) levels have a strong genetic component and are difficult to treat. LDL particles differ in size and density, and people with a high proportion of small, dense LDL particles—a condition called LDL pattern B—also appear to be at greater risk for CVD. Exercise, a low-fat diet, and certain lipid-lowering drugs may help lower CVD risk in people with LDL pattern B.

Terms   **glycemic index** A measure of how the ingestion of a particular food affects blood glucose levels.

Is reducing the total amount of fat you eat always a good idea? Are you better off replacing saturated and trans fats with carbohydrates or with unsaturated fats? The answers to these hotly debated questions are not necessarily what you might think based on current dietary recommendations.

A diet with 30% or less of total calories from fat is recommended by most major health organizations. However, some experts feel that the total amount of fat we consume is much less important than the type of fat we consume—and that we may benefit from eating more fat, as long as it's the right kind. Research has shown that people from Mediterranean countries whose diets are rich in olive oil (a monounsaturated fat) have low rates of CVD, even though their total fat intake is high. Since monounsaturated fats raise HDL levels, increasing the amount of these fats in our diets may be a good CVD prevention strategy, even if it raises total fat intake above 30% of daily calories. Omega-3 fatty acids from fish are also considered heart-healthy.

Most experts agree that reducing intake of saturated and trans fat is important for CVD prevention. There is less agreement, however, on whether it's best to replace saturated and trans fats with carbohydrates or with unsaturated fats. (For those trying to lose weight, the best strategy may be simply to cut back on saturated and trans fats without replacing them with anything else.) In some people, a diet high in carbohydrate and low in fat has a negative effect—lowering HDL levels and raising levels of triglycerides and glucose. These effects occur in part due to the high **glycemic index** of some carbohydrate-rich foods. Glycemic index refers to how quickly and how high a food causes blood glucose levels to rise. For example, white rice and potatoes have high glycemic indices and cause a dramatic rise in glucose and insulin levels a few hours after eating; legumes have a low index, and they break down more slowly and produce a more gradual rise in glucose and

insulin levels. Eating lots of foods that rapidly raise glucose levels may contribute to the development or worsening of diabetes and CVD in some people, including those with syndrome X. For this group, then, a diet relatively high in unsaturated and total fat might be a better choice than a diet high in carbohydrates.

Another consideration, however, is that carbohydrate-rich foods typically have a lower calorie density than fat-rich foods, so substituting carbohydrates for fats can be helpful if it means consuming fewer total calories. If one chooses to substitute carbohydrates for fats, it's important to focus on healthy choices— fruits, vegetables, and whole grains—rather than low-fat or fat-free foods that are high in added sugars and calories and low in other nutrients. For people with insulin resistance or diabetes, choosing foods based on glycemic index may be a helpful strategy. Consuming high-fiber foods has also been shown to improve cholesterol and glucose levels.

The 2001 NCEP guidelines for people with elevated cholesterol allow total fat intake of up to 35% of total daily calories, with up to 10% of total calories from polyunsaturated fat, up to 20% from monounsaturated fat, and less than 7% as saturated fat. This slightly higher intake of total fat, primarily as unsaturated fat, can help raise HDL and lower triglycerides in people with syndrome X. However, simply adding unsaturated fats to the typical American diet is unlikely to yield all the benefits associated with the Mediterranean diet. In addition to being rich in olive oil, the Mediterranean diet is also low in saturated and trans fats, meats, and dairy products and rich in grains, fresh fruits and vegetables, and fish.

Ongoing research should help clarify the effects of different types and amounts of dietary fat. It may be that in the future, each of us will get individualized advice based on our particular risk profile—diets high in unsaturated fats for some people, diets high in healthy carbohydrates for others. Until that time,

Several infectious agents, including *Chlamydia pneumoniae, cytomegalovirus,* and *Helicobacter pylori,* have also been identified as possible risk factors. Infections may damage arteries and lead to chronic inflammation, another potential risk factor for CVD. When an artery is injured by smoking, cholesterol, infectious agents, or other factors, the body responds with inflammation. A substance called C-reactive protein is released into the bloodstream during the inflammatory response; high levels of C-reactive protein may indicate an elevated risk of heart attack and stroke. Another marker for higher risk is fibrinogen, a protein involved in blood clotting. Aspirin, which reduces both clotting and inflammation, is often recommended for people at high risk for heart attacks and strokes. Other possible risk factors under investigation are blood viscosity (thickness), excess stored iron, high blood levels of uric acid

and a cluster of risk factors—including high blood pressure, high triglycerides, low HDL, abdominal obesity, and insulin resistance—that appear together in some individuals and are known as syndrome X or metabolic syndrome.

MAJOR FORMS OF CARDIOVASCULAR DISEASE

Collectively, the various forms of CVD kill more Americans than the next four leading causes of death combined (Figure 12-3). The financial burden of CVD, including the costs of medical treatments and lost productivity, exceeds $300 billion annually. Although the main forms of CVD are interrelated and have elements in common, we treat them separately here for the sake of clarity.

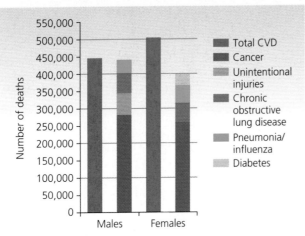

(a) Leading causes of death

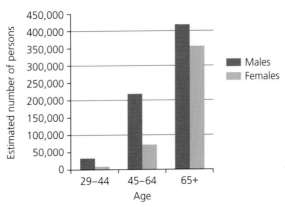

(b) Annual incidence of heart attack

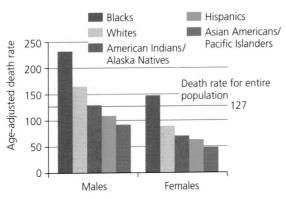

(c) Heart disease death rates

Figure 12-3 A statistical look at cardiovascular disease in the United States. (a) The leading causes of death. CVD causes more deaths than the next four causes combined. (b) Estimated numbers of Americans who have a heart attack each year. Among heart attack victims under age 65, men significantly outnumber women; after age 65, women start to catch up. (c) Heart disease death rates by gender and ethnicity.   SOURCES: American Heart Association. 2001. *2001 Heart and Stroke Facts Statistical Update.* Dallas, Tex.: American Heart Association. National Center for Health Statistics. 2000. *Health, United States, 2000.* Hyattsville, Md.: U.S. Public Health Service, DHHS Pub. No. (PHS) 00–1232.

Hypertension

Blood pressure, the force exerted by the blood on blood vessel walls, is created by the pumping action of the heart. When the heart contracts (systole), blood pressure increases; when the heart relaxes (diastole), pressure decreases. Short periods of high blood pressure are normal, but blood pressure that is continually at an abnormally high level is known as hypertension.

Blood pressure is measured with a stethoscope and an instrument called a sphygmomanometer. It is expressed as two numbers—for example, 120 over 80—and measured in millimeters of mercury. The first and larger number is the systolic blood pressure; the second is the diastolic blood pressure. Average blood pressure readings for young adults in good physical condition are 110–120 systolic over 70–80 diastolic. High blood pressure in adults is defined as equal to or greater than 140 over 90 (Table 12-2).

High blood pressure results from either an increased output of blood by the heart or, most often, increased resistance to blood flow in the arteries. When a person has high blood pressure, the heart must work harder than normal to force blood through the narrowed arteries, thereby straining both the heart and arteries. High blood pressure is often called a "silent killer," because it usually has no symptoms. A person may have high blood pressure for years without realizing it. But during that time, it damages vital organs and increases the risk of heart attack, congestive heart failure, stroke, kidney failure, and blindness.

Hypertension is common, occurring in about 1 in 4 adults. In most cases, hypertension cannot be cured, but it can be controlled. The key to avoiding the complications of hypertension is to have your blood pressure checked regularly and to follow your physician's advice about lifestyle changes and medication.

People with mild hypertension can frequently lower their blood pressure through lifestyle changes, including quitting smoking, exercising regularly, and improving diet. Controlling total calorie intake is important for achieving and maintaining a healthy body weight. Increasing intake of fruits, vegetables, and whole grains is recommended because these foods are rich in potassium and fiber, both of which may reduce blood pressure. About half of all people with hypertension are "salt-sensitive," meaning that their blood pressure will decrease significantly when salt intake is restricted. Most experts feel that restricting sodium intake to about 2400 mg per day is a good strategy for all people—whether they have hypertension or not. Recent research has shown that lowering your blood pressure through healthy lifestyle changes improves cardiovascular health even if your current blood pressure is already below 140 over 90. For people whose blood pressure isn't adequately controlled with lifestyle changes, many different types of antihypertensive drugs are available.

Table 12-2	Blood Pressure Classification for Healthy Adults			
Category[a]	Systolic (mm Hg)			Diastolic (mm Hg)
Optimal[b]	below 120	and		below 80
Normal	below 130	and		below 85
High-normal	130–139	or		85–89
Hypertension[c]				
Stage 1	140–159	or		90–99
Stage 2	160–179	or		100–109
Stage 3	180 and above	or		110 and above

[a]When systolic and diastolic pressure fall into different categories, the higher category should be used to classify blood pressure status.
[b]Optimal blood pressure with respect to cardiovascular risk is below 120/80 mm Hg; however, unusually low readings should be evaluated.
[c]Based on the average of two or more readings taken at different physician visits.

SOURCE: *The Sixth Report of the Joint National Committee on Prevention, Detection, Evaluation, and Treatment of High Blood Pressure.* 1997. Bethesda, Md.: National Heart, Lung, and Blood Institute. National Institutes of Health (NIH Publication No. 98-4080).

Atherosclerosis

Atherosclerosis is a slow, progressive hardening and narrowing of the arteries that can begin in childhood. Arteries become narrowed by deposits of fat, cholesterol, and other substances. The process begins when the cells that line the arteries (endothelial cells) become damaged, most likely through a combination of factors such as smoking, high blood pressure, and deposits of oxidized LDL particles. The body's response to this damage results in inflammation and changes in the artery lining. Deposits, called **plaques,** accumulate on artery walls, and the arteries lose their elasticity and their ability to expand and contract, restricting blood flow. Once narrowed by a plaque, an artery is vulnerable to blockage by blood clots (Figure 12-4).

If the heart, brain, and/or other organs are deprived of blood, and thus the vital oxygen it carries, the effects of atherosclerosis can be deadly. Coronary arteries, which supply the heart with blood, are particularly susceptible to plaque buildup, a condition called **coronary heart disease (CHD),** or *coronary artery disease.* The blockage of a coronary artery causes a heart attack. If a cerebral artery (leading to the brain) is blocked, the result is a stroke. If an artery in a limb becomes narrowed or blocked, it causes *peripheral vascular disease,* a condition that causes pain and sometimes loss of the affected limb.

The main risk factors for atherosclerosis are cigarette smoking, physical inactivity, high levels of blood cholesterol, high blood pressure, and diabetes.

Heart Disease and Heart Attacks

Although a **heart attack,** or myocardial infarction (MI), may come without warning, it is usually the end result of a long-term disease process. When one of the coronary arteries becomes blocked, a heart attack results. A heart attack caused by a clot is called a **coronary thrombosis.** During a heart attack, part of the heart muscle (myocardium) may die from lack of oxygen. If an MI is not fatal, the heart muscle may sometimes partially repair itself.

Angina   Arteries narrowed by disease may still be open enough to deliver blood to the heart. At times, however—primarily during emotional excitement, stress, or physical exertion—the heart requires more oxygen than narrowed arteries can accommodate. When the need for oxygen exceeds the supply, chest pain, called **angina pectoris,** may occur. Angina pain is felt as an extreme tightness in the chest and heavy pressure behind the breastbone or in the shoulder, neck, arm, hand, or back. Angina may be controlled with drugs or surgical procedures, but over a period ranging from hours to years, the narrowing may go on to full blockage and a heart attack.

Arrhythmias and Sudden Cardiac Death   The pumping of the heart is controlled by electrical impulses that maintain a regular heartbeat of 60–100 beats per minute. If this electrical conduction system is disrupted, the heart may beat too quickly, too slowly, or in an irregular fashion, a condition known as **arrhythmia.** The symptoms of arrhythmia range from imperceptible to severe and even fatal.

Sudden cardiac death is most often caused by an arrhythmia called ventricular fibrillation, a kind of "quivering" of the ventricle that makes it ineffective in pumping blood. If ventricular fibrillation continues for more than a few minutes, it is fatal. Cardiac defibrillation, in which an electrical shock is delivered to the heart, can be effective in jolting the heart into a more efficient

plaque A deposit of fatty (and other) substances on the inner wall of the arteries.

coronary heart disease (CHD) Heart disease caused by atherosclerosis in the arteries that supply oxygen to the heart muscle; also called *coronary artery disease.*

heart attack Damage to, or death of, heart muscle, sometimes resulting in a failure of the heart to deliver enough blood to the body; also known as myocardial infarction (MI).

coronary thrombosis A clot in a coronary artery, often causing sudden death.

angina pectoris A condition in which the heart muscle does not receive enough blood, causing severe pain in the chest and often in the left arm and shoulder.

arrhythmia A change in the normal pattern of the heartbeat.

sudden cardiac death A nontraumatic, unexpected death from sudden cardiac arrest, most often due to arrhythmia; in most instances, victims have underlying heart disease.

Terms

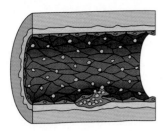 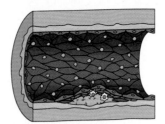 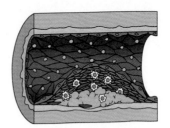 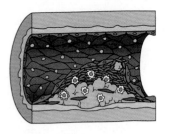

Plaque buildup begins when endothelial cells lining the arteries are damaged by smoking, high blood pressure, oxidized LDL, and other causes; excess cholesterol particles collect beneath these cells.

In response to the damage, platelets and other types of cells collect at the site; a fibrous cap forms, isolating the plaque within the artery wall. An early-stage plaque is called a fatty streak.

Chemicals released by cells in and around the plaque cause further inflammation and buildup; an advanced plaque contains LDL, white blood cells, connective tissue, smooth muscle cells, platelets, and other compounds.

The narrowed artery is vulnerable to blockage by clots. The risk of blockage and heart attack rises if the fibrous cap cracks (probably due to destructive enzymes released by white blood cells within the plaque).

Figure 12-4 Stages of plaque development.

rhythm. Some arrhythmias cause no problems and resolve without treatment; more serious arrhythmias are usually treated with medication or a surgically implanted pacemaker.

Helping a Heart Attack Victim   Most people who die from a heart attack do so within 2 hours of experiencing the first symptoms. If you or someone you are with has any of the warning signs of heart attack listed in the box "What to Do in Case of a Heart Attack or Stroke," take immediate action. Call your emergency medical service immediately or get to the nearest hospital emergency room or clinic that offers 24-hour emergency cardiac care. Get help even if the person denies there is something wrong. One additional step recommended by many experts is for the affected individual to chew and swallow one adult aspirin tablet (325 mg); aspirin has an immediate anticlotting effect.

If the person loses consciousness, emergency **cardiopulmonary resuscitation (CPR)** should be initiated by a qualified person. If the victim receives emergency care quickly enough, a clot-dissolving agent can be injected to break up a clot in the coronary artery. These "clot-busting" drugs are being used successfully to treat not only heart attacks but also some types of stroke.

Detecting and Treating Heart Disease   Currently, the most common initial screening tool for heart disease is the stress, or exercise, test, in which a patient runs or walks on a treadmill or pedals a stationary cycle while being monitored for abnormalities with an **electrocardiogram (ECG or EKG)**. Certain characteristic changes in the heart's electrical activity while under stress can reveal particular heart problems, such as restricted blood flow. Exercise testing can also be performed in conjunction with techniques such as ultrasonography and X ray.

Other tests for evaluating CVD include electron-beam computed tomography (EBCT), used to detect calcium in the arteries, a marker for atherosclerosis; echocardiographic equipment, which uses sound waves to examine the heart; and magnetic resonance imaging, which uses powerful magnets to look inside the body. If these tests suggest coronary artery disease, the next step is usually a coronary angiogram. In this test, a special dye is injected into the bloodstream, and X rays are used to trace the flow of blood through the coronary arteries and heart.

Various treatments are available if a problem is detected. Along with a low-fat diet, regular exercise, and smoking cessation, one frequent nonsurgical recommendation for people at high risk for CVD is to take half an aspirin tablet a day. Aspirin has an anticlotting effect and reduces inflammation. Various prescription drugs can help control heart rate, lower blood pressure, reduce the strain on the heart, and lower cholesterol levels.

A common surgical procedure for treating heart disease is *balloon angioplasty.* This technique involves threading a catheter with an inflatable balloon tip through the artery until it reaches the area of blockage. The balloon is then inflated, flattening the fatty plaque and widening the arterial opening. However, repeat clogging of the artery, known as *restenosis,* is common. To keep arteries open following angioplasty, many surgeons also permanently implant coronary stents—flexible, stainless steel mesh tubes that remain in place as a framework to prop the artery open and prevent restenosis.

Every year, coronary bypass surgery is performed on well over 300,000 men and women, about half of whom are under age 65. Surgeons remove a healthy blood vessel, usually a vein from one of the patient's legs, and graft it to one or more coronary arteries to bypass a blockage.

Stroke

For brain cells to function as they should, they must have a continuous and ample supply of oxygen-rich blood. If brain cells are deprived of blood for more than a few minutes, they die. A **stroke,** also called a *cerebrovascular accident (CVA),* occurs when the blood supply to the brain is cut off. Prompt treatment of stroke can greatly decrease the risk of permanent disability.

Heart Attack Warning Signs

The American Heart Association says these are the most common warning signs of a heart attack:

- Uncomfortable pressure, fullness, squeezing, or pain in the center of the chest lasting more than a few minutes
- Pain spreading to the shoulders, neck, or arms
- Chest discomfort with light-headedness, fainting, sweating, nausea, or shortness of breath

Less-common warning signs of a heart attack are . . .

- Atypical chest pain or stomach or abdominal pain
- Nausea or dizziness
- Shortness of breath and difficulty breathing
- Unexplained anxiety, weakness, or fatigue
- Palpitations, cold sweat, or paleness

Stroke Warning Signs

The American Stroke Association says these are the warning signs of stroke:

- Sudden weakness or numbness of the face, arm, or leg, especially on one side of the body
- Sudden confusion or trouble speaking or understanding
- Sudden trouble seeing in one or both eyes
- Sudden trouble walking, dizziness, or loss of balance or coordination
- Sudden, severe headache with no known cause

Dial 9-1-1 Fast

Heart attack and stroke are life-and-death emergencies—every second counts. If you see or have any of these symptoms, immediately call 9-1-1. Not all these signs occur in every attack. Sometimes they go away and return. If some occur, get help fast! Treatment is more effective when given quickly.

Types of Strokes   There are two major types of strokes: **ischemic strokes,** which are caused by blockages in blood vessels, and **hemorrhagic strokes,** which are caused by rupture of blood vessels, leading to bleeding into the brain (Figure 12-5). One type of ischemic stroke, the *thrombotic stroke,* is caused by a **thrombus,** a blood clot that forms in a cerebral artery that has been narrowed or damaged by atherosclerosis. The second type of ischemic stroke, called an *embolic stroke,* is caused by an **embolus,** a wandering blood clot that is carried in the bloodstream and may become wedged in one of the cerebral arteries. Many embolic strokes are linked to a type of abnormal heart rhythm called atrial fibrillation.

The other, less common but more severe, type of stroke is the hemorrhagic stroke. It occurs when a blood vessel in the brain bursts, spilling blood into the surrounding tissue. Cells normally nourished by the artery are deprived of blood and cannot function. In addition, accumulated blood from the burst vessel may put pressure on surrounding brain tissue, causing damage and even death. Hemorrhages can be caused by head injuries or the bursting of an **aneurysm,** a blood-filled pocket that bulges out from a weak spot in an artery wall. Aneurysms in the brain may remain stable and never break. But when they do, the result is a stroke. Aneurysms may be caused or worsened by high blood pressure.

The Effects of a Stroke   The interruption of the blood supply to any area of the brain prevents the nerve cells there from functioning—in some cases, causing death. Of the 600,000 Americans who have strokes each year, nearly one-third die within a year. Those who survive usually have some lasting disability. A stroke may cause paralysis, walking disability, speech impairment, memory loss, and changes in behavior. The severity of the stroke and its long-term effects depend on which brain cells have been injured, how widespread the damage is, how effectively the body can restore the blood supply, and how rapidly other areas of the brain can take over.

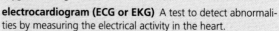

cardiopulmonary resuscitation (CPR) A technique involving mouth-to-mouth breathing and chest compression to keep oxygen flowing to the brain.

electrocardiogram (ECG or EKG) A test to detect abnormalities by measuring the electrical activity in the heart.

stroke An impeded blood supply to some part of the brain resulting in the destruction of brain cells; also called *cerebrovascular accident.*

ischemic stroke Impeded blood supply to the brain caused by the obstruction of a blood vessel by a clot.

hemorrhagic stroke Impeded blood supply to the brain caused by the rupture of a blood vessel.

thrombus A blood clot in a blood vessel that usually occurs at the point of its formation.

embolus A blood clot that breaks off from its place of origin in a blood vessel and travels through the bloodstream.

aneurysm A sac formed by a distention or dilation of the artery wall.

Terms

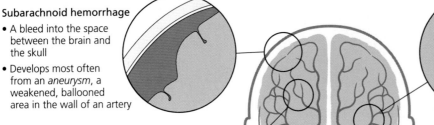

HEMORRHAGIC STROKE
- 20% of strokes
- Caused by ruptured blood vessels followed by blood leaking into tissue
- Usually more serious than ischemic stroke

ISCHEMIC STROKE
- 80% of strokes
- Caused by blockages in brain blood vessels; potentially treatable with clot-busting drugs
- Brain tissue dies when blood flow is blocked

Subarachnoid hemorrhage
- A bleed into the space between the brain and the skull
- Develops most often from an *aneurysm*, a weakened, ballooned area in the wall of an artery

Embolic stroke
- Caused by *emboli*, blood clots that travel from elsewhere in the body to the brain blood vessels
- 25% of embolic strokes are related to atrial fibrillation

Intracerebral hemorrhage
- A bleed from a blood vessel inside the brain
- Often caused by high blood pressure and the damage it does to arteries

Thrombotic stroke
- Caused by *thrombi*, blood clots that form where an artery has been narrowed by atherosclerosis
- Most often develops when part of a thrombus breaks away and causes a blockage in a "downstream" artery

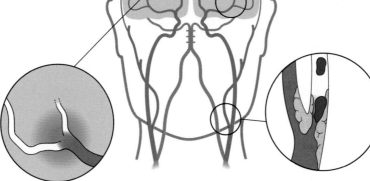

 Figure 12-5 **Types of stroke.** SOURCE: Types of stroke. 2000. *Harvard Health Letter,* April.

Detecting and Treating Stroke Effective treatment of a stroke requires the prompt recognition of symptoms and correct diagnosis of the type of stroke that has occurred. Some stroke victims have a **transient ischemic attack (TIA),** or ministroke, days, weeks, or months before they have a full-blown stroke. A TIA produces temporary strokelike symptoms, such as weakness or numbness in an arm or a leg, speech difficulty, or dizziness, but these symptoms are brief, often lasting just a few minutes, and do not cause permanent damage. However, TIAs should be taken as warning signs of a stroke, and anyone with a suspected TIA should get immediate medical help.

Strokes should be treated with the same urgency as heart attacks. A person with stroke symptoms should be rushed to the hospital. A **computed tomography (CT)** scan, which uses a computer to construct an image of the brain from X rays, can assess brain damage and determine the type of stroke. Newer diagnostic techniques using MRI and ultrasound are becoming increasingly available and should improve the speed and accuracy of stroke diagnosis.

If tests reveal that a stroke is caused by a blood clot—and if help is sought within a few hours of the onset of symptoms—the person can be treated with the same kind of clot-dissolving drugs that are used to treat coronary artery blockages. If the clot is dissolved quickly enough, brain damage is minimized and symptoms may disappear. (The longer the brain goes without oxygen, the greater the risk of permanent damage.) People who are at high risk for stroke due to narrowing of the carotid arteries may undergo a procedure called *carotid endarterectomy,* in which plaque is surgically removed.

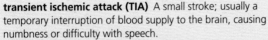

Terms

transient ischemic attack (TIA) A small stroke; usually a temporary interruption of blood supply to the brain, causing numbness or difficulty with speech.

computed tomography (CT) The use of computerized X ray images to create a cross-sectional depiction (scan) of tissue density.

congestive heart failure A condition resulting from the heart's inability to pump out all the blood that returns to it; blood backs up in the veins leading to the heart, causing an accumulation of fluid in various parts of the body.

congenital heart disease A defect or malformation of the heart or its major blood vessels, present at birth.

hypertrophic cardiomyopathy An inherited condition in which there is an enlargement of the heart muscle, especially between the two ventricles.

rheumatic fever A disease, mainly of children, characterized by fever, inflammation, and pain in the joints; often damages the heart muscle, a condition called rheumatic heart disease.

mitral valve prolapse (MVP) A condition in which the mitral valve "billows" out during ventricular contraction, possibly allowing leakage of blood from the left ventricle into the left atrium; often asymptomatic and usually only requiring treatment in cases of significant leakage.

If tests reveal that a stroke was caused by a cerebral hemorrhage, drugs may be prescribed to lower the blood pressure, which will usually be high. Careful diagnosis is crucial, because administering clot-dissolving drugs to a person suffering a hemorrhagic stroke would cause more bleeding and potentially more brain damage.

If detection and treatment of stroke come too late, rehabilitation is the only treatment. Although damaged or destroyed brain tissue does not normally regenerate, nerve cells in the brain can make new pathways, and some functions can be taken over by other parts of the brain. Some people recover completely in a matter of days or weeks, but most stroke victims who survive must adapt to a lifelong disability.

Congestive Heart Failure

A number of conditions—high blood pressure, heart attack, atherosclerosis, rheumatic fever, birth defects—can damage the heart's pumping mechanism. When the heart cannot maintain its regular pumping rate and force, fluids begin to back up. When extra fluid seeps through capillary walls, edema (swelling) results, usually in the legs and ankles, but sometimes in other parts of the body as well. Fluid can collect in the lungs and interfere with breathing, particularly when a person is lying down. This condition is called *pulmonary edema,* and the entire process is known as **congestive heart failure.** Treatment includes reducing the workload on the heart, modifying salt intake, and using drugs that help the body eliminate excess fluid.

Other Forms of Heart Disease

Other, less common forms of heart disease include congenital heart disease, rheumatic heart disease, and heart valve disorders.

About 40,000 children born each year in the United States have a defect or malformation of the heart or major blood vessels. These conditions are collectively referred to as **congenital heart disease,** and they cause about 5000 deaths a year. The most common congenital defects are holes in the wall that divides the chambers of the heart and *coarctation of the aorta,* a narrrowing, or constriction, of the aorta. Most of the common congenital defects can now be accurately diagnosed and treated with medication or surgery.

The congital condition **hypertrophic cardiomyopathy** is the most common cause of sudden death among athletes younger than 35 years of age. It causes the heart muscle to become enlarged, primarily in the area between the two ventricles; it generally develops gradually between the ages of 5 and 15. People with hypertrophic cardiomyopathy are at high risk for sudden death, mainly due to serious arrhythmias. Individuals with this condition should usually not participate in competitive sports.

Rheumatic fever, a result of certain types of streptoccal throat infections, can damage the heart muscle and heart valves. Symptoms of strep throat are the sudden onset of a sore throat, painful swallowing, fever, swollen glands, headache, nausea, and vomiting. Rheumatic fever can be prevented by treating strep throat, when it occurs, with antibiotics.

Congenital defects and certain types of infections can cause heart valve disorders, abnormalities in the valves between the chambers of the heart. The most common heart valve disorder is **mitral valve prolapse (MVP),** which occurs in about 4% of the population. MVP is characterized by a "billowing" of the mitral valve, which separates the left ventricle and left atrium, during ventricular contraction; in some cases, blood leaks from the ventricle into the atrium. Most people with MVP have no symptoms, and treatment is usually unnecessary.

WW. PROTECTING YOURSELF AGAINST CARDIOVASCULAR DISEASE

There are several important steps you can take now to lower your risk of developing CVD in the future. Reducing CVD risk factors when you are young can pay off with many extra years of life and health.

Eat Heart-Healthy

For most Americans, changing to a heart-healthy diet involves cutting total fat intake, substituting unsaturated fats for saturated and trans fats, and increasing fiber.

Decreased Fat and Cholesterol Intake The National Cholesterol Education Program (NCEP) recommends that all Americans over the age of 2 adopt a diet in which total fat consumption is no more than 30% of total daily calories. No more than 10% of total daily calories (7% for those with heart disease or high LDL levels) should be from saturated fat. Saturated fat is found in animal products; palm and coconut oil; and hydrogenated vegetable oils, which are also high in trans fats. Saturated and trans fats influence the production and excretion of cholesterol by the liver, so decreasing intake of these fats is the most important dietary change you can make to improve cholesterol levels. Animal products contain cholesterol as well as saturated fat, and the NCEP recommmends that most Americans limit dietary cholesterol intake to no more than 300 mg per day; for people with heart disease or high LDL levels, the suggested daily limit is 200 mg.

Increased Fiber Intake Soluble fiber traps the bile acids the liver needs to manufacture cholesterol and carries them to the large intestine, where they are excreted. It also slows the production of proteins that promote blood clotting. Insoluble fiber may interfere with the absorption of dietary fat and may also help you cut total food intake

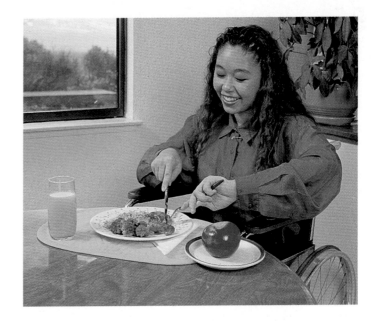

A diet high in fiber and low in saturated and trans fats can help lower levels of total cholesterol and LDL. This young woman is enjoying a healthy dinner of baked chicken, broccoli, rice, fruit, and juice.

because foods rich in insoluble fiber tend to be filling. A high-fiber diet is associated with a 40–50% reduction in the risk of heart attack and stroke. To obtain the recommended 20–35 grams of dietary fiber per day, choose a diet rich in whole grains, fruits, and vegetables. Good sources of fiber include oatmeal, some breakfast cereals, barley, legumes, and most fruits and vegetables.

Alcohol The *Dietary Guidelines for Americans* state that moderate alcohol consumption may lower the risk of CHD among men over 45 and women over 55. (Moderate means no more than one drink per day for women and two drinks per day for men.) For most people under age 45, however, the risks of alcohol use probably outweigh any health benefit. If you do drink, do so moderately, with food, and at times when drinking will not put you or others at risk.

Other Dietary Factors Researchers have identified other dietary factors that may affect CVD risk:

• *Omega-3 fatty acids* may reduce clotting and inflammation and have other heart-healthy effects. They are found in fish, shellfish, and some plant foods (nuts and canola, soybean, and flaxseed oils). The American Heart Association recommends eating fish two or more times a week.

• *Vitamin E*—found in nuts, vegetable oils, wheat germ, margarine, avocados, and leafy green vegetables—may help prevent CVD by inhibiting the buildup of fatty plaques on artery walls.

• *Plant sterols* reduce the absorption of cholesterol in the body and may help lower LDL levels.

• *Folic acid, vitamin B-6, and vitamin B-12* affect homocysteine levels.

• *Salt* raises blood pressure in salt-sensitive people, and high intake is not recommended for anyone. Consume no more than 2400 mg of sodium per day.

• *Patassium and calcium* are helpful in preventing and treating hypertension; they may also decrease the risk of stroke.

• *Soy protein* may lower LDL cholesterol. Soy-based foods include tofu and tempeh.

• *Total calorie intake* may be as important as fat intake in affecting cholesterol and triglyceride levels; lowering calorie intake may reduce these risk factors.

DASH A dietary plan that reflects many of the suggestions described here was released as part of a study called Dietary Approaches to Stop Hypertension, or DASH. The DASH diet plan is as follows:

• 7–8 servings per day of grains and grain products
• 4–5 servings per day of vegetables
• 4–5 servings per day of fruits
• 2–3 servings per day of low-fat or nonfat dairy products
• 2 or fewer servings per day of meats, poultry, and fish
• 4–5 servings per *week* of nuts, seeds, and legumes
• 2–3 servings per day of added fats, oils, and salad dressings
• 5 servings per *week* of snacks and sweets

Exercise Regularly

You can significantly reduce your risk of CVD with a moderate amount of physical activity. Try to accumulate at least 30 minutes of moderate-intensity physical activity

There are many products on the market that claim to improve cholesterol levels. Do any of these products work? Are they worth the cost?

Perhaps the most widely advertised functional foods for improving cholesterol are margarine spreads that contain plant sterol or plant stanol esters. Studies show that if these spreads are used on a regular basis, they can help decrease LDL cholesterol by about 10%. The 2001 NCEP guidelines recommend up to 2 grams per day of plant sterols or stanols for people with high LDL levels. However, these spreads are relatively high in calories, and are meant to replace margarine or butter, not supplement them. They also cost much more than standard butter or margarine.

Another popular product is a food bar that contains L-arginine, an amino acid typically found in protein-rich foods such as meat. The body uses L-arginine to make nitric oxide, a chemical that promotes dilation of blood vessels. A few small studies suggest that L-arginine may help improve blood flow in people with congestive heart failure or constricted arteries. However, the FDA has expressed concerns about this product, and the safest approach may be to wait until further research clarifies the benefits and risks of L-arginine supplementation.

Garlic supplements have also received attention for their possible health benefits. Allacin, a component of garlic, may inhibit cholesterol production by the liver. Research findings on the effects of garlic supplements have been mixed, however, and it's likely that if there is a positive effect, it is minimal.

Dietary supplements containing red rice yeast also claim to support healthy cholesterol levels. One of the substances in red rice yeast is chemically identical to lovastatin, the active ingredient in a prescription cholesterol-lowering medication. Various legal actions have been undertaken by the FDA relating to the marketing of these supplements and to their classification as supplements (rather than drugs).

Most functional foods and dietary supplements carry structure-function claims, which are not evaluated by the FDA; "promotes healthy cholesterol levels" is an example of a structure-function claim. The FDA *does* evaluate health claims, and those that have been approved can be considered to be based on solid science. As of 2001, these claims included the following:

- Foods low in saturated fat and cholesterol and reduced risk of coronary heart disease (CHD)
- Low-sodium foods and reduced risk of hypertension
- Soluble fiber and reduced risk of CHD
- Foods high in potassium and low in sodium and reduced risk of hypertension and stroke
- Soy protein and reduced risk of CHD
- Foods and supplements with plant sterol and plant stanol esters and reduced risk of CHD

For more strategies for evaluating supplements and functional foods, refer to Chapter 9 and visit the FDA Web site listed in For More Information at the end of the chapter.

---

each day through such activities as brisk walking and stair climbing. A formal exercise program can provide even greater benefits. The American Heart Association recently recommended strength training in addition to aerobic exercise for building and maintaining cardiovascular health.

Avoid Tobacco

Remember: The number one risk factor for CVD that you can control is smoking. If you smoke, quit. If you don't, don't start. If you live or work with people who smoke, encourage them to quit—for their sake and yours. If you find yourself breathing in smoke, take steps to prevent or stop this exposure. Quitting smoking will significantly reduce your CVD risk, but studies show that smoking and exposure to ETS may permanently increase the rate of plaque formation in arteries. Quitting smoking is highly beneficial, but abstaining from smoking and avoiding ETS throughout your life is even better.

Know and Manage Your Blood Pressure

If you have no CVD risk factors, have your blood pressure measured by a professional at least once every 2 years; yearly tests are recommended if you have other risk factors. If your blood pressure is high, follow your physician's advice on how to lower it.

Know and Manage Your Cholesterol Levels

Everyone age 20 and over should have a lipoprotein profile—which measures total cholesterol, HDL, LDL, and triglyceride levels—at least once every five years. Your goal for LDL depends in part on how many of the following major risk factors you have: cigarette smoking, high blood pressure, low HDL cholesterol (less than 40 mg/dl), a family history of heart disease, and age above 45 years for men and 55 years for women. (An HDL level of 60 mg/dl or higher is protective and removes one risk factor from your total count of risk factors.)

If you have two or fewer risk factors, the NCEP sets an LDL goal of less than 160 mg/dl. If your LDL is above that level, begin the "Therapeutic Lifestyle Changes," or TLC, recommended by the NCEP, including weight management, increased physical activity, and the TLC diet, which suggests total fat intake of 25–35% of total daily calories, saturated fat intake less than 7% of daily calories, and, for some people, 10–25 grams per day of soluble fiber and 2 grams per day of plant stanols and sterols. If your LDL level is 190 mg/dl or higher, medication may also be recommended.

If you have two or more risk factors for heart disease, the NCEP sets an LDL goal of less than 130 mg/dl. If your LDL level is 130 or above, you should begin TLC. Depending on other factors, your physician may also suggest drug therapy.

If you have CVD or diabetes, your goal for LDL is less than 100 mg/dl. TLC is recommended for all people in this risk category, and a vareity of medications is available to lower LDL and improve other blood fat levels.

Develop Effective Ways to Handle Stress and Anger and Manage Medical Conditions

Develop effective strategies for handling the stress in your life: Shore up your social support network, and try some of the techniques described in Chapter 2 for managing stress. If anger and hostility are problems for you, try some of the tips on p. 47 for defusing your anger.

Know your CVD risk factors and follow your physician's advice for testing, lifestyle modification, and any drug treatments. If you are at high risk for CVD, consult a physician about taking small doses of aspirin, which can reduce the risk of CVD for some people. If you are a postmenopausal woman, discuss hormone replacement therapy with your physician.

COMMUNICATE! Expressing chronic anger can put you at risk for heart disease, but suppressing and internalizing anger and resentment can also be dangerous. If someone is inconsiderate, rude, manipulative, or abusive toward you, you have the right to demand respect and fair treatment. Practice being assertive—defined as the ability to communicate your thoughts and feelings with confidence and skill—without being aggressive: Be specific about the behavior that bothers you, say how you feel about it, and specify how you would like it to change. For example, "I'm very upset that you forgot to tell me my brother called. This is the third time people have asked me why I haven't returned their calls. I feel as if you don't consider my calls important. In the future, can you please write it down when someone calls me and leave the message here by the phone?"

WHAT IS CANCER?

Cancer, the second leading cause of death in the United States, is a disease of abnormal and uncontrolled cellular growth.

Benign Versus Malignant Tumors

Most cancers take the form of tumors, although not all tumors are cancerous. A tumor is simply a mass of tissue that serves no physiological purpose. It can be benign, like a wart, or malignant, like most lung cancers. The term **malignant tumor** (or *neoplasm*) is synonymous with cancer.

Benign tumors are made up of cells similar to the surrounding normal cells and are enclosed in a membrane that prevents them from penetrating neighboring tissues. They are dangerous only if their physical presence interferes with body functions. A benign brain tumor, for example, may block the blood supply to the brain.

A malignant tumor, or cancer, is capable of invading surrounding structures, including blood vessels, the **lymphatic system,** and nerves. It can also spread to distant sites via the blood and lymphatic circulation, thereby producing invasive tumors in almost any part of the body. A few cancers, like leukemia, cancer of the blood, do not produce a mass and therefore are not properly called tumors. But since leukemia cells do have the fundamental property of rapid, uncontrolled growth, they are still malignant and therefore cancers.

Every case of cancer begins as a change in a cell that allows it to grow and divide when it should not. Normally (in adults), cells divide and grow at a rate just sufficient to replace dying cells. In contrast, a malignant cell divides without regard for normal control mechanisms and gradually produces a mass of abnormal cells, or a tumor. It takes about a billion cells to make a mass the size of a pea, so a single tumor cell must go through many divisions, often taking years, before the tumor grows to a noticeable size.

Eventually a tumor produces a sign or symptom of its presence. In the breast, a tumor may be felt as a lump and diagnosed as cancer by an X ray or **biopsy.** In less accessible locations, like the lung, ovary, or intestine, a tumor may be detected only by an indirect symptom—for instance, a persistent cough or unexplained bleeding or pain. In the case of leukemia, the changes in the blood will eventually be noticed as increasing fatigue, infection, or abnormal bleeding.

How Cancer Spreads: Metastasis

Metastasis, the spreading of cancer cells, occurs because cancer cells can break away from the *primary tumor* and pass through the lining of lymph or blood vessels to invade nearby tissue. They can also drift to distant parts of the body, where they establish new colonies of cancer cells. This traveling and seeding process is called metastasizing, and the new tumors are called *secondary tumors,* or *metastases.* The ability of cancer cells to metastasize makes early cancer detection critical. To control the cancer and prevent death, every cancerous cell must be removed. Once cancer cells enter either the lymphatic system or the bloodstream, it is extremely difficult to stop their spread.

Types of Cancer

The behavior of tumors is characteristic of the tissue in which they originated. (Figure 12-6 shows the major cancer sites and the incidence of each type.) Malignant tumors are classified as follows:

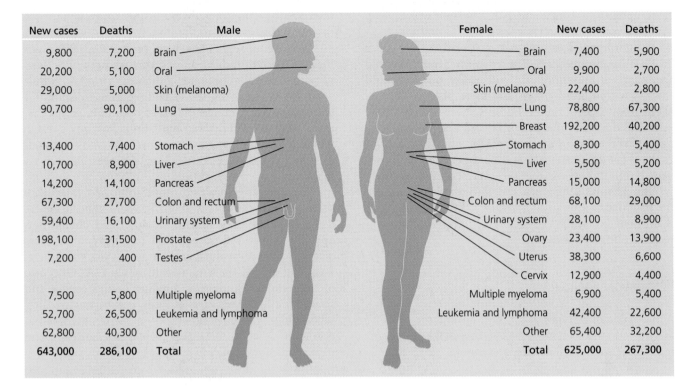

New cases	Deaths	Male	Female	New cases	Deaths
9,800	7,200	Brain	Brain	7,400	5,900
20,200	5,100	Oral	Oral	9,900	2,700
29,000	5,000	Skin (melanoma)	Skin (melanoma)	22,400	2,800
90,700	90,100	Lung	Lung	78,800	67,300
			Breast	192,200	40,200
13,400	7,400	Stomach	Stomach	8,300	5,400
10,700	8,900	Liver	Liver	5,500	5,200
14,200	14,100	Pancreas	Pancreas	15,000	14,800
67,300	27,700	Colon and rectum	Colon and rectum	68,100	29,000
59,400	16,100	Urinary system	Urinary system	28,100	8,900
198,100	31,500	Prostate	Ovary	23,400	13,900
7,200	400	Testes	Uterus	38,300	6,600
			Cervix	12,900	4,400
7,500	5,800	Multiple myeloma	Multiple myeloma	6,900	5,400
52,700	26,500	Leukemia and lymphoma	Leukemia and lymphoma	42,400	22,600
62,800	40,300	Other	Other	65,400	32,200
643,000	286,100	Total	Total	625,000	267,300

 VITAL STATISTICS

Figure 12-6 Cancer cases and deaths by site and sex. The Incidence column indicates the number of cancers that occurred in each site; the Death column indicates the number of cancer deaths were that attributed to each type. SOURCE: American Cancer Society. 2001. *Cancer Facts and Figures, 2001.* Atlanta: American Cancer Society.

- *Carcinomas* arise from epithelia, tissues that cover external body surfaces, line internal tubes and cavities, and form the secreting portion of glands. They are the most common type of cancers; major sites include the skin, breast, uterus, prostate, lungs, and gastrointestinal tract.

- *Sarcomas* arise from connective and fibrous tissues like muscle, bone, cartilage, and the membranes covering muscles and fat.

- *Lymphomas* are cancers of the lymph nodes, part of the body's infection-fighting system.

- *Leukemias* are cancers of the blood-forming cells, which reside chiefly in the **bone marrow.**

There is a great deal of variation in how easily different cancers can be detected and how well they respond to treatment. For example, certain types of skin cancer are easily detected, grow slowly, and are very easy to remove; virtually all of the 1 million cases that occur each year in the United States are cured. Cancer of the pancreas, on the other hand, is very difficult to detect or treat, and very few patients survive the disease.

 The Incidence of Cancer

Each year, about 1.3 million people in the United States are diagnosed with cancer. More than half will be cured, but about 40% will eventually die as a result of their cancer. These grim statistics exclude more than 1 million cases of the curable types of skin cancer. At current U.S.

cancer Abnormal, uncontrolled cellular growth.

malignant tumor A tumor that is cancerous and capable of spreading.

benign tumor A tumor that is not cancerous.

lymphatic system A system of vessels that returns proteins, lipids, and other substances from fluid in the tissues to the circulatory system.

biopsy The removal and examination of a small piece of body tissue; a needle biopsy uses a needle to remove a small sample; some biopsies require surgery.

metastasis The spread of cancer cells from one part of the body to another.

bone marrow Soft vascular tissue in the interior cavities of bones that produces blood cells.

Terms

rates, about 1 in 2 men and 1 in 3 women will develop cancer at some point in their lives.

The death rate from cancer began to fall in 1991; since 1990, it has dropped 3%. This promising trend suggests that efforts at prevention, early detection, and improved therapy are all bearing fruit. But more people could be saved from cancer. The American Cancer Society (ACS) estimates that 90% of skin cancer could be prevented by protecting the skin from the rays of the sun. Thousands of cases of colon, breast, and uterine cancer could be prevented by improving the diet and controlling body weight. Regular screenings and self-examinations have the potential to save an additional 100,000 lives per year. Many concrete actions you can take today can help you reduce your risk of cancer.

WW. COMMON CANCERS

A discussion of all types of cancer is beyond the scope of this book. In this section we look at some of the most common cancers and their causes, prevention, and treatment.

Lung Cancer

Lung cancer is the most common cause of cancer death in the United States; it is responsible for about 157,000 deaths each year. For over 40 years, breast cancer was the major cause of cancer death in women, but since 1987, lung cancer has surpassed breast cancer as a killer of women.

Risk Factors The chief risk factor for lung cancer is tobacco smoke, which accounts for 87% of lung cancers. (Other negative effects of tobacco smoke on the lungs were discussed in Chapter 8.) When smoking is combined with exposure to other **carcinogens,** such as asbestos particles, the risk of lung cancer can be multiplied by a factor of 10 or more. Long-term exposure to ETS increases risk of lung cancer for nonsmokers. Secondhand smoke, the smoke from the burning end of the cigarette, has significantly higher concentrations of the toxic and carcinogenic compounds found in mainstream smoke.

Detection and Treatment Lung cancer is difficult to detect at an early stage and hard to cure even when de-

tected early. Symptoms do not usually appear until the disease has advanced to the invasive stage. Signals such as a persistent cough, chest pain, or recurring bronchitis may be the first indication of a tumor's presence. Diagnosis can usually be made by chest X ray, or, where available, by studying the cells in sputum by spiral CT (computerized tomography) scans. Tumors can sometimes be visualized by fiber-optic bronchoscopy, a test in which a flexible lighted tube is inserted into the windpipe and the surfaces of the lung passages are directly inspected.

If caught early, localized cancers can be treated with surgery. But because only about 15% of lung cancers are detected before they spread, radiation and **chemotherapy** are often used in addition to surgery. For cases detected early, 49% of patients are alive 5 years after diagnosis, but overall, the survival rate is only 14%. One form of lung cancer, known as small-cell lung cancer and accounting for about 20% of cases, can be treated fairly successfully with chemotherapy—alone or in combination with radiation. A large percentage of cases respond with **remission,** which in some cases lasts for years.

Colon and Rectal Cancer

Colon and rectal cancer (also called colorectal cancer) is the second leading cause of cancer death.

Risk Factors Age is a key risk factor for colon and rectal cancer, with more than 90% of cases diagnosed in people age 50 and older. Heredity also plays a role: Many cancers arise from preexisting polyps, small growths on the wall of the colon that may gradually develop into malignancies. The tendency to form colon polyps appears to be determined by specific genes, and 15–30% of colon cancers may be due to inherited gene mutations. Chronic inflammation of the colon as a result of disorders such as ulcerative colitis also increases the risk of colon cancer.

Lifestyle is another risk factor for colon and rectal cancer. Regular physical activity appears to reduce a person's risk, while obesity increases risk. A diet rich in red meat is thought to increase risk, although it is unclear whether fat or some other component of meat is the culprit. A diet rich in fruits, vegetables, and whole grains is associated with lower risk. However, recent findings have contradicted the long-standing view that dietary fiber prevents colon cancer. Studies have suggested that folic acid and calcium may have a protective role; in contrast, high intake of simple sugars and smoked meats and fish may increase risk.

Other lifestyle factors that may increase the risk of colon and rectal cancer include excessive alcohol consumption and smoking. Use of oral contraceptives or hormone replacement therapy may reduce risk in women. Regular use of nonsteroidal anti-inflammatory drugs such as aspirin and ibuprofen may decrease the risk of colon cancer and other cancers of the digestive tract.

Terms   **carcinogen** Any substance that causes cancer.

chemotherapy The treatment of cancer with chemicals that selectively destroy cancerous cells.

remission A period during the course of cancer in which there are no symptoms or other evidence of disease.

mammograms Low-dose X rays of the breasts used to check for early signs of breast cancer.

Detection and Treatment If identified early, precancerous polyps and early-stage cancers can be removed before they become malignant or spread. Because polyps may bleed as they progress, the standard warning signs of colon cancer are bleeding from the rectum and a change in bowel habits. Regular screening tests are recommended beginning at age 50 (earlier for people with a family history of the disease). A stool blood test, which should be performed every year, can detect small amounts of blood in the stool long before obvious bleeding would be noticed. More involved screening tests are recommended at 5- or 10-year intervals. In sigmoidoscopy or colonoscopy, a flexible fiber-optic device is inserted through the rectum; part or all of the colon can be examined, and polyps can be biopsied or even removed without major surgery.

Surgery is the primary treatment for colon and rectal cancer. Radiation and chemotherapy may be used before surgery to shrink a tumor or after surgery to destroy any remaining cancerous cells. The survival rate is 90% for colon and rectal cancers detected early and 61% overall.

Breast Cancer

Breast cancer is the most common cancer in women and causes almost as many deaths in women as lung cancer. In men, breast cancer occurs only rarely. About one American woman in nine will develop breast cancer during her lifetime, each year, about 190,000 American women are diagnosed with breast cancer. Although mortality rates declined during the early 1990s, about 40,000 women die from breast cancer each year. Less then 1% of breast cancer cases occur in women under age of 30, but a woman's risk doubles every 5 years between the ages of 30 and 45 and then increases more slowly, by 10–15% every 5 years after age 45. More than 75% of breast cancers are diagnosed in women over 50.

Risk Factors There is a strong genetic factor in breast cancer. A woman who has two close relatives with breast cancer is four to six times more likely to develop the disease than a woman who has no close relatives with it. However, only about 15% of cancers occur in women with a family history of breast cancer.

Other risk factors include early onset of menstruation, late onset of menopause, having no children or having a first child after age 30, current use of hormone replacement therapy, obesity, and alcohol use. The unifying factor for many of these risk factors may be the female sex hormone estrogen, which circulates in a woman's body in high concentrations between puberty and menopause. Fat cells also produce estrogen, and estrogen levels are higher in obese women. Alcohol can interfere with estrogen metabolism in the liver and increase estrogen levels in the blood. Estrogen promotes the growth of cells in responsive sites, including the breast and the uterus, so any factor that increases estrogen exposure may raise breast cancer risk. In addition, pregnancy and breastfeeding trigger changes in breast cells that make them less susceptible to cancerous changes.

Recent studies indicate that certain types of dietary fat may be important in increasing or decreasing risk. Monounsaturated fats have been linked with reduced risk, while certain types of polyunsaturated fat may increase risk. Dietary fiber may also have a protective effect. Regular exercise is extremely important. Vigorous exercise may reduce estrogen levels in the blood, and physical activity of all intensities helps control body weight. Both obesity and significant weight gain during adulthood are linked to increased risk of breast cancer. Although some of the risk factors for breast cancer cannot be changed, minimizing lifestyle risk factors reduces the chance of developing breast cancer, even for women at risk from family history or other factors.

Early Detection A cure is most likely if breast cancer is detected early, so regular screening is a good investment, even for younger women. The ACS advises a three-part personal program for the early detection of breast cancer:

1. Monthly breast self-examination (BSE) for all women over age 20.

2. A clinical breast exam by a physician every 3 years for women between 20 and 39 and every year for women 40 and older.

3. **Mammograms** (low-dose breast X rays) every year for most women over 40.

Treatment If a lump is detected, it may be scanned by ultrasonography and biopsied to see if it is cancerous. The biopsy may be done either by needle in the physician's office or surgically. In 90% of cases, the lump is found to be a cyst or other harmless growth, and no further treatment is needed. If the lump does contain cancer cells, a variety of surgeries may be called for, ranging from a lumpectomy (removal of the lump and surrounding tissue) to a mastectomy (removal of the breast). If the tumor is discovered early, before it has spread to the adjacent lymph nodes, the patient has about a 97% chance of surviving more than 5 years. The survival rate for all stages is 85% at 5 years, 71% at 10 years, and 57% at 15 years.

New Strategies for Treatment and Prevention Several new drugs have been developed for the treatment or prevention of breast cancer. A family of drugs called selective estrogen-receptor modulators, or SERMs, act like estrogen in some tissues of the body but block estrogen's effects in others. One SERM, tamoxifen, has long been used in breast cancer treatment because it blocks the action of estrogen in breast tissue. In 1998, the FDA approved the use of tamoxifen to reduce the risk of breast cancer in healthy women who are at high risk for the disease. Another SERM currently being tested as a potential

The best time to do a breast self-exam is right after your period, when breasts are not tender or swollen. If you do not have regular periods or sometimes skip a month, do it on the same day every month.

1. Lie down and put a pillow under your right shoulder. Place your right arm behind your head.

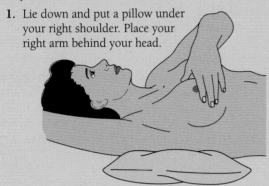

2. Use the finger pads of your three middle fingers on your left hand to feel for lumps or thickening in your right breast. Your finger pads are the top third of each finger.

3. Press firmly enough to know how your breast feels. If you're not sure how hard to press, ask your health care provider. Or try to copy the way your health care provider uses the finger pads during a breast exam. Learn what your breast feels like most of the time. A firm ridge in the lower curve of each breast is normal.

4. Move around the breast in a set way. You can choose either the circle (A), the up and down (B), or the wedge (C). Do it the same way every time. It will help you to make sure that you've gone over the entire breast area, and to remember how your breast feels.

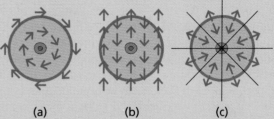

(a)   (b)   (c)

5. Now examine your left breast using right hand finger pads.

6. Repeat the examination of both breasts while standing, with one arm behind your head. The upright position makes it easier to check the upper and outer part of the breasts (toward your armpit). You may want to do the standing part of the BSE while you are in the shower. Some breast changes can be felt more easily when your skin is wet and soapy.

For added safety, you can also check your breasts for any dimpling of the skin, changes in the nipple, redness, or swelling while standing in front of a mirror right after your BSE each month.
   If you find any changes, see your doctor right away.

SOURCE: *How to Do Breast Self-Examination.* © 2001 American Cancer Society, Inc. Reprinted by the permission of the American Cancer Society, Inc.

---

preventive agent is raloxifene, a drug used to treat oseto-porosis that has fewer side effects than tamoxifen.
   A new therapy for advanced breast cancer is Herceptin (trastuzumab), a monoclonal antibody; monoclonal antibodies are produced in the laboratory and designed to bind to a specific cancer-related target. About 30% of metastatic breast cancer tumors produce excess amounts of a growth-promoting protein called HER2. Herceptin binds to the excess HER2, thus blocking its action and slowing tumor growth.

Prostate Cancer

The prostate gland is situated at the base of the bladder in men. It produces seminal fluid; if enlarged, it can block the flow of urine. Prostate cancer is the most common cancer in men and, after lung cancer, the cause of the most deaths. More than 190,000 new cases are diagnosed each year, and about 32,000 American men die from the disease each year.

Risk Factors   Age is the strongest predictor of the risk, with about 75% of cases of prostate cancer diagnosed in men over age 65. Inherited genetic predisposition may be responsible for 5–10% of cases. African American men have the highest rate of prostate cancer of any group in the world; both genetic and lifestyle factors may be involved. Diets high in calories, dairy products, and animal fats and low in plant foods have also been implicated as possible culprits. Compounds in soy foods and cruciferous vegetables are being investigated for their possible protective effects.

Detection and Treatment   Warning signs of prostate cancer include changes in urinary frequency, weak or interrupted urine flow, painful urination, and blood in the urine. Screening tests for early detection are recommended annually for men age 50 and over—earlier for African Americans and those with a strong family history of the disease. Most cases of prostate cancer are first detected during a digital rectal exam.

The **PSA blood test,** which measures the amount of prostate-specific antigen (PSA) in the blood, can also be used to help diagnose prostate cancer. An elevated level or a rapid increase in PSA can signal trouble. Ultrasound can be used as a follow-up to detect small lumps, and a needle biopsy can be performed to determine if the cells are malignant.

Treatments vary based on the stage of the cancer and the age of the patient. A small, slow-growing tumor in an older man may be treated with "watchful waiting" because he is more likely to die from another cause before his cancer becomes life threatening. More aggressive treatment would be indicated for younger men or those with more advanced cancers. Treatment usually involves radical prostatectomy, in which the prostate is removed surgically. While radical surgery has an excellent cure rate, it is major surgery and often results in incontinence and impotence. A less-invasive alternative under study involves radiation of the tumor using radioactive seeds implanted in the prostate. Alternative or additional treatments include external radiation, hormones, cryotherapy, and anticancer drugs. Survival rates for all stages of this cancer have improved steadily since 1940; the 5-year survival rate is currently about 93%.

Cancers of the Female Reproductive Tract

Because the uterus, cervix, and ovaries are subject to similar hormonal influences, the cancers of these organs can be discussed as a group.

Cervical Cancer   Cervical cancer is at least in part a sexually transmitted disease. Probably more than 80% of cervical cancer stems from infection by the human papillomavirus (HPV), which causes both common warts and genital warts. When certain types of HPV infect the cervix, the infection can develop into cervical cancer. Cervical cancer is associated with multiple sex partners, risk can be reduced by the regular use of condoms. Smoking and herpes infection are additional risk factors; both can cause cancerous changes in cells in the laboratory and can speed and intensify the cancerous changes begun by HPV. Some studies show that exposure to the STD chlamydia may also be a risk factor for cervical cancer, independent of HPV (STDs are discussed in Chapter 13).

Screening for the changes in cervical cells that precede cancer is done chiefly by means of the **Pap test.** During a pelvic exam, loose cells are scraped from the cervix, spread on a slide, stained for easier viewing, and examined under a microscope to see whether they are normal in size and shape. If cells are abnormal, a condition commonly referred to as *cervical dysplasia,* the Pap test is repeated at intervals. Sometimes cervical cells spontaneously return to normal, but in about one-third of cases, the cellular changes progress toward malignancy. If this

happens, the abnormal cells must be removed, either surgically or by destroying them with a cryoscopic (ultracold) probe or localized laser treatment. Without surgery, the malignant patch of cells goes on to invade the wall of the cervix and spreads to adjacent lymph nodes and to the uterus. At this stage, chemotherapy may be used with radiation, but chances for a complete cure are lower.

Because the Pap test is highly effective, all sexually active women and women between the ages of 18 and 65 should be tested annually. Unlike most cancers, cancer of the cervix occurs frequently in women in their thirties or even twenties. Although screening can clearly save lives, *Healthy People 2010* reports lower-than-average rates of Pap testing for certain groups, including women of low socioeconomic status and women with less than a high school education.

Uterine, or Endometrial, Cancer   Cancer of the lining of the uterus, or endometrium, most often occurs after the age of 55. The risk factors are similar to those for breast cancer: prolonged exposure to estrogen, early onset of menstruation, late menopause, never having been pregnant, and other medical conditions, including obesity. The use of oral contraceptives, which combine estrogen and progestin, appears to provide protection.

Endometrial cancer is usually detectable by pelvic examination. It is treated surgically, commonly by hysterectomy, or removal of the uterus; radiation treatment and chemotherapy may be used in addition to surgery. When the tumor is detected at an early stage, about 96% of patients are alive and disease-free 5 years later. When the disease has spread beyond the uterus, the 5-year survival rate is less than 64%.

Ovarian Cancer   Although ovarian cancer is rare compared with cervical or uterine cancer, it causes more deaths than the other two combined. It cannot be detected by Pap tests or any other simple screening method, and there are often no warning signs. The risk factors are similar to those for breast and endometrial cancer: increasing age, never having been pregnant, a family history of breast or ovarian cancer, and specific genetic mutations. A high number of ovulations appears to increase the chance that a cancer-causing genetic mutation will occur, so anything that lowers the number of lifetime ovulation cycles—pregnancy, breastfeeding, or use of oral contraceptives—reduces a woman's risk of ovarian cancer.

PSA blood test A diagnostic test for prostate cancer that measures blood levels of prostate-specific antigen (PSA).

Pap test A scraping of cells from the cervix for examination under a microscope to detect cancer.

Terms

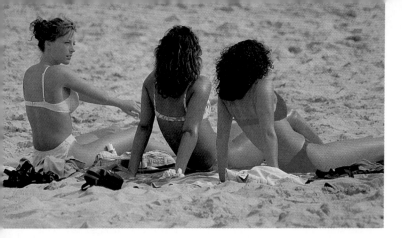

Cumulative exposure to sunlight, beginning in childhood, increases the risk of skin cancer later in life. Blistering sunburns are particularly dangerous, but tanning also poses a hazard. Sunscreens help protect the skin from the sun's radiation.

Women at high risk should have thorough pelvic exams at regular intervals, perhaps with ultrasound imaging of the ovaries. Ovarian cancer is treated by surgical removal of both ovaries, the fallopian tubes, and the uterus. Radiation and chemotherapy are sometimes also used.

Other Female Reproductive Tract Cancers   Daughters born to women who took DES (diethylstilbestrol) to prevent miscarriage have an increased risk, about 1 in 1000, of a vaginal or cervical cancer called clear cell cancer. There is also some risk to DES sons, who may have an increased risk of abnormalities of the reproductive tract, including undescended testicles, a risk factor for testicular cancer. A DES daughter should find a physician who is familiar with the problems of DES exposure; more frequent and more thorough pelvic exams are recommended. A recent animal study suggested the possibility of an increased third-generation cancer risk from DES, but further research is needed to determine if the finding applies to DES granddaughters.

Skin Cancer

Skin cancer is the most common cancer of all when cases of the highly curable forms are included in the count. Of the more than 1 million cases of skin cancer diagnosed

Terms

melanoma A malignant tumor of the skin that arises from pigmented cells, usually a mole.

ultraviolet (UV) radiation Light rays of a specific wavelength emitted by the sun; most UV rays are blocked by the ozone layer in the upper atmosphere.

basal cell carcinoma Cancer of the deepest layers of the skin.

squamous cell carcinoma Cancer of the surface layers of the skin.

each year, 51,000 are of the most serious type, **melanoma.** Treatments are usually simple and successful when the cancers are caught early.

Risk Factors   Almost all cases of skin cancer can be traced to excessive exposure to **ultraviolet (UV) radiation** from the sun, including longer-wavelength ultraviolet A (UVA) and shorter-wavelength ultraviolet B (UVB) radiation. UVB radiation causes sunburns and can damage the eyes and the immune system. UVA is less likely to cause an immediate sunburn, but by damaging connective tissue, it leads to premature aging of the skin. (Tanning lamps and tanning-salon beds emit mostly UVA radiation.) Both UVA and UVB radiation have been linked to the development of skin cancer, and the National Toxicology Program has declared both solar and artificial sources of UV radiation to be known human carcinogens.

Both severe, acute sun reactions (sunburns) and chronic low-level sun reactions (suntans) can lead to skin cancer. People with fair skin have less natural protection against skin damage from the sun and a higher risk of developing skin cancer than people with naturally dark skin: Caucasians are about 20 times more likely than African Americans to develop melanoma. Severe sunburns in childhood have been linked to a greatly increased risk of skin cancer in later life, so children in particular should be protected. Damage to the ozone layer of the atmosphere may be increasing exposure to UV radiation and thus the risk of skin cancer for everyone. Other risk factors for skin cancer include having many moles, particularly large ones, spending time at high altitudes, and a family history of the disease.

Types of Skin Cancer   There are three main types of skin cancer, named for the types of skin cell from which they develop. **Basal cell** and **squamous cell carcinomas** together account for about 95% of the skin cancers diagnosed each year. They are usually found in chronically sun-exposed areas, such as the face, neck, hands, and arms. They usually appear as pale, waxlike, pearly nodules or red, scaly, sharply outlined patches. These cancers are often painless, although they may bleed, crust, and form an open sore on the skin.

Melanoma is by far the most dangerous skin cancer because it spreads so rapidly. It is the most common cancer among women age 25–29 years. It can occur anywhere on the body, but the most common sites are the back, chest, abdomen, and lower legs. A melanoma usually appears at the site of a preexisting mole. The mole may begin to enlarge, become mottled or varied in color (colors can include blue, pink, and white), or develop an irregular surface or irregular borders. Tissue invaded by melanoma may also itch, burn, or bleed easily.

Prevention   One of the major steps you can take to protect yourself against all forms of skin cancer is to avoid

- Wear long-sleeved shirts and long pants made of tightly woven fabric. Wear a wide-brimmed hat to protect your ears and face.

- Wear UV-blocking sunglasses to protect your eyes. A dark color does not imply UV protection; check the label.

- Use a sunscreen and lip balm with a sun protection factor (SPF) of 15 or higher. (An SPF rating refers to the amount of time you can stay out in the sun before you burn, compared to using no sunscreen; for example, a product with an SPF of 15 would allow you to remain in the sun without burning 15 times longer, on average, than if you didn't apply sunscreen.) If you're fair-skinned or will be outdoors for long hours, use a sunscreen with a high (30+) SPF.

- Choose a "broad-spectrum" sunscreen that protects against both UVA and UVB radiation. The SPF rating of a sunscreen currently applies only to UVB, but a number of ingredients, including avobenzone (Parsol 1789), benzophenone, oxybenzone, titanium dioxide, and zinc oxide, are effective at blocking most UVA radiation. Use a water-resistant sunscreen if you swim or sweat quite a bit.

- Apply sunscreen 30 minutes before exposure to allow it time to penetrate the skin; shake it before applying.

- Reapply sunscreen frequently and generously to all sun-exposed areas, including the temples, ears, and sides and back of the neck). Most people use less than half as much as they would need to attain the full SPF rating. One ounce of sunscreen—one-fourth of a 4-ounce container—is about enough to cover an average-size adult in a swimsuit.

- If you're taking medication, ask your physician or pharmacist about possible reactions to sunlight or interactions with sunscreens. Medications for acne (Retin-A), allergies, and diabetes are just a few of the products that can trigger reactions. If you're using sunscreen and an insect repellent containing DEET, use extra sunscreen (research has suggested that DEET may decrease sunscreen effectiveness).

- Avoid sun exposure between 10 A.M. and 4 P.M., when the sun's rays are most intense. Clouds allow as much as 80% of UV rays to reach your skin.

- Consult the day's UV Index, which predicts UV levels on a 0–10+ scale, to get a sense of the sun protection you'll need; take special care on days with a rating of 5 or above.

- UV rays can penetrate at least 3 feet in water, so swimmers should wear water-resistant sunscreen.

- Locations near the equator or at high altitudes have more intense sunlight, so stronger sunscreens should be used.

- Snow reflects the sun's rays, so don't forget to apply sunscreen before skiing and other snow activities. Sand and water also reflect the sun's rays, so you still need to apply a sunscreen if you are under a beach umbrella. Concrete and white-painted surfaces are also highly reflective.

- Don't let sunscreens give you a false sense of security. The effectiveness of sunscreens in preventing skin cancer has not been firmly established, so even if you wear sunscreen, sun exposure may increase your cancer risk.

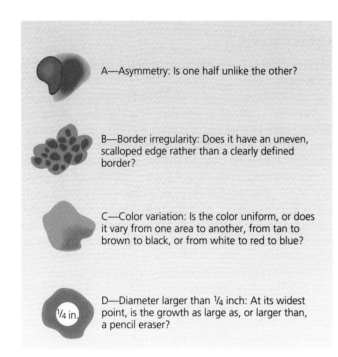

A—Asymmetry: Is one half unlike the other?

B—Border irregularity: Does it have an uneven, scalloped edge rather than a clearly defined border?

C—Color variation: Is the color uniform, or does it vary from one area to another, from tan to brown to black, or from white to red to blue?

D—Diameter larger than ¼ inch: At its widest point, is the growth as large as, or larger than, a pencil eraser?

Figure 12-7   The ABCD test for melanoma.

lifelong overexposure to sunlight. Blistering, peeling sunburns from unprotected sun exposure are particularly dangerous, but suntans—whether from sunlight or tanning lamps—also increase your risk of developing skin cancer later in life. People of every age, including babies and children, need to be protected from the sun with sunscreens and protective clothing.

Detection and Treatment   Make it a habit to examine your skin regularly. Most of the spots, freckles, moles, and blemishes on your body are normal; you were born with some of them, and others appear and disappear throughout your life. But if you notice an unusual growth, discoloration, sore that does not heal, or mole that undergoes a sudden or progressive change, see your physician or a dermatologist immediately.

The characteristics that may signal that a skin lesion is a melanoma are asymmetry, border irregularity, color change, and a diameter greater than ¼ inch (Figure 12-7). If someone in your family has had numerous skin cancers or melanomas, you may want to consult a dermatologist for a complete skin examination and discussion of your

The best time to perform a testicular self-exam is after a warm shower or bath, when the scrotum is relaxed. First, stand in front of a mirror and look for any swelling of the scrotum. Then, examine each testicle with both hands. Place the index and middle fingers under the testicle and the thumbs on top; roll the testical gently between the fingers and thumbs. Don't worry if one testicle seems slightly larger than the other—that's common. Also, expect to feel the epididymis, the soft, sperm-carrying tube at the rear of the testicle.

Perform the self-exam each month. If you find a lump, swelling, or nodule, consult a physician right away. The abnormality may not be cancer, but only a physician can make a diagnosis. Other possible signs of testicular cancer include a change in the way a testicle feels, a sudden collection of fluid in the scrotum, a dull ache in the lower abdomen or groin, a feeling of heaviness in the scrotum, or pain in a testicle or the scrotum.

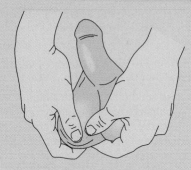

SOURCES: Testicular Cancer Resource Center. 2001. *How to Do a Testicular Self Examination* (http://www.acor.org/TCRC/tcexam.html; retrieved February 14, 2001). National Cancer Institute. 2000. *Questions and Answers About Testicular Cancer* (http://cis.nci.nih.gov/fact/6_34.htm; retrieved February 14, 2001).

particular risk. If you do have an unusual skin lesion, your physician will examine it and possibly perform a biopsy. If the lesion is cancerous, it is usually removed surgically, a procedure that can almost always be performed in the physician's office using a local anesthetic.

> **COMMUNICATE!**   The media often portray beautiful people with a "healthy tan." Yet research studies as well as everyday experience confirm that the sun irreparably damages the skin and causes skin cancer. Both sunlight and tanning salons are human carcinogens. What messages are the media communicating with their images of tanned skin? Are you influenced by these messages? Can you look at the messages critically and counter them with scientific information and common sense?

Oral Cancer

Oral cancer—cancers of the lip, tongue, mouth, and throat—can be traced principally to cigarette, cigar, or pipe smoking, the use of spit tobacco, and the excess use of alcohol. The incidence of oral cancer is twice as great in men as in women and most frequent in men over 40. Oral cancers are fairly easy to detect but often hard to cure. The primary methods of treatment are surgery and radiation.

Testicular Cancer

Testicular cancer is relatively rare, accounting for only 1% of cancer in men (about 7200 cases per year), but it is the most common cancer in men age 20–35. It is much more common among white Americans than Latinos, Asian

Americans or African Americans and among men whose fathers had testicular cancer. Men with undescended testicles are at increased risk for testicular cancer, and for this reason the condition should be corrected in early childhood. Men whose mothers took DES during pregnancy have an increased risk of undescended testicles and other genital anomalies. For this reason, they may have a higher risk of testicular cancer. Self-examination may help in the early detection of testicular cancer. Tumors are treated by surgical removal of the testicle and, if the tumor has spread, by chemotherapy.

Other Cancers

Several other cancers affect a significant number of people each year. Some have identifiable risk factors, but the causes of others are still under investigation.

Pancreatic cancer is the fifth leading cause of cancer death in the United States. Because of the pancreas's location deep within the abdomen, behind the stomach, the disease is usually well advanced before symptoms become noticeable. No effective cure is available. About 3 out of 10 cases are linked to smoking. Other risk factors include being male, African American, or over age 60; having a family hisory of pancreatic cancer; having diabetes; and eating a diet high in fat and meat and low in vegetables.

Stomach cancer is relatively rare in the United States, but it is the most common form of cancer in many parts of the world. It tends to occur after the age of 50 and is twice as common in men as in women. Risk factors include infection with the bacterium *Helicobacter pylori,* which has also been linked to the development of ulcers, and a diet high in smoked, salted, or pickled fish or meat.

There is no screening test for stomach cancer; it is usually recognized only after it has spread.

Bladder cancer is twice as common in men as in women, and smoking is the key risk factor. The first symptoms are likely to be blood in the urine and/or increased frequency of urination. These symptoms can also signal a urinary infection but should trigger a visit to a physician, who can evaluate the possibility of cancer. With early detection, more than 90% of cases are curable.

Kidney cancer usually occurs in people over 50; smoking and obesity are mild risk factors, as is a family history of the disease. Symptoms may include fatigue, pain in the side, and blood in the urine. Kidney cancer has been difficult to treat, with a 5-year survival rate of only 61% for all stages.

Brain tumors can develop almost anywhere in the brain. One of the few established risk factors for brain cancer is ionizing radiation, such as X rays of the head. Symptoms of a brain tumor are often nonspecific and include headaches, fatigue, behavioral changes, and sometimes seizures. Some brain tumors are curable by surgery or by radiation and chemotherapy, but most are not. Survival time varies, depending on the type of the tumor, from 1 to 8 years.

Leukemia, cancer of the white blood cells, starts in the bone marrow but can then spread to the lymph nodes, spleen, liver, other organs, and central nervous system. Like brain cancer, it is a complex disease with many different types and subtypes. Most people with leukemia have no known risk factors. About 20% of cases of adult leukemia are related to smoking; other possible risk factors include radiation and certain chemicals and infections. Most symptoms occur because leukemia cells crowd out the production of normal blood cells; the result can be fatigue, anemia, weight loss, and increased risk of infection. Treatment and survival rates vary, depending on the exact type and other factors.

Lymphoma is a form of cancer that begins in the lymph nodes and then may spread to almost any part of the body. There are two types—Hodgkin's disease and non-Hodgkin's lymphoma (NHL). NHL is the more common and more deadly form of the disease. It is the fifth most common cancer in the U.S., with about 56,000 people diagnosed annually; about half of all patients will eventually die from the disease. Risk factors for NHL are not well understood but may include genetic factors, radiation, and certain chemicals and infections. Rates of Hodgkin's disease have fallen by more than 50% since the early 1970s.

Multiple myeloma (MM) is a cancer in which malignant plasma cells produce tumors in multiple sites, particularly in the bone marrow. By crowding out normal bone marrow cells, MM can lead to anemia, excessive bleeding, and decreased resistance to infection. Age is the most significant risk factor; the average age at diagnosis is about 70. The disease is slow in its progression but usually fatal.

THE CAUSES OF CANCER

Although scientists do not know everything about what causes cancer, they have identified genetic, environmental, and lifestyle factors. There are usually several steps in the transformation of a normal cell into a cancer cell, and in many cases, different factors may work together in the development of cancer.

The Role of DNA

Almost daily, the mass media report on some new link between heredity and cancer. But how exactly do genes influence cancer? And what do these links mean for you and your risk of developing particular cancers?

DNA Basics   The nucleus of each cell in your body contains 23 pairs of **chromosomes,** which are made up of tightly packed coils of **DNA** (deoxyribonucleic acid). Each chromosome contains hundreds and, in some cases, thousands of **genes;** you have about 30,000–40,000 genes in all. Each of your genes controls the production of a particular protein. By making different proteins at different times, genes can act as switches to alter the ways a cell works. Genes that control the rate of cell division often play a critical role in the development of cancer.

DNA Mutations and Cancer   A mutation is any change in the makeup of a gene. Some mutations are inherited; others occur during cell division; and still others are caused by environmental agents known as *mutagens.* Mutagens include radiation, certain viruses, and chemical substances in the air. (When a mutagen also causes cancer, it is called a carcinogen.)

A mutated gene no longer contains the proper code for producing its protein. It requires several mutational changes over a period of years before a normal cell takes on the properties of a cancer cell. Genes in which mutations are associated with the conversion of a normal cell into a cancer cell are known as **oncogenes.** In their undamaged form, many oncogenes play a role in controlling or restricting cell growth; they are called tumor suppressor genes. Mutational damage to these genes releases the brake on

chromosomes The threadlike bodies in a cell nucleus that contain molecules of DNA; most human cells contain 23 pairs of chromosomes.

DNA Deoxyribonucleic acid, a chemical substance that carries genetic information.

gene A section of a chromosome that contains the nucleotide base sequence for making a particular protein; the basic unit of heredity.

oncogene A gene involved in the transformation of a normal cell into a cancer cell.

Terms

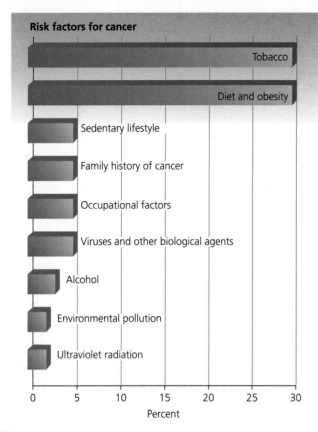

Risk factors for cancer

(Bar chart, Percent 0 to 30)

- Tobacco
- Diet and obesity
- Sedentary lifestyle
- Family history of cancer
- Occupational factors
- Viruses and other biological agents
- Alcohol
- Environmental pollution
- Ultraviolet radiation

0   5   10   15   20   25   30
Percent

W VITAL STATISTICS

Figure 12-8 Percentage of all cancer deaths linked to risk factors. SOURCE: Harvard Center for Cancer Prevention. 1996. Harvard Report on Cancer Prevention. Vol. 1: Causes of Human Cancer. *Cancer Causes and Control* 7 (Supplement).

growth and leads to rapid and uncontrolled cell division—a precondition for the development of cancer.

An example of an inherited mutated oncogene is an alteration in a suppressor gene vital for controlling the growth of color cells. Children who inherit the altered gene are thought to face a 70%–80% chance of developing the disease. Using information from the Human Genome Project, scientists have been able to identify the genes responsible for the condition. Another example is BRCA1 (breast cancer gene 1): Women who inherit a damaged copy of this suppressor gene face a significantly increased risk of breast and ovarian cancer.

In most cases, however, mutational damage occurs after birth. For example, only about 5–10% of breast cancer cases can be traced to inherited copies of a damaged BRCA1 gene. In addition, lifestyle is important even for those who have inherited a damaged suppressor gene: Eating a high-fiber diet, exercising regularly, and maintaining a healthy body weight may protect against breast cancer. Testing and identification of hereditary cancer risks can be helpful for some people, especially if it leads

to increased attention to controllable risk factors and better medical screening.

Cancer Promoters Substances known as cancer promoters make up another important piece of the cancer puzzle. Although they don't directly produce DNA mutations, they accelerate the growth of cells, leaving less time for a cell to repair DNA damage caused by other factors. Estrogen, which stimulates cellular growth in the female reproductive organs, is an example of a cancer promoter.

Although much still needs to be learned about the role of genetics in cancer, it's clear that minimizing mutation damage to our DNA will lower our risk of many cancers. Unfortunately, a great many substances produce cancer-causing mutations, and we can't escape them all. By identifying the important carcinogens and understanding how they produce their effects, we can help keep our DNA intact and avoid activating "sleeping" oncogenes.

W. Dietary Factors

Diet is one of the most important factors in cancer prevention (Figure 12-8). It is also one of the most complex and controversial. Diets high in meat, fast food, refined carbohydrates, and simple sugars and low in fruits and vegetables are associated with a higher risk of cancer than are plant-based diets rich in whole grains, fruits, and vegetables. The picture becomes less clear, however, when researchers attempt to identify the particular constituents of foods that affect cancer risk.

Dietary Fat and Meat In general, diets high in fat and meat have been associated with higher rates of certain cancers, including those of the colon and prostate. Dietary fat may promote colon cancer by stimulating the production of bile acids, which are necessary to break down and digest material in the colon. Once produced, these bile acids remove layers of cells from the intestinal epithelium, which in turn are replaced by new cells. Newly formed and rapidly growing cells are particularly susceptible to carcinogens. Diets high in animal fats and low in plant fats may also increase the risk of aggressive forms of prostate cancer, possibly by affecting hormone levels.

Some studies suggest that diets favoring omega-6 polyunsaturated fats over the omega-3 forms commonly found in fish may be associated with a higher risk of certain cancers, while monounsaturated fats may have a protective effect. Omega-3 fatty acids appear to slow the growth of colon cancer cells and may have protective factors against breast, prostate, and pancreatic cancers. Particular fatty acids found in meat as well as nonfat constituents of meat such as iron may also help explain the association between meat and cancer. In addition, curing, smoking, and grilling and other cooking methods utilizing a direct flame or high temperatures may produce carcinogenic compounds.

Alcohol   Alcohol is associated with an increased incidence of several cancers. An average alcohol intake of three drinks per day is associated with a doubling in the risk of breast cancer. Alcohol and tobacco interact as risk factors of oral cancer.

Fiber   Determining the effects of fiber intake on cancer risk is complicated by the fact that fiber is found in foods that also contain many other potential anti-cancer agents—fruits, vegetables, and whole grains. Various potential cancer-fighting actions have been proposed for fiber, but none of these actions has been firmly established. Experts recommend a high-fiber diet for its possible effect on cancer risk and for its overall positive effect on health.

Fruits and Vegetables   A massive number of epidemiological studies provide evidence that high consumption of fruits and vegetables reduces the risk of many cancers. Exactly which constituents of fruits and vegetables are responsible for this reduction in risk is less certain. Some essential nutrients have been found to act against cancer. For example, vitamin C, vitamin E, selenium, and the **carotenoids** (vitamin A precursors) may help block the initiation of cancer by acting as **antioxidants.** Antioxidants prevent **free radicals** from damaging DNA. Vitamin C may also block the conversion of nitrates (food preservatives) into cancer-causing agents. Folic acid may inhibit the transformation of normal cells into malignant cells and strengthen immune function. Calcium inhibits the growth of cells in the colon and may slow the spread of potentially cancerous cells.

Many other anti-cancer agents in the diet fall under the broader heading of **phytochemicals,** substances in plants that help protect against chronic diseases. One of the first to be identified was sulforaphane, a compound found in broccoli. To increase your intake of phytochemicals, eat a wide variety of fruits, vegetables, legumes, and grains. Don't try to rely on supplements. Like many vitamins and minerals, isolated phytochemicals may be harmful if taken in high doses. Beta-carotene pills, for example, may increase smokers' risk of lung cancer. In addition, it is likely that the anticancer effects of many foods are the result of many chemical substances working in combination.

Inactivity and Obesity

Several common types of cancer are associated with an inactive lifestyle, and research has shown a relationship between increased physical activity and a reduction in cancer risk. There is good evidence that exercise reduces the risk of colon cancer.

Exercise is also important because it helps prevent obesity, an independent risk factor for cancers of the prostate, breast, female reproductive tract, and kidney and possibly the colon and gallbladder.

Microbes

It is estimated that about 15% of the world's cancers are caused by microbes, including viruses, bacteria, and parasites, although the percentage is much lower in developed countries like the United States. The Epstein-Barr virus, best known for causing mononucleosis, is also suspected of contributing to Hodgkin's disease, cancer of the pharynx, and some stomach cancers. Human herpesvirus 8 has been linked to Kaposi's sarcoma and certain types of lymphoma. Hepatitis virus B and C together cause as many as 80% of the world's liver cancers. (See Chapter 13 for more information on hepatitis.)

Carcinogens in the Environment

Some carcinogens occur naturally in the environment, like the sun's UV rays. Others are synthetic substances that show up occasionally in the general environment but more often in the work environments of specific industries.

Ingested Chemicals   The food industry uses preservatives and other additives to prevent food from becoming spoiled or stale. Some of these compounds are antioxidants and may actually decrease any cancer-causing properties the food might have. Other compounds, like the nitrates and nitrites found in beer and ale, ham, bacon, hot dogs, and lunch meats are potentially more dangerous. Although nitrates and nitrites are not themselves carcinogenic, they can combine with dietary substances in the stomach and be converted to nitrosamines, highly potent carcinogens. Foods cured with nitrites, as well as those cured by salt or smoke, have been linked to esophageal and stomach cancer, and they should be eaten only in modest amounts.

Terms

carotenoid Any of a group of yellow-to-red plant pigments that can be converted to vitamin A by the liver; many act as antioxidants or have other anticancer effects. The carotenoids include beta-carotene, lutein, lycopene, and zeaxanthin.

antioxidant A substance that can lessen the breakdown of food or body constituents; actions include binding oxygen and donating electrons to free radicals.

free radicals Electron-seeking compounds that can react with fats, proteins, and DNA, damaging cell membranes and mutating genes in their search for electrons; produced through chemical reactions in the body and by exposure to environmental factors such as sunlight and tobacco smoke.

phytochemical A naturally occurring substance found in plant foods that may help prevent chronic diseases such as cancer and heart disease; *phyto* means plant.

Table 12-3

Tests Recommended by the American Cancer Society for the Early Detection of Cancer in Asymptomatic People

Site	Recommendation
Cancer-related checkup	A cancer-related checkup is recommended every 3 years for people age 20–40 and every year for people age 40 or older. This exam should include health counseling and, depending on a person's age, might include examination for cancers of the thyroid, oral cavity, skin, lymph nodes, testes, and ovaries, as well as for some nonmalignant diseases.
Breast	Women age 20–39 should have a clinical breast exam (CBE) performed by a health care professional every 3 years and should perform monthly breast self-examination. Women 40 or older should have an annual mammogram, an annual CBE by a health care professional, and should perform monthly breast self-examination. The CBE should be conducted close to and preferably before the scheduled mammogram.
Colon and rectum	Beginning at age 50, men and women at average risk should follow one of these five examination schedules: (1) fecal occult blood test (FOBT) every year, (2) flexible sigmoidoscopy every 5 years, (3) FOBT every year and flexible sigmoidoscopy every 5 years, (4) double-contrast barium enema every 5 years, or (5) colonoscopy every 10 years. (Among the first three options, the ACS prefers option 3.) A digital rectal exam should be done at the same time as sigmoidoscopy, colonoscopy, or double-contrast barium enema. People who are at increased or high risk for colorectal cancer should talk with a physician about a different testing schedule.
Prostate	Beginning at age 50, the prostate-specific antigen (PSA) test and the digital rectal exam should be offered annually to men who have a life expectancy of at least 10 years. Men at high risk (African American men and men who have a first-degree relative who was diagnosed with prostate cancer at a young age) should begin testing at age 45.
Skin	All men and women should perform a monthly skin self-exam to look for early signs of skin cancer. A skin examination by a physician is recommended as part of a cancer-related checkup.
Testes	Men who choose to perform testicular self-exams should do so once a month.
Uterus	*Cervix:* All women who are or have been sexually active or who are 18 or older should have an annual Pap test and pelvic examination. After three or more consecutive satisfactory examinations with normal findings, the Pap test may be performed less frequently. Discuss the matter with your physician. *Endometrium:* Beginning at age 35, women with or at risk for hereditary non-polyposis colon cancer should be offered endometrial biopsy annually to screen for endometrial cancer.

SOURCES: American Cancer Society, 2001. *Cancer Facts and Figures, 2001.* Atlanta: American Cancer Society. Reprinted by permission of the American Cancer Society, Inc. American Cancer Society. 2000. *Testicular Cancer Detection and Symptoms* (http://www3.cancer.org/cancerinfo/load_cont.asp?st=ds&ct=41&language=english; retrieved April 20, 2001).

Environmental and Industrial Pollution Urban air pollution appears to have a measurable but limited role in causing lung cancer. Fossil fuels and their combustion products, such as complex hydrocarbons, have been of special concern. Data indicate, however, that less than 2% of cancer deaths are caused by general environmental pollution, such as substances in the air and water. Exposure to carcinogenic materials in the workplace is a more serious problem. Occupational exposure to specific carcinogens may account for up to 5% of cancer deaths. For example, diesel exhaust may contribute to lung cancer in truck operators and railroad workers. With increasing industry and government regulations, industrial sources of cancer risk should continue to diminish.

Radiation All sources of radiation are potentially carcinogenic, including medical X rays, radioactive substances (radioisotopes), and UV rays from the sun. Most physicians and dentists are quite aware of the risk of radiation, and successful efforts have been made to reduce the amount of radiation needed for mammograms, dental X rays, and other necessary medical X rays.

Another source of environmental radiation is radon gas. Radon is a radioactive decomposition product of radium, which is found in small quantities in some rocks and soils. Fortunately, in most of our homes and classrooms, radon is rapidly dissipated into the atmosphere, and very low levels of radon do not appear to increase cancer risk. But in certain kinds of enclosed spaces, such as mines, some basements, and airtight houses built of brick or stone, it can rise to dangerous levels.

Sunlight is a very important source of radiation, but because its rays penetrate only a millimeter or so into the skin, it could be considered a "surface" carcinogen. Most cases of skin cancer are the relatively benign and highly curable basal cell carcinomas, but a substantial minority are the potentially deadly malignant melanomas.

DETECTING, DIAGNOSING, AND TREATING CANCER

Early cancer detection often depends on our willingness to be aware of changes in our own body and to make sure we keep up with recommended diagnostic tests.

Detecting Cancer

Self-monitoring is the first line of defense against cancer: the American Cancer Society recommends that you watch for the seven major warning signs, which you can remember with the acronym CAUTION:

- Change in bowel or bladder habits
- A sore that does not heal
- Unsual bleeding or discharge
- Thickening or lump in the breasts or elsewhere
- Indigestion or difficulty in swallowing
- Obvious change in a wart or mole
- Nagging cough or hoarseness

Although none of the warning signs is a sure indication of cancer, the appearance of any one should send you to see your physician. By being aware of the risk factors in your own life, including the cancer history of your immediate family and your own past history, you can often bring a problem to the attention of a physician long before it would have been detected at a routine physical. In addition to self-monitoring, the ACS recommends routine tests to screen for common cancers (Table 12-3).

Diagnosing and Treating Cancer

A biopsy or exploratory surgery may be performed to identify a cancer's *stage*—a designation based on a tumor's size, location, and spread that helps determine appropriate treatment. New diagnostic imaging techniques have replaced exploratory surgery for some patients. In magnetic resonance imaging (MRI), a huge electromagnet is used to detect hidden tumors by mapping, on a computer screen, the vibrations of different atoms in the body. Computed tomography (CT) scanning uses X rays to examine the brain and other parts of the body. The process allows the construction of cross sections, which show a tumor's shape and location more accurately than is possible with conventional X rays. Ultrasonography has also been used increasingly in the past few years to view tumors.

The primary treatment methods for cancer are surgery, chemotherapy, and radiation therapy. In chemotherapy, cancer cells that can't be surgically removed are killed by interfering chemically with their growth; in radiation therapy they are killed directly with concentrated ionizing radiation. Newer and still experimental methods are also showing promise. In gene therapy, for example, based on findings from the Human Genome Project, scientists can compare normal DNA sequences with the sequences found in the tumor cells. Using this approach, they hope to develop a variety of powerful, targeted therapies for use in treatment of specific cancers. Bone marrow and stem cell transplants are used in cancers of the blood-forming cells or lymph cells. Biological therapies are used to enhance the immune system's reaction to a tumor. New drugs are being developed to block cancer cells' ability to invade normal tissue and metastasize, to prevent their growth, and to keep them from dividing.

Because of successful treatment of cancer, survival has become the norm. However, cancer survivors must live with the fear of recurrence. They may also suffer from discrimination from insurers, although several states have passed legislation to prevent this.

For cancer patients, psychological support is an important part of treatment and recovery. Family and friends, concerned health care providers, and organized support groups can all play roles in the lives of cancer patients. Support groups can have an especially positive impact on the emotional wellness of both patients and families.

PREVENTING CANCER

Lifestyle choices can radically lower your cancer risks, so you *can* take a very practical approach to cancer prevention. Here are some guidelines:

- *Avoid tobacco.* People who smoke two or more packs of cigarettes a day have lung cancer mortality rates 15–25 times greater than those of nonsmokers. The carcinogenic chemicals in smoke are transported throughout the body in the bloodstream, making smoking a carcinogen for many forms of cancer other than lung cancer. The use of spit tobacco increases the risk of cancers of the mouth, larynx, throat, and esophagus.

- *Control diet and weight.* About one-third of all cancers are in some way linked to what we eat. Choose a low-fat, plant-based diet containing a wide variety of fruits, vegetables, and whole grains rich in phytochemicals. Drink alcohol only in moderation, if at all. Maintain a healthy weight.

- *Exercise regularly.* Regular exercise is linked to lower rates of colon and other cancers. It also helps control weight.

- *Protect skin from the sun.* Almost all cases of skin cancer are considered to be sun-related. Wear protective clothing when you're out in the sun, and use a sunscreen with an SPF rating of 15 or higher. Don't go to tanning salons.

• *Avoid environmental and occupational carcinogens.* Try to avoid occupational exposure to carcinogens, and don't smoke; the cancer risks of many of these agents increase greatly when combined with smoking.

• *Have recommended screening tests done.* Stay alert for the signs and symptoms that could indicate cancer, and follow the American Cancer Society screening guidelines listed in Table 12-3. Both lifestyle changes and a program of early detection are important to your long-term health.

SUMMARY

• The cardiovascular system pumps and circulates blood throughout the body. The heart pumps blood to the lungs via the pulmonary artery and to the body via the aorta.

• The six major risk factors for CVD that can be changed are smoking, high blood pressure, unhealthy cholesterol levels, inactivity, obesity, and diabetes.

• Contributing risk factors that can be changed include high triglyceride levels and psychological and social factors.

• Risk factors for CVD that can't be changed include being over 65, being male, being African American, and having a family history of CVD.

• Hypertension occurs when blood pressure exceeds normal limits most of the time.

• Atherosclerosis is a progressive hardening and narrowing of arteries that can lead to restricted blood flow and even complete blockage.

• Heart attacks are usually the result of a long-term disease process.

• A stroke occurs when the blood supply to the brain is cut off by a blood clot or hemorrhage.

• Congestive heart failure occurs when the heart's pumping action becomes less efficient and fluid collects in the lungs or in other parts of the body.

• Dietary changes that can protect against CVD include decreasing your intake of fat, saturated fat, trans fat, and cholesterol; increasing your intake of fiber; by eating more fruits, vegetables, and whole grains.

• CVD risk can also be reduced by engaging in regular exercise, not smoking cigarettes and avoiding ETS, knowing and managing your blood pressure and cholesterol levels, developing effective ways of handling stress and anger, and managing other risk factors and medical conditions.

• Cancer is a disease of abnormal and uncontrolled cellular growth.

• A malignant tumor can invade surrounding structures and spread to distant sites via the blood and lymphatic system, producing additional tumors.

• A malignant cell divides without regard for normal growth.

• Lung cancer kills more people than any other type of cancer. Tobacco smoke is the primary cause.

• Colon and rectal cancer is linked to age, heredity, obesity, and a diet rich in red meat and low in fruits and vegetables.

• Although there is a genetic component to breast cancer, diet and hormones are also risk factors.

• Prostate cancer is chiefly a disease of aging; diet and lifestyle probably are factors in its occurrence.

• Cancers of the female reproductive tract include cervical, uterine, and ovarian cancer. The Pap test is an effective screening test for cervical cancer.

• Skin cancers occur as basal cell carcinoma, squamous cell carcinoma, and melanoma.

• Oral cancer is caused primarily by smoking, excess alcohol consumption, and use of spit tobacco.

• Testicular cancer can be detected early through self-examination.

• Mutational damage to a cell's DNA, either inherited or environmental, can lead to cancer.

Gradually modifying your diet to include less saturated and trans fat and more fruits and vegetables can help you avoid both CVD and cancer in the future. Begin by assessing your current diet: Keep a record in your health journal of everything you eat for a week. At the end of the week, you can evaluate your diet and start taking steps to modify it.

Reducing Saturated and Trans Fat in Your Diet

The American Heart Association recommends that no more than 10% of the calories in your diet come from saturated and trans fat. Food high in these fats include meat, poultry skin, full-fat dairy products, coconut and palm oils, and products made with hydrogenated vegetable oils, such as deep-fried fast food and packaged baked goods. To find out if your diet is within the 10% recommendation, at the end of the week, record the grams of saturated and trans fat next to the foods you've listed in your health journal. This information is available on many food labels, in books, and on the Internet. For fast foods, use the Appendix. Trans fat content may be more difficult to determine. Here are the average values per serving for a few trans fat–rich foods: french fries (large), 5 g; pound cake, 5 g; doughnut, 4 g; fried breaded chicken, 3 g; Danish pastry, 3 g; vegetable shortening, 3 g; sandwich cookies, 2 g; crackers, 2 g; margarine (stick), 2 g; margarine (tub), 1g.

Once you have the grams of fat listed, add up what you consumed each day. For a 1600-calorie diet, the 10% limit corresponds to 18 grams of saturated and trans fat; for a 2200-calorie diet, it corresponds to 24 grams; and for a 2800-calorie diet, it corresponds to 31 grams. (If you have high cholesterol, you may want to follow the 7% limit set by the NCEP, which corresponds to 12 grams of saturated and trans fat in a 1600-calorie diet, 17 grams in a 2200-calorie diet, and 22 grams in a 2800-calorie diet.) If you're not able to get all the data you need, estimate by looking at the number of servings of food high in saturated or trans fat you consume in a day.

If your diet is higher in these fats than it should be, look at your food record to see if you are choosing high-fat foods more often than you should. To reduce your intake of saturated and trans fats, try making healthy substitutions:

- Vegetable oils or trans fat–free tub margarine rather than butter, stick margarine, or vegetable shortening

- Fruits, vegetables, rice cakes, unbuttered popcorn, or pretzels instead of chips, crackers, or cheese puffs

- Low-fat or fat-free milk, cheese, yogurt, or mayonnaise instead of the full-fat versions

- Fruit or a low-fat sweet (angel food cake, frozen yogurt, sorbet) instead of cakes, cookies, pastries, or regular ice cream

- Whole-grain breads and rolls, English muffins, or bagels instead of croissants, muffins, or coffee cake

- Lean meat, skinless poultry, or a veggie burger instead of ground beef, fried chicken, or lunch meats

- Baked potato or rice instead of french fries or onion rings

- Vegetarian chili or pasta with vegetables instead of pizza or macaroni and cheese

When you do eat high-fat foods, eat smaller portions, and balance your higher-fat choices with low-fat choices over the course of the day.

Increasing Fruits and Vegetables in Your Diet

Many fruits and vegetables contain phytochemicals, compounds that help slow, stop, or even reverse the process of cancer. For this reason, the National Cancer Institute (NCI) has developed the "5 a Day for Better Health" program to help Americans increase their consumption of fruits and vegetables to health-promoting levels. Take a look at the foods you've listed in your health journal for a week. Have you included five fruits and vegetables each day? If not, here are some tips from the NCI:

- Drink 100% juice every morning.

- Add raisins, berries, or sliced fruit to cereal; top bagels with tomato slices.

- Make a fruit smoothie from fresh or frozen fruit and orange juice or low-fat yogurt.

- Have vegetable soup or a salad with your lunch.

- Replace french fries or potato chips with cut-up vegetables.

- At dinner, choose a vegetarian main dish, such as stir-fry, or include two servings of vegetables.

- Substitute vegetables for meat in pasta, chili, and casseroles.

- Keep raw fruits and vegetables (apples, plums, carrots) on hand for snacks.

- Try buying a new fruit or vegetable at the store every week.

Some fruits and vegetables are particularly rich in phytochemicals; choose them as often as you can. They include cruciferous vegetables (e.g., broccoli, cauliflower, cabbage, bok choy, brussels sprouts); citrus fruits (e.g., oranges, lemons, grapefruit); berries (e.g., strawberries, raspberries); dark-green leafy vegetables (e.g., spinach, chard, romaine lettuce); and deep-yellow, orange, and red fruits and vegetables (e.g., carrots, red and yellow bell peppers, winter squash, cantaloupe, apricots).

With a little attention and effort, you can modify your diet now, with steps like these, to help safeguard yourself from CVD and cancer in the future.

SOURCES: American Heart Association. 2000. *An Eating Plan for Healthy Americans: The New 2000 Food Guidelines.* Dallas, Tex.: American Heart Association. Food and Drug Administration. 1999. *Questions and Answers on Trans Fat Proposed Rule* (http://vm.cfsan.fda.gov/~dms/qa-trans.html). Center for Science in the Public Interest. 1997. The sat fat switch. *Nutrition Action Healthletter,* January/February. National Cancer Institute. 2000. *Eating 5 a Day: Steps to Sure Success* (http://www.5aday.gov/serving.html; retrieved November 2, 2000). Welland, D. 1999. Fruits and vegetables: Easy ways to five-a-day. *Environmental Nutrition,* June.

- Cancer-promoting dietary factors include meat, certain types of fats, and alcohol.
- Other possible causes of cancer include inactivity and obesity, certain types of infections and chemicals, and radiation.
- Self-monitoring and regular screening tests are essential to early cancer detection.
- Methods of cancer diagnosis include magnetic resonance imaging, computed tomography, and ultra-

sound. Treatment methods usually consist of some combination of surgery, chemotherapy, and radiation.
- Strategies for preventing cancer include avoiding tobacco; eating a varied, moderate diet and controlling weight; exercising regularly; protecting skin from the sun; avoiding exposure to environmental and occupational carcinogens; and getting recommended cancer screening tests.

TAKE ACTION

1. The CPR courses given by the American Red Cross and other groups provide invaluable training that may help you save a life some day. Anyone can take these courses and become qualified to perform CPR. Investigate CPR courses in your community, and sign up to take one.

2. Do some research into your family medical history. Is there cardiovascular disease or cancer in your family, as indicated by premature deaths from heart attack, stroke,

congestive heart failure, or any form of cancer? Take these factors into account as you consider whether you need to make lifestyle changes to avoid CVD or cancer.

3. Devise a plan for incorporating regular self-examinations for cancer (breast self-examination or testicle self-examination) into your life. What strategies will help you remember to do your monthly exam? How can you keep yourself motivated?

JOURNAL ENTRY

1. If the quiz in the box "Anger, Hostility, and Heart Disease" indicates that you may have a quick temper, examine your thoughts and behavior more carefully. In your health journal, keep track of your cynical thoughts, angry feelings, and aggressive acts. For each entry, include the time, place, and cause of your cynical thoughts; what thoughts actually went through your head; the emotions you felt; and any actions you took. Review your journal at the end of a week to learn more about the frequency and kinds of situations that trigger these thoughts and behaviors.

2. In your health journal, list the positive behaviors that help you avoid CVD and cancer. How can you strengthen these behaviors? Also list the behaviors that tend to increase your risk, and plan ways to change them.

3. *Critical Thinking*   Are tobacco companies in any way responsible for the high number of deaths from lung cancer each year? Or is each person entirely responsible for his or her own behavior and health? In your health journal, write a brief essay outlining your position on this issue. Then write a brief essay that supports the opposite viewpoint.

4. *Critical Thinking*   Should people who inherit a genetic defect that increases their risk of cancer pay higher insurance premiums? Should companies be able to deny them employment or health, life, or disability insurance? Should people be held responsible for risk factors like heredity that they cannot control or only for risk factors they can control, such as smoking? What about risk factors like obesity that are due to a combination of heredity and lifestyle? Write an essay explaining your position.

FOR MORE INFORMATION

Books

American Heart Association and American Cancer Society. 1999. *Living Well, Staying Well: The Ultimate Guide to Help Prevent Heart Disease and Cancer.* New York: Times Books. *Provides practical, easy-to-follow guidelines to help you reduce your risk of developing CVD and cancer.*

American Institute for Cancer Research. 2000. *Stopping Cancer Before It Starts.* New York: Griffin. *Suggests research-based changes in diet and lifestyle to help prevent cancer.*

Cooper, G. M. 2001. *Elements of Human Cancer.* Sudbury, Mass.: Jones and Bartlett. *Provides a general overview of the biology and causes of cancer as well as information on specific types of cancers.*

Farquhar, J. W., and G. A. Spiller. 2001. *Diagnosis: Heart Disease.* New York: Norton. *Provides information about heart disease treatment and recovery for patients and their families.*

Gersh, B. J., ed. 2000. *The Mayo Clinic Heart Book.* New York: Morrow. *Covers risk factors, major forms of CVD, diagnosis, and treatment.*

Holland, J. C., and S. Lewis. 2000. *The Human Side of Cancer: Living with Hope, Coping with Uncertainty.* New York: HarperCollins. *A resource for dealing with the stresses and fears brought on by a serious illness.*

W. Organizations and Web Sites

American Academy of Dermatology. Provides information on skin cancer prevention.

888-462-DERM

http://www.aad.org

American Cancer Society. Provides a wide range of free materials on the prevention and treatment of cancer.

800-ACS-2345

http://www.cancer.org

American Heart Association. Provides information on hundreds of topics relating to the prevention and control of cardiovascular disease; sponsors a general Web site as well as several sites focusing on specific topics.

800-AHA-USA1 (general information)

888-MY-HEART (women's health information)

888-4-STROKE (Stroke Connection)

http://www.americanheart.org (general information)

http://www.deliciousdecisions.org (dietary advice)

http://www.justmove.org (fitness advice)

http://women.americanheart.org (women and CVD)

American Institute for Cancer Research. Provides information of lifestyle and cancer prevention, especially nutrition.

800-843-8114

http://www.aicr.org

Cancer Guide: Steve Dunn's Cancer Information Page. Links to many good cancer resources on the Internet and advice about how to make best use of information.

http://www.cancerguide.org

Cardiology Compass. An index and links to cardiovascular information on the Internet.

http://www.cardiologycompass.com

Clinical Trials. Information about clinical trials for new cancer treatments can be accessed at the following sites:

http://cancertrials.nci.nih.gov

http://www.centerwatch.com

Dietary Approaches to Stop Hypertension (DASH). Provides information about the design, diets, and results of the DASH study, including tips on how to follow the DASH diet at home.

http://dash.bwh.harvard.edu

EPA/UV Index. Information about the UV Index and the effects of sun exposure, with links to sites with daily UV Index ratings for cities in the United States and other countries.

http://www.epa.gov/ozone/uvindex/uvover.html

Franklin Institute Science Museum/The Heart: An On-Line Exploration. An online museum exhibit containing information on the structure and function of the heart, how to monitor your heart's health, and how to maintain a healthy heart.

http://www.fi.edu/biosci/heart.html

Harvard Center for Cancer Prevention: Your Cancer Risk. Includes interactive risk assessments as well as tips for preventing common cancers.

http://www.yourcancerrisk.harvard.edu

HeartPoint. Presents news, information, and tips relating to heart health.

http://www.heartpoint.com

National Cancer Institute. Provides information on treatment options, screening, and clinical trials and on the national "5 a Day for Better Health Program" that promotes greater consumption of fruits and vegetables.

800-4-CANCER; 800-624-2511 (Cancer Fax)

http://www.nci.nih.gov

http://cancernet.nci.nih.gov

http://5aday.nci.nih.gov

National Heart, Lung, and Blood Institute. Provides information on a variety of topics relating to cardiovascular health and disease, including cholesterol, smoking, obesity, and hypertension; Web site has special fact sheets covering women and heart disease.

800-575-WELL

http://www.nhlbi.nih.gov

http://rover.nhlbi.nih.gov/chd

National Stroke Association. Provides information and referrals for stroke victims and their families; the Web site has a stroke risk assessment.

800-STROKES

http://www.stroke.org

Oncolink/The University of Pennsylvania Cancer Center Resources. Contains information on different types of cancer and answers to frequently asked questions.

http://www.oncolink.org

See also the listings for Chapters 2, 3, and 9–11.

SELECTED BIBLIOGRAPHY

American Cancer Society. 2001. *Cancer Facts and Figures, 2001.* Atlanta: American Cancer Society.

American Heart Association. 2000. *An Eating Plan for Healthy Americans: The New 2000 Food Guidelines.* Dallas, Tex.: American Heart Association.

American Heart Association. 2001. *Heart and Stroke Statistical Update, 2001.* Dallas, Tex.: American Heart Association.

American Heart Association Nutrition Committee. 2000. AHA Dietary Guidelines: Revision 2000. *Circulation* 102: 2296–2311.

Anttila, T., et al. 2001. Serotypes of *Chlamydia trachomatis* and risk for development of cervical squamous cell carcinoma. *Journal of the American Medical Association* 285(1): 47–51.

Aranow, W., et al. 2000. Aiming for lower than 140/90 mm Hg. *Patient Care* 34(7): 160–176.

Ayanian, J. Z. 2001. Increased mortality among middle-aged women after myocardial infarction: Searching for mechanisms and solutions. *Annals of Internal Medicine* 134(3): 239–241.

Canto, J. 2000. Prevalence, clinical characteristics, and mortality among patients with myocardial infarction presenting without chest pain. *Journal of the American Medical Association* 283(24): 3223–3229.

Cohen, J. H., A. R. Kristal, and J. L. Stanford. 2000. Fruit and vegetable intakes and prostate cancer risk. *Journal of the National Cancer Institute* 92(1): 61–68.

Cooper, R. S., C. N. Rotimi, and R. Ward. 1999. The puzzle of hypertension in African-Americans. *Scientific American* 280(2): 56–63.

Fernandez, E., et al. 2001. Oral contraceptives and colorectal cancer risk: A meta-analysis. *British Journal of Cancer* 84(5): 722–727.

Garcia-Rodriguez, L. A., and C. Huerta-Alvarez. 2001. Reduced risk of colorectal cancer among long-term users of aspirin and nonaspirin nonsteroidal anti-inflammatory drugs. *Epidemiology* 12(1): 88–93.

Goldberg, I. J., et al. 2001. Wine and your heart: A science advisory for healthcare professionals from the Nutrition Committee, Council on Epidemiology and Prevention, and Council on Cardiovascular Nursing of the American Heart Association. *Circulation* 103: 472–475.

Goldstein, L. B., et al. 2001. Primary prevention of ischemic stroke: A statement for healthcare professionals from the Stroke Council of the American Heart Association. *Circulation* 103(1): 163–182.

Ibarren, C., et al. 2000. Association of hostility with coronary artery calcification in young adults. *Journal of the American Medical Association* 283(19): 2546–2551.

Iso, H., et al. 2001. Intake of fish and omega-3 fatty acids and risk of stroke in women. *Journal of the American Medical Association* 285(3): 304–312.

Lee, I-Min, et al. 2001. Physical activity and coronary heart disease in women. *Journal of the American Medical Association* 285(11): 1447–1454.

Lewis, C. 2000. Health claims for foods that lower heart disease risk. *FDA Consumer,* November/December.

Liu, S., et al. 2000. Fruit and vegetable intake and risk of cardiovascular disease: The Women's Health Study. *American Journal of Clinical Nutrition* 72(4): 922–928.

Murphy, M. E., et al. 2000. The effect of sunscreen on the efficacy of insect repellent: A clinical trial. *Journal of the American Academy of Dermatology* 43(2 Pt 1): 219–222.

National Human Genome Research Institute. 2000. *Hereditary Colon Cancer: Genetic Discoveries Offer Hope for Prevention* (http://www.nhgri. nih.gov/Policy_and_public_affairs/Communications/Publications/Maps_to_medicine/colon.html; retrieved May 10, 2000).

National Toxicology Program. 2000. *Ninth Report on Carcinogens.* Research Triangle Park, N.C.: U.S. Department of Health and Human Services.

Ostir, G. V., et al. 2001. The association between emotional well-being and the incidence of stroke in older adults. *Psychosomatic Medicine* 63(2): 210–215.

Pollock, M. L., et al. 2000. AHA Science Advisory: Resistance exercise in individuals with and without cardiovascular disease. *Circulation* 101: 828–833.

Raeini-Sarjaz, M., et al. 2001. Comparison of the effect of dietary fat restriction with that of energy restriction on human lipid metabolism. *American Journal of Clinical Nutrition* 73: 262–267.

Rosenberg, L., et al. 2001. Low-dose oral contraceptive use and the risk of myocardial infarction. *Archives of Internal Medicine* 161(8): 1065–1070.

Sacks, F. M., et al. 2001. Effects on blood pressure of reduced dietary sodium and the Dietary Approaches to Stop Hypertension (DASH) diet. *New England Journal of Medicine* 344(1): 3–10.

Strohsnitter, W. C., et al. 2001. Cancer risk in men exposed in utero to diethylstilbestrol. *Journal of the National Cancer Institute* 93(7): 545–551.

Vaccarino, V., et al. 2001. Sex differences in 2-year mortality after hospital discharge for myocardial infarction. *Annals of Internal Medicine* 134(3): 173–181.

Verloop, J., M. A. Rookus, and F. E. van Leeuwen. 2000. Prevalence of gynecologic cancer in women exposed to diethylstilbestrol in utero. *New England Journal of Medicine* 342(24): 1838–1839.

Vita, J., and J. Keaney. 2000. Exercise—Toning up the endothelium? *New England Journal of Medicine* 342(7): 503–505.

Vogel, R. 2000. The Mediterranean diet and endothelial function: Why some dietary fats may be healthy. *Cleveland Clinic Journal of Medicine* 67(4): 232–236.

Immunity and Infection

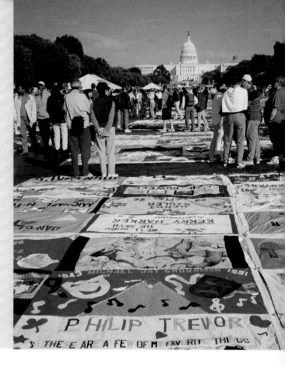

13

LOOKING AHEAD

After reading this chapter, you should be able to

- Describe the step-by-step process by which infectious diseases are transmitted
- Explain how the immune system responds to an invading microorganism
- List the major types of pathogens and describe the common diseases they cause
- Explain the transmission, diagnosis, and treatment of the major STDs, including HIV infection
- List strategies for protecting yourself against STDs

The immune system works continuously to keep the body from being overwhelmed by external invaders that cause **infections** and from internal changes, such as cancer. Most people don't pay much attention to these internal skirmishes unless they become sick and find themselves deprived of their usual feelings of well-being. But many people today are more knowledgeable about the complexities of immunity because they have heard about, or had experience with, HIV infection, which directly attacks the immune system. This chapter provides information that will help you understand immunity, infection, and how to keep yourself well in a world of disease-causing microorganisms.

THE CHAIN OF INFECTION

Infectious diseases are transmitted from one person to another through a series of steps—a chain of infection. The infectious disease cycle begins with a **pathogen**, a microorganism that causes disease. HIV, the virus that causes AIDS, and the tuberculosis bacterium are examples of pathogens. The pathogen has a natural environment in which it typically resides. This so-called *reservoir* can be a person, an animal, or an environmental component like soil or water.

To transmit infection, the pathogen must leave the reservoir through some *portal of exit*. In the case of a human reservoir, portals of exit include saliva (for mumps, for example), the mucous membranes (for many sexually

> **infection** Invasion of the body by a microorganism.
> **pathogen** An organism that causes disease.

Terms

293

transmitted diseases), blood (for HIV and hepatitis), feces (for intestinal infections), and nose and throat discharges (for colds and influenza). *Transmission* can occur directly—from one person to another—or indirectly—through an insect or animal, through contaminated soil or water, or from inanimate objects, such as eating utensils.

To infect a new host, a pathogen must have a *portal of entry* into the body. Pathogens can enter via penetration of the skin or direct contact, inhalation through the mouth or nose, or ingestion of contaminated food or water. Pathogens that enter the skin or mucous membranes can cause a local infection of the tissue, or they may penetrate into the bloodstream or **lymphatic system**, thereby caus-

ing a more extensive **systemic infection.** Agents that cause STDs usually enter the body through the mucous membranes lining the urethra (in males) or the cervix (in females). Organisms that are transmitted via respiratory secretions may cause upper respiratory infections or pneumonia, or they may enter the bloodstream and cause systemic infection. Foodborne and waterborne organisms enter the mouth and may attack the cells of the small intestine or the colon, causing diarrhea, or they may enter the bloodstream via the digestive system and travel to other parts of the body.

Once a pathogen enters the *new host,* a variety of factors determine whether the pathogen will be able to establish itself and cause infection. People with a strong immune system or resistance to a particular pathogen will be less likely to become ill than people with poor immunity. If conditions are right, the pathogen will multiply and produce disease in the new host. In such a case, the new host may become a reservoir from which a new chain of infection can be started.

Interruption of the chain of infection at any point can prevent disease. Strategies for breaking the chain include a mix of public health measures and individual action. For example, a pathogen's reservoir can be isolated or destroyed, as when a sick individual is placed under quarantine or when insects or animals carrying pathogens are killed. Public sanitation practices, such as sewage treatment and the chlorination of drinking water, can also kill pathogens. Transmission can be disrupted through strategies like hand washing, and immunization can stop the pathogen from being passed on to a new host.

THE BODY'S DEFENSE SYSTEM

Our bodies have very effective ways of protecting themselves against invasion by pathogens. The body's first line of defense is a formidable array of physical and chemical barriers. When these barriers are breached, the body's immune system comes into play.

Physical and Chemical Barriers

The skin, the body's largest organ, prevents many microorganisms from entering the body. Although many bacterial and fungal organisms live on the surface of the skin, very few can penetrate it except through a cut or break. Wherever there is an opening in the body, or an area without skin, other barriers exist. The mouth, the main entry to the gastrointestinal system, is lined with mucous membranes, which contain cells designed to prevent the passage of unwanted organisms and particles. Body openings and the fluids that cover them (for example, tears, saliva, and vaginal secretions) are rich in antibodies (discussed in detail later in the chapter) and in enzymes that break down and destroy many microorganisms.

Terms

lymphatic system A system of vessels and organs that picks up excess fluid, proteins, lipids, and other substances from the tissues; filters out pathogens and other waste products; and returns the cleansed fluid to the general circulation.

systemic infection An infection spread by the blood or lymphatic system to large portions of the body.

neutrophil A type of white blood cell that engulfs foreign organisms and infected, damaged, or aged cells; particularly prevalent during the inflammatory response.

macrophage A large phagocytic (cell-eating) cell that devours foreign particles.

natural killer cell A type of white blood cell that directly destroys virus-infected cells and cancer cells.

lymphocytes A white blood cell continuously made in lymphoid tissue as well as in bone marrow.

T cell A lymphocyte that arises in bone marrow and matures in the thymus (thus its name).

B cell A lymphocyte that matures in the bone marrow and produces antibodies.

helper T cell A lymphocyte that helps activate other T cells and may help B cells produce antibodies.

killer T cell A lymphocyte that kills body cells that have been invaded by foreign organisms; also can kill cells that have turned cancerous.

suppressor T cell A lymphocyte that inhibits the growth of other lymphocytes.

antibody A specialized protein, produced by white blood cells, that can recognize and neutralize specific microbes.

memory T and B cells Lymphocytes generated during an initial infection that circulate in the body for years, "remembering" the specific antigens that caused the infection and quickly destroying them if they appear again.

autoimmune disease A disease in which the immune system attacks the person's own body.

antigen A marker on the surface of a foreign substance that immune system cells recognize as nonself and that triggers the immune response.

histamine A chemical responsible for the dilation and increased permeability of blood vessels in allergic reactions.

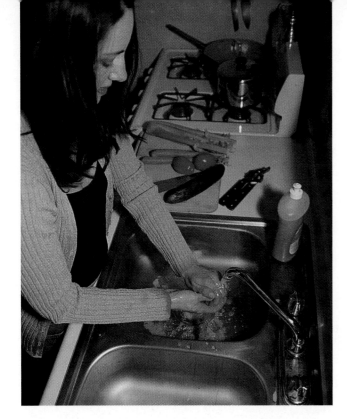

Hand washing is one of the best ways to prevent the spread of infectious diseases. Always wash your hands before, during, and after preparing food; before eating; and after using the bathroom. Wet your hands, apply soap, and rub vigorously for 10–20 seconds.

The respiratory tract is lined not only with mucous membranes but also with cells having hairlike protrusions called cilia. The cilia sweep foreign matter up and out of the respiratory tract. Particles that are not caught by this mechanism may be expelled from the system by a cough. If the ciliated cells are damaged or destroyed, as they are by smoking, a cough is the body's only way of ridding the airways of foreign particles.

The Immune System

Once the body has been invaded by a foreign organism, an elaborate system of responses is activated. We discuss here two of them: the inflammatory response and the immune response. But before we cover these specific defenses, we'll briefly describe the defenders themselves and the mechanisms by which they work.

Immunological Defenders   The immune response is carried out by different types of white blood cells, all of which are continuously being produced in the bone marrow. **Neutrophils,** one type of white blood cell, travel in the bloodstream to areas of invasion, attacking and ingesting pathogens. **Macrophages,** or "big eaters," take up stations in tissues and act as scavengers, devouring pathogens and worn-out cells. **Natural killer cells**

directly destroy virus-infected cells and cells that have turned cancerous. **Lymphocytes,** of which there are several types, are white blood cells that travel in both the bloodstream and the lymphatic system. At various places in the lymphatic system there are lymph nodes (or glands), where macrophages congregate and filter bacteria and other substances from the lymph. When these nodes are actively involved in fighting an invasion of microorganisms, they fill with cells; physicians use the location of swollen lymph nodes as a clue to the location and cause of an infection.

The two main types of lymphocytes are known as **T cells** and **B cells.** T cells are further differentiated into **helper T cells, killer T cells,** and **suppressor T cells.** B cells are lymphocytes that produce **antibodies.** The first time T cells and B cells encounter a specific invader, some of them are reserved as **memory T and B cells,** enabling the body to mount a rapid response should the same invader appear again in the future.

The immune system is built on a remarkable feature of these defenders: the ability to distinguish foreign cells from the body's own cells. Because lymphocytes are capable of great destruction, it is essential that they not attack the body itself. When they do, they cause **autoimmune diseases,** such as lupus and rheumatoid arthritis.

How do lymphocytes know when they have encountered foreign substances? All the cells of an individual's body display markers on their surfaces—tiny molecular shapes—that identify them as "self" to lymphocytes that encounter them. Invading microorganisms also display markers on their surface; lymphocytes identify these as foreign, or "nonself." Nonself markers that trigger the immune response are known as **antigens.** Antibodies have complementary surface markers that work with antigens like a lock and key. When an antigen appears in the body, it eventually encounters an antibody with a complementary pattern; the antibody locks onto the antigen, triggering a series of events designed to destroy the invading pathogen.

The Inflammatory Response   When the body has been injured or infected, one of the body's responses is the inflammatory response. Special cells in the area of invasion or injury release **histamine** and other substances that cause blood vessels to dilate and fluid to flow out of capillaries into the injured tissue. This produces increased heat, swelling, and redness in the affected area. White blood cells, including neutrophils and macrophages, are drawn to the area and attack the invaders—in many cases, destroying them.

The Immune Response   Another body reaction to infection is the immune response (Figure 13-1). For convenience, we can think of the immune response as having four phases: (1) recognition of the invading pathogen, (2) amplification of defenses, (3) attack, and (4) slowdown.

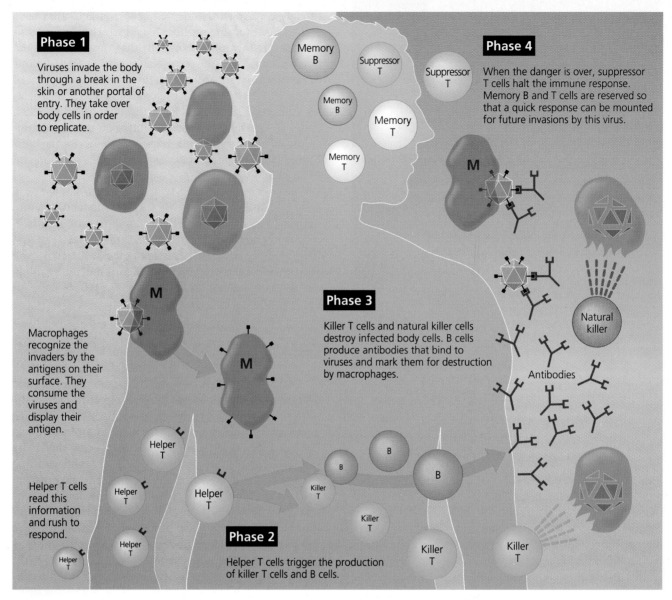

Phase 1

Viruses invade the body through a break in the skin or another portal of entry. They take over body cells in order to replicate.

Memory B

Suppressor T

Memory B

Memory T

Memory T

Memory T

Phase 4

Suppressor T

When the danger is over, suppressor T cells halt the immune response. Memory B and T cells are reserved so that a quick response can be mounted for future invasions by this virus.

M

Macrophages recognize the invaders by the antigens on their surface. They consume the viruses and display their antigen.

M

M

Phase 3

Killer T cells and natural killer cells destroy infected body cells. B cells produce antibodies that bind to viruses and mark them for destruction by macrophages.

Natural killer

Antibodies

Helper T cells read this information and rush to respond.

Helper T

Helper T

Helper T

Helper T

Helper T

Killer T

B

B

B

Killer T

Killer T

Killer T

Killer T

Phase 2

Helper T cells trigger the production of killer T cells and B cells.

Figure 13-1 The immune response. Once invaded by a pathogen, the body mounts a complex series of reactions to eliminate the invader. Pictured here are the principal elements of the immune response to a virus; not shown are the many types of cytokines that help coordinate the actions of different types of defenders.

- *Phase 1.* Macrophages are drawn to the site of the injury and consume the foreign cells; they then provide information about the pathogen by displaying its antigen on their surfaces. Helper T cells "read" this information and rush to respond.

- *Phase 2.* Helper T cells multiply rapidly and trigger the production of killer T cells and B cells in the spleen and lymph nodes. Cytokines, chemical messengers secreted by lymphocytes, help regulate and coordinate the immune response; *interleukins* and *interferons* are two examples of cytokines. They stimulate increased production of T cells, B cells, and antibodies;

promote the activities of natural killer cells; produce fever; and have special antipathogenic properties themselves.

- *Phase 3.* Killer T cells strike at foreign cells and body cells that have been invaded and infected, identifying them by the antigens displayed on the cell surfaces. Puncturing the cell membrane, they sacrifice body cells in order to destroy the foreign organism within. This type of action is known as a *cell-mediated immune response,* because the attack is carried out by cells.

B cells work in a different way. Stimulated to multiply by helper T cells, they produce large quantities of antibody molecules, which are released in the bloodstream and tissues. Antibodies are Y-shaped protein molecules that bind to antigen-bearing targets and mark them for destruction by macrophages. This type of response is known as an *antibody-mediated immune response*. Antibodies work against pathogens when they are in the body but outside cells.

- *Phase 4.* The last phase of the immune response is a slowdown of activity. When the danger is over, suppressor T cells halt the immune response and restore stability, or homeostasis. Dead cells, killed pathogens, and other debris that result from the immune response are filtered out of circulation and excreted from the body.

Immunity   In many infections, survival confers immunity; that is, an infected person will never get the same illness again. This is because some of the lymphocytes created during the amplification phase of the immune response are reserved as memory T and B cells. If the same antigen enters the body again, the memory T and B cells recognize and destroy it before it can cause illness. This subsequent response takes only a day or two, whereas the original response lasted several days, during which time the individual suffered the symptoms of illness. The ability of memory lymphocytes to remember previous infections is known as *acquired immunity*.

Symptoms and Contagion   The immune system is operating at the cellular level within your body all the time, maintaining its vigilance when you're well and fighting invaders when you're sick. During **incubation,** when pathogens are actively multiplying before the immune system has gathered momentum, you may not have any symptoms of the illness, but you may be contagious. During the second and third phases of the immune response, you may still be unaware of the infection, or you may "feel a cold coming on." Symptoms first appear during the **prodromal period,** which follows incubation. If the infected host has prior immunity, the infection may be eradicated during the incubation period or prodromal period. In this case, although you may have felt you were coming down with a cold, for example, it does not develop into a full-blown illness.

Many of the symptoms of an illness are actually due to the immune response of the body rather than to the actions or products of the invading organism. For example, fever is thought to be caused by the release and activation of certain cytokines by macrophages and other cells during the immune response. Cytokines travel in the bloodstream to the brain, where they cause the body's thermostat to be "reset" to a higher level. The resulting elevated temperature is thought to help the body in its fight against pathogens by enhancing immune responses. (During an illness, it is necessary to lower a fever only if it

is uncomfortably high [over 101.5°F] or if it occurs in an infant who is at risk for seizures from fever.)

Similarly, you get a runny nose when your lymphocytes destroy infected mucosal cells, leading to increased mucus production. You get a sore throat when your lymphocytes destroy infected throat cells, and the malaise and fatigue of the flu may be caused by interferons.

You are contagious when there are active microbes replicating in your body and they can gain access to another person. This may be before a vigorous immune response has occurred, so at times you may be contagious before experiencing any symptoms. This means that you can transmit an illness without knowing you're infected or catch an illness from someone who doesn't appear to be sick. On the other hand, your symptoms may continue after the pathogens have been mostly destroyed, when you are no longer infectious.

> **COMMUNICATE!**   A person who "feels a cold coming on" may be highly contagious, as may be the person sitting next to you in a meeting sneezing, blowing her nose, and leaving wadded-up tissues on the table. What can you do to protect yourself from being infected by another person? Offer information—"Did you know you're probably contagious even before you start sneezing?"—and assert your right to stay healthy—"Don't be offended, but I'm moving to the other side of the table. I can't afford to catch a cold right now."

Immunization

The ability of the immune system to remember previously encountered organisms and retain its strength against them is the basis for immunization. When a person is immunized against a disease, the immune system is "primed" with an antigen similar to the pathogenic organism but not as dangerous. The body responds by producing antibodies to the organism, which prevent serious infection when and if the person is exposed to the disease itself. These preparations used to manipulate the immune system are known as **vaccines.** Most vaccines are made from microbes that have been weakened or killed in the laboratory but still retain their ability to stimulate the production of antibodies.

---

incubation The period when bacteria or viruses are actively multiplying inside the body's cells; usually a period without symptoms of illness.

prodromal period The stage of an infection, following incubation, during which initial symptoms begin to appear but the host does not feel ill; a highly contagious period.

vaccine A preparation of killed or weakened microorganisms, inactivated toxins, or components of microorganisms that is administered to stimulate an immune response; a vaccine protects against future infection by the pathogen.

Terms

Vaccines confer what is known as *active immunity*—that is, the vaccinated person produces his or her own antibodies to the microorganism. Another type of injection confers *passive immunity*. In this case, a person exposed to a disease is injected with the antibodies themselves, produced by other human beings or animals who have recovered from the disease. Injections of gamma globulin—a product made from the blood plasma of many individuals, containing all the antibodies they have ever made—are sometimes given to people exposed to a disease against which they have not been immunized. Such injections create a rapid but temporary immunity and are useful against certain viruses, such as hepatitis A.

Allergy: The Body's Defense System Gone Haywire

Are you among the estimated 50 million Americans affected by **allergies?** Allergies result from a hypersensitive and overactive immune system. The immune system typically defends the body against only genuinely harmful pathogens such as viruses and bacteria. However, in someone with an allergy, the immune system also mounts a response to a harmless substance such as pollen or animal dander. The unpleasant and potentially serious symptoms of an allergy—stuffy nose, sneezing, wheezing, skin rashes, and so on—result primarily from the immune response rather than from the **allergens**, the substances that provoke the response. Different people have allergic reactions to different substances. Common allergens include pollen, animal dander, dust mites, cockroaches, molds, mildew, foods, and insect stings. People may also be allergic to certain medications, plants such as poison oak, metals such as nickel, latex, and compounds found in cosmetics.

Terms

allergy A disorder caused by the body's exaggerated response to foreign chemicals and proteins; also called hypersensitivity.

allergen A substance that triggers an allergic reaction.

anaphylaxis A severe systemic hypersensitive reaction to an allergen characterized by difficulty breathing, low blood pressure, heart arrhythmia, seizure, and sometimes death.

bacterium (plural, **bacteria**) A microscopic single-celled organism; about 100 bacterial species can cause disease in humans.

pneumonia Inflammation of the lungs, typically caused by infection or exposure to chemical toxins or irritants.

meningitis Infection of the membranes covering the brain and spinal cord (meninges).

streptococcus Any of a genus (*Streptococcus*) of spherical bacteria; streptococcal species can cause skin infections, strep throat, rheumatic fever, pneumonia, scarlet fever, and other diseases.

staphylococcus Any of a genus (*Staphylococcus*) of spherical, clustered bacteria commonly found on the skin or in the nasal passages; staphylococcal species may enter the body and cause such conditions as boils, pneumonia, and toxic shock syndrome.

The Allergic Response   Most allergic reactions are due to the production of a special type of antibody known as immunoglobulin E (IgE). Initial exposure to a particular allergen may cause little response, but it sensitizes the immune system. When the body is subsequently exposed to the allergen, the allergen binds to IgE, causing the release of large amounts of histamine and other compounds into surrounding tissues. Histamine has many effects, including increasing the inflammatory response and stimulating mucus production. In the nose, histamine may cause congestion and sneezing; in the eyes, itchiness and tearing; in the skin, redness, swelling, and itching; in the intestines, bloating and cramping; and in the lungs, coughing, wheezing, and shortness of breath. In some people, an allergen can trigger an asthma attack.

The most serious, but rare, kind of allergic reaction is **anaphylaxis**, which results from a release of histamine throughout the body. Anaphylactic reactions can be life-threatening because symptoms may include swelling of the throat, extremely low blood pressure, fainting, heart arrhythmia, and seizures. Anaphylaxis is a medical emergency, and treatment requires immediate injection of epinephrine.

Dealing with Allergies   If you suspect you might have an allergy, visit your physician or an allergy specialist. You may be asked to keep a diary to help identify allergens to which you are susceptible, or you may undergo allergy skin tests or blood tests. There are three general strategies for dealing with allergies:

• *Avoidance:* You may be able to avoid or minimize exposure to allergens by making changes in your environment or behavior. For example, removing carpets from the bedroom and using special bedding can reduce dust mite contact.

• *Medication:* Many over-the-counter (OTC) antihistamines are effective at controlling symptoms, but the side effect of sedation may limit your daytime use of these medications; nonsedating antihistamines are available with a prescription. Corticosteroids markedly reduce allergy symptoms, but they have significant side effects.

• *Immunotherapy:* Referred to as "allergy shots," immunotherapy desensitizes a person to a particular allergen through the administration of gradually increasing doses of the allergen over a period of months or years.

THE TROUBLEMAKERS: PATHOGENS AND DISEASE

Now that we've discussed the intricate system that protects us from disease, let's consider some pathogens, the disease-producing organisms that live within us and around us. When they succeed in gaining entry to body

Table 13-1	Top Infectious Diseases Worldwide

Disease	Approximate Number of Deaths per Year
Pneumonia	3,963,000
HIV/AIDS	2,673,000
Diarrheal diseases	2,213,000
Tuberculosis	1,669,000
Malaria	1,086,000
Measles	875,000
Tetanus	377,000
Pertussis (whooping cough)	295,000
Meningitis	171,000
Syphilis	153,000

In addition, many of the 589,000 deaths from liver cancer each year can be traced to viral hepatitis. Overall, infectious diseases kill more than 14 million people each year, representing nearly 25% of all deaths.

SOURCE: World Health Organization. 2000. *The World Health Report 2000: Health Systems: Improving Performance.* Geneva: World Health Organization.

tissue, they can cause illness and sometimes death to the unfortunate host. Worldwide, infectious diseases are responsible for more than 13 million deaths each year (Table 13-1). Pathogens include bacteria, viruses, fungi, protozoa, parasitic worms, and prions (Figure 13-2).

Bacteria

The most abundant living things on earth are **bacteria,** single-celled organisms that usually reproduce by splitting in two to create a pair of identical cells. Bacteria are often classified according to their shape: they may be rod-shaped (bacilli), spherical (cocci), spiral-shaped (spirochete), or comma-shaped (vibrios).

We harbor both helpful and harmful bacteria on our skin and in our gastrointestinal and reproductive tracts. The human colon contains "friendly" bacteria that produce certain vitamins and help digest nutrients. (A large portion of human feces consists of bacteria). Friendly bacteria also keep harmful bacteria in check by competing for food and resources and secreting substances toxic to pathogenic bacteria. Not all bacteria found in the body are beneficial, however. Some bacterial infections of concern are described below.

Pneumonia   Inflammation of the lungs, called **pneumonia,** may be caused by infection with bacteria, viruses, or fungi or by contact with chemical toxins or irritants. Pneumonia often follows another illness, such as a cold or the flu, but the symptoms are typically more severe—

fever, chills, shortness of breath, increased mucus production, and cough. Pneumonia ranks sixth among the leading causes of death for Americans.

Pneumococcus bacteria are the most common cause of bacterial pneumonia; a vaccine is available and recommended for all adults age 65 and older and others at risk. Other bacteria that may cause pneumonia include *Streptococcus pneumoniae, Chlamydia pneumoniae,* and mycoplasmas. Outbreaks of infection with mycoplasmas are relatively common among young adults, especially in crowded settings such as dormitories. Legionnaires' disease is a severe form of pneumonia caused by the rod-shaped bacterium *Legionella pneumophila.*

Meningitis   Infection of the *meninges,* the membranes covering the brain and spinal cord, is called **meningitis.** Viral meningitis is usually mild and goes away on its own; bacterial meningitis, however, can be life-threatening and requires immediate treatment with antibiotics. Symptoms of meningitis include fever, a severe headache, stiff neck, sensitivity to light, and confusion. The disease is fatal in 10–15% of cases, and about 10% of people who recover have permanent hearing loss or other serious effects.

A vaccine is available, but it is not effective against all strains of meningitis-causing bacteria. First-year college students who live in dormitories have been found to be at a modestly increased risk for meningitis compared to other people their age. For this reason, the CDC recommended in 2000 that first-year college students be given information about meningitis and the benefits of vaccination and be offered the vaccine.

Strep Throat and Other Streptococcal Infections   The **streptococcus** bacterium is spherical-shaped and often grows in chains. Streptococcal pharyngitis, or strep throat, is characterized by a red, sore throat with white patches on the tonsils, swollen lymph nodes, fever, and headache. It is typically spread through close contact with an infected person via respiratory droplets (sneezing or coughing). If left untreated, strep throat can develop into the more serious rheumatic fever.

A particularly virulent type of streptococcus can invade the bloodstream, spread to other parts of the body, and produce dangerous systemic illness. It can also cause a serious but rare infection of the deeper layers of the skin, a condition called necrotizing fascitis or "flesh-eating strep." This dangerous infection is characterized by tissue death and is treated with antibiotics and removal of the infected tissue or limb.

Toxic Shock Syndrome and Other Staphylococcal Infections   The spherical-shaped **staphylococcus** bacterium often appears in small clusters when viewed under a microscope. Staphylococci cause infections ranging from minor skin infections such as boils to very serious conditions such as blood infections or pneumonia. A particular

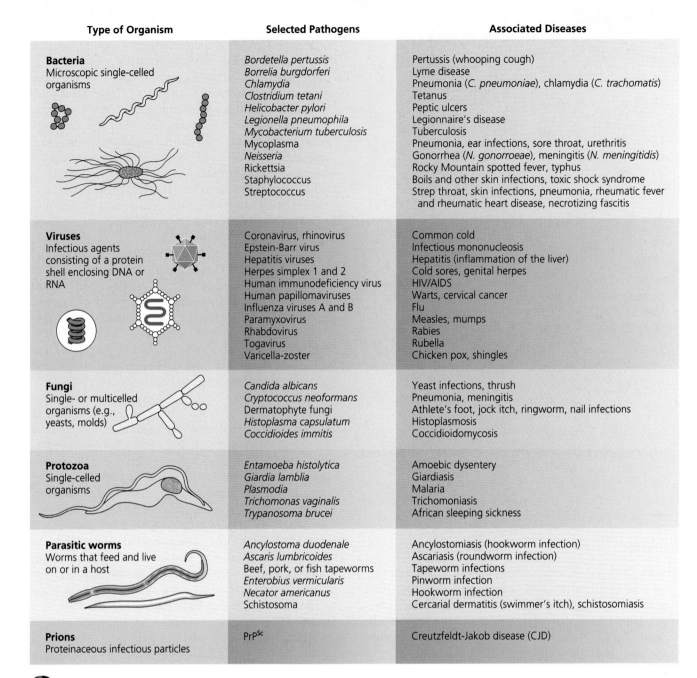

Type of Organism	Selected Pathogens	Associated Diseases
Bacteria Microscopic single-celled organisms	*Bordetella pertussis* *Borrelia burgdorferi* *Chlamydia* *Clostridium tetani* *Helicobacter pylori* *Legionella pneumophila* *Mycobacterium tuberculosis* Mycoplasma *Neisseria* Rickettsia Staphylococcus Streptococcus	Pertussis (whooping cough) Lyme disease Pneumonia (*C. pneumoniae*), chlamydia (*C. trachomatis*) Tetanus Peptic ulcers Legionnaire's disease Tuberculosis Pneumonia, ear infections, sore throat, urethritis Gonorrhea (*N. gonorroeae*), meningitis (*N. meningitidis*) Rocky Mountain spotted fever, typhus Boils and other skin infections, toxic shock syndrome Strep throat, skin infections, pneumonia, rheumatic fever and rheumatic heart disease, necrotizing fascitis
Viruses Infectious agents consisting of a protein shell enclosing DNA or RNA	Coronavirus, rhinovirus Epstein-Barr virus Hepatitis viruses Herpes simplex 1 and 2 Human immunodeficiency virus Human papillomaviruses Influenza viruses A and B Paramyxovirus Rhabdovirus Togavirus Varicella-zoster	Common cold Infectious mononucleosis Hepatitis (inflammation of the liver) Cold sores, genital herpes HIV/AIDS Warts, cervical cancer Flu Measles, mumps Rabies Rubella Chicken pox, shingles
Fungi Single- or multicelled organisms (e.g., yeasts, molds)	*Candida albicans* *Cryptococcus neoformans* Dermatophyte fungi *Histoplasma capsulatum* *Coccidioides immitis*	Yeast infections, thrush Pneumonia, meningitis Athlete's foot, jock itch, ringworm, nail infections Histoplasmosis Coccidioidomycosis
Protozoa Single-celled organisms	*Entamoeba histolytica* *Giardia lamblia* *Plasmodia* *Trichomonas vaginalis* *Trypanosoma brucei*	Amoebic dysentery Giardiasis Malaria Trichomoniasis African sleeping sickness
Parasitic worms Worms that feed and live on or in a host	*Ancylostoma duodenale* *Ascaris lumbricoides* Beef, pork, or fish tapeworms *Enterobius vermicularis* *Necator americanus* Schistosoma	Ancylostomiasis (hookworm infection) Ascariasis (roundworm infection) Tapeworm infections Pinworm infection Hookworm infection Cercarial dermatitis (swimmer's itch), schistosomiasis
Prions Proteinaceous infectious particles	PrP^{Sc}	Creutzfeldt-Jakob disease (CJD)

Figure 13-2 Pathogens and associated infectious diseases.

species of the bacteria, *Staphylococcus aureus*, is responsible for many cases of **toxic shock syndrome (TSS)**. The bacteria produce a deadly toxin that causes shock (potentially life-threatening low blood pressure), high fever, a peeling skin rash, and inflammation of several organ systems.

Tuberculosis   Caused by the rod-shaped bacterium *Mycobacterium tuberculosis*, **tuberculosis (TB)** is a chronic bacterial infection that usually affects the lungs. TB is spread via the respiratory route through prolonged contact with someone who has the disease in its active form.

Symptoms include coughing, fatigue, night sweats, weight loss, and fever. Ten to 15 million Americans have been infected with, and therefore continue to carry, *M. tuberculosis*. However, only about 10% of people with so-called latent TB infections actually develop an active case of the disease during their lifetime. In the United States, active TB is most common among people infected with HIV, recent immigrants from countries where TB is **endemic**, and those who live in the inner cities.

Lyme Disease   Each year in the United States more than 15,000 cases of Lyme disease are reported. The disease is

Avoid Tick Habitats

When possible, avoid areas that are likely to be infested with ticks, particularly in spring and summer, when the immature ticks, called nymphs, are most likely to feed. Ticks favor moist, shaded habitats, especially as provided by leaf litter and low-lying vegetation in wooded, brushy, or overgrown grassy habitats. State and local health departments, park personnel, and agricultural extension services can provide information on the distribution of ticks in your area.

Wear Protective Clothing and Apply Insect Repellent

Wear light-colored clothing so that ticks can be spotted more easily. Wear long-sleeved shirts and tuck pants into socks or the tops of boots to help keep ticks from reaching your skin. Ticks are usually located close to the ground, so wearing high boots may provide additional protection. Application of insect repellents containing DEET (n,n-diethyl-m-toluamide) to clothes and exposed skin, and permethrin to clothes, should also help reduce the risk of tick attachment. DEET can be used safely on adults and children, but it should be applied according to Environmental Protection Agency guidelines to reduce the possibility of toxicity.

Remove Attached Ticks

Transmission of an infectious agent is unlikely to occur until a tick has fed on you for several hours (36 hours in the case of Lyme dis-

ease), so daily checks for ticks and their prompt removal will help prevent infection. Search your entire body for ticks, using a handheld or full-length mirror; also check children and pets. Ticks are small; in the nymph phase, they may resemble poppy seeds.

Deer tick (actual size)

larva   nymph   female   male

1   2

To remove a tick, use fine-tipped tweezers and shield your fingers with rubber gloves or a paper towel. Grasp the tick as close to the skin surface as possible and pull upward (away from the skin) with steady, even pressure. Do not twist or jerk the tick, as this may cause the mouthparts to break off and remain in the skin. If this happens, remove the mouthparts with tweezers. Do not squeeze, crush, or puncture the body of the tick because its fluids may contain infectious organisms. After removing the tick, disinfect the bite site and wash your hands with soap and water. Save ticks for identification in case you become ill. Place the tick in a plastic bag in your freezer, and note the date of the bite.

SOURCES: Centers for Disease Control and Prevention. 2000. *Lyme Disease: Prevention and Control* (http://www.cdc.gov/ncidod/dvbid/lymeprevent.htm; retrieved December 5, 2000). Centers for Disease Control and Prevention. 2000. *Rocky Mountain Spotted Fever: Questions and Answers* (http://www.cdc.gov/ncidod/dvrd/rmsf/q&a.htm; retrieved

spread by the bite of a tick of the genus *Ixodes* that is infected with the spiral-shaped bacterium *Borrelia burgdorferi*. Symptoms of Lyme disease vary but typically occur in stages, beginning with a bull's-eye-shaped rash in the area of the bite; later symptoms can include impaired coordination and chronic or recurrent arthritis. Lyme disease is preventable by avoiding contact with ticks or by removing a tick before it has had the chance to transmit the infection. A vaccine is available for people age 15–70 years who are at high risk, but it is not 100% effective against the disease. Lyme disease is treatable at all stages, although arthritis symptoms may not completely resolve.

Ulcers   About 25 million Americans suffer from ulcers, sores or holes in the lining of the stomach or the first part of the small intestine (duodenum). It used to be thought that spicy food and stress were major causes of ulcers, but it is now known that as many as 90% of ulcers are caused by infection with *Helicobacter pylori*. Ulcer symptoms include gnawing or burning pain in the abdomen, nausea, and loss of appetite. If tests show the presence of *H. pylori*, treatment with antibiotics often cures the infection and the ulcers.

Antibiotic Treatments   Antibiotics are both naturally occurring and synthetic substances having the ability to

kill bacteria. Most antibiotics work in a similar fashion: They interrupt the production of new bacteria by damaging some part of their reproductive cycle or by causing faulty parts of new bacteria to be made. When antibiotics inhibit a specific bacterial strain's growth, these bacteria are said to be "sensitive." Unfortunately, antibiotic-resistant strains (types) of many common bacteria have developed, including strains of gonorrhea (an STD), salmonellosis (a foodborne illness), and tuberculosis. Antibiotic resistance is a major factor contributing to the recent rise in problematic infectious diseases.

You can help prevent the development of antibiotic-resistant strains of bacteria by using antibiotics properly:

- Don't expect to take an antibiotic every time you get sick. They are mainly helpful for bacterial infections; against viruses, they are ineffective.

Terms

toxic shock syndrome (TSS) Sudden onset of fever, aches, vomiting, and peeling rash, followed in some cases by shock and inflammation of multiple organs; often caused by a toxin produced by *Staphylococcus aureus*.

tuberculosis (TB) A chronic bacterial infection that usually affects the lungs.

endemic Persistent and relatively widespread in a given population.

Prevention

Colds are usually spread by hand-to-hand contact with another person or with objects such as doorknobs and telephones, which an infected person may have handled. The best way to avoid transmission is to wash your hands frequently with warm water and soap. Keeping your immune system strong is another good prevention strategy.

Home Treatments

- Get some extra rest. It isn't usually necessary to stay home in bed, but you will need to slow down a little from your usual routine to give your body a chance to fight the infection.

- Drink plenty of liquids to prevent dehydration. Hot liquids such as herbal tea and clear chicken soup will soothe a sore throat and loosen secretions; gargling with a glass of slightly salty water may also help. Avoid alcoholic beverages when you have a cold.

- Hot showers or the use of a humidifier can help eliminate nasal stuffiness and soothe inflamed membranes.

Over-the-Counter Treatments

Avoid multisymptom cold remedies. Because these products include drugs to treat symptoms you may not even have, you risk suffering from side effects from medications you don't need. It's better to treat each symptom separately:

- *Analgesics*—aspirin, acetaminophen (Tylenol), ibuprofen (Advil or Motrin), and naproxen sodium (Aleve)—all help lower fever and relieve muscle aches. Use of aspirin is associated with an increased risk of a serious condition called Reye's syndrome in children and teenagers; for this reason, aspirin should be given only to adults.

- *Decongestants* shrink nasal blood vessels, relieving swelling and congestion. However, they may dry out mucous membranes in the throat and make a sore throat worse.

- *Cough medicines* may be helpful when your cough is nonproductive (not bringing up mucus) or if it disrupts your sleep or work. Expectorants make coughs more productive by increasing the volume of mucus and decreasing its thickness, thereby helping remove irritants from the respiratory airways. Suppressants (antitussives) reduce the frequency of coughing.

- *Antihistamines* decrease nasal secretions caused by the effects of histamine, so they are much more useful in treating allergies than colds. *Caution:* Many antihistamines can make you drowsy.

Antibiotics will not help a cold unless a bacterial infection such as strep throat is also present, and overuse of antibiotics leads to the development of drug resistance. The jury is still out on whether other remedies, including zinc gluconate lozenges, echinacea, and vitamin C, will relieve symptoms or shorten the duration of a cold. Researchers are also studying antiviral drugs that target the most common types of cold viruses.

Sometimes a cold leads to a more serious complication, such as bronchitis, pneumonia, or strep throat. If a fever of 102°F or higher persists, or if cold symptoms don't get better after 2 weeks, see your physician.

- Use antibiotics as directed, and finish the full course of medication even if you begin to feel better. This helps ensure that all targeted bacteria are killed off.

- Never take an antibiotic without a prescription. If you take an antibiotic for a viral infection, take the wrong one, or take an insufficient dose, your illness will not improve, and you'll give bacteria the opportunity to develop resistance.

Viruses

Viruses are on the borderline between living and nonliving matter. They lack all the enzymes essential to energy production and protein synthesis in normal animal cells, and they cannot grow or reproduce by themselves; they use what they need for growth and reproduction from the cells they invade. Once a virus is inside the host cell, it sheds its protein covering and its genetic material takes control of the cell and manufactures more viruses like itself. The normal functioning of the host cell is thereby disrupted. Illnesses caused by viruses are the most common forms of **contagious disease.**

The Common Cold   Although generally brief, lasting only 4–7 days, colds are nonetheless irritating and often interfere with one's normal activities. A cold may be caused by any of more than 200 different viruses that attack the lining of the nasal passages. Cold viruses are almost always transmitted by hand-to-hand contact. To lessen your risk of contracting a cold, wash your hands frequently; if you touch someone else, avoid touching your face until after you've washed your hands. If you do catch a cold, over-the-counter cold remedies may help treat your symptoms but do not directly attack the viral cause.

Influenza   Commonly called "the flu," **influenza** is an infection of the respiratory tract caused by the influenza virus. Compared to the common cold, influenza is a more serious illness, usually including a fever and extreme fatigue. Most people who get the flu recover within 1–2 weeks, but some develop potentially life-threatening complications, such as pneumonia. Influenza is highly contagious and is spread via respiratory droplets. The influenza virus is responsible for **epidemics** of respiratory illness that occur almost every winter.

The most effective way of preventing the flu is through annual vaccination, which is recommended for anyone age 6 months or older who is at increased risk for complications of influenza, who has close contact with people in high-risk groups, or who wants to reduce his or her risk of the flu. There are also a number of medications that can treat influenza.

Chicken Pox, Cold Sores, and Other Herpesvirus Infections

The **herpesviruses** are a large and important group of viruses. Once infected, the host is never free of the virus. The virus lies latent within certain cells and becomes active periodically, producing symptoms. The family of herpesviruses includes varicella-zoster virus, which causes chicken pox and shingles; herpes simplex virus (HSV) types 1 and 2, which cause cold sores and the STD herpes; and Epstein-Barr virus (EBV), which causes infectious mononucleosis. Two herpesviruses that can cause severe infections in people with a suppressed immune system are cytomegalovirus (CMV), which infects the lungs, brain, colon, and eyes, and human herpesvirus 8 (HHV-8), which has been linked to Kaposi's sarcoma.

Viral Hepatitis

Viral **hepatitis** is a term used to describe several different infections that cause inflammation of the liver. Hepatitis is usually caused by one of the three most common hepatitis viruses. Hepatitis A virus (HAV) causes the mildest form of the disease and is usually transmitted by food or water contaminated by sewage or an infected person. Hepatitis B virus (HBV) is usually transmitted sexually (see p. 317). Hepatitis C virus (HCV) can also be transmitted sexually, but it is much more commonly passed through direct contact with infected blood via injection drug use or, prior to the development of screening tests, blood transfusions. HBV and, to a lesser extent, HCV, can also be passed from a pregnant woman to her child. There are effective vaccines for hepatitis A and B.

Most people recover from hepatitis A within a month or so. However, 5–10% of people infected with HBV and 85–90% of people infected with HCV become chronic carriers of the virus, capable of infecting others for the rest of their lives. Some chronic carriers remain asymptomatic, while others slowly develop chronic liver disease, cirrhosis, or liver cancer. An estimated 5 million Americans and 500 million people worldwide may be chronic carriers of hepatitis.

The extent of HCV infection has only recently been recognized, and most infected people are unaware of their condition. To ensure proper treatment and prevention, testing for HCV may be recommended for people at risk, including people who have ever injected drugs (even once), who received a blood transfusion or a donated organ prior to July 1992, who have engaged in high-risk sexual behavior, or who have had body piercing, tattoos, or acupuncture involving unsterile equipment.

Warts

Infection by the human papillomavirus (HPV), which causes cell proliferation, can cause warts (noncancerous skin tumors). The more than 100 different types of HPV cause a variety of warts, including common warts on the hands, plantar warts on the soles of the feet, and genital warts around the genitalia. Depending on their location, warts may be removed using over-the-counter preparations or professional methods such as laser surgery or cryosurgery. Because HPV infection is chronic, warts can reappear despite treatment.

Treating Viral Illnesses

Although many viruses cannot be treated medically, researchers have recently begun to develop antiviral drugs. These typically work by interfering with some part of the viral life cycle; for example, they may prevent a virus from entering body cells or from successfully reproducing. Antivirals are available to fight infections caused by HIV, influenza, herpes simplex, varicella-zoster, HBV, and HCV. Most other viral diseases must simply run their course.

Fungi

A **fungus** is a primitive plant. Mushrooms and the molds that form on bread and cheese are all examples of fungi. Only about 50 fungi out of many thousands of species cause disease in humans, and these diseases are usually restricted to the skin, mucous membranes, and lungs.

Candida albicans is a common fungus found naturally in the vagina of most women. In normal amounts, it causes no problems, but when excessive growth occurs, the result is itching and discomfort, commonly known as a yeast infection. Other common fungal conditions, including athlete's foot, jock itch, and ringworm, a disease

> **Terms**
>
> **virus** A very small infectious agent composed of nucleic acid (DNA or RNA) surrounded by a protein coat; lacks an independent metabolism and reproduces only within a host cell.
>
> **contagious disease** A disease that can be transmitted from one person to another; most are viral diseases, such as the common cold and flu.
>
> **influenza** Infection of the respiratory tract by the influenza virus, which is highly infectious and adaptable; the form changes so easily that every year new strains arise, making treatment difficult; commonly known as the flu.
>
> **epidemic** The occurrence in a particular community or region of more than the expected number of cases of a particular disease.
>
> **herpesvirus** A family of viruses responsible for cold sores, mononucleosis, chicken pox, and the STD known as herpes; frequently cause latent infections.
>
> **hepatitis** Inflammation of the liver, which can be caused by infection, drugs, or toxins.
>
> **fungus** A single-celled or multicelled organism that absorbs food from living or dead organic matter; examples include molds, mushrooms, and yeasts. Fungal diseases include yeast infections, athlete's foot, and ringworm.

of the scalp, affect the skin. Fungi can also cause systemic diseases that are severe, life-threatening, and extremely difficult to treat. Fungal infections can be especially deadly in people with an impaired immune system.

Protozoa

Another group of pathogens are **protozoa,** single-celled organisms that often cause recurrent diseases: The pathogen remains in the body, alternating between activity and inactivity. Hundreds of millions of people in developing countries suffer from protozoal infections; for example, each year, there are 300–500 million new cases of malaria and more than 1 million deaths, mostly among infants and children. Other protozoal diseases include giardiasis, an intestinal infection characterized by nausea and diarrhea; trichomoniasis ("trich"), a treatable vaginal infection; trypanosomiasis, known as African sleeping sickness; and amoebic dysentery.

Parasitic Worms

The **parasitic worms** are the largest organisms that can enter the body to cause infection. The tapeworm, for example, can grow to a length of many feet. Worms cause a great variety of relatively mild infections. Pinworm, the most common worm infection in the United States, primarily affects young children. Generally speaking, worm infections originate from contaminated food or drink and can be controlled by careful attention to hygiene.

Prions

In recent years, several fatal degenerative disorders of the central nervous system have been linked to "proteinaceous infectious particles," or **prions.** Unlike all other infectious agents, prions appear to lack DNA or RNA and to consist only of protein. Prions have an abnormal shape and form deposits in the brain. They are associated with a class of diseases known as *transmissible spongiform encephalopathies (TSEs),* which are characterized by spongelike holes in the brain. Known prion diseases include Creutzfeldt-Jakob disease (in humans), bovine spongiform encephalopathy

("mad cow disease" in cattle), and scrapie (in sheep). Some prion diseases are inherited or the result of spontaneous genetic mutations; others are the result of eating infected tissue or being exposed to prions during medical procedures such as organ or tissue transplants.

Emerging Infectious Diseases

The reduction in deaths from infectious diseases in the United States is one of the major public health achievements of the past century. Improvements in sanitation, hygiene, and water quality and the development of antibiotics all contributed to reduced death rates from infections. However, after decades of decline, the U.S. death rate from infectious disease began to climb in 1981, largely due to the AIDS epidemic. Globally, infectious diseases remain a major killer, and new areas of concern have emerged in the past 20 years. Emerging infectious diseases are diseases of infectious origin whose incidence in humans has increased or threatens to increase in the near future. They include both known diseases that have experienced a resurgence and diseases that were previously unknown or confined to specific areas.

What's behind this rising tide of infectious diseases? Contributing factors are complex and interrelated. They include the following:

- *Drug resistance.* New or increasing drug resistance has been found in organisms that cause malaria, tuberculosis, gonorrhea, influenza, AIDS, and pneumococcal and staphylococcal infections. Some bacterial strains now appear to be resistant to all available antibiotics.

- *Poverty.* More than 1 billion people live in extreme poverty, and half the world's population has no regular access to essential drugs. Population growth, urbanization, overcrowding, and migration (including the movement of refugees) also contribute to the spread of infectious diseases.

- *The breakdown of public health measures.* A poor public health infrastructure is often associated with poverty and social upheaval, but problems such as contaminated water supplies and inadequate vaccination can occur even in industrial countries.

- *Environmental changes.* Changes in land use—deforestation, the damming of rivers, the spread of ranching and farming—alter the distribution of disease vectors and bring people into contact with new pathogens. A shift in rainfall patterns caused by global warming may allow mosquito-borne diseases such as malaria to spread from the tropics into the temperate zones.

- *Travel and commerce.* International tourism and trade open the world to infectious agents. For example, the reintroduction of cholera into the Western hemisphere is thought to have occurred through the dis-

Terms

protozoan A microscopic single-celled organism that often produces recurrent, cyclical attacks of disease.

parasitic worm A pathogen that causes intestinal and other infections; includes tapeworms, hookworms, pinworms, and flukes.

prion Proteinaceous infectious particles thought to be responsible for a class of neurodegenerative diseases known as transmissible spongiform encephalopathies; Creutzfeldt-Jakob disease in humans and bovine spongiform encephalopathy ("mad cow disease") are examples of prion diseases.

pandemic A disease epidemic that is unusually severe or widespread; often used to refer to worldwide epidemics affecting a large proportion of the population.

The appearance of West Nile virus in New York in 1999–2000 brought the issue of emerging infectious diseases back into the headlines. Although the chances of the average American contracting an exotic infection are very low, emerging infections are a concern to public health officials and represent a challenge to all nations in the future. Some of the emerging infections that concern scientists include the following:

• *West Nile virus.* A mini-outbreak of encephalitis in New York in 1999 led to identification of this virus, which had previously been restricted to Africa, the Middle East, and parts of Europe. Since that time, the virus has spread to more than 12 states and resulted in at least 8 deaths. Experts believe it arrived in this country in an infected bird or person from a country where the virus is common. West Nile virus is carried by birds and then passed to humans when mosquitoes bite first an infected bird and then a person. Most people who are bitten have few or no symptoms, but the virus can cause permanent brain damage or death in some cases.

• *Escherichia coli O157: H7.* This potentially deadly strain of *E. coli,* transmitted in contaminated food, can cause bloody diarrhea and kidney damage. The first major outbreak occurred in 1993, when over 600 people became ill and four children died after eating contaminated and undercooked fast-food hamburgers. Additional outbreaks have been linked to lettuce, alfalfa sprouts, unpasteurized juice, and contaminated public swimming pools. An estimated 70,000 cases and 6 deaths occur in the United States each year.

• *Hantavirus.* Since first being recognized in 1993, over 500 cases of hantavirus pulmonary syndrome (HPS) have been reported in the United States and South America. HPS is caused by the rodent-borne Sin Nombre virus (SNV) and is spread primarily through airborne viral particles from rodent urine, droppings, or saliva. It is characterized by a dangerous fluid buildup in the lungs and is fatal in about 45% of cases.

• *Necrotizing fasciitis.* The "flesh-eating bacteria" that cause necrotizing fasciitis are a virulent strain of streptococci

that also cause scarlet fever, toxic shock syndrome, and the lethal type of pneumonia that killed Muppets creator Jim Henson in 1990. The bacteria break down tissue and damage blood vessels at the site of a wound, sometimes leading to gangrene, shock, and, in about 20% of cases, death. The disease is rare (about 500–1500 cases per year in the United States).

• *Mad cow disease.* By 2001, more than 90 cases of a new variant of a rare, incurable brain affliction called Creutzfeldt-Jakob disease (CJD) had been reported in the United Kingdom. The new variant of CJD has affected younger people, average age 29 years, and has several unique features. Researchers suspect that this new variant of CJD is caused by people eating beef contaminated with central nervous system tissue from cows infected with bovine spongiform encephalopathy (BSE), commonly called mad cow disease. No cases have been reported in the United States.

• *Ebola.* So far, outbreaks of the often fatal Ebola hemorrhagic fever (EHF) in humans have occurred only in Africa. The Ebola virus is transmitted by direct contact with infected blood or other body secretions, and many cases of EHF have been linked to unsanitary conditions in medical facilities. Because symptoms appear quickly and 75% of victims die, usually within a few days, the virus tends not to spread widely (unlike HIV or hepatitis, which can infect a person for years before any symptoms appear).

• *Influenza A(H5N1).* An outbreak in 1997–1998 of this unusual strain of influenza killed 6 people in Hong Kong. Local authorities contained the outbreak quickly by tracing its source to infected chickens, ducks, and geese and then ordering the slaughter of all domestic poultry. Although small, the outbreak raised the specter of the 1918–1919 influenza **pandemic.** A strain like A(H5N1) is so unique that few, if any, people have immunity from past exposure; had it mutated into a form that more easily infects humans, influenza A(H5N1) could conceivably have killed as many as 30% of the world's people.

charge of bilge water from a Chinese freighter into the waters off Peru.

• *Mass food production and distribution.* Food now travels long distances to our table, and microbes are transmitted along with it. Mass production of food increases the likelihood that a chance contamination can lead to mass illness.

• *Human behaviors.* Changes in patterns of human behavior also have an impact on the spread of infectious diseases. The widespread use of injectable drugs rapidly transmits HIV infection and hepatitis. Changes in sexual behavior over the past 30 years have led to a proliferation of new and old STDs. The use of day-care facilities for children has led to increases in the incidence of several infections that cause diarrhea.

International efforts at monitoring, preventing, and controlling their spread are underway. These efforts require worldwide coordination because microbes do not respect national borders. Only a global response can make the world a safer and healthier place for everyone.

Other Immune Disorders: Cancer and Autoimmune Diseases

Sometimes, as in the case of cancer, the body comes under attack by its own cells. The immune system can often detect cells that have recently become cancerous and then destroy them just as it would a foreign microorganism. But if the immune system breaks down, the cancer cells may multiply out of control before the immune system recognizes the danger.

Another type of immune disorder occurs when the body confuses its own cells with foreign organisms. In autoimmune diseases, the immune system seems to be a bit too sensitive and begins to misapprehend itself as "nonself." Rheumatoid arthritis and systemic lupus erythematosus are examples of autoimmune diseases. For reasons not well understood, these conditions are much more common in women than men.

GIVING YOURSELF A FIGHTING CHANCE: HOW TO SUPPORT YOUR IMMUNE SYSTEM

Public health measures protect people from many diseases that are transmitted via water, food, or insects. A clean water supply and adequate sewage treatment help control typhoid fever and cholera, for example; and mosquito eradication programs control malaria and encephalitis. Proper food inspection and preparation prevent illness caused by foodborne pathogens.

What can you do as an individual to strengthen your immune system to help prevent infection? The most important thing you can do is to take good care of your body, with adequate nutrition, exercise (but not while you're sick), rest (6–8 hours sleep per night), and moderation in lifestyle. Don't smoke, and drink alcohol only in moderation; both smoking and drinking interfere with immunefunction. Wash your hands frequently; don't eat raw meat or unpasteurized dairy products; and try to avoid ticks, rodents, and other disease vectors.

One factor that is known to influence the immune response and that can also be affected by lifestyle and attitudes is stress. Research has shown that the actual number of helper T cells rises and falls inversely with stress; that is, the higher the stress, the lower the T-cell count. Developing effective ways of coping with stress can improve many of the dimensions of wellness.

WW. SEXUALLY TRANSMITTED DISEASES

Acquired immunodeficiency syndrome (AIDS) is a leading cause of death in many parts of the world. Most of the more than 36 million people around the world who are infected with **human immunodeficiency virus (HIV),** the virus that causes AIDS, will likely die within the next 10 years. Although the death rate from AIDS in the United States began to decline in 1996, more than 430,000 of the 750,000 Americans who had been diagnosed with AIDS by 2000 had died from the disease, and it remains a major killer of Americans. Recent public education campaigns have focused primarily on HIV infection, but rates of all the **sexually transmitted diseases (STDs)** continue to be high among Americans. The United States has the highest rate of STDs of any developed nation. Worldwide, nearly 300 million people are affected by STDs each year.

In general, seven different STDs pose major health threats: HIV/AIDS, hepatitis, syphilis, chlamydia, gonorrhea, herpes, and genital warts. These diseases are considered major because they are serious in themselves, cause serious complications if left untreated, and/or pose risks to a fetus or newborn. Pelvic inflammatory disease (PID), a common complication of gonorrhea and chlamydia, also merits discussion as a separate disease.

The bacterial STDs, including chlamydia, gonorrhea, and syphilis, are curable with antibiotics. Unfortunately, previous infection does not confer immunity, so a person can be reinfected despite treatment. The viral STDs—herpes, genital warts, hepatitis, and HIV infection—are not curable with current therapies. Although antiviral drugs and other medications can help target the effects of these STDs, the virus remains in the body and may cause chronic or recurrent infection. A further risk of all STDs is that the associated sores and inflammation allow HIV to pass more easily from one person to another.

HIV Infection and AIDS

HIV infection is one of the most serious and challenging problems facing the United States and the world today. Worldwide, it is estimated that more than 57 million people have been infected since the epidemic began—nearly 1% of the world's population—and that more than 21 million have died. About 10 people are infected every minute, and half of these new infections are in people age 15–24. By 2000, an estimated 650,000–1,000,000 Americans were believed to be living with HIV—about 1 in 160 males and 1 in 800 females over age 12. Although the death rate from AIDS among Americans has declined, new infections are holding steady at about 40,000 per year, meaning the number of Americans living with HIV infection is growing.

What Is HIV Infection? **HIV infection** is a chronic disease that progressively damages the body's immune system, making an otherwise healthy person less able to resist a variety of infections and disorders. Under normal conditions, when a virus or other pathogen enters the body, it is targeted and destroyed by the immune system. But the human immunodeficiency virus (HIV) attacks the

Terms

acquired immunodeficiency syndrome (AIDS) A generally fatal, incurable, sexually transmitted viral disease.

human immunodeficiency virus (HIV) The virus that causes HIV infection and AIDS.

sexually transmitted disease (STD) A disease that can be transmitted by sexual contact; some STDs can also be transmitted by other means.

HIV infection A chronic, progressive disease that damages the immune system.

Since the AIDS epidemic began, nearly 60 million people worldwide have been infected with HIV, and more than 21 million have died. The vast majority of cases—95%—have occurred in developing countries, where heterosexual contact is the primary means of transmission, responsible for 75–85% of all adult infections. In the developed world, HIV is increasingly becoming a disease that disproportionately affects the poor and ethnic minorities, especially women, youth, and children. Worldwide, women are the fastest-growing group of newly infected people. In addition, an estimated 1.4 million children are living with HIV infection and about 13.2 million children are AIDS orphans.

Currently, more than 25 million of those infected with HIV are in Africa, where AIDS has become the leading cause of death and in some countries, 20–35% of adults carry the virus. However, because the epidemic started about 10 years later in Asia than in Africa, experts expect an explosion of new cases in Asia, where already nearly 6 million people are infected. HIV is also spreading rapidly in Eastern Europe, where injection drug use and commercial sex are increasing.

Efforts to combat AIDS are complicated by political, economic, and cultural barriers in many parts of the world. Educa-tion and prevention programs are often hampered by resistance from social and religious institutions and by the taboo on openly discussing sexual issues. Condoms are unfamiliar in many countries, and women in many societies do not have sufficient control over their lives to demand that men use condoms during sex. Prevention approaches that have had success include STD treatment and education, public education campaigns about safer sex, and syringe exchange programs for injection drug users.

In developed nations such as the United States, new drugs are reversing AIDS symptoms and lowering viral levels dramatically for some patients. But these drugs are almost entirely unavailable in the developing world. Until vaccines or a low-cost cure is developed, efforts must continue to focus on widespread educational campaigns and prevention through behavior change.

SOURCES: Joint United Nations Programme on HIV/AIDS (UNAIDS). 2000. *AIDS Epidemic Update: December 2000*. Geneva: UNAIDS/WHO. Centers for Disease Control and Prevention. 2000. World AIDS Day—December 1, 2000. *Morbidity and Mortality Weekly Report* 49(47): 1061.

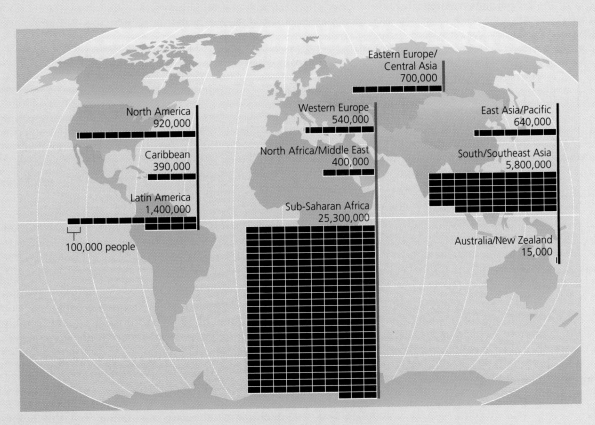

Approximate number of people with HIV/AIDS at the beginning of 2001.

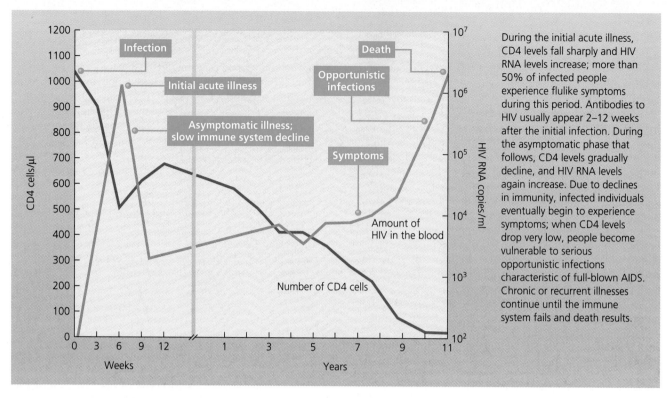

Figure 13-3   The general pattern of untreated HIV infection.   The purple line represents the number of CD4 cells in the blood, a marker for the status of the immune system. The orange line shows the amount of HIV RNA in the blood.   SOURCE: Adapted from Fauci, A. S., et al. 1996. Immunopathogenic mechanisms of HIV infection. *Annals of Internal Medicine* 124: 654–663. Reprinted with permission of the publisher.

immune system itself, invading and taking over **CD4 T cells,** monocytes, and macrophages. HIV enters a human cell and converts its own genetic material, RNA, into DNA. It then inserts this DNA into the chromosomes of the host cell. The viral DNA takes over the CD4 cell, causing it to produce new copies of HIV; it also makes the CD4 cell incapable of performing its immune functions.

The destruction of the immune system is signaled by the loss of CD4 T cells (Figure 13-3). As the number of CD4 cells declines, an infected person may begin to experience mild to moderately severe symptoms. A person is diagnosed with fullblown AIDS when he or she develops one of the conditions defined as a marker for AIDS or when the number of CD4 cells in the blood drops below a certain level (200/μl). People with AIDS are vulnerable to a number of serious, often fatal, secondary, or opportunistic, infections.

Shortly after being infected with HIV, about 50% of people develop flulike symptoms that disappear after a few days or weeks. Once the initial symptoms resolve, most people feel generally well. This asymptomatic (symptom-free) period of HIV infection can last from 2 to 20 years, with an average of 11 years in untreated adults.

During this time the virus is progressively infecting and destroying the cells of the immune system. People infected with HIV can pass the virus to others—even if they have no symptoms and even if they do not know they have been infected.

Transmitting the Virus   HIV lives only within cells and body fluids, not outside the body. It is transmitted by blood and blood products, semen, vaginal and cervical secretions, and breast milk. The HIV infection cannot live in air, in water, or on objects or surfaces such as toilet seats, eating utensils, or telephone handsets. The three main routes of HIV transmission are (1) from specific kinds of sexual contact, (2) from direct exposure to infected blood, and (3) from an HIV-infected woman to her fetus during pregnancy or childbirth or to her infant during breastfeeding.

Of the different types of sexual contact, HIV is more likely to be transmitted by unprotected anal or vaginal intercourse than by other sexual activities. Being the receptive partner during unprotected anal intercourse is the riskiest of all sexual activities. Oral-genital contact carries some risk of transmission, although less than anal or vaginal intercourse. Oral sex is responsible for a small but significant number of cases of HIV transmission. HIV can be transmitted through tiny tears in the fragile lining of the vagina, cervix, penis, anus, and mouth and through direct infection of cells in some of these areas.

The presence of lesions, blisters, or inflammation from other STDs in the genital, anal, or oral areas makes it two to nine times easier for the virus to be passed. In addition, any trauma or irritation of tissues, such as might occur from rough or unwanted intercourse or the overuse of spermicides, increases the risk. The risk of HIV transmission during oral sex increases if a person has poor oral hygiene, has oral sores, or has brushed or flossed just before or after oral sex. During vaginal intercourse, male-to-female transmission is more likely to occur than female-to-male transmission. HIV has been found in preejaculatory fluid, so transmission can occur before ejaculation.

Direct contact with the blood of an infected person is the second major route of HIV transmission. Needles used to inject drugs (including heroin, cocaine, and anabolic steroids) are routinely contaminated by the blood of the user. If needles are shared, small amounts of one person's blood are directly injected into another person's bloodstream. HIV may be transmitted through subcutaneous and intramuscular injection as well, from needles or blades used in acupuncture, tattooing, ritual scarring, and piercing of the earlobes, nose, lip, nipple, navel, or other body part.

HIV has been transmitted in blood and blood products used in the medical treatment of injuries, serious illnesses, and **hemophilia**, resulting in about 14,000 cases of AIDS in the United States. The blood supply in all licensed blood banks and plasma centers in the United States is now screened for HIV. The odds are less than 1 in 650,000 that a unit of HIV-infected donated blood will fail to be detected with today's testing methods, and new genetic tests may further reduce the risk.

The final major route of HIV transmission is mother-to-child, also called *vertical, or perinatal transmission,* which can occur during pregnancy, childbirth, or breast-feeding. Twenty-five to 30% of infants born to untreated HIV-infected mothers are also infected with the virus; treatment, discussed later in the chapter, can dramatically lower this infection rate. Worldwide, about two-thirds of vertical transmission occurs during pregnancy and childbirth and one-third through breast feeding. An estimated 600,000 infants are infected with HIV each year, 90% of them in developing countries.

A person is *not* at risk of getting HIV infection by being in the same classroom, dining room, or even household with someone who is infected. Before this was generally known, many people with HIV infection, including children, were the targets of ostracism, hysteria, and outright violence. Today, it is an acknowledged responsibility of everyone to treat people with HIV infection with respect and compassion, regardless of their age or how they became infected.

Populations of Special Concern for HIV Infection

Among Americans with AIDS, the most common means of exposure to HIV has been sexual activity between men; injection drug use (IDU) and heterosexual contact are the next most common (Figure 13-4). Changes in the sexual behavior of homosexual men and the screening of all donated blood have slowed the rate of infection from these sources, and HIV in the United States is increasingly becoming a disease that disproportionately affects minorities, women, children, and the poor.

The rate of HIV infection is eight times higher in African Americans than it is in whites, and the rate among Hispanics is twice that of whites. African American and Hispanic women account for nearly 80% of new HIV cases among women in the United States. In 2000, about 85% of children reported with AIDS were African American or Hispanic. AIDS incidence and deaths have declined since 1996 among all groups of Americans, but these declines have been smaller among women and minorities compared to other groups. Another group of concern is younger homosexual men; surveys indicate that younger gay and bisexual men are much more likely to engage in unsafe sexual activity than older men.

More than 90% of all cases of HIV infection in children are the result of transmission from infected mothers. In the United States, new treatments to reduce vertical transmission are in use, and the number of new cases of HIV infection in children has declined significantly. The situation worldwide is bleak, however: By 2000 fewer than 1 in 20 children born to HIV-positive women in the United States became infected with HIV; in developing countries, the average was about 1 in 3.

These patterns of HIV infection reflect complex social, economic, and behavioral factors. Reducing the rates of HIV transmission and AIDS death in minorities, women, and other groups at risk will require dealing with the difficult problems of drug abuse, poverty, and discrimination. HIV prevention programs must be tailored to meet the special needs of minority communities.

Symptoms of HIV Infection

Within a few days or weeks of infection with HIV, about half of people will develop flulike symptoms associated with acute HIV infection. Diagnosis of HIV at this very early stage of infection, although uncommon, is extremely beneficial; people who have engaged in behavior that places them at

---

CD4 T cell A type of white blood cell that helps coordinate the activity of the immune system; the primary target for HIV infection. A decrease in the number of these cells correlates with the risk and severity of HIV-related illness.

hemophilia A hereditary blood disease in which blood fails to clot and abnormal bleeding occurs, requiring transfusions of blood products with a specific factor to aid coagulation.

Terms

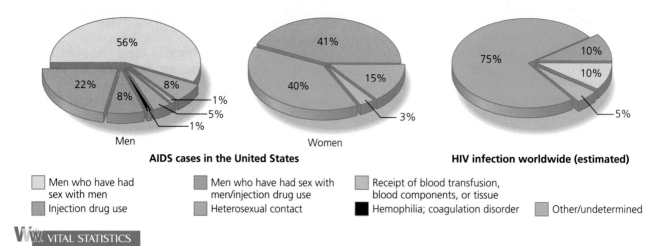

Men

56%

22%

8%

8%

1%

5%

1%

Women

41%

40%

15%

3%

AIDS cases in the United States

75%

10%

10%

5%

HIV infection worldwide (estimated)

Men who have had sex with men

Injection drug use

Men who have had sex with men/injection drug use

Heterosexual contact

Receipt of blood transfusion, blood components, or tissue

Hemophilia; coagulation disorder

Other/undetermined

Figure 13-4   Routes of HIV transmission among adults.   SOURCES: Centers for Disease Control and Prevention. 2000. *HIV/AIDS Surveillance Report* 12(1). Joint United Nations Programme on HIV/AIDS (UNAIDS). 2000. *AIDS Epidemic Update: December 2000.* Geneva: UNAIDS/WHO.

risk for HIV infection and who then experience symptoms should immediately inform their physician of their risk status. Standard tests for HIV will usually be negative in the very early stages of infection, so specialized tests such as the HIV RNA assay, which directly measures the amount of virus in the body, must be used.

Other than the initial flulike symptoms associated with acute HIV infection, most people in the first months or years of HIV infection have few if any symptoms. As the immune system weakens, however, a variety of symptoms can develop—ranging from persistent swollen lymph nodes and night sweats to seizures and memory loss. Because the immune system is weakened, people with HIV infection are highly susceptible to infections, both common and uncommon. The infection most often seen among people with HIV is *Pneumocystis carinii* pneumonia, a protozoal infection. Kaposi's sarcoma, a rare form of cancer, is common in HIV-infected men. Women with HIV infection often have frequent and difficult-to-treat vaginal yeast infections. Cases of tuberculosis (TB) are also increasingly being reported in people with HIV.

Diagnosing HIV Infection and AIDS   Early diagnosis of HIV infection is important to minimize the impact of the disease. The most common tests are **HIV antibody tests,** which consist of an initial test, called an ELISA, and a second, confirmatory test called a Western blot. Not every-

one with HIV infection will test positive on antibody tests, however. Antibodies may not appear in the blood for weeks or months after infection, so people who are newly infected are likely to have a negative antibody test. The infection can be detected with a more expensive test that directly measures the presence of the virus, such as an HIV RNA test.

If a person is diagnosed as **HIV-positive,** the next step is to determine the current severity of the disease. The status of the immune system can be gauged by taking CD4 T-cell measurements every few months. The infection itself can be monitored by tracking the amount of virus in the body (the "viral load") through HIV RNA assay. The CDC's criteria for a diagnosis of AIDS reflect the stage of HIV infection at which a person's immune system becomes dangerously compromised. Since January 1993, a diagnosis of AIDS has been made if a person is HIV-positive and either has developed an infection defined as an AIDS indicator or has a severely damaged immune system (as measured by CD4 T-cell counts).

Treatment   Although there is no known cure for HIV infection, medications can significantly alter the course of the disease and extend life. The drop in the number of U.S. AIDS deaths in recent years is in large part due to the increasing use of combinations of new drugs.

ANTIVIRAL DRUGS AND TREATMENTS FOR OPPORTUNISTIC INFECTIONS   Current antiviral drugs to combat HIV fall into two major categories: reverse transcriptase inhibitors and protease inhibitors. Both types of medications inhibit the ability of the virus to replicate itself. Treatment with a combination of drugs, referred to as *highly active antiretroviral therapy,* or HAART, can reduce HIV in the blood to undetectable levels in some people. However, latent virus is still present in the body, and HIV-infected men on HAART carry potentially transmissible HIV in their se-

Terms

HIV antibody test A blood test to determine whether a person has been infected by HIV; becomes positive within weeks or months of exposure.

HIV-positive A diagnosis resulting from the presence of HIV in the bloodstream; also referred to as *seropositive.*

seroconversion The appearance of antibodies to HIV in the blood of an infected person; usually occurs 1–6 months after infection.

Getting an early diagnosis of HIV infection is more important than ever, but many people with HIV do not know they are infected. You should consider being tested if you have had unprotected sex (vaginal, anal, or oral) with more than one partner or with a partner who was not in a mutually monogamous relationship with you; if you have used or shared needles, syringes, or other paraphernalia for injecting drugs (including steroids); if you received a transfusion of blood or blood products prior to 1985; or if you have been diagnosed with an STD.

Testing Options

If you decide to get an HIV test, either you can visit a physician or health clinic or you can take a home test. A big advantage to having the test performed by a physician or clinician is that you will get one-on-one counseling about the test, your results, and ways to avoid future infection or spreading the disease. The home test is a good alternative for people at low risk who just want to be sure.

Physician or Clinic Testing

Your physician, student health clinic, Planned Parenthood, public health department, or local AIDS association can arrange your HIV test. It usually costs $50–$100, but public clinics often charge little or nothing. The test itself is fairly simple. A sample of blood will be drawn and sent to a laboratory for analysis for the presence of antibodies to HIV. If the first stage of testing, the ELISA test, proves positive, it is followed by a confirmatory test, the Western blot. You'll be asked to phone or come in personally to get your results, which should include appropriate counseling. (Some clinics now also offer "rapid tests" that yield results within 10–30 minutes; positive results must still be confirmed with the standard antibody tests and may require an additional week or two.)

Alternative tests may be used in some circumstances. The Orasure test uses oral fluid, which is collected by placing a treated cotton pad in the mouth for several minutes. Urine tests are also available. Oral fluid and urine tests may be helpful for people who avoid blood tests because of fear of needles. If you are ill and have reason to think your symptoms could be due to acute (very recent) HIV infection, see your physician and request an HIV RNA test.

Before you get an HIV test, be sure you understand what will be done with the results. Results from confidential tests may still become part of your medical record and/or reported (with your name or some other identifier) to state and federal public health agencies. If you decide you want to be tested anonymously—in which case the results will not be reported to anyone but yourself—check with your physician or counselor about how to obtain an anonymous test or use a home test.

Home Testing

Home test kits for HIV are now available; they cost about $40. (Take care to avoid testing kits that are not FDA-approved; many such unapproved kits are being sold over the Internet.) To use a home test, you prick a finger with a supplied lancet, blot a few drops of blood onto blotting paper, and mail it to the company's laboratory. There the sample is tested for HIV by the same methods used for samples collected by physicians. In about a week, you call a toll-free number to find out your results. Anyone testing positive is routed to a trained counselor, who can provide emotional and medical support.

The results of home test kits are completely anonymous. Your blood sample is assigned an identification number, and you never give your name or address. Even if you test positive and receive counseling, your conversation will be anonymous.

Understanding the Results

A negative test result means that no antibodies were found in your sample. However, it usually takes at least a month (and possibly as long as 6 months in some people) after exposure to HIV for antibodies to appear, a process called **seroconversion**. Therefore, an infected person may get a false-negative result. If you think you've been exposed to HIV, get a test immediately; if it's negative but your risk of infection is high, ask about obtaining an HIV RNA assay, which allows very early diagnosis.

A positive result means that you are infected. It is important to seek medical care and counseling immediately. Rapid progress is being made in treating HIV, and treatments are potentially much more successful when begun early.

---

men. In addition to antiviral drugs, most patients with low CD4 T-cell counts also take a variety of antibiotics to help prevent opportunistic infections. A person with advanced HIV infection may need to take 20 or more pills every day.

Researchers are looking for different ways to attack HIV. People who carry a particular genetic mutation have been found to be resistant to infection, and scientists hope to develop a drug that will mimic the effect of this mutation. Another new approach to treatment is *structured intermittent therapy,* in which HAART is used for a

period of time, discontinued, and then restarted. Researchers hope that drug-free intervals will help stimulate the patient's own immune response against HIV.

HIV AND PREGNANCY   Early-stage HIV infection does not appear to significantly affect a woman's chance of becoming pregnant. Without treatment, 25–30% of infants born to HIV-infected women are themselves infected with the virus. But treatment with antiviral drugs during pregnancy, labor, and early infancy has been shown to decrease a child's chance of contracting HIV by as much as

90%. Cesarean delivery can lower the risk of infection in women who have high blood levels of HIV; and HIV-infected women are usually advised not to breastfeed because this has been shown to transmit HIV.

TREATMENT CHALLENGES   The cost of treatment for HIV infection—more than $18,000 per year in the United States—is much too high for the vast majority of people around the world who are infected with HIV. For those who can afford the drugs, toxicity is a key concern. Long-term use of HAART can cause a number of serious side effects, and the treatment guidelines issued by the National Institutes of Health in 2001 recommend that asymptomatic patients hold off on treatment until they are at a more advanced stage of the disease. Even for people who have access to the drugs and can tolerate the side effects, treatment is difficult and involves taking dozens of pills every day at precise times. The medications are more effective for some people than others, and they do not eliminate the virus from the body. Even for those people who are treated, it is unclear to what degree their damaged immune systems can rebound from the effects of long-term HIV infection.

The best hope for preventing the spread of HIV worldwide rests with the development of a safe, effective, and inexpensive vaccine. Many different approaches to the development of an AIDS vaccine are currently under investigation, and human trials have begun on several vaccines. However, no vaccine is likely to be ready for widespread use within the next 5 years.

Prevention   Although AIDS is currently incurable, it is preventable. You can protect yourself by avoiding behaviors that may bring you into contact with HIV. This means making careful choices about sexual activity and not sharing needles if you inject drugs.

MAKE CAREFUL CHOICES ABOUT SEXUAL ACTIVITY   In a sexual relationship, the current and past behaviors of you and your partner determine the amount of risk involved. If you are uninfected and in a mutually monogamous relationship with another uninfected person, you are not at risk for HIV. Of course, it is often hard to know for sure whether your partner is completely faithful and is truly uninfected. Having a series of monogamous relationships is not a safe prevention strategy.

For anyone not involved in a long-term, mutually monogamous relationship, abstinence from any sexual activity that involves the exchange of body fluids is the only sure way to prevent HIV infection. Safer sex includes many activities that carry virtually no risk of HIV infection, like hugging, massaging, closed-lip kissing, rubbing clothed bodies together, kissing your partner's skin, and mutual masturbation.

Anal and vaginal intercourse are the sexual activities associated with the highest risk of HIV infection. If you have intercourse, always use a latex condom. Condoms are not perfect, and they do not provide risk-free sex; however, used properly, a latex condom provides a high level of protection against HIV. Condoms should also be worn during oral sex. Some experts also suggest the use of latex squares and dental dams, rubber devices that can be used as barriers during oral-genital or oral-anal sexual contact.

Limiting the number of partners you have—particularly those who have engaged in risky sexual behaviors in the past—can also lower your risk of exposure to HIV. Take the time to talk with a potential new partner about HIV and safer sex. Talking about sex may seem embarrassing and uncomfortable, but good communication is critical for your health. Asking a partner about past sexual experiences can also be helpful, but you cannot always depend on that information.

Removing alcohol and other drugs from sexual activity is another crucial component of safer sex. The use of alcohol and mood-altering drugs may lower inhibitions and affect judgment, making you more likely to engage in unsafe sex. The use of drugs is also associated with sexual activity with multiple partners.

Surveys of college students indicate that the majority of students are not engaging in safer sex. Although most students know that condom use can protect against HIV infection, this knowledge is often not translated into action. Many students also report a willingness to lie about past sexual activity in order to obtain sex. In addition, many students believe their risk of contracting HIV depends on "who they are" rather than on their sexual behavior. These attitudes and behaviors place college students at continued high risk for contracting HIV.

DON'T SHARE DRUG NEEDLES   People who inject any drug should avoid sharing needles, syringes, or anything that might have blood on it. Needles can be decontaminated with a solution of bleach and water, but it is not a foolproof procedure and HIV can survive in a syringe for a month or longer. (Boiling needles and syringes does not necessarily destroy HIV either.) If you are an injection drug user, your best protection against HIV is to obtain treatment and refrain from using drugs.

COMMUNICATE!   How can you find out whether your partner could expose you to a sexually transmitted disease? The simplest and most direct way is to ask. You can say something like, "It seems as if we're getting to a point in our relationship where we should talk about STDs and safer sex." If your partner is agreeable, you might continue, "I'm wondering whether you've had other partners, and if you have, whether any of them ever had an STD, or if you've ever had an STD." Remember that your partner has a right to know your health status as well, so be prepared to answer his or her questions.

For those who don't have a long-term monogamous relationship with an uninfected partner, abstinence is the only truly safe option. Individuals should remember that it's OK to say no to sex and drugs.

Safer sexual activities that allow close person-to-person contact with almost no risk of contracting STDs or HIV include fantasy, hugging, massage, rubbing clothed bodies together, self-stimulation by both partners, and kissing with lips closed.

If you choose to be sexually active, talk with potential partners about HIV, safer sex, and the use of condoms before you begin a sexual relationship. The following behaviors will help lower your risk of exposure to HIV during sexual activities:

- Limit the number of partners. Avoid sexual contact with people who have HIV or an STD or who have engaged in risky behaviors in the past, including unprotected sex and injection drug use.

- Use latex condoms during every act of intercourse and oral sex. Even if your partner claims to have been tested for HIV and STDs, there is no guarantee that he or she is uninfected. Many STDs are not easy to diagnose in their asymptomatic stage, which can last for years; and asymptomatic individuals can still infect others. No matter what your partner says, you have no guarantee that you will not contract an STD during any sexual encounter. If you choose to have intercourse, your best protection is to *always* use a condom. They do not provide perfect protection, but they greatly reduce your risk of contracting an infection.

- Use condoms properly to obtain maximum protection (refer to the instructions for condom use in Chapter 6). Use a water-based lubricant; don't use oil-based lubricants such as petroleum jelly or baby oil or any vaginal product containing mineral or vegetable oil. Unroll condoms gently to avoid tearing them, and smooth out any air bubbles.

- Avoid sexual contact that could cause cuts or tears in the skin or tissue. Using extra lubricant (water-based) can help prevent damage to delicate tissues.

- Get periodic screening tests for STDs and HIV, and get prompt treatment for any STDs you contract. Young women need yearly pelvic exams and Pap tests.

- Get vaccinated for hepatitis B.

- Don't drink or use drugs in sexual situations. Mood-altering drugs can affect your judgment and make you more likely to engage in risky behaviors.

If you inject drugs of any kind, don't share needles, syringes, or anything that might have blood on it. If your community has a syringe exchange program, use it. Seek treatment; stop using injectable drugs.

If you are at risk for HIV infection, don't donate blood, sperm, or body organs. Don't have unprotected sex or share needles or syringes. Get tested for HIV soon, and get treated.

Chlamydia

Chlamydia trachomatis causes **chlamydia,** the most prevalent bacterial STD in the United States. About 3 million new cases occur each year. An estimated 5–10% of all sexually active American women are infected with chlamydia; rates among men are similar. The highest rates of infection occur in single people between ages 18 and 24. *C. trachomatis* can be transmitted by oral sex as well as by other forms of sexual intercourse.

Both men and women are susceptible to chlamydia, but, as with most STDs, women bear the greater burden because of possible complications and consequences of the disease. If left untreated, chlamydia can lead to pelvic inflammatory disease (PID), a serious infection involving the oviducts (fallopian tubes) and uterus that can lead to infertility. Chlamydia also greatly increases a woman's risk for ectopic (tubal) pregnancy. Because rates of infection are high and most women with chlamydia have no symptoms, many physicians screen sexually active women at the time of their routine pelvic exam; for young sexually active women, some experts recommend screening every 6 months.

Chlamydia can also lead to infertility in men, although not as often as in women. In men under age 35, chla-mydia is the most common cause of *epididymitis,* inflammation of the sperm-carrying ducts. And up to half of all cases of *urethritis,* inflammation of the urethra, in men are caused by chlamydia. Despite these statistics, many infected men have no symptoms.

Infants of infected mothers can acquire the infection during delivery. Every year, over 150,000 newborns suffer from eye infections and pneumonia as a result of untreated maternal chlamydial infections.

Symptoms Most people experience few or no chlamydia symptoms, increasing the likelihood that they will inadvertently spread the infection to their partners. In men, symptoms include painful urination, a slight watery discharge from the penis, and sometimes pain around the testicles. Women may notice increased vaginal discharge, burning with urination, pain or bleeding with intercourse, and lower abdominal pain.

> **chlamydia** An STD transmitted by the pathogenic bacterium *Chlamydia trachomatis.*

Terms

Diagnosis and Treatment   Chlamydia is typically diagnosed through laboratory tests on a urine sample or a small amount of fluid from the urethra or cervix. Once chlamydia has been diagnosed, the infected person and his or her partner(s) are given antibiotics—usually doxycycline, erythromycin, or a newer drug, azithromycin, which can cure infection in one dose.

Gonorrhea

In the United States, an estimated 700,000 new cases of **gonorrhea** are diagnosed every year. The highest incidence is among 15–24-year-olds. Like chlamydia, untreated gonorrhea can cause PID in women and urethritis and epididymitis in men. It can also cause arthritis, rashes, and eye infections, and it occasionally involves internal organs. A woman who is infected during pregnancy is at risk for preterm delivery and for having a baby with life-threatening gonorrheal infection of the blood or joints. An infant passing through the birth canal of an infected mother may contract an infection in the eyes that can cause blindness if not treated. Gonorrhea is caused by the bacterium *Neisseria gonorrhoeae,* which flourishes in mucous membranes.

Symptoms   In males, the incubation period for gonorrhea is brief, generally 2–7 days. The first symptoms are due to urethritis, which causes urinary discomfort and a thick, yellowish white or yellowish green discharge from the penis. The lips of the urethral opening may become inflamed and swollen. In some cases, the lymph glands in the groin become enlarged and swollen. Up to half of males have very minor symptoms or none at all.

Most females with gonorrhea are asymptomatic. Those who do have symptoms often experience pain with urination, increased vaginal discharge, and severe menstrual cramps. Up to 40% of women with untreated gonorrhea develop PID. Women may also develop painful abscesses in the Bartholin's glands, a pair of glands located on either side of the opening of the vagina.

Gonorrhea can also infect the throat or rectum of people who engage in oral or anal sex. Gonorrhea symptoms in the throat may be a sore throat or pus on the tonsils, and those in the rectum may be pus or blood in the feces or rectal pain and itching.

Diagnosis and Treatment   Several tests—gram stain, detection of bacterial genes or DNA, or culture—may be performed; depending on the test, samples of urine or cervical, urethral, throat, or rectal fluids may be collected. A variety of new and relatively expensive antibiotics are usually effective in curing gonorrhea. Older, less expensive antibiotics such as penicillin and tetracycline are not currently recommended for treating gonorrhea because of widespread drug resistance.

Pelvic Inflammatory Disease

A major complication in 10–40% of women who have been infected with either gonorrhea or chlamydia and have not received adequate treatment is **pelvic inflammatory disease (PID).** PID occurs when the initial infection with gonorrhea and/or chlamydia travels upward, often along with other bacteria, beyond the cervix into the uterus, oviducts, ovaries, and pelvic cavity. PID is often serious enough to require hospitalization and sometimes surgery. Even if the disease is treated successfully, about 25% of affected women will have long-term problems such as a continuing susceptibility to infection, ectopic pregnancy, infertility, and chronic pelvic pain. PID is the leading cause of infertility in young women. Infertility occurs in 8% of women after one episode of PID, 20% after two episodes, and 40% after three episodes.

Young women under age 25 are much more likely to develop PID than older women. As with all STDs, the more sex partners a woman has had, the greater her risk of PID. Smokers have twice the risk of PID as nonsmokers. Using IUDs for contraception and vaginal douching also increases the risk of PID. In general, women should avoid douching because this practice may actually force bacteria up through the cervix and into the uterus and oviducts. Research into whether the use of other contraceptives protects against PID has yielded mixed results; OC use may reduce the severity of PID symptoms.

Symptoms   Symptoms of PID vary greatly. Some women, especially those with PID from chlamydia, may be asymptomatic; others may feel very ill with abdominal pain, fever, chills, nausea, and vomiting. Early symptoms are essentially the same as those described earlier for chlamydia and gonorrhea. Symptoms often begin or worsen during or soon after a woman's menstrual period. Many women have abnormal vaginal bleeding—either bleeding between periods or heavy and painful menstrual bleeding.

Diagnosis and Treatment   Diagnosis of PID is made on the basis of symptoms, physical examination, ultrasound, and laboratory tests. Laparoscopy may be used to confirm

Terms

gonorrhea A sexually transmitted bacterial infection that usually affects mucous membranes.

pelvic inflammatory disease (PID) An infection that progresses from the vagina and cervix to the uterus, oviducts, and pelvic cavity.

genital warts A sexually transmitted viral infection characterized by growths on the genitals; also called *genital HPV infection.*

human papillomavirus (HPV) The pathogen that causes human warts, including genital warts.

genital herpes A sexually transmitted infection caused by the herpes simplex virus.

the diagnosis and obtain material for cultures. Treatment of PID should begin as quickly as possible to minimize damage to the reproductive organs. Antibiotics are usually started immediately; in severe cases, the woman may be hospitalized and antibiotics given intravenously. It is especially important that an infected woman's partners be treated. As many as 60% of the male contacts of women with PID are infected but asymptomatic.

Genital Warts

Genital warts, also known as condyloma, are caused by infection with **human papillomavirus (HPV).** The CDC estimates that more than 20 million people in the United States have this persistent viral infection, and another 5.5 million people are infected each year. Approximately 15% of Americans age 15–49 years have HPV infection and are contagious. The vast majority of these people have no visible warts and have no idea that they are infected. Rates are even higher among college students.

A precancerous condition known as cervical dysplasia often occurs among women with genital HPV infection. If untreated, women with this condition sometimes develop cervical cancer. Recent evidence suggests that HPV infection also speeds the progression of HIV/AIDS.

Human papillomaviruses cause many types of human warts. There are more than 100 different strains of HPV, and different strains infect specific locations. More than 20 types are likely to cause genital infections, and 5 of these are often implicated in cervical cancer; other strains are linked to anal, penile, and other genital cancers.

Genital HPV infection is quite contagious. Condoms and other barrier methods can help prevent the transmission of HPV, but HPV infection frequently occurs in areas where condoms are not fully protective. These areas are the labia in women, the base of the penis and the scrotum in men, and around the anus in both men and women.

Symptoms   Genital warts are often dry, painless growths, rough in texture and gray or pink in color. They can be flat or raised, and they vary in size. Early on, genital warts look like small, barely noticeable bumps. Untreated warts can grow together to form a cauliflowerlike mass. In males, they appear on the penis and often involve the urethra, appearing first at the opening and then spreading inside. The growths may cause irritation and bleeding, leading to painful urination and a urethral discharge. Warts may also appear around the anus or within the rectum. In women, warts may appear on the labia or vulva and may spread to the perineum, the area between the vagina and the rectum. If warts occur only on the cervix, the woman will generally have no symptoms or awareness that she has HPV.

The incubation period ranges from 1 month to 2 years from the time of contact. People can be infected with the virus and be capable of transmitting it to their sex partners without having any symptoms at all. The vast major-

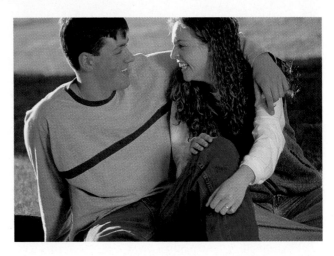

By taking a responsible attitude toward STDs, people show respect and concern for themselves and their partners. This couple's plans for the future could be seriously disrupted if one of them contracted an STD like gonorrhea or chlamydia. Either of these diseases, if untreated, could result in PID, the leading cause of infertility in young women.

ity of people with HPV infection have no visible warts or symptoms of any kind.

Diagnosis and Treatment   Genital warts are usually diagnosed based on the appearance of the lesions. Sometimes examination with a special magnifying instrument or biopsy is done to evaluate suspicious lesions. Frequently, HPV infection of the cervix is detected on routine Pap tests.

Treatment of genital warts focuses on reducing the number and size of warts. The currently available treatments do not eradicate HPV infection. Warts may be removed by cryosurgery (freezing), electrocautery (burning), or laser surgery. Direct applications of podophyllin or other cytotoxic acids may be used. Two treatments may be applied by patients at home: imiquimod, an immune system enhancer, and podofilox, a drug that destroys warts.

HPV infection often resolves on its own after an number of months, although this is unpredictable. Even after treatment and the disapearance of visible warts, the individual may continue to carry HPV in healthy-looking tissue and can probably still infect others. Anyone who has ever had HPV should inform all partners. Condoms should be used, even though they do not provide total protection. Because of the relationship between HPV and cervical cancer, women who have had genital warts should have Pap tests at least every 12 months.

Genital Herpes

Genital herpes affects about 45 million people in the United States. Two types of herpes simplex viruses, HSV-1 and HSV-2, cause genital herpes and oral-labial herpes

For decades, patients and health care workers alike have suspected that stress and genital herpes outbreaks are related. Research studies that have investigated this potential link have yielded mixed results. There is no doubt that having genital herpes is a considerable stress to many people, but does stress itself make a person with herpes infection more likely to have an outbreak? A recent study of women with genital herpes found that persistent stressors (those lasting more than a week) and persistent high levels of anxiety were associated with increased genital herpes outbreaks. Short-term stress, mood changes, and brief negative life experiences did not influence the rate of herpes outbreaks.

Why should persistent stress make a person with genital herpes have more frequent outbreaks? No one knows for sure, but experts suspect that stress has a negative impact on the immune system. Studies have shown that cell-mediated immune function and antibody levels may drop in response to psychological stress. Perhaps herpesviruses that are usually dormant in nervous system tissue become activated when immune function declines due to stress.

The next logical step is to investigate whether stress-reduction techniques such as meditation or exercise result in reduced rates of herpes outbreaks. Until such research becomes available, it makes sense for people who suffer recurrent genital herpes outbreaks to do what they can to reduce stress, especially long-term stress and anxiety (see Chapter 2). If you have herpes, joining a support group may help reduce your stress and improve your ability to cope with this chronic disease (see For More Information at the end of the chapter). If you have more than six outbreaks a year, consider taking an antiviral medication. Keep in mind that regardless of stress level, genital herpes outbreaks naturally tend to become less and less frequent over time. Knowing that your outbreaks are likely to diminish can, in and of itself, help reduce your feelings of stress.

SOURCE: Rein, M. 2000. Stress and genital herpes recurrences in women: Commentary. *Journal of the American Medical Association* 283(11): 1394.

(cold sores). Genital herpes is usually caused by HSV-2, and oral-labial herpes is usually caused by HSV-1, although both virus types can cause either genital or oral-labial lesions. HSV can also cause rectal lesions, usually transmitted through anal sex.

HSV-1 infection is so common that 50–80% of U.S. adults have antibodies to HSV-1 (indicating previous exposure to the virus); most were exposed to HSV-1 during childhood. HSV-2 infection usually occurs between ages 18 and 25. Approximately 22% of adults—nearly one in four—have antibodies to HSV-2; about a million are infected each year.

HSV-2 is almost always sexually transmitted. It is theoretically possible, but much less common, to become infected through contaminated clothing, towels, or other objects. The infection is more easily transmitted when people have active sores, but HSV-2 can be transmitted to a sex partner even when no lesions are present. Because HSV is asymptomatic in 80–90% of people, the infection is often acquired from a person who has no awareness that he or she is infected. If you have ever had an outbreak of genital herpes, you must always consider yourself contagious and inform your partners. Avoid intimate contact when any sores are present, and use condoms during all sexual contact.

Newborns can occasionally be infected with HSV, usually during passage through the birth canal of an infected mother or due to HSV infection acquired by the mother during the third trimester of pregnancy. Without treatment, 65% of newborns with HSV will die, and most who survive will have some degree of brain damage. The risk of mother-to-child HSV transmission during pregnancy and delivery is low (less than 1%) in women with long-standing herpes infection. However, a woman who acquires the infection during pregnancy, especially in the third trimester, has a much higher risk of transmitting the infection to her infant. Infected pregnant women sometimes deliver by cesarean section if active lesions are present at the time of delivery. Fortunately, most babies born to mothers with a history of genital herpes do not acquire the infection, and most women are able to have normal vaginal deliveries.

Symptoms   Up to 90% of people who are infected with HSV have no symptoms. Those that do develop symptoms often first notice them within 2–20 days of having sex with an infected partner. (However, it is not unusual for the first outbreak to occur months or even years after initial exposure.) The first episode of genital herpes frequently causes flulike symptoms in addition to genital lesions. The lesions usually heal within 3 weeks, but the virus remains alive in an inactive state within nerve cells. A new outbreak of herpes can occur at any time. On average, newly diagnosed people will experience 5–8 outbreaks per year, with a decrease in the frequency of outbreaks over time. Recurrent episodes are usually less severe than the initial one, with fewer and less painful sores that heal more quickly. Outbreaks can be triggered by stress, illness, fatigue, sun exposure, sexual intercourse, and menstruation.

Diagnosis and Treatment   Genital herpes is often diagnosed on the basis of symptoms. A new blood test that can determine if a person is infected with HSV-1 or HSV-

2 is now available and may potentially alert many asymptomatic people to the fact that they are infected.

There is no cure for herpes. Once infected, a person carries the virus for life. Antiviral drugs such as acyclovir can be taken at the beginning of an outbreak to shorten the severity and duration of symptoms. People who have frequent outbreaks, more than six per year, can take acyclovir or other similar drugs on a daily basis to suppress outbreaks. Support groups are available to help people learn to cope with herpes.

Hepatitis B

Hepatitis (inflammation of the liver) can cause serious and sometimes permanent damage to the liver, which can result in death in severe cases. One of the many types of hepatitis is caused by hepatitis B virus (HBV). HBV is somewhat similar to HIV; it is found in most body fluids, and it can be transmitted sexually, by injection drug use, and during pregnancy and delivery. However, HBV is much more contagious than HIV, and it can also be spread through nonsexual close contact. Hepatitis B is a potentially fatal disease with no cure, but fortunately there is an effective vaccine. Vaccination is recommended for everyone under age 19 and for all adults at increased risk for hepatitis B.

Transmission HBV is found in all body fluids, including blood and blood products, semen, saliva, urine, and vaginal secretions. It is easily transmitted through any sexual activity that involves the exchange of body fluids, the use of contaminated needles, and any blood-to-blood contact, including the use of contaminated razor blades, toothbrushes, and eating utensils. The primary risk factors for acquiring HBV are sexual exposure and injection drug use; having multiple partners greatly increases risk. A pregnant woman can transmit HBV to her unborn child during pregnancy or delivery.

Symptoms Many people infected with HBV never develop symptoms; they have what are known as "silent" infections. Mild cases of hepatitis cause flulike symptoms; as the illness progresses, there may be nausea, vomiting, dark-colored urine, abdominal pain, and jaundice.

People with hepatitis B sometimes recover completely, but they can also become chronic carriers of the virus, capable of infecting others for the rest of their lives. Some chronic carriers remain asymptomatic, while others develop chronic liver disease. Chronic hepatitis can cause cirrhosis of the liver, liver failure, and a deadly form of liver cancer. Hepatitis kills some 6000 Americans each year; worldwide, the annual death toll exceeds 700,000.

Diagnosis and Treatment Blood tests can be used to diagnose hepatitis through analysis of liver function and detection of the specific organism causing the infection.

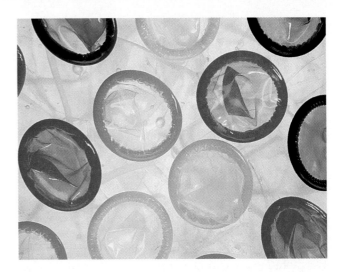

The use of condoms declined as more advanced methods of contraception, such as birth control pills and IUDs, became available. But condoms are once again gaining in popularity because of the protection they provide against STDs.

There is no cure for hepatitis B and no specific treatment for acute infections; antiviral drugs may be used for cases of chronic HBV infection. For people exposed to HBV, treatment with hepatitis B immunoglobulin can provide protection against the virus.

Prevention Preventive measures for hepatitis B are similar to those for HIV infection: Avoid sexual contact that involves sharing body fluids, including saliva; use condoms during sexual intercourse; and don't share needles. If you choose to have tattooing or body piercing done, make sure all needles and equipment are sterile. The vaccine for hepatitis B is safe and highly effective.

Syphilis

Syphilis, a disease that once caused death and disability for millions, can now be effectively treated with antibiotics. Each year, there are about 7000–10,000 new cases of early syphilis in the United States, and about 70,000 people are diagnosed at all stages of the disease. The number of new cases hit an all-time low in 1999, and most were clustered in a few counties in the south and Northeast. Some experts feel that aggressive public health measures could eliminate syphilis in the United States.

Syphilis is caused by *Treponema pallidum*, a thin, corkscrew-shaped bacterium. The disease is usually acquired through sexual contact, although infected pregnant women

hepatitis Inflammation of the liver, which can be caused by infection, drugs, or toxins; some forms of infectious hepatitis can be transmitted sexually.

syphilis A sexually transmitted bacterial infection caused by the spirochete *Treponema pallidum*.

can transmit it to the fetus. The pathogen passes through any break or opening in the skin or mucous membranes and can be transmitted by kissing, vaginal or anal intercourse, or oral-genital contact.

Symptoms Syphilis progresses through several stages. *Primary syphilis* is characterized by an ulcer called a **chancre** that appears within, 10–90 days after exposure. Chancres contain large numbers of bacteria and make the disease highly contagious when present; they are often painless and typically heal on their own within a few weeks. If the disease is not treated during the primary stage, about a third of infected individuals progress to chronic stages of infections.

Secondary syphilis is usually marked by mild, flulike symptoms and a skin rash that appears 3–6 weeks after the chancre. The rash may cover the entire body or only a few areas, but the palms of the hands and soles of the feet are usually involved. Areas of skin affected by the rash are highly contagious but usually heal within several weeks or months. If the disease remains untreated, the symptoms of secondary syphilis may recur over a period of several years. In about a third of cases of untreated secondary syphilis, the individual develops *late,* or *tertiary, syphilis.* Late syphilis can damage many organs of the body, possibly causing severe dementia, cardiovascular damage, blindness, and death.

In infected pregnant women, the syphilis bacterium can cross the placenta. If the mother is not treated, the probable result is stillbirth, prematurity, or congenital deformity. In many cases, the infant is also born infected (*congenital syphilis*) and requires treatment.

Diagnosis and Treatment Syphilis is diagnosed by examination of infected tissues and with blood tests. All stages can be treated with antibiotics, but damage from late syphilis can be permanent.

OTHER STDS

Although less serious than the diseases already described, a few other diseases are transmitted sexually or linked to sexual activity. They include trichomoniasis, bacterial vaginosis, chancroid, pubic lice, and scabies.

Trichomoniasis, often called "trich," is a common STD, with about 5 million new cases per year. The single-celled organism that causes trich, *Trichomonas vaginalis,* thrives in warm, moist conditions, making women particularly susceptible to these infections in the vagina. Women who become symptomatic with trich develop a greenish, foul-smelling vaginal discharge and severe itching and irritation of the vagina and vulva. Treatment with metronidazole (Flagyl) is important because studies suggest that trich may increase the risk of HIV transmission and, in pregnant women, premature delivery.

Bacterial vaginosis (BV) is the most common cause of abnormal vaginal discharge in women of reproductive age. BV involves a shift in the makeup of the bacteria that normally inhabit the vagina: Instead of *Lactobacillus* being most numerous, there is an overgrowth of anaerobic microorganisms and bacteria such as *Gardnerella vaginalis.* BV is clearly associated with sexual activity, but research on the degree to which BV is sexually transmitted is ongoing. Recent research suggests that a sexually transmitted virus that infects and kills *Lactobacillus* may be the underlying cause of BV.

Symptoms of BV include a vaginal discharge with a fishlike odor and, in some cases, vaginal irritation; many women with BV have no symptoms. Some studies have shown an association between BV and increased risk of PID, HIV transmission, infection following childbirth or gynecological surgery (including abortion), and in pregnant women, premature delivery. The CDC recommends that any pregnant woman who has symptoms of BV or who is at risk for premature delivery be screened and, if necessary, treated for BV with antibiotics.

Chancroid is a sexually transmitted bacterial infection caused by *Haemophilus ducreyi.* Prevalent in some parts of the world, chancroid is relatively uncommon in the United States, although there are periodic outbreaks. The infection is characterized by painful open sores in the genital area that may resemble the sores associated with herpes or syphilis. Chancroid is treated with antibiotics.

Pubic lice, commonly known as "crabs," and scabies are highly contagious parasitic infections. Treatment is generally easy, although lice infestation may require repeated applications of medication.

WHAT YOU CAN DO ABOUT STDS

You can take responsibility for your health and help reduce the incidence of STDs in three major areas: education, diagnosis and treatment, and prevention.

Education

Education efforts targeted at increasing public awareness about AIDS through the media have included public service announcements, dramatic presentations, and support from well-known public figures. Colleges offer courses in human sexuality. Free pamphlets and other literature are available from public health departments, health clinics, physicians' offices, student health centers, and Planned Parenthood; and easy-to-understand books are available in libraries and

Terms   **chancre** The sore produced by syphilis in its earliest stage.

bookstores. Several national hotlines have been set up to provide free, confidential information and referral services to callers anywhere in the country.

Although information about STDs is widely disseminated, learning about STDs is still up to every person individually. You must assume responsibility for learning about the causes and nature of STDs and their potential effects on you, the children you may have, and others with whom you have sexual relationships.

Diagnosis and Treatment

Early diagnosis and treatment of STDs can help you and your sex partner(s) avoid unnecessary complications and help prevent the spread of STDs. If you are sexually active, be alert for any sign or symptom of disease, such as a rash, a discharge, sores, or unusual pain, and don't hesitate to have a professional examination if you notice such a symptom. Be alert for these signs or symptoms in your partner too, and don't hesitate to question him or her if you notice something unusual.

Remember that almost all STDs—including HIV infection—can be asymptomatic for long periods of time. Sexually active young women should have pelvic exams and Pap tests at least once a year with chlamydia and gonorrhea screening in most cases. Sexually active men, especially if they have had more than one partner, should receive periodic STD and HIV screening. If you have a risky sexual encounter, see a physician as soon as possible.

Testing for STDs is done through private physicians, public health clinics, community health agencies, and most student health services. If you are diagnosed as having an STD, you should begin treatment as quickly as possible. Inform your partner(s), and avoid any sexual activity until your treatment is complete and testing indicates that you are cured. If your partner tells you that he or she has contracted an STD, get tested immediately, even if you don't have any symptoms. Asymptomatic partners are often treated to ensure that an infection will not spread or recur.

Telling a partner that you have exposed him or her to an STD isn't easy. Despite the awkwardness and difficulty, it is crucial that your sex partner or partners be informed and urged to seek testing and/or treatment as quickly as possible. In asymptomatic cases, the only way infected people can find out they have a disease is by being told they need to be tested. Uninformed partners can go on to spread the disease, contributing to anguish for others as well as spiraling public health problems. The responsibility of informing partners is an ethical task too important to shirk.

With the exception of AIDS treatments, treatments for STDs are safe and generally inexpensive. If you are being treated, follow instructions carefully and complete all the medication as prescribed. Don't stop taking the medication just because you feel better or your symptoms have disappeared, and don't give any of your medication to your partner or to anyone else. Being cured of an STD does not mean that you will not get it again, and exposure does not confer lasting immunity, nor does it prevent you from getting any other STD.

> **COMMUNICATE!** Talking with your health care provider is a critical step in protecting yourself from STDs and their potentially lasting effects. Don't wait for your provider to bring up the topic; if you have concerns or questions, it's important to ask, even if you feel embarrassed or uncomfortable. For example, "My girlfriend thinks she may have genital warts. I'd like to be examined for warts and other STDs," or "I have a new sexual partner who thinks he may have been exposed to herpes in the past. Should I be checked for herpes?" Make sure you understand what your provider tells you about your health status and any treatments prescribed for you. If there are medical terms you don't understand, ask for clarification; you have the right to fully understand issues related to your health.

Prevention

The only sure way to avoid exposure to STDs is to abstain from sexual activity. But if you do choose to be sexually active, the key is to think about prevention *before* you have a sexual encounter or find yourself in the "heat of the moment." Remember, you can become infected with an STD from just one unprotected encounter.

All your good intentions are likely to fly out the window if you enter into a sexual situation when you are intoxicated. If you or your partner (or both of you) is drunk, you are likely to be less cautious about sex than you would be if you were sober. Many people use alcohol and drugs as a way to deal with their anxiety in social and sexual situations. However, being intoxicated leaves you vulnerable to sexual assault and greatly increases your risk of acquiring a serious STD.

Plan ahead for safer sex. Find out about your partner's sexual history and practices. Be honest, and ask your partner to do the same, but don't stake your health and life on assumptions about your partner's honesty. Even if your partner's past seems low-risk, still insist on using a condom every time you have sex. Many honest people are simply unaware that they have an STD.

Aside from abstinence, the next most effective approach to preventing STDs is having sex only with one mutually monogamous uninfected partner. If you are sexually active, use a condom during every act of intercourse to reduce your risk of contracting a disease. Although not foolproof, a properly used condom provides an effective barrier against pathogens, including HIV. A disease can be transmitted if there is contact with an infected area that isn't protected by the condom, however.

The only sure way to prevent STDs, including HIV infection, is to abstain from sexual activity. If you choose to be sexually active, you should do everything possible to protect yourself from STDs. This includes good communication with your sex partner(s).

The time to talk about safer sex is before you begin a sexual relationship. However, even if you've been having unprotected sex with your partner, it is still worth it to start practicing safer sex now. If you're nervous about initiating a conversation about safer sex, rehearse what you will say first. Practice in front of a mirror or with a friend.

There are many ways to bring up the subject of safer sex and condom use with your partner. Be honest about your concerns and stress that protection against STDs means that you care about yourself and your partner. Here are a few suggestions:

- "I heard on the news that more and more people are buying and using condoms. I think it shows that people are being more responsible about sex. What do you think?"

- "I'm worried about the diseases we can get from having sex because so many don't have symptoms. I want to protect both of us by using condoms whenever we have sex."

- "I've been thinking about making love with you. But first we need to talk about how to have safer sex and be protected."

You may find that your partner shares your concerns and also wants to use condoms. He or she may be happy and relieved that you have brought up the subject of safer sex. However, if he or she resists the idea of using condoms, you may need to negotiate. Stress that you both deserve to be protected and that sex will be more enjoyable when you aren't worrying about STDs (see the suggestions to the right). If you and your partner haven't used condoms before, buy some and familiarize yourselves with how to use them. Once you feel more comfortable handling condoms, you'll be able to use them correctly and incorporate them into your sexual activity in fun ways.

If your partner still won't agree to use condoms, think carefully about whether you want to have a sexual relationship with him or her. Safer sex is part of a responsible, caring sexual relationship, and it's smart to say "no" to a partner who won't use a condom. It's up to you to protect yourself.

If your partner says . . .	Try saying . . .
"They're not romantic."	"Worrying about AIDS isn't romantic, and with condoms we won't have to worry." OR "If we put one on together, a condom could be fun."
"You don't trust me."	"I do trust you, but how can I trust your former partners or mine?" OR "It's important to me that we're both protected."
"I don't have any diseases. I've been tested."	"I'm glad you've been tested, but tests aren't foolproof for all diseases. To be safe, I always use condoms."
"I forgot to bring a condom. But it's OK to skip it just this once."	"I'd really like to make love with you, but I never have sex without a condom. Let's go get some."
"I don't like the way they feel."	"They might feel different, but let's try." OR "Sex won't feel good if we're worrying about diseases."
"I don't use condoms."	"I use condoms every time." OR "I don't have sex without condoms."
"But I love you."	"Being in love can't protect us from diseases." OR "I love you, too. We still need to use condoms."
"But we've been having sex without condoms."	"I want to start using condoms now so we won't be at any more risk." OR "We can still prevent infection or reinfection."

The use of a barrier over the cervix (diaphragm or cervical cap) in addition to a condom may provide women with some additional protection against the organisms that cause gonorrhea, genital warts, and chlamydia.

Approaches to STD prevention that do not work include urinating or douching after intercourse, engaging in oral sex, and genital play without full penetration. Birth control pills and sterilization protect you against conception and unwanted pregnancy but not against STDs.

Caring about yourself and your partner means asking questions and being aware of signs and symptoms. It may be a bit awkward, but the temporary embarrassment of asking intimate questions is a small price to pay to avoid contracting or spreading disease. Concern about STDs is part of a sexual relationship, not an intrusion into it, just as sexuality is part of life, not separate from it.

The immune system is a remarkable information network; it operates continuously on the cellular level to keep you well. You can support your immune system by practicing a wellness lifestyle—getting enough sleep, managing stress, eating well, exercising, and protecting yourself against infectious agents, including those that are transmitted sexually.

Right now you can

- Go wash your hands, and count out 20 seconds while doing so; you can estimate 20 seconds by singing "Twinkle, Twinkle, Little Star" slowly or "Happy Birthday" twice.

- Plan to move your bedtime up by 15 minutes, starting tonight.

- Put a small pack of tissues in your bag or coat pocket to use when you sneeze or cough, to avoid transmitting infection to others.

- Resolve to discuss condom use with your partner if you are sexually active and are not already using condoms.

- Call to make an appointment with your health care provider if you need or want to see someone about possible STD infection.

SUMMARY

- The step-by-step process by which infections are transmitted from one person to another includes the pathogen, its reservoir, a portal of exit, a means of transmission, a portal of entry, and a new host.

- The immune response is carried out by white blood cells that are continuously produced in the bone marrow. It has four stages: recognition of the invading pathogen; rapid replication of killer T cells and B cells; attack by killer T cells and macrophages; suppression of the immune response.

- Immunization is based on the body's ability to remember previously encountered organisms and retain its strength against them.

- Allergic reactions occur when the immune system responds to harmless substances as if they were dangerous antigens.

- Bacterial infections include pneumonia, meningitis, strep throat, toxic shock syndrome, tuberculosis, Lyme disease, and ulcers; they can be treated with antibiotics.

- Different viruses cause the common cold, influenza, chicken pox, cold sores, hepatitis, and warts.

- Other diseases are caused by certain types of fungi, protozoa, parasitic worms, and prions.

- Autoimmune diseases occur when the body identifies its own cells as foreign.

- HIV affects the immune system, making an otherwise healthy person less able to resist a variety of infections.

- HIV is carried in blood and blood products, semen, vaginal and cervical secretions, and breast milk. HIV is transmitted through the exchange of these fluids.

- There is currently no cure or vaccine for HIV infection. Drugs have been developed to slow the course of the disease and to prevent or treat certain secondary infections.

- Chlamydia and gonorrhea cause epididymitis and urethritis in men; in women, they can lead to PID and infertility if untreated.

- Pelvic inflammatory disease (PID) is an infection of the uterus and oviducts that may extend to the ovaries and pelvic cavity.

- Genital warts, caused by the human papillomavirus (HPV), are associated with cervical cancer. Treatment does not eradicate the virus, which can be passed on even by asymptomatic people.

- Genital herpes is a common incurable infection that can be fatal to newborns. After an initial infection, outbreaks may recur at any time.

- Hepatitis B is a viral infection of the liver transmitted through sexual and nonsexual contact.

- Syphilis is a highly contagious bacterial infection that can be treated with antibiotics. If left untreated, it can lead to deterioration of the central nervous system and death.

- All STDs are preventable; the key is practicing responsible sexual behaviors. Those who are sexually active are safest with one mutually monogamous uninfected partner. Using a condom with every act of sexual intercourse helps protect against STDs.

TAKE ACTION

1. Find out from your parents or your health records which immunizations you have had, including when you last had a tetanus shot. Are your immunizations up to date? If they aren't, or if you're not sure, check with your school health center about what they recommend.

2. Go to your local pharmacy and examine the cold and cough remedies. Exactly which symptoms does each one claim to alleviate, and with what active ingredient? If possible, ask the pharmacist which ones he or she recommends for various symptoms.

3. If you have ever engaged in unprotected sex or another behavior that puts you at risk for STDs, talk with your health care provider about being screened for common STDs. What tests are available and useful for your situation?

1. In your health journal, list the positive behaviors that help you avoid or resist infection, including sexually transmitted diseases. Consider how you can strengthen those behaviors. Then list the behaviors that tend to block your positive behaviors and put you at risk for contracting an infection. Consider which of these you can change.

2. *Critical Thinking* What responsibility do you think the federal government has for funding programs for the prevention and treatment of HIV infec-

tion? Do you think the government should pay for national prevention programs or increase financial aid to cities bearing the medical costs of caring for people with HIV? Or should these costs be borne by individuals, families, communities, or private insurance companies? Should the expensive drugs be available only to people who can afford them or who have private insurance? Write an essay describing what role, if any, you think the government should play.

FOR MORE INFORMATION

Books

Kolata, G. 2001. *Flu: The Story of the Great Influenza Pandemic of 1918 and the Search for the Virus That Caused It.* New York: Touchstone Books. *A fascinating look at the 1918 flu pandemic.*

Marr, L. 1999. *Sexually Transmitted Disease: A Physician Tells You What You Need to Know.* Baltimore, Md.: Johns Hopkins University Press. *Provides practical information about protecting oneself against infection and obtaining appropriate medical care.*

Matthews, D. D., ed. 2000. *Sexually Transmitted Diseases Sourcebook.* Detroit, Mich.: Omnigraphics. *Includes consumer-oriented information on a wide variety of topics.*

Postgate, J. R. 2000. *Microbes and Man,* 4th ed. New York: Cambridge University Press. *An updated introduction to microbes and how they affect people's everyday lives.*

Smith, R. A., ed. 2001. *Encyclopedia of AIDS.* New York: Penguin. *An overview of the scientific, medical, and social aspects of HIV/AIDS.*

Sompayrac, L. M. 1999. *How the Immune System Works.* Malden, Mass.: Blackwell Science. *A highly readable overview of basic concepts of immunity.*

VW. Organizations, Hotlines, and Web Sites

American Academy of Allergy, Asthma, and Immunology. Provides information and publications; pollen counts are available from the hotline and Web site.
> 800-822-2662; 800-9-POLLEN
> http://www.aaaai.org

American College of Allergy, Asthma, and Immunology. Provides information for patients and physicians; Web site includes an extensive glossary of terms related to allergies and asthma.
> http://allergy.mcg.edu

American Social Health Association (ASHA). Provides written information and referrals on STDs; sponsors support groups for people with herpes and HPV.
> 800-230-6039
> http://www.ashastd.org

ASHA/CDC STD and AIDS Hotlines. ASHA operates several hotlines related to STDs, including those sponsored by the CDC; callers can obtain information, counseling, and referrals for testing and treatment. The general hotline offers information on more than 20 STDs and includes Spanish and TTY service. Specific hotlines for herpes and HPV infection are also available.
> 800-342-AIDS or 800-227-8922
> 800-344-SIDA (Spanish)
> 800-243-7889 (TTY, deaf access)
> 919-361-8488 (herpes)
> 919-361-4848 (HPV infection)

The Body/A Multimedia AIDS and HIV Information Resource. Provides basic information about HIV—prevention, testing, treatment—and links to related sites.
> http://www.thebody.com

Bugs in the News! Provides information about microbiology—allergies, antibodies, antibiotics, mad cow disease, and more—in easy-to-understand language.
> http://falcon.cc.ukans.edu/~jbrown/bugs.html

CDC National Center for Infectious Diseases. Provides extensive information on infectious diseases, including emerging infections.
> 888-CDC-FAXX
> http://www.cdc.gov/ncidod

CDC National Immunization Program. Information and answers to frequently asked questions about immunizations.
> 800-CDC-SHOT
> http://www.cdc.gov/nip
> 877-FYI-TRIP (international travel information)
> http://www.cdc.gov/travel

CDC National Prevention Information Network. Provides extensive information and links on HIV/AIDS and other STDs.
> 800-458-5231
> http://www.cdcnpin.org

Cells Alive: Includes micrographs of immune cells and pathogens at work.
> http://www.cellsalive.net

HIV InSite: Gateway to AIDS Knowledge. Provides information about prevention, education, treatment, and clinical trials.

http://hivinsite.ucsf.edu

Joint United Nations Programme on HIV/AIDS (UNAIDS). Provides statistics and information on the international HIV/AIDS situation.

http://www.unaids.org

Latex Love. Sponsored by the makers of Trojan condoms, this site includes directions for condom use and sample dialogues for overcoming excuses for not using condoms.

http://www.trojancondoms.com/quizzes/safer_sex

National Institute of Allergy and Infectious Diseases. Includes fact sheets about many topics relating to allergies and infectious diseases, including tuberculosis and STDs.

http://www.niaid.nih.gov

Safer Sex Page. Provides information on a variety of topics related to safer sex and STD prevention; includes audio of sample dialogues for talking about safer sex and condom use with partners. (Information is geared to people of all sexual orientations, and some is explicit.)

http://www.safersex.org/safer.sex

World Health Organization: Infectious Diseases. Provides fact sheets about many emerging and tropical diseases as well as information about current outbreaks.

http://www.who.int/health-topics/idindex.htm

See also the listings in Chapter 6 (contraception) and Chapter 9 (food safety).

SELECTED BIBLIOGRAPHY

American Academy of Pediatrics Committee on Infectious Diseases. 2000. Meningococcal disease prevention and control strategies for practice-based physicians (Addendum: Recommendations for college students). *Pediatrics* 106(6): 1500–1504.

Barroso, P. F., et al. 2000. Effect of antiretroviral therapy on HIV shedding in semen. *Annals of Internal Medicine* 133(4): 280–284.

Bren, L. 2001. Trying to keep "mad cow disease" out of U.S. herds. *FDA Consumer,* March–April.

Burstein, G. R., et al. 2001. Predictors of repeat *Chlamydia trachomatis* infections diagnosed by DNA amplification testing among inner city females. *Sexually Transmitted Infections* 77(1): 26–32.

Centers for Disease Control and Prevention. 1998. 1998 guidelines for treatment of sexually transmitted diseases. *MMWR Recommendations and Reports* 47(RR-1).

Centers for Disease Control and Prevention. 2000. CDC statement on study results of product containing nonoxynol-9. *Morbidity and Mortality Weekly Report* 49(31): 717–718.

Centers for Disease Control and Prevention. 2001. Primary and secondary syphilis—United States, 1999. *Morbidity and Mortality Weekly Report* 50(7): 113–117.

Centers for Disease Control and Prevention. 2001. Serosurveys for West Nile virus infection. *Morbidity and Mortality Weekly Report* 50(3): 37–39.

Centers for Disease Control and Prevention, National Immunization Program. 2000. *Epidemiology and Prevention of Vaccine-Preventable Diseases,* 6th ed. Washington, D.C.: Public Health Foundation.

Corey, L., and H. Handsfield. 2000. Genital herpes and public health: Addressing a global problem. *Journal of the American Medical Association* 283(6): 791–794.

Daar, E. S., et al. 2001. Diagnosis of primary HIV-1 infection. *Annals of Internal Medicine* 134(1): 25–29.

Deeks, S. G., et al. 2001. Virologic and immunologic consequences of discontinuing combination antiretroviral-drug therapy in HIV-infected patients with detectable viremia. *New England Journal of Medicine* 344(7): 472–480.

Delves, P. J., and I. M. Roitt. 2000. The immune system. *New England Journal of Medicine* 343(1): 37–49.

Friedrich, M. 2000. HAART stopping news: Experts examine structured therapy interrruption for HIV. *Journal of the American Medical Association* 283(2): 2917–2918.

Gonzales, R., et al. 2001. Principles of appropriate antibiotic use for treatment of acute respiratory tract infections in adults: Background, specific aims, and methods. *Annals of Internal Medicine* 134(6): 479–486.

Hader, S. L., et al. 2001. HIV infection in women in the United States. *Journal of the American Medical Association* 285(9): 1186–1112.

Kirchner, J., and D. Emmert. 2000. Sexually transmitted diseases in women: *Chlamydia trachomatis* and herpes simplex infection. *Postgraduate Medicine* 107(1): 55–65.

Marsland, A. L., et al. 2001. Associations between stress, trait negative affect, acute immune reactivity, and antibody response to hepatitis B injection in healthy young adults. *Health Psychology* 20(1): 4–11.

Miller, K., and J. Graves. 2000. Update on the prevention and treatment of sexually transmitted diseases. *American Family Physician* 61(2): 379–386.

Moore, P. S. 2000. The emergence of Kaposi's sarcoma–associated herpesvirus (human herpesvirus 8). *New England Journal of Medicine* 343(19):1411–1413.

National Institute of Allergy and Infectious Diseases. 2000. *Fact Sheet: Group A Streptococcal Infections* (http://www.niaid.nih.gov/factsheets/strep.htm; retrieved July 24, 2000).

Ness, R. B., et al. 2001. Douching and endometritis: Results from the PID evaluation and clinical health (PEACH) study. *Sexually Transmitted Diseases* 28(4): 240–245.

Sparrer, H. E., et al. 2000. Evidence for the prion hypothesis. *Science* 289(5479): 595–599.

Stephenson, J. 2000. HIV risk from oral sex higher than many realize. *Journal of the American Medical Association* 283(10): 1279.

Super-germ alert: How to avoid antibiotic misuse and overuse. 2001. *Consumer Reports,* January.

U.S. Department of Health and Human Services and the Henry J. Kaiser Foundation. 2001. *Guidelines for the Use of Antiretroviral Agents in HIV-Infected Adults and Adolescents* (http://www.hivatis.org/trtgdlns.html; retrieved February 10, 2001).

Wald, A., et al. 2000. Reactivation of genital herpes simplex virus type 2 infection in asymptomatic seropositive persons. *New England Journal of Medicine* 342(12): 844–850.

World Health Organization. 2000. *Fact Sheet: Variant Creutzfeldt–Jakob Disease* (http://www.who.int/inf-fs/en/fact180.html; retrieved December 4, 2000).

World Health Organization. 2000. *Overcoming Antimicrobial Resistance.* Geneva: World Health Organization.

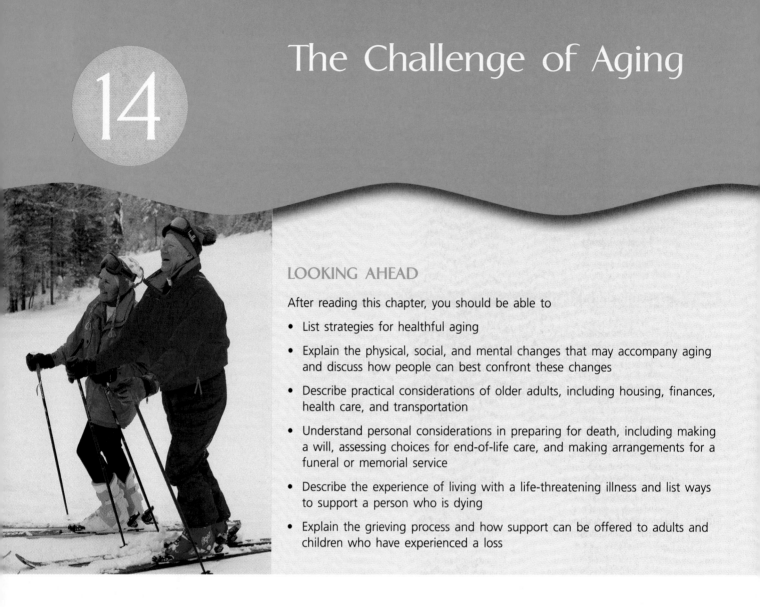

The Challenge of Aging

14

LOOKING AHEAD

After reading this chapter, you should be able to

- List strategies for healthful aging

- Explain the physical, social, and mental changes that may accompany aging and discuss how people can best confront these changes

- Describe practical considerations of older adults, including housing, finances, health care, and transportation

- Understand personal considerations in preparing for death, including making a will, assessing choices for end-of-life care, and making arrangements for a funeral or memorial service

- Describe the experience of living with a life-threatening illness and list ways to support a person who is dying

- Explain the grieving process and how support can be offered to adults and children who have experienced a loss

Many people would like to live for a long time and never grow old. When we see that old age has taken us in its grip, we're stunned. We regard old age as something foreign. But aging is a normal process of development that occurs over the entire lifetime. It happens to everyone, but at different rates for different people. Some people are "old" at 25, and others are still "young" at 75.

Learning to accept and deal with aging and death is a difficult but important part of life, a process that requires information, insight, and commitment. If you optimize wellness during young adulthood, you can exert great control over the physical and mental aspects of aging, and you can better handle your response to events that might be out of your control. With foresight and energy you will be able to shape a creative, graceful, and even triumphant old age.

GENERATING VITALITY AS YOU AGE

As we age, we experience both gains and losses. Physical and mental changes occur gradually, over a lifetime. Biological aging includes all the normal, progressive, irreversible changes to one's body that begin at birth and continue until death. Psychological and social aging usually involve more abrupt changes in circumstance and emotion: relocating, changing homes, losing a spouse and friends, retiring, having a lower income, and changing roles and social status. These changes represent opportunities for growth throughout life.

Successful aging requires preparation. People need to establish good health habits in their teens and twenties. During their twenties and thirties, they usually develop important relationships and settle into a particular lifestyle. By their mid-forties, they must assess their financial

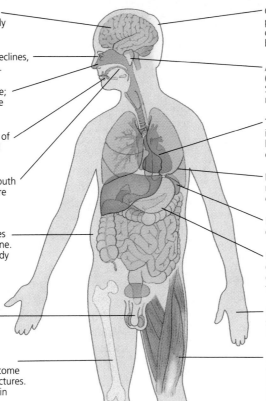

Blood flow to the brain decreases and nerve cells atrophy. Neuron loss does not necessarily mean a decline in mental ability.

The ability to focus on objects close to you declines, and night driving may become more difficult.

Many of the sensory receptors in the nose die; long-term exposure to smoke also lessens the ability to smell.

Teeth can last a lifetime; however, a buildup of plaque can lead to tooth loss if brushing and flossing are neglected.

About two-thirds of the taste buds in the mouth die by age 70; some medications can interfere with taste.

Body fat increases and muscle mass decreases as activity levels drop and calorie needs decline. Regular exercise helps maintain a healthy body composition

Men take longer to attain an erection and it may not be as firm or as large as when they were younger. Enlargement of the prostate gland is common. In women, menopause occurs and estrogen levels drop.

Women in particular are prone to bone loss, especially after menopause, when bones become weaker, more porous, and more likely to fractures. Calcium intake and weight-bearing exercise in younger years can slow bone loss later.

Cells at the base of hair follicles produce progressively less pigment and eventually die, causing hair to turn gray and some men to go bald. Hair also becomes finer.

Ability to hear high-pitched and sibilant (hissing) sounds such as s, z, sh, and ch declines. Some losses may be due to damage from loud music or machinery.

The heart pumps less blood with each beat; this is particularly noticeable during exercise. A healthy diet and regular exercise can often counteract potential cardiovascular problems.

Lung capacity stays steady or even increases with regular exercise. Colds are fewer and less severe due to a buildup in immunity.

Kidneys filter waste more slowly, affecting drug clearance and increasing frequency of urination.

Decreases in acid production and digestive enzymes make digestion take longer; constipation may become more common unless fiber intake increases.

Long-term sun exposure produces wrinkles and spotty pigmentation ("age spots"). Skin gets looser, stretches more easily, and is less resilient.

Muscle fibers atrophy and lose their ability to contract as more protein is broken down and less is synthesized. Regular exercise can slow this process. Muscles are also less flexible and more susceptible to injury.

Figure 14-1 Age-related changes in the body. The body changes in predictable ways as we age. Many of these changes can be slowed by choices we make throughout our lives.

status and perhaps adjust their savings in order to continue enjoying the lifestyle they've chosen after retirement. In their mid-fifties, they need to reevaluate their health insurance plans and may want to think about retirement housing. In their seventies, eighties, and nineties, they need to consider ways of sharing their legacy with the next generation. Throughout life, people should cultivate interests and hobbies they enjoy, both alone and with others, so they can continue to live an active and rewarding life in their later years.

What Happens As You Age?

Many of the characteristics associated with aging are not due to aging at all. Rather, they are the result of neglect and abuse of our bodies and minds. These assaults lay the foundation for later problems like arthritis, heart disease, diabetes, hearing loss, and hypertension. We sacrifice our optimal health by smoking, having poor nutrition, overeating, abusing alcohol and drugs, bombarding our ears with excessive noise, and exposing our bodies to too much ultraviolet radiation from the sun. We also jeopardize our bodies through inactivity, and we endure abuse from the toxic chemicals in our environment.

But even with the healthiest behavior and environment, aging inevitably occurs. It results from biochemical processes we don't yet fully understand. Figure 14-1 shows some of the changes that are a part of aging.

Life-Enhancing Measures: Age-Proofing

You can prevent, delay, lessen, or even reverse some of the changes associated with aging through good health habits. A few simple things you can do every day will make a vast difference to your appearance, level of energy, and vitality—your overall wellness. The following suggestions have been mentioned throughout this text. But because they are profoundly related to health in later life, we highlight them here.

Challenge Your Mind Creativity and intelligence remain stable in healthy individuals. Develop interests and hobbies you can enjoy throughout your life. Staying involved in learning as a lifelong process can help you remain alert and keep your mental abilities.

Develop Physical Fitness Exercise enhances both psychological and physical health. The benefits of an active lifestyle include the following:

- Lower blood pressure and healthier cholesterol levels

- Better protection against heart attacks and an increased chance of survival should one occur
- Sustained capacity of the lungs and respiratory reserves
- Weight control through less accumulation of fat
- Maintenance of strength, flexibility, and balance
- Protection against osteoporosis and Type 2 diabetes
- Increased effectiveness of the immune system
- Maintenance of mental agility and flexibility, response time, memory, and hand-eye coordination

The stimulus that exercise provides also seems to protect against the loss of fluid intelligence, the ability to find solutions when confronted with a new problem. Fluid intelligence depends on rapidity of responsiveness, memory, and alertness. Individuals who exercise regularly have also been found to be less susceptible to depression than those whose level of physical activity has declined.

Find a variety of activities that you enjoy and can do regularly. Accumulate at least 30 minutes of moderate-intensity physical activity every day, and begin a formal exercise program to develop cardiorespiratory endurance, muscular strength and endurance, and flexibility. Studies have shown that it's never too late to start exercising. Even in people over 80, endurance and strength training can improve balance, flexibility, and physical functioning and reduce the potential for dangerous falls.

Eat Wisely   Good health at any age is enhanced by eating a varied diet, paying special attention to lower fat and calorie intake. A new version of the Food Guide Pyramid has been developed to address the changing dietary concerns of people age 70 and older; it differs from the original pyramid in several ways:

- The new pyramid contains the same food groups and range of recommended servings as in the original pyramid, but because of decreased energy levels, most individuals only need the number of servings at the low end of the range.
- A new base includes eight 8-ounce glasses a day of water or any other nonalcoholic or caffeine-free beverages. Decreased sensitivity to thirst and changes in fluid needs from medications and kidney function make it important to monitor fluid intake.
- Recommended choices within groups emphasize foods that are high in nutrient density and fiber.
- Fiber-rich whole fruits and vegetables are recommended instead of juices, especially a variety of fruits and vegetables for vitamin C, beta-carotene, and folate content and cruciferous vegetables for the phytochemicals they contain.
- Three key supplements are mentioned: calcium, vitamin D, and vitamin B-12, which are the nutrients most often lacking in seniors' diets.

Maintain a Healthy Weight   Weight management is especially difficult if you have been overweight most of your life. A sensible program of expending more calories through exercise, cutting calorie intake, or a combination of both will work for most people who want to lose weight, but there is no magic formula. Obesity is not physically healthy, and it leads to premature aging.

Control Drinking and Overdependence on Medications   Alcohol abuse ranks with depression as a common hidden mental health problem, affecting about 10% of older adults. (The ability to metabolize alcohol decreases with age.) The problem is often not identified because the effects of alcohol or drug dependence can mimic disease, such as Alzheimer's disease. Signs of potential alcohol or drug dependence include unexplained falls or frequent injuries, forgetfulness, depression, and malnutrition. Problems can be avoided by not using alcohol to relieve anxiety or emotional pain and not taking medication when safer forms of treatment are available. Women taking hormone replacements should use alcohol cautiously because it appears to raise blood levels of estrogen to more than three times the intended dose.

Don't Smoke   The average pack-a-day smoker can expect to live about 12 years less than a nonsmoker. Furthermore, smokers suffer more illnesses that last longer, and they are subject to respiratory disabilities that limit their total vigor for many years before their death. Premature balding, skin wrinkling, and osteoporosis have been linked to cigarette smoking.

Schedule Physical Examinations to Detect Treatable Diseases   When detected early, many diseases, including hypertension, diabetes, and many types of cancer, can be successfully controlled by medication and lifestyle changes. Regular testing for **glaucoma** after age 40 can prevent blindness from this eye disease. Recommended immunizations, including those for influenza and pneumococcus, can protect you from preventable infectious diseases.

Recognize and Reduce Stress   Stress-induced physiological changes increase wear and tear on your body. Cut down on the stresses in your life. Don't wear yourself out through lack of sleep, substance abuse or misuse, or overwork. Practice relaxation, using the techniques described in Chapter 2. If you contract a disease, consider it your body's attempt to interrupt your life pattern; reevaluate your lifestyle, and perhaps slow down.

CONFRONTING THE CHANGES OF AGING

The changes that occur with aging have repercussions that must be grappled with and resolved. Just as you can act now to limit the physical changes of aging, you can also begin preparing yourself psychologically, socially, and financially for changes that may occur later in life.

W. Planning for Social Changes

Retirement marks a major change in the second half of life. As the longevity of Americans has increased, people spend a larger proportion of their lives in retirement.

Changing Roles and Relationships   Changes in social roles are a major feature of middle age. Children become young adults and leave home, putting an end to daily parenting. Parents experiencing this "empty nest syndrome" must adapt to changes in their customary responsibilities and personal identities. And while retirement may be a desirable milestone for most people, it may also be viewed as a threat to prestige, purpose, and self-respect—the loss of a valued or customary role—and will probably require a period of adjustment.

Retirement and the end of child rearing also bring about changes in the relationship between marriage partners. The amount of time a couple spend together will increase and activities will change. Couples may need a period of adjustment, in which they get to know each other as individuals again. Discussing what types of activities each partner enjoys can help couples set up a mutually satisfying routine of shared and independent activities.

Increased Leisure Time   Planning ahead for retirement is crucial. What kinds of things do you enjoy doing? How will you spend your days? If you have developed diverse interests, retirement can be a joyful and fulfilling period of your life. It can provide opportunities for expanding your horizons by giving you the chance to try new activities, take classes, and meet new people. Volunteering in your community can enhance self-esteem and allow you to be a contributing member of society.

The Economics of Retirement   Financial planning for retirement should begin early in life. People in their twenties and thirties should estimate how much money they need to support their standard of living, calculate their projected income, and begin a savings program. The earlier such a program is begun, the more money they will have at retirement.

Financial planning for retirement is especially critical for women. American women are much less likely than men to be covered by pension plans, reflecting the fact that many women have lower-paying jobs or work part-time during their childbearing years. They tend to have less money vested in other types of retirement plans as well. Although the gap is narrowing, women currently outlive men by about 7 years, and they are more likely to develop chronic conditions that impair their daily activities later in life. The net result of these factors is that older women are almost twice as likely as older men to live in poverty. Women should investigate their retirement plans and take charge of their finances to be sure they will be provided for as they get older.

W. Adapting to Physical Changes

Some changes in physical functioning are inevitable, and successful aging involves anticipating and accommodating these changes. Decreased energy and changes in health mean that older people have to develop priorities for how to use their energy. Rather than curtailing activities to conserve energy, they need to learn how to generate energy. This usually involves saying "yes" to enjoyable activities and paying close attention to the need for rest and sleep. Adapting, rather than giving up, favorite activities may be the best strategy for dealing with physical limitations. For example, if **arthritis** interferes with piano playing, a person can continue to enjoy music by attending concerts or checking out music from the local library.

Hearing Loss   The loss of hearing is a common physical disability that can have a particularly strong effect on the lives of older adults. Hearing loss affects a person's ability to interact with others and can lead to a sense of isolation and depression. Hearing loss should be assessed and treated by a health care professional; in some cases, hearing can be completely restored by dealing with the underlying cause of hearing loss. In other cases, hearing aids may be prescribed.

Vision Changes   Vision usually declines with age. For some individuals this can be traced to conditions such as glaucoma or **age-related macular degeneration (AMD)** that can be treated medically. Glaucoma is caused by increased pressure within the eye due to built-up fluid. The optic nerve can be damaged by this increased pressure, resulting in a loss of side vision and, if untreated, blindness. Medication can relieve the pressure by decreasing the amount of fluid produced or by helping it drain more efficiently. Laser and conventional surgery are other options.

AMD is a slow disintegration of the macula, the tissue at the center of the retina where fine, straight-ahead detail is distinguished. It is not known what causes the 90% of AMD cases known as "dry," in which usually one eye is gradually

glaucoma A disease in which fluid inside the eye is under abnormally high pressure; can lead to the loss of peripheral vision and blindness.

arthritis Inflammation of a joint or joints, causing pain and swelling.

age-related macular degeneration (AMD) A deterioration of the macula (the central area of the retina) leading to blurred vision and sensitivity to glare; some cases can lead to blindness.

Terms

Choosing to help others—whether as a volunteer for a community organization or through spontaneous acts of kindness—can enhance emotional, social, spiritual, and physical wellness. In a national survey of volunteers from all fields, helpers reported the following benefits:

- "Helper's high"—physical and emotional sensations such as sudden warmth, a surge of energy, and a feeling of euphoria that occur immediately after helping

- Feelings of increased self-worth, calm, and relaxation

- A perception of greater physical health

- Fewer colds and headaches, improved eating and sleeping habits, and some relief from the pain of chronic diseases such as asthma and arthritis

Just how might helping benefit the health of the helper? By helping others, we focus on things other than our own problems. Helping others can be effective at banishing a bad mood or a case of the blues. Helping may block physical pain because we can pay attention only to a limited number of things at a given time. Helping others can also expand our perspective and enhance our appreciation for our own lives. Helping may benefit physical health by providing a temporary boost to the immune system and by combating stress and hostile feelings linked to the development of chronic diseases.

Helping others doesn't require a huge time commitment or a change of career. To get the most out of helping, keep the following guidelines in mind:

- *Make contact.* Choose an activity that involves personal contact.

- *Help as often as possible.*

- *Volunteer with others.* Working with a group enables you to form bonds with other helpers who can support your interests and efforts.

- *Focus on the process, not the outcome.* We can't always measure or know the results of our actions.

- *Practice random acts of kindness.* Smile, let people go ahead of you in line, pick up litter, and so on.

- *Adopt a pet.* Several studies suggest that pet owners enjoy better health, perhaps by feeling needed or by having a source of unconditional love and affection.

- *Avoid burnout.* Recognize your own limits, pace yourself, and try not to feel guilty or discouraged.

In addition to the benefits for you, volunteering has the added bonus of having a positive impact on the wellness of others. It fosters a sense of community and can provide some practical help for many of the problems facing our society today.

SOURCES: Musick, M. A., A. R. Herzog, and J. S. House. 1999. Volunteering and mortality among older adults: Findings from a national sample. *Journal of Gerontology: Social Sciences* 54B(3): 5173. Adapted with permission from Sobel, D. S., M.D., and R. Ornstein, Ph.D. 1996. *The Healthy Mind, Healthy Body Handbook* (Los Altos, Calif.: DRx).

---

affected. About 10% of AMD cases are the more serious "wet" type, in which new blood vessels in the eye grow toward the macula and leak fluid, quickly causing serious damage. Although dry AMD cannot be treated, it progresses so gradually that many people can adjust to it. Some cases of wet AMD can be treated with laser surgery. Both glaucoma and AMD can be detected with regular screening.

Vision can also be affected by conditions that are products of aging. By the time they reach their forties, many people have developed **presbyopia**, a gradual decline in the ability to focus on objects close to them. This occurs because the lens of the eye no longer expands and contracts as readily. **Cataracts,** a clouding of the lens caused by lifelong oxidation damage (a by-product of normal body chemistry) may dim vision by the sixties.

Whether vision is affected by disease or simply as a function of aging, there are many strategies to deal with reduced vision: Increasing light sources and painting rooms in a lighter color can help. Wearing a hat and sunglasses outside helps reduce glare. If visual losses are more severe, large-print books, talking clocks, magnifying mirrors, large numbers on telephone keypads, and a variety of electronic devices are available to help.

Arthritis   Half of all people over the age of 65 have some form of arthritis. This degenerative disease causes joint inflammation leading to chronic pain, swelling, and loss of mobility. There are more than 100 different types of arthritis; osteoarthritis (OA) is by far the most common. In a person with OA, the cartilage that caps the bones in joints wears away, forming sharp spurs. It most often affects the hands and weight-bearing joints of the body—knees, ankles, and hips. OA is second only to heart disease in disabling people so that they cannot work; 74% of those it affects are women.

Terms

presbyopia The inability of the eyes to focus sharply on nearby objects, caused by a loss of elasticity of the lens that occurs with advancing age.

cataracts Opacity of the lens of the eye that impairs vision and can cause blindness.

Parkinson's disease A neurological disorder caused by a deficiency of the neurotransmitter dopamine; symptoms include muscle rigidity, tremors, and difficulty walking.

osteoporosis The loss of bone density, causing bones to become weak, porous, and more prone to fractures.

The news that television actor Michael J. Fox has **Parkinson's disease** brought increased attention to a disease that is usually associated with older adults. Parkinson's is a degenerative illness caused by a decrease in the production of dopamine, a chemical in the brain crucial for muscle control and movement.

The early signs and symptoms of Parkinson's usually develop on one side of the body. They include shaking or trembling; changes in handwriting (which becomes smaller or more cramped, for example); problems with movement, such as hands, arms, or legs not moving as smoothly as they have in the past; and diminished facial expression. A person with these symptoms should see a physician for evaluation. As the disease progresses, other symptoms appear. The most common include rigidity of muscles, tremor, postural instability, and bradykinesia (a slowing down of movement and loss of the ability to move automatically and spontaneously).

The main risk factor for developing Parkinson's disease is age. Although 15% of patients are diagnosed before age 50, it is more common among older adults, affecting 1 out of every 100 persons over the age of 60. It is estimated that up to 1.5 million Americans have the disease. A recent study suggests that men may be at higher risk of developing the disease than women. The reasons for this are not clear, although estrogen may be a protective factor for women. Other than age, risk factors for the disease are unclear.

As researchers continue to search for a cure, Parkinson's can be treated and managed with medication. The most common drug used is levodopa (called L-dopa for short), which can mask symptoms of the disease for several years. Brain cells convert L-dopa into dopamine and release it as needed to allow the body to move normally. This regained mobility comes at the price of side effects that can include hallucinations and agitation caused by overstimulation of other brain cells by the dopamine and, after prolonged use, dyskinesias, or wild involuntary movements. Other drugs may be used to postpone the effects of L-dopa.

Patients may turn to surgery as their drug regimen becomes more problematic. Treatments that have had some success include destroying a small mass of cells within the brain to calm tremors and implanting an electrode to stimulate targeted parts of the brain. A controversial area of research, but one that has held out some promise, is fetal-cell implantation, in which dopamine-producing fetal cells are implanted in the brain.

SOURCES: Parkinson disease. 2000. *Journal of the American Medical Association* 284(5). The National Parkinson Foundation. 2000. *What the Patient Should Know* (http://www.parkinson.org/pdedu.htm; retrieved December 21, 2000). Perry, P. 2000. Understanding Parkinson's disease. *Saturday Evening Post* 272 (6). Baldereschi, M., et al. 2000. Parkinson's disease and Parkinsonism in a longitudinal study: Two-fold higher incidence in men. ILSA Working Group. Italian Longitudinal Study on Aging. *Neurology.* 55(9): 1358–1363.

Strategies for reducing the risk of arthritis and, for those who already have OA, for managing it include exercise, weight control, and avoidance of heavy or repetitive muscle use. Exercise lubricates joints and strengthens the muscles around them, protecting them from further damage. Swimming, walking, and t'ai chi are good low-impact exercises. Maintaining an appropriate weight is important to avoid placing stress on the hips, knees, and ankles. Many people with OA also take nonsteroidal anti-inflammatory drugs to reduce pain and swelling.

Menopause   A special concern for women is menopause and the changes accompanying it. During their forties or fifties, women's ovaries gradually stop functioning and menstruation ceases. About 85% of women experience symptoms related to menopause, such as hot flashes, vaginal dryness, and emotional changes. Health care providers agree that menopause is not an illness but a natural part of a woman's life cycle, a time that provides the opportunity for new energy, self-discovery, and growth.

One important decision that women need to make after menopause is whether to start hormone replacement therapy (HRT). The advantages of HRT include a reduction in hot flashes and vaginal dryness, improvement in short-term memory, reduced stress incontinence, and lowered risk of osteoporosis. HRT's effect on heart disease is less clear; recent studies have shown that it may reduce cholesterol levels but may not slow the progression of heart disease. There are drawbacks to HRT including an increase in breast density and cancer risk for some women. Women should carefully review their personal risk factors with their physician before deciding whether to begin HRT.

Osteoporosis   As described in Chapter 9, **osteoporosis** is a condition in which bones become dangerously thin and fragile over time. The possible consequences of osteoporosis include fractures, loss of height, stooped posture, back and hip pain, and breathing problems.

Women are at greater risk than men for osteoporosis because they have 10–25% less bone in their skeleton and because bone loss accelerates in women during the first 5–10 years after the onset of menopause due to the drop in estrogen production. Black women have higher bone density and fewer fractures than white or Asian women. Other risk factors include a family history of osteoporosis, early menopause (before age 45), abnormal or

Alzheimer's disease (AD) is a fatal brain disorder that causes physical and chemical changes in the brain. As the brain's nerve cells are destroyed, the system that produces the neurotransmitter acetylcholine breaks down, and communication among parts of the brain deteriorates. Autopsies reveal that the interiors of the affected neurons are filled with clusters of proteins known as tangles; the spaces between the neurons are filled with protein deposits called amyloid plaques. More than 4 million Americans have Alzheimer's disease, and that number is expected to quadruple in the next 50 years, as more people live into their eighties and nineties. AD usually occurs in people over 60 but can occur in people as young as 40.

Symptoms

The first symptoms of AD are forgetfulness and inability to concentrate. A person may have difficulty performing familiar tasks at home and work and have problems with abstract thinking. As the disease progresses, people experience severe memory loss, especially for recent events. They may vividly remember events from their childhood but be unable to remember the time of day or their location. Depression and anxiety are also common. In the later stages, people with AD are disoriented and may even hallucinate; some experience personality changes—becoming very aggressive or very docile. Eventually, they lose control of physical functioning and are completely dependent on caregivers. On average, a person will survive 8 years after the development of the first symptoms.

Causes

Scientists do not yet know what causes Alzheimer's disease. Age is the main risk factor, although about 10% of cases seem tied to inherited gene mutations. Inherited familial AD generally strikes people before age 65, while the more common late-onset AD occurs in people 65 and older. Other possible clues are provided by substances that appear to delay the onset or progression of the disease. People who regularly take nonsteroidal anti-inflamma-

tory drugs (NSAIDS) like ibuprofen (often to control arthritis), and people who regularly consume fish rich in omega-3 fatty acids appear to have lower rates of AD, indicating a possible protective effect of substances that reduce inflammation. Some studies indicate that vitamin E and other antioxidants may reduce risk for AD or slow the progress of the disease, suggesting that oxidative stress caused by free radicals may play a role. (As described in Chapter 12, antioxidants block damage by free radicals.) Other possible risk factors include a high-fat diet, high blood levels of homocysteine, a history of head injuries, brain damage from small strokes, and a sedentary lifestyle.

Diagnosis and Treatment

Currently, the only certain way to diagnose AD is to examine brain tissue during an autopsy. In most cases, physicians use physical, psychological, and neurological tests. A recent study that combined a positron emission tomography (PET) scan of the brain with a blood test for a genetic disposition for AD diagnosed the disease in people without symptoms. Often a 7-minute pencil-and-paper test is given to evaluate whether memory and related mental functions are appropriate for a person of a particular age. A behavior diary can also aid in diagnosis.

For people with mild to moderate AD, there are several drugs that provide modest improvements in memory. Several medications help maintain cognitive function by inhibiting the breakdown of the neurotransmitter acetylcholine but do not alter the course of the disease. They include donepezil, rivastigmine, physostigmine, and metrifonate. People with AD may also be prescribed antidepressant or antianxiety medications. Many new treatments are under study, including selegiline, a drug used to treat Parkinson's disease; high doses of the antioxidant vitamin E; and the herbal compound ginkgo biloba, which may improve blood flow to the brain and act as an antioxidant. As scientists gain more insight into Alzheimer's disease, they hope to develop more effective treatments that will ease the burden of AD for both families and society.

---

irregular menstruation, a history of anorexia, and a thin, small frame. Thyroid medication and corticosteroid drugs for arthritis or asthma can also have a negative impact on bone mass.

Terms

dementia Deterioration of mental functioning (including memory, concentration, and judgment) resulting from a brain disorder; often accompanied by emotional disturbances and personality changes.

Alzheimer's disease A disease characterized by a progressive loss of mental functioning (dementia), caused by a degeneration of brain cells.

Preventing osteoporosis requires building as much bone as possible during your young years and then maintaining it as you age. Diet and exercise play key roles in this process; see Chapter 9 for recommendations for calcium, vitamin D, and vitamin K intake. Weight-bearing aerobic activities must be performed regularly throughout life to have lasting effects. Strength training improves bone density, muscle mass, strength, and balance, protecting against both bone loss and falls, a major cause of fractures. Even for women in their seventies, low-intensity strength training has been shown to improve bone density. It is also important to avoid tobacco use and manage depression and stress.

Bone mineral density testing can be used to gauge an individual's risk of fracture and help determine if any treatment is needed. HRT and a variety of other drug treatments are effective in treating and preventing osteoporosis.

Handling Psychological and Mental Changes

Many people associate old age with forgetfulness, and slowly losing one's memory was once considered an inevitable part of growing old. However, we now know that most older adults in good health remain mentally alert and retain their full capacity to learn and remember new information. Many people become smarter as they become older and more experienced.

Dementia   Severe and significant brain deterioration in elderly individuals, termed **dementia,** affects about 7% of people under age 80 (the incidence rises sharply for people in their eighties and nineties). Early symptoms include slight disturbances in a person's ability to grasp the situation he or she is in. As dementia progresses, memory failure becomes apparent, and the person may forget conversations, the events of the day, or how to perform simple tasks. It is important to have any symptoms evaluated by a health care professional because some of the over 50 known causes of dementia are treatable. The two most common forms of dementia among older people—**Alzheimer's disease** and multi-infarct dementia—are irreversible. Alzheimer's disease is characterized by changes in brain nerve cells. Multi-infarct dementia results from a series of small strokes or changes in the brain's blood supply that destroy brain tissue.

Repeatedly telling stories about the past—something older people often do—doesn't necessarily indicate dementia. Reminiscence is a normal part of development and allows an older person to integrate life by making past events meaningful in the present. Reminiscing can be of great significance to members of the younger generations because it is a rich source of social, cultural, and family history.

Grief   Another psychological and emotional challenge of aging is dealing with grief and mourning. Aging is associated with loss—the loss of friends, peers, physical appearance, possessions, and health. Grief is the process of getting through the pain of loss, and it can be one of the loneliest and most intense times in a person's life. It can take a year or two or more to completely come to terms with the loss of a loved one. Unresolved grief can have serious physical and psychological or emotional health consequences and may require professional help.

Depression   Unresolved grief can lead to depression, a common problem in older adults (see Chapter 3). If you notice the signs of depression in yourself or someone you

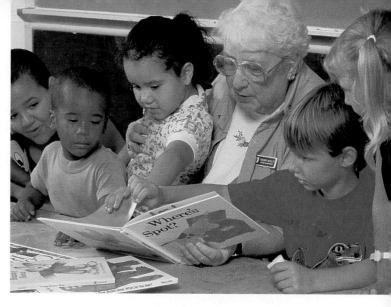

One of the challenges of aging is finding satisfying activities that provide meaningful connections with others. This retired woman reads to a group of children as part of a foster grandparent program.

know, consult a mental health professional. Both professional treatment and support groups can help people deal successfully with major life changes, such as retirement, moving, health problems, or loss of a spouse. If someone refuses help, be reassuring and emphasize that treatment helps make people feel better.

Depression is probably the single most significant factor associated with suicidal behavior among older adults. Suicide is relatively common among the elderly, especially white males over the age of 65. One explanation for this is that because white men generally have greater power and status in our society, aging and retirement represent a relatively greater loss for them. Women, more accustomed to "secondary" status, are not as threatened by the loss of economic and social power. Another theory is that white men tend to have weaker social ties than women or than men from other cultural groups, and as they retire, their increasing social isolation leads to depression and suicide. Some cultural groups, particularly Latinos and Native Americans, afford greater respect and status to older people, who are valued for their wisdom and experience. Cultural groups that emphasize family and social ties also seem to have lower rates of suicide.

One of the most important ways of dealing with the changes associated with aging is to adopt a flexible attitude toward whatever life brings you. Self-acceptance can help make the later years more meaningful and enjoyable. Accepting limitations, having an optimistic outlook, and having a sense of humor are tools that can help you cope with all of life's changes.

COMMUNICATE!   Communicating with a person who suffers from dementia requires patience and compassion. Here are some tips that may help: Approach the person from the front, and wait to make eye contact before talking. Turn off the television or radio to reduce distraction. Communicate in a calm, clear, and supportive way. Speak slowly to give the person more time to process information, and simplify your message. If you can't understand what the person is saying, listen for the feeling, tone, or basic meaning behind the person's communication. If the person talks about an event that happened long ago as if it were happening now, accept that perception of reality. Ask the person to tell you more. Don't make corrections; the person can't help making mistakes in memory or cognition, and you will not be able to "talk sense" into him or her. Reassure and support the person if he or she feels confused, lost, abandoned, or disoriented.

LIFE IN AN AGING AMERICA

Life expectancy is the average length of time we can expect to live. It is calculated by averaging mortality statistics, the ages of death of a group of people over a certain period of time. A female born in the United States in 2000 has a longer life expectancy (79.4 years) than her male counterpart (73.6 years). Individuals who reach their sixty-fifth birthday can expect to live even longer—17 more years or longer—because they have already survived hazards to life in the younger years.

As life expectancy increases, a larger proportion of the population will be in their later years. This change will necessitate new government policies and changes in our general attitudes toward older adults.

America's Aging Minority

People over 65 are a large minority in the American population—over 35 million people, about 13% of the total population in 2000 (Figure 14-2). As birth rates drop, the percentage increases dramatically. Today the status of older adults is improving more than ever before. The enormous increase in the over-55 population is markedly affecting our stereotypes of what it means to grow old. The misfortunes associated with aging—frailty, forgetfulness, poor health, isolation—occur in fewer people in their sixties and seventies and are shifting instead to burden the very old, those over 85.

In general, today's older adults are better off than they have ever been in the past. They have more money than they did 20 years ago. The poverty rate of the elderly has dropped from 28.5% to 11% since the 1960s, largely from the effects of Social Security payments and health care benefits from Medicare. About 78% of older Americans own their homes. Their living expenses are lower after retirement because they no longer support children and have fewer work-related expenses; they consume and buy less food. They receive greater amounts of assistance, such as Medicare, pay proportionately lower taxes, and have greater net worth from life time savings.

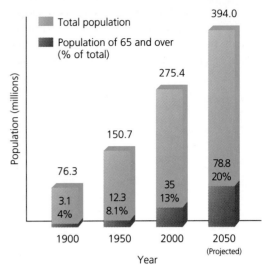

(a) Population growth over age 65 as a proportion of the total population.

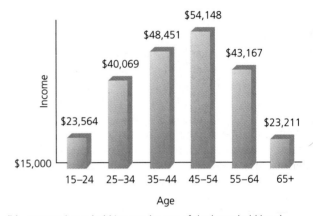

(b) Average household income by age of the household head.

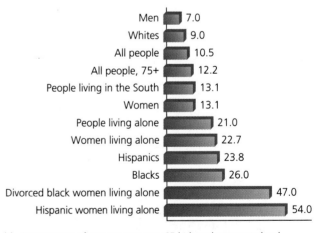

(c) Percentages of groups over age 65 below the poverty level.

VITAL STATISTICS

Figure 14-2   A statistical look at older Americans.   SOURCES: U.S. Bureau of the Census. U.S. Administration on Aging.

As the aging population increases proportionately, however, the number of older people who are ill and dependent rises. Health care remains the largest expense for older adults. Tens of thousands of older Americans live in poverty, particularly minorities and women living alone. These other elderly—poverty-stricken, isolated, lonely—are just as ignored as they ever were, and their numbers are increasing.

Retirement finds many older people with their incomes reduced to subsistence levels. The majority of older Americans live with fixed sources of income, such as pensions, that are eroded by inflation. Many Americans rely on Social Security payments as their only source of income; they are not covered by other types of retirement plans. **Social Security** was intended to serve as a supplement to personal savings and private pensions, not as a sole source of income. It is vital that people plan early for an adequate retirement income.

Family and Community Resources for Older Adults

With help from friends, family members, and community services, people in their later years can remain active and independent. About 66% of noninstitutionalized older Americans live with a spouse or other family member; the other 34% live alone or with a nonrelative. Only 4% live in nursing homes or other institutional settings at any point in time. In about three out of four cases, a grown daughter or daughter-in-law assumes a caregiving role for elderly relatives. Recent surveys indicate that the average woman will spend about 17 years raising children and 18 years caring for an aging relative.

Caregiving can be rewarding, but it is also hard work. Caregivers should use available community services and consider their own needs for relaxation and relief from caregiving duties. Corporations are increasingly responsive to the needs of their employees who are family caregivers by providing such services as referrals, flexible schedules and leaves, and on-site adult care. Professional health care advice is another critical part of successful home care.

The best thing a family can do to prepare for the task of caring for aging parents is to talk frankly about the future. Open communication and planning ahead can reduce the stress on everyone involved and help ease difficult transitions.

Government Aid and Policies

The federal government helps older Americans through several programs, such as food stamps, housing subsidies, Social Security, Medicare, and Medicaid. Social Security, the life insurance and old-age pension plan, has saved many from destitution, although it is intended not as a sole source of income but as a supplement to other income.

Medicare is a major health insurance program for the elderly and the disabled, paying about 30% of the medical costs of older Americans. It provides basic health care coverage for acute episodes of illness that require skilled professional care; it does not pay for custodial or preventive care. When their financial resources are exhausted, older people may apply for Medicaid, which provides medical insurance to low-income people of any age.

Health care policy planners hope that rising medical costs for older adults will dwindle dramatically through education and prevention. Health care professionals are beginning to advise older people about how to avoid and, if necessary, how to manage disabilities. They try to instill an ethic of physical and psychological maintenance that will prevent chronic disease and enable older people to live long, healthy, vigorous lives.

There can be benefits to aging, but they don't come automatically. They require planning and wise choices earlier in life. One octogenarian, Russell Lee, founder of a medical clinic in California, perceived the advantages of aging as growth: "The limitations imposed by time are compensated by the improved taste, sharper discretion, sounder mental and esthetic judgment, increased sensitivity and compassion, clearer focus—which all contribute to a more certain direction in living. . . . The later years can be the best of life for which the earlier ones were preparation."

WHAT IS DEATH?

Death, like life, is change. When the body is no longer able to resist unhealthy changes in itself or is mechanically broken beyond repair, it ceases to function and dies. Ultimately, no answer to the question of why death exists is completely satisfying. We may acknowledge the fact that all living things eventually die, that this is nature's way of renewal, but this recognition offers little comfort when death touches our own lives.

Questions about the meaning of death and what happens when we die are central concerns of the great religions and philosophies. Some promise a better life after death. Others teach that everyone is evolving toward perfection or divinity, a goal reached after successive rounds of death and rebirth. There are also those who suggest that it is not possible to know what happens—

life expectancy The average length of time a person is expected to live.

Social Security A government program that provides financial assistance to people who are unemployed, disabled, or retired (and over a certain age); financed through taxes on business and workers.

Terms

In contrast to the solemn attitude toward death so prevalent in the United States, a familiar and even ironic attitude is more common among Mexicans and Mexican Americans. In the Mexican worldview, death is another phase of life, and those who have passed into it remain accessible. Ancestors are not forever lost, nor is the past dead. This sense of continuity has its roots in the culture of the Aztecs, for whom regeneration was a central theme. When the Spanish came to Mexico in the sixteenth century, their beliefs about death, along with such symbols as skulls and skeletons, were absorbed into the native culture.

Mexican artists and writers confront death with humor and even sarcasm, depicting it as the inevitable fate that all—even the wealthiest—must face. At no time is this attitude toward death livelier than at the beginning of each November on the holiday known as Día de los Muertos, "the Day of the Dead." This holiday coincides with All Souls' Day, the Catholic commemoration of the dead, and represents a unique blending of indigenous ritual and religious dogma.

Festive and gay, the celebration in honor of the dead typically spans two days—one day devoted to dead children, one to adults. It reflects the belief that the dead return to Earth in spirit once a year to rejoin their families and partake of holiday foods prepared especially for them. The fiesta usually begins at mid-day on October 31, with flowers and food—candies, cookies, honey, milk—set out on altars in each house for the family's dead. The next day, family groups stream to the grave-yards, where they have cleaned and decorated the graves of their loved ones, to celebrate and commune with the dead. They bring games, music, and special food—chicken with *mole* sauce, enchiladas, tamales, and *pan de muertos*, the "bread of the dead," sweet rolls in the shape of bones. People sit on the graves, eat, sing, and talk with the departed ones. Tears may be shed as the dead are remembered, but mourning is tempered by the festive mood of the occasion.

Does this more familiar attitude toward death help people accept death and come to terms with it? Keeping death in the forefront of consciousness may provide solace to the living, reminding them of their loved ones and assuring them that they themselves will not be forgotten when they die. Yearly celebrations and remembrances may help people keep in touch with their past, their ancestry, and their roots. The festive atmosphere may help dispel the fear of death, allowing people to look at it more directly. Although it is possible to deny the reality of death even when surrounded by images of it, such practices as Día de los Muertos may help people face death with more equanimity.

SOURCES: Adapted from DeSpelder, L., and A. Strickland. 2002. *The Last Dance*, 6th ed. New York: McGraw-Hill. Puente, T. 1991. Día de los Muertos. *Hispanic*, October, Milne, J. 1965. *Fiesta Time in Latin America*. Los Angeles: Ward Ritche Press. Azcentral. 2000. *Dia de los Muertos* (http://www.azcentral.com/rep/dead; retrieved March 8, 2001).

---

if anything—after death, that any judgment about whether life is worth living must be made on the basis of satisfactions or rewards that we create for ourselves in this life. Dying and death are more than biological events; they have social and spiritual dimensions. Our beliefs—religious or philosophical—can be a key to how we relate to the prospect of our own death, as well as the deaths of others.

Terms

brain death A medical determination of death as the cessation of brain activity indicated by various diagnostic criteria, including a flat EEG reading.

electroencephalogram (EEG) A record of the electrical activity of the brain (brain waves).

clinical death A determination of death made according to accepted medical criteria.

cellular death The breakdown of metabolic processes at the level of the cell.

will A legal instrument expressing a person's intentions and wishes for the disposition of his or her property after death.

testator The person who makes a will.

intestate Referring to the situation in which a person dies without having made a legal will.

Defining Death

Traditionally, death has been defined as cessation of the flow of vital bodily fluids. This occurs when the heart stops beating and breathing ceases. These traditional signs are adequate for determining death in most cases. However, the use of respirators and other life-support systems in modern medicine allows some body functions to be artificially sustained. The concept of **brain death** has been developed to determine whether a person is alive or dead when the traditional signs are inadequate because of supportive medical technology.

According to the standards published in 1968 by a Harvard Medical School committee, brain death involves the following four characteristics: (1) lack of receptivity and response to external stimuli, (2) absence of spontaneous muscular movement and spontaneous breathing, (3) absence of observable reflexes, and (4) absence of brain activity, as signified by a flat **electroencephalogram (EEG)**. The Harvard criteria require a second set of tests to be performed after 24 hours have elapsed, and they exclude cases of hypothermia (body temperature below 90°F), as well as situations involving central nervous system depressants, such as barbiturates.

In contrast to **clinical death**, which is determined by either the cessation of heartbeat and breathing or the criteria for establishing brain death, **cellular death** refers to a gradual process that occurs when heartbeat, respiration, and brain activity have stopped. It encompasses the breakdown of metabolic processes and results in complete nonfunctionality at the cellular level.

The way in which death is defined has potential legal and social consequences in a variety of areas, including criminal prosecution, inheritance, taxation, treatment of the corpse, even mourning. It also affects the practice of organ transplantation because some organs—hearts, most obviously—must be harvested from a human being who is legally determined to be dead.

Learning About Death

Our understanding of death changes as we grow and mature, as do our attitudes toward it. Very young children view death as an interruption and an absence, but their lack of a mature time perspective means that they do not understand death as final and irreversible. A child's understanding of death evolves greatly from about age 5 to age 9. During this period, most children come to understand that death is final, universal, and inevitable. A child who consciously recognizes these facts is said to possess a mature understanding of death. This understanding of death is further refined during the years of adolescence and young adulthood by considering the impact of death on close relationships and contemplating the value of religious or philosophical answers to the enigma of death.

It is important to add, however, that individuals who possess a mature understanding of death commonly hold nonempirical ideas about it as well. Such nonempirical ideas—that is, ideas not subject to scientific proof—deal mainly with the notion that human beings survive in some form beyond the death of the physical body. What happens to an individual's "personality" after he or she dies? Does the self or soul continue to exist after the death of the physical body? If so, what is the nature of this "afterlife"? Developing personally satisfying answers to such questions is also part of the process of acquiring a mature understanding of death.

Denying Versus Welcoming Death

Our ability to find meaning and comfort in the face of mortality depends not only on our having an understanding of the facts of death, but also on our attitudes toward it. Many people seek to avoid any thought or mention of death. The sick and old are often isolated in hospitals and nursing homes. Relatively few Americans have been present at the death of a loved one. Where the reality of death is concerned, "out of sight, out of mind" often appears to be the rule of the day. Instead of facing death directly, we tend to amuse ourselves with unrealistic portrayals on television and movie screens. The fictitious deaths of characters we barely know do not cause us to confront the reality of death as it is experienced in real life.

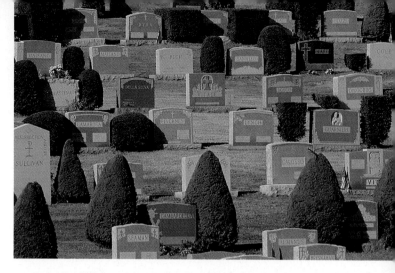

Death awaits all of us at the end of our lives, and accepting and dealing with death are difficult but important tasks. Some people have found that facing the prospect of death makes them more aware of the preciousness of life.

Although some commentators characterize the predominant attitude toward death in the United States as "death denying," others are reluctant to paint society as a whole with such a broad brush. Individuals often maintain conflicting or ambivalent attitudes toward death. Those who come to view death as a relief or release from insufferable pain may have at least a partial sense of welcoming death. Few people wholly avoid or wholly welcome death.

PLANNING FOR DEATH

Acknowledging the inevitability of death allows us to plan for it. Adequate planning can help ensure a death is not made even more difficult for survivors. Although some decisions cannot be made until one is actually in a particular situation, many decisions relating to dying and death can be anticipated, considered, and discussed with close relatives and friends.

Making a Will

Statistics indicate that seven out of ten Americans die without leaving a will. A **will** is a legal instrument expressing a person's intentions and wishes for the disposition of his or her property after death. It is a declaration of how one's estate—that is, money, property, and other possessions—will be distributed after death. During the life of the **testator** (the person making the will), a will can be changed, replaced, or revoked. Upon the testator's death, it becomes a legal instrument governing the distribution of the testator's estate.

When a person dies **intestate**—that is, without having left a valid will—property is distributed according to rules set up by the state. The failure to execute a will may result in a distribution of property that is not compatible with a person's wishes nor best suited to the interests and needs of heirs. In making a will, it is generally advisable to involve close family members to prevent problems that can arise when actions are taken without the knowledge of those who will be affected.

Considering Options for End-of-Life Care

If you were facing the prospect of dying soon, would you prefer to spend your last days or weeks at home, cared for by relatives and friends? Or would you rather have access to the sophisticated medical technologies available in the hospital? By becoming aware of our options, we and our families are empowered to make informed, meaningful choices.

Home Care   Many people express a preference to be cared for at home during the end stage of a terminal illness. An obvious advantage of home care is the fact that the dying person is in a familiar setting, ideally in the company of family and friends. For home care to be an option, however, support generally must be provided not only by family and friends, but also by skilled, professional caregivers.

Hospital-Based Palliative Care   Although hospitals are primarily organized to provide short-term intensive treatment for acute injury and illness, they are also adopting the principles of **palliative care** for patients who require comprehensive care at the end of life. Unlike acute care, which involves taking active measures to sustain life, palliative care focuses on controlling pain and relieving suffering by caring for the physical, psychological, spiritual, and existential needs of the patient. Although the emphasis is generally placed on comfort care, palliative

therapies can be combined with cure-oriented treatment approaches in some cases. In all cases, the goal of palliative care is to achieve the best possible quality of life for patients and their families.

Hospice Programs   As a comprehensive program of care offering a set of services designed to support terminally ill patients and their families, **hospice** is a well-known form of palliative care. Although the term *hospice* sometimes refers to a freestanding medical facility to which terminally ill patients are admitted, most hospice care takes place in patients' homes with family members as primary caregivers. Hospice (and palliative care generally) seeks to provide state-of-the-art care to prevent or relieve pain and other distressing symptoms, as well as to offer emotional and spiritual support to both patient and family.

Deciding to Prolong Life or Hasten Death

Modern medicine can keep the human organism alive despite the cessation of normal heart, brain, respiratory, or kidney function. But should a patient without any hope of recovery be kept alive by means of artificial life support? At what point does such treatment become futile? What if a patient has fallen into a **persistent vegetative state**, a state of profound unconsciousness, lacking any sign of normal reflexes and unresponsive to external stimuli, with no reasonable hope of improvement?

Ethical questions about the "right to die" have become prominent since the landmark case of Karen Ann Quinlan in 1975. Following a respiratory arrest, she was left in a permanent vegetative state. Her family asked the court for permission to discontinue artificial respiration and were eventually granted the right to do so. Since then, courts have ruled on removing other types of life-sustaining treatment. Most notable was the case of Nancy Beth Cruzan, who was in a persistent vegetative state and kept alive with an artificial feeding mechanism. The U.S. Supreme Court ruled in 1990 that the right to refuse unwarranted treatment, even if it is life-sustaining, is constitutionally protected.

Withholding or Withdrawing Treatment   The right of a competent patient to refuse unwanted treatment is now generally established in both law and medical practice. The consensus is that there is no medical or ethical distinction between withholding (not starting) a treatment and withdrawing (stopping) a treatment once it has been started. The choice to forgo life-sustaining treatment involves refusing treatments that would be expected to extend life. The right to refuse treatment remains constitutionally protected even when a patient is unable to communicate. Although specific requirements vary, all of the states authorize some type of written advance directive to honor the decisions of individuals unable to speak

Terms

palliative care A form of medical care aimed at reducing the intensity or severity of a disease by controlling pain and other discomforting symptoms.

hospice a program of care for dying patients and their families.

persistent vegetative state A condition of profound unconsciousness in which a person lacks normal reflexes and is unresponsive to external stimuli, lasting for an extended period with no reasonable hope of improvement.

passive euthanasia The practice of withholding (not starting) or withdrawing (stopping) treatment that could potentially sustain a person's life, with the recognition that, without such treatment, death is likely to occur.

physician-assisted suicide (PAS) The practice of a physician intentionally providing, at the patient's request, lethal drugs or other means for a patient to hasten death with the understanding that the patient plans to use them to end his or her life.

What does it mean to die a "good death"? Participants in a recent study were asked to discuss the deaths of family members, friends, or patients and reflect on what made those deaths good or bad. From these discussions and interviews, six major themes emerged as components of a good death.

The first component was pain and symptom management. Many people fear dying in pain, and portrayals of bad deaths usually included inadequate pain management. Every health care provider in the study told regret-filled stories of patients who died in pain. Patients were concerned with both current and future pain control; when reassured that pain could be managed with drugs, they were less anxious.

The second major component of a good death was clear decision making. Patients and families who had good communication with health care providers and had discussed treatment decisions ahead of time felt empowered, and providers felt they were giving good care. Researchers noted that although all uncertainty about end-of-life decisions cannot be eliminated, tolerance for uncertainty may increase if values and preferences are clarified.

The third component was preparation for death. Patients expressed satisfaction when they had adequate time to prepare their wills and help plan the events that would follow their death, such as funeral arrangements. Many times, providers avoided end-of-life discussions to prevent their patients from losing hope, thus depriving them of the opportunity to plan ahead. Patients and families also wanted to know what to expect during the course of the illness and what physical and psychosocial changes would take place as death approached.

The fourth element was completion, the opportunity to review one's life, to resolve conflicts, to spend time with loved ones, and to say good-bye. Participants confirmed the deep importance of spirituality or meaningfulness at the end of life. Many times, patients were able to view their experience of dying as part of a broader life trajectory and thus continue to grow emotionally and spiritually in their last days. Issues of faith were often mentioned as important to healing.

The fifth component was contributing to others. Patients wanted to know that they still had something to offer to others, whether it was making someone laugh or lightening the load of someone closer to death. Many patients found that as they reflected on their lives, what they valued most was their personal relationships with family and friends, and they were anxious to impart this wisdom to others.

The last component of a good death was affirmation of the whole person. Patients appreciated empathic health care providers, and family members were comforted by those who treated their loved ones as unique and whole people, rather than as a "disease." The quality of dying is related to the acknowledgment that people die "in character," that is, as an extension of who they have been in their lives.

The study affirmed that most people think of death as a natural part of life, not as a "failure of technology." Although the biomedical aspects of end-of-life care are crucial, they merely provide a point of departure toward a good death. When pain is properly managed and the practical aspects of dying are taken care of, patients and their families have the opportunity to address the important emotional, psychological, and spiritual issues that all human beings face at the end of life.

SOURCE: Steinhauser, K. S., et al. 2000. In search of a good death: Observations of patients, families, and providers. *Annals of Internal Medicine* 132(10): 825–832.

for themselves, but who have previously recorded their wishes in an appropriate legal document.

The practice of withholding or withdrawing a treatment that could potentially sustain life is sometimes termed **passive euthanasia**, although many people consider this term a misnomer because it tends to confuse the widely accepted practice of withholding or withdrawing treatment with the generally unacceptable and unlawful practice of taking active steps to cause death.

Assisted Suicide and Active Euthanasia   In contrast to withdrawing or withholding treatment, assisted suicide and active euthanasia refer to practices that intentionally hasten the death of a person. Assisted suicide refers to providing someone with the means to commit suicide, knowing that the recipient intends to use them to end his or her life. In **physician-assisted suicide (PAS),** a physician provides lethal drugs or other interventions—at the patient's explicit request—with the understanding that the patient plans to use them to end his or her life. The patient, not the doctor, administers the fatal dose.

In 1997, the Supreme Court reviewed two cases relating to physician-assisted suicide. The decisions in these cases (*Washington v. Glucksberg* and *Vacco v. Quill*) are important for several reasons. First, the Court upheld the distinction between, on the one hand, withholding or withdrawing treatment, and, on the other hand, physician-assisted suicide. Second, the Court affirmed the rights of states to craft policy concerning physician-assisted suicide, prohibiting it, as most states now do, or permitting it under some regulatory system, as is now happening in Oregon.

Oregon is currently the only state where PAS is permitted. The Death with Dignity Act, a ballot initiative, was passed by Oregon voters in 1994 and, after surviving judicial challenges, was reaffirmed in 1997. During its first three years of implementation, 70 people were reported to have legally committed suicide with the assistance of their physicians. These patients exhibited strong beliefs in personal autonomy and determination to control the end of their lives. The decision to request a prescription for

Some of the following tasks must be attended to soon after a death occurs, others take weeks or months to complete. Many of these tasks, especially those that need to be dealt with in the first hours and days following the death, can be taken care of by friends and relatives of the immediate survivors.

- Prepare a list of relatives, close friends, and business colleagues, and arrange to telephone them about the death as soon as possible. Friends can help with the notification process.

- Find out whether the deceased left instructions or made plans for disposition of the body or for a funeral or memorial service.

- If no prior plan exists, contact a mortuary or memorial society for help in making arrangements. Clergy, friends, and other family members can be asked to help decide what is most appropriate.

- If flowers are to be omitted from the funeral or memorial service, choose an appropriate charity or other memorial to which gifts can be made.

- Write the obituary. Include the deceased's age, place of birth, cause of death, occupation, academic degrees, memberships, military service record, accomplishments, names and relationships of nearest survivors, and an announcement of the time and place of the funeral or memorial service.

- Arrange for family members or close friends to take turns welcoming those who come to express their condolences in person and responding to those who telephone their condolences.

- Ask friends to help coordinate the supplying of meals for the first few days following the death, as well as the management of other household tasks and child care, if necessary.

- Arrange hospitality for relatives and friends who are visiting from out of town.

- If a funeral ceremony is planned, choose the individuals who are to be pallbearers, and notify them that you would like their participation.

- Notify the lawyer, accountant, and other personal representatives who will be helping to settle the deceased's estate.

- Send handwritten or printed notes of acknowledgment to the people who have provided assistance or who have sent flowers, contributions, or their condolences.

- With the help of a lawyer or an accountant, review all insurance policies as well as other sources of potential death benefits, such as Social Security, military service, fraternal organizations, and unions.

- Review all debts, mortgages, and installment payments. Some may carry clauses that cancel debt in the event of death. If payments must be delayed, contact creditors to arrange for a grace period.

---

lethal medication was associated mainly with concerns about loss of autonomy and control.

A third finding of importance in the Supreme Court's 1997 rulings about PAS relates to the concept of double effect in the medical management of pain. The doctrine of double effect states that a harmful effect of treatment, even if it results in death, is permissible if the harm is not intended and occurs as a side effect of a beneficial action. Sometimes the dosages of medication needed to relieve a patient's pain must be increased to levels that can cause respiratory depression, resulting in the patient's death. The Court said that such medication for pain, even if it hastens death, is not physician-assisted suicide if the intent is to relieve pain. (Many people believe that the emphasis on a "right to die," along with the movement to legalize physician-assisted suicide, results from inattention to the needs of the dying, including inadequate pain management, by the health care system.)

Unlike physician-assisted suicide, **active euthanasia** involves a deliberate act to end another person's life. Voluntary euthanasia (also known as voluntary active euthanasia or VAE) is the intentional termination of life at the patient's request by someone other than the patient. In practice, this generally means that a competent patient requests direct assistance to die, and he or she receives assistance from a qualified medical practitioner. Voluntary active euthanasia is currently unlawful in the United States, and it is for this practice that Michigan physician Dr. Jack Kevorkian was convicted of second-degree murder in 1999. Taking active steps to end someone's life is a crime—even if the motive for doing so results from good intentions as an act of mercy.

WW. Completing an Advance Directive

To make our opinions about medical preferences known to health care providers and others who should be aware of them, it is important to document them through a written **advance directive.** Two forms of advance directives are legally important. First is the **living will,** which enables individuals to provide instructions about the kind of medical care they wish to receive if they become incapacitated or otherwise unable to participate in treatment decisions (Figure 14-3). The second important form of advance directive is the **health care proxy,** which is also known as a durable power of attorney for health care. This document makes it possible to appoint another person to make decisions about medical treatment if you be-

INSTRUCTIONS

NEW YORK LIVING WILL

This Living Will has been prepared to conform to the law in the State of New York, as set forth in the case *In re* Westchester County Medical Center, *72 N.Y.2d 517 (1988)*. In that case the Court established the need for "clear and convincing" evidence of a patient's wishes and stated that the "ideal situation is one in which the patient's wishes were expressed in some form of writing, perhaps a 'living will.'"

PRINT YOUR NAME

I, _____, being of sound mind, make this statement as a directive to be followed if I become permanently unable to participate in decisions regarding my medical care. These instructions reflect my firm and settled commitment to decline medical treatment under the circumstances indicated below:

I direct my attending physician to withhold or withdraw treatment that merely prolongs my dying, if I should be in an **incurable or irreversible mental or physical condition with no reasonable expectation of recovery,** including but not limited to: (a) **a terminal condition;** (b) a **permanently unconscious condition;** or (c) **a minimally conscious condition in which I am permanently unable to make decisions or express my wishes.**

I direct that my treatment be limited to measures to keep me comfortable and to relieve pain, including any pain that might occur by withholding or withdrawing treatment.

While I understand that I am not legally required to be specific about future treatments **if I am in the condition(s) described above I feel especially strongly about the following forms of treatment:**

CROSS OUT ANY STATEMENTS THAT DO NOT REFLECT YOUR WISHES

I do not want cardiac resuscitation.
I do not want mechanical respiration.
I do not want artificial nutrition and hydration.
I do not want antibiotics.

However, I **do want** maximum pain relief, even if it may hasten my death.

© 2000
PARTNERSHIP FOR CARING, INC.

NEW YORK LIVING WILL — PAGE 2 OF 2

ADD PERSONAL INSTRUCTIONS (IF ANY)

Other directions:

These directions express my legal right to refuse treatment, under the law of New York. I intend my instructions to be carried out, unless I have rescinded them in a new writing or by clearly indicating that I have changed my mind.

SIGN AND DATE THE DOCUMENT AND PRINT YOUR ADDRESS

Signed _____ Date _____

Address _____

WITNESSING PROCEDURE

I declare that the person who signed this document appeared to execute the living will willingly and free from duress. He or she signed (or asked another to sign for him or her) this document in my presence.

YOUR WITNESSES MUST SIGN AND PRINT THEIR ADDRESSES

Witness 1 _____

Address _____

Witness 2 _____

Address _____

© 2000
PARTNERSHIP FOR CARING, INC.

Courtesy of **Partnership for Caring, Inc.** 12/00
1035 30th Street, NW Washington, DC 20007 800-989-9455

Figure 14-3 Sample living will. Because of differences in state law, each state has its own format for advance directives. SOURCE: Partnership for Caring, 1035 30th St., Washington, DC 20007 (800-989-9455; http://www.partnershipforcaring.org).

come unable to do so. This decision maker is expected to act in accordance with your wishes as stated in an advance directive or as otherwise made known.

Becoming an Organ Donor

Each day about 60 people receive an organ transplant while another 18 people on the waiting list die because not enough organs are available. If you decide to become a donor, the first step is to indicate your wish by completing a **Uniform Donor Card;** alternately, you can indicate your wish on your driver's license. (In 2001, federal officials announced plans for a national organ donor card that would carry more legal weight than the current versions.) Because relatives are called upon to make decisions about organ and tissue donation at the time of a loved one's death, your second step is to discuss your decision with your family.

Planning a Funeral or Memorial Service

Funerals and memorial services are rites of passage that commemorate a person's life in a community and acknowledge his or her passing from that community. They provide a framework that allows survivors to support one

another as they cope with the fact of their loss and express their grief.

Terms

active euthanasia A deliberate act intended to end another person's life; voluntary active euthanasia involves the practice of a physician administering—at the request of a patient—medication or other intervention that causes death.

advance directive Any statement made by a competent person about his or her choices for medical treatment should he or she become unable to make such decisions or communicate them in the future.

living will A type of advance directive that allows individuals to provide instructions about the kind of medical care they wish to receive if they become unable to participate in treatment decisions.

health care proxy A type of advance directive that allows an individual to appoint another person as an agent in making health care decisions in the event he or she becomes unable to participate in treatment decisions; also known as a durable power of attorney for health care.

Uniform Donor Card A consent form authorizing the use of the signer's body parts for transplantation or medical research upon his or her death.

Disposition of the Body   People generally have a preference about the final disposition of their body. For must Americans, the choice is either burial or cremation. *Burial* usually involves a grave dug into the soil or entombment in a mausoleum. *Cremation* involves subjecting a body to intense heat. Cremated remains can be buried, placed in a columbarium niche, put into an urn kept by the family or interred in an urn garden, or scattered at sea or on land. A body destined for burial or cremation may or may not be embalmed. If the body is to be viewed during a wake or will be present at the funeral, **embalming** is generally done.

Arranging a Service   Bereaved relatives and friends usually derive important benefits from having an opportunity to honor the deceased and express their grief through ceremony. Decisions about one's own last rites are ideally made with a view to the needs and wishes of one's survivors. Religious and cultural or ethnic traditions play a major role in shaping the way people honor their dead. The diversity of life and death in the United States calls for a diversity of rites. A meaningful funeral or memorial service can be designed in many different ways.

Costs also may influence the choices people make for last rites. According to the latest available figures, the average cost of a funeral, not including cemetery costs, is $5800. People who prefer a no-frills approach may have the option of arranging economic burial or cremation through a non-profit memorial society. Veterans are eligible for burial in a national cemetery, an option that can also reduce costs.

COPING WITH DYING

There is no one right way to live with or die of a life-threatening illness. Every disease has its own set of problems and challenges, and each person copes with these problems and challenges in his or her own way. Living with an illness that is life-threatening and incurable can be described as a "living-dying" experience. Hope and honesty are often delicately balanced—honesty to face reality as it is, hope for a positive outcome. The object of hope changes. The early hope that the symptoms are not really serious gives way to hope that a cure is possible. When the illness is deemed incurable, there is hope for more time. As time begins to run out, one hopes for a pain-free death, a good death.

The Tasks of Coping

In her 1969 book *On Death and Dying* Elisabeth Kübler-Ross suggested that the response to an awareness of imminent death involves five psychological stages: denial, anger, bargaining, depression, and acceptance. The notion that these "five stages" occur in a linear progression has since become a kind of modern myth of how people *ought* to cope with dying. Unfortunately, this can lead to the idea that it is a person's "task" to move sequentially through these stages, one after another; and, if this is not accomplished, the person has somehow failed. In fact, however, Kübler-Ross said that individuals go back and forth among the stages during the course of an illness and different stages can occur simultaneously.

The notion of sequential stages has been deemphasized in favor of highlighting the *tasks* that deserve attention in coping with a life-threatening illness. Charles Corr, for example, distinguishes four primary dimensions in coping with dying:

1. *Physical:* Satisfying bodily needs and minimizing physical distress
2. *Psychological:* Maximizing a sense of security, self-worth, autonomy, and richness in living
3. *Social:* Sustaining significant relationships and addressing the social implications of dying
4. *Spiritual:* Identifying, developing, or reaffirming sources of meaning and fostering hope

Contemplating these dimensions gives us a framework for considering the specific tasks that need to be addressed in coping with dying. However, to avoid mistaking the map for the territory, we must remember that a person's death is as unique as his or her life. Each person's pathway through life-threatening illness is determined by such factors as the specific disease and its course, his or her personality, and the available supportive resources.

Patterns of Coping

The threat of a potentially fatal illness evokes a variety of responses to make the threat somehow manageable. The main aim of the mental processes and behaviors involved in coping is to establish control over a stressful situation. People who apparently cope best with life-threatening illness often exhibit a "fighting spirit" that views the illness not only as a threat, but also as a challenge. These people strive to inform themselves about their illness and take an active part in treatment decisions. They are optimistic and have a capacity to discover positive meaning in ordinary events. Holding to a positive outlook despite distressing circumstances involves creating a sense of meaning that is bigger than the threat. In the context of life-threatening illness, this includes a person's ability to accomplish goals, maintain relationships, and sustain a sense of personal vitality, competence, and power.

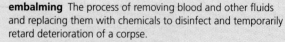

Terms

embalming The process of removing blood and other fluids and replacing them with chemicals to disinfect and temporarily retard deterioration of a corpse.

grief A person's reaction to loss as manifested physically, emotionally, mentally, and behaviorally.

bereavement The objective event of loss.

mourning The process whereby a person actively copes with grief in adjusting to a loss and integrating it into his or her life.

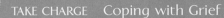

- Recognize and acknowledge the loss.
- React to grief by accepting and expressing it.
- Take time for nature's process of healing.
- Know that powerful, overwhelming feelings will change with time.
- Review and remember the relationship with the deceased.
- Share your pain by accepting support from others.
- Surround yourself with life: plants, animals, friends.
- Make use of mementos to promote your mourning, not to live in the past.

- Avoid major decisions, if possible, and give yourself time to readjust.
- Adapt to a new world without forgetting the old.
- Prepare for change, new interests, new friends, creativity, and growth.
- Reinvest in life.

SOURCES: The Centre for Living with Dying (554 Mansion Park Dr., Santa Clara, CA 95054; 408-980-9801). Rando, T. A. 1993. *The Treatment of Complicated Mourning.* Champaign, Ill.: Research Press.

COMMUNICATE! If someone you know tells you that he or she is facing a life-threatening illness, you may not be sure what to say. Give the person the opportunity to express his or her concerns and needs, and respond with questions, such as "Can you tell me more?" Practice active, empathic listening, avoiding statements such as "Everything will be OK" or "You should see another doctor." Stay present with the person, and offer practical assistance if you feel comfortable doing so ("Do you need anything right now?"). Keep in mind that you don't have to have answers or make things better; all you need to offer is your caring presence.

Supporting a Dying Person

People often feel uncomfortable in the presence of a person who is close to dying. What can we say? How should we act? It may seem that any attempt to be comforting could only result in words that are little more than stale platitudes. Yet we want to express concern and establish meaningful contact with the person who is facing the major loss of his or her life. In such circumstances, the most important gift we can bring is the gift of listening. Offering the person opportunities to speak openly and honestly about his or her experience can be crucial, even when such conversation is initially painful.

We tend to place dying persons in a special category, but the reality is that their needs are not fundamentally different from anyone else's, although their situation is perhaps more urgent. Dying people need to know that they are valued, that they are not alone, that they are not being unfairly judged, and that those closest to them are also striving to come to terms with a difficult situation. As with any relationship, there are opportunities for growth on both sides.

COPING WITH LOSS

Even if we have not experienced the death of someone close, we are all survivors of losses that occur in our lives because of changes and endings. The loss of a job, the ending of a relationship, transitions from one school or neighborhood to another—these are examples of the kinds of losses that occur in all our lives. Such losses are sometimes called "little deaths," and, in varying degrees, they all involve grief.

Experiencing Grief

Grief is the reaction to loss. It encompasses thoughts and feelings, as well as physical and behavioral responses. Mental distress may involve disbelief, confusion, anxiety, disorganization, and depression. The emotions that can be present in normal grief include not only sorrow and sadness, but also relief, anger, and self-pity, among others. Common behaviors associated with grief include crying, "searching" for the deceased, and talking incessantly about the deceased and the circumstances of the death. Bereaved people may be restless, as if not knowing what to do with themselves. Physically, grief may involve frequent sighing, insomnia, and loss of appetite. Grief may also evoke a reexamination of religious or spiritual beliefs as a person struggles to make meaning of the loss. All such manifestations of grief can be present as part of one's total response to **bereavement**—that is, the event of loss.

Mourning is closely related to grief and is often used as a synonym for it. However, mourning refers not so much to the *reaction* to loss, but to the *process* by which a bereaved person adjusts to loss and incorporates it into his or her life. How this process is managed is determined, at least partly, by cultural norms for the expression of grief. Considered jointly, grief and mourning are the means to healing the pain of loss.

Tasks of Mourning   Experiencing grief is part of the process by which a bereaved person integrates a significant loss into his or her life. Psychologist William Worden has identified four tasks that must be attended to:

1. *Accepting the reality* of the loss
2. *Working through the pain* of grief
3. *Adjusting to a changed environment* in which the deceased is absent
4. *Emotionally relocating the deceased and moving on with life*

Accomplishing the fourth task does not mean dishonoring the deceased's memory or denying normal feelings of connection that persist beyond death. Making the journey of grief and attending to the various tasks along the way, we come to a place where we learn how to keep a special place for the deceased in our heart and memory while moving forward with our lives.

The Course of Grief   Grieving, like dying, is highly individual. In the first hours or days following a death, a bereaved person is likely to experience overwhelming shock and numbness, as well as a sense of disbelief. The cause or mode of death—natural, accidental, homicide, or suicide—has an impact on how grief is experienced. Even when a death is anticipated, grief is not necessarily diminished when the loss becomes real.

The sense of disorganization experienced by survivors during the early period of grief is set against the need to attend to decisions and actions surrounding the disposition of the deceased's body. As family and friends gather to offer mutual support, funeral ceremonies are held. Engaging in such activities promotes accepting the reality of the death and moving beyond the initial shock and numbness.

In its middle phase, the course of grief is characterized by anxiety, apathy, and pining for the deceased. The "pangs of grief" are felt as the bereaved person deeply experiences the pain of separation. There is often a sense of despair as a person repeatedly goes over the events surrounding the loss, perhaps fantasizing that somehow everything could be undone and be as it was before. During this period, the bereaved also begins looking toward the future and taking the first steps toward building a life without the deceased.

The last phase of "active" grief involves coming to a sense of resolution. The acute pain and emotional turmoil of grief subsides. Physical and mental balance is reestablished. The bereaved becomes increasingly reintegrated into his or her social world. Sadness doesn't go away completely, but it recedes into the background. Although reminders of the loss stimulate active grieving from time to time, the main focus is the present, not the past. Adjusting to loss may sometimes feel like a betrayal of our deceased loved one, but it is healthy to engage again in our ongoing lives and our future.

Supporting a Grieving Person

In experiencing a significant loss, a person initially may feel and behave much like a frightened, helpless child. He or she may respond best to the kind of loving support that is given by a parent. A hug may be more comforting than any words. Also, because talking about a loss is an important way that survivors cope with the changed reality, simply listening can be very helpful. The key to being a good listener is to refrain from making judgments about whether the feelings expressed by a survivor are "right" or "wrong," "good" or "bad."

Funerals and other leave-taking ceremonies generally help survivors gain a sense of closure and begin to integrate a loss into their lives. For some, funerals are occasions of weeping and wailing; for others, stoic and subdued emotions are the rule. Different styles of mourning behavior can be equally valid and appropriate.

Social support is as critical during the later course of grief as it is during the first days after a loss. Besides continuing support from individuals who are part of their social network, bereaved people may want to share their stories and concerns through organized support groups.

> **COMMUNICATE!**   Few of us know just what to say to a friend who has lost a loved one. Some things to *avoid* are making references to the deceased person's advanced age, declaring that the death was "for the best," asking the widow or widower to let you introduce him or her to new people, suggesting the adoption of a pet, saying "I know how you feel," and expecting the person to be consoled by the presence of his or her remaining family. Very often, the most appreciated expression of sympathy is just "I'm so sorry."

Children tend to cope with loss in a healthier fashion when they are included as part of their family's experience of grief and mourning. In talking about death with children, the most important guideline is to be honest. Set the explanation you are offering at the child's level of understanding. A child's readiness for more details can usually be assessed by paying attention to his or her questions.

COMING TO TERMS WITH DEATH

We may wish we could keep death out of view and not make a place for it in our lives. But this wish cannot be fulfilled. With the death of a beloved friend or relative, we are confronted with emotions and thoughts that relate not only to the immediate loss but also to our own mortality.

Our encounters with dying and death teach us that relationships are more important than things and that life offers no guarantees. In discovering the meaning of death in our own lives, we find that life is both precious and precarious. Allowing ourselves to make room for death, we discover that it touches not only the dying or bereaved person and his or her family and friends, but also the wider community of which we are all part. We recognize that dying and death offer opportunities for extraordinary growth in the midst of loss. Denying death, it turns out, results in denying life.

Tips for Today

Cultivating physical and mental wellness in your earlier years can help you both to age gracefully and to develop a healthy attitude toward loss and death. Facing the natural processes of aging and dying clear-sightedly, despite your fears and discomfort, can deepen your appreaction of life.

Right now you can

- Start a list of the books you'd like to read for pleasure, and get one of them from the library or bookstore.

- Get in the habit of volunteering by contacting a nonprofit group in your community and offering your time and talent; consider a literacy campaign, a soup kitchen, a youth mentoring program, or Habitat for Humanity.

- Consider asking your parents or grandparents what their wishes are for end-of-life care and for funeral arrangements, if you don't already know.

- Think about whether you want to be an organ donor; if you do, look into filling out a donor card (see Take Action at the end of the chapter).

SUMMARY

- People who take charge of their health during their youth have greater control over the physical and mental aspects of aging.

- Age-proofing strategies include challenging your mind, developing physical fitness, eating wisely, maintaining a healthy weight, controlling drinking and medication overuse, avoiding tobacco use, recognizing and reducing stress, and obtaining regular screening tests.

- Retirement can be a fulfilling and enjoyable time of life for those who adjust to their new roles, enjoy participating in a variety of activities, and have planned ahead for financial stability.

- Slight confusion and forgetfulness are not signs of a serious illness; severe symptoms may indicate Alzheimer's disease or another from of dementia.

- Resolving grief and mourning and dealing with depression are important tasks for older adults.

- Life expectancy, which has risen dramatically since the 1900s, is generally longer for women.

- Government aid to the elderly includes food stamps, housing subsidies, Social Security, Medicare, and Medicaid.

- Dying and death are more than biological events; they have social and spiritual dimensions.

- The traditional criteria for determining death focus on vital signs such as breathing and heartbeat. Brain death is characterized by a lack of physical responses other than breathing and heartbeat.

- A will is a legal instrument that governs the distribution of a person's estate after death.

- End-of-life care may involve a combination of home care, hospital stays, and hospice or palliative care.

- The practice of withholding or withdrawing potentially life-sustaining treatment is sometimes termed passive euthanasia.

- Physician-assisted suicide occurs when a physician provides lethal drugs or other interventions, at a patient's request, with the understanding that the patient plans to use them to end his or her life. Voluntary active euthanasia refers to the intentional ending of a patient's life, at his or her request, by someone other than the patient.

- Advance directives, such as living wills and health care proxies, are used to express one's wishes about the use of life-sustaining treatment.

- People can donate their bodies or specific organs for transplantation and other medical uses after death.

- Bereaved people usually benefit from participating in a funeral or memorial service to commemorate a loved one's death.

- Coping with dying involves physical, psychological, social, and spiritual dimensions.

- In offering support to a dying person, the gift of listening can be especially important.

- Grief encompasses thoughts and feelings, as well as physical and behavioral responses.

- Mourning, the process by which a person integrates a loss into his or her life, is determined partly by social and cultural norms for expressing grief.

1.   Interview your parents or grandparents to find out how they want to spend their later years. Do they want to live at home, in a retirement community, with a relative? Do they plan to live on a pension, retirement account, Social Security? Have they made any concrete plans, or have they not yet confronted those decisions?

2.   In most states, the Department of Motor Vehicles provides organ donor forms. You can also request a donor form or download one from the National Kidney Foundation (800-622-9010; http://www.kidney.org), the Coalition on Donation (800-355-7427; http://www.shareyourlife.org), or the Department of Health and Human Services (http://www.organdonor.gov). When you receive your donor form, consider the advantages and disadvantages of becoming a donor. If you decide to be a donor, fill out the card and keep it with your driver's license. Discuss your decision with members of your family.

3.   Obtain sample copies of advance directives that are appropriate for the state you live in. Check with your local hospital or health services organization for these forms, or request them from Partnership for Caring (800-989-9455; http://www.partnershipforcaring.org). Review the forms and consider the advantages and disadvantages of using them. If you decide to execute a living will or health care proxy, discuss your decision with members of your family and anyone else who might become involved in your health care.

JOURNAL ENTRY

1.   Imagine that you are very old and are looking back on your life. What will have given you satisfaction—a successful career, parenthood, happiness, travel, self-knowledge? Make a list in your health journal of your life goals and priorities. What actions can you take now to work toward your goals? Choose one goal, and take an action this week that moves you toward it.

2.   *Critical Thinking*   Research the issue of physician-assisted suicide. Write a brief essay that presents the main arguments on both sides of the issue, and conclude with a statement of your own opinion. Be sure to explain your reasoning. What are the most important factors in your decision? Why do you think you have the opinion you do?

FOR MORE INFORMATION

Books

Brannigan, M. C., and J. A. Boss. 2000. *Healthcare Ethics in a Diverse Society.* Mountain View, Calif.: Mayfield. *A comprehensive overview of U.S. health care ethics that introduces a cross-cultural perspective on many issues.*

Cassel, C. K., and G. A. Vallasi. 2001. *The Practical Guide to Aging: What Everyone Needs to Know.* New York: New York University Press. *A practical, comprehensive reference to many aspects of aging.*

Cohen, D., and C. Eisdorfer. 2001. *The Loss of Self: A Family Resource for the Care of Alzheimer's Disease and Related Disorders.* Rev. ed. New York: Norton. *A resource for caregivers of people with dementia that addresses biological, emotional, medical, and social issues.*

Cohen, H. J. 2000. *Taking Care After 50: A Self-Care Guide for Seniors.* New York: Three Rivers Press. *Addresses a variety of issues for older adults, including nutrition, mental health, safety, and sexuality.*

DeSpelder, L. A., and A. L. Strickland. 2002. *The Last Dance: Encountering Death and Dying,* 6th ed. New York: McGraw-Hill. *A comprehensive and readable text highlighting a broad range of topics related to dying and death.*

Kessler, D. 2000. *The Needs of the Dying: A Guide for Bringing Hope, Comfort, and Love to Life's Final Chapter.* New York: HarperCollins. *A compassionate and honest guide for people facing life-threatening illness and those caring for them.*

Organizations and Web Sites

AARP. Provides information on all aspects of aging, including health promotion, health care, and retirement planning.
    800-424-2277
    http://www.aarp.org

Access America for Seniors. A gateway to government resources on the Internet for older Americans.
    http://www.seniors.gov

Aging Well. A practical resource for seniors that includes information on diet, exercise, safety, and medical care.
    http://agingwell.state.ny.us

Alzheimer's Association. Offers tips for caregivers and patients, as well as information on research into the causes and treatment of Alzheimer's disease.
    800-272-3900
    http://www.alz.org

Arthritis Foundation. Provides information about arthritis, including free brochures, referrals to local services, and research updates.
    800-283-7800
    http://www.arthritis.org

Association for Death Education and Counseling (ADEC). Provides resources for education, bereavement counseling, and care of the dying.

860-586-7503
http://www.adec.org

Exercise: A Guide from the National Institute on Aging. Provides practical advice on fitness for seniors; includes animated instructions for specific exercises.
http://www.nih.gov/nia/health/pubs/nasa-exercise

Growth House. Offers an extensive directory of Internet resources relating to life-threatening illness and end-of-life care.
http://www.growthhouse.org

Longwood College Library: Doctor Assisted Suicide—A Guide to Web Sites and the Literature. Information on physician-assisted suicide and links to related sites.
http://web.lwc.edu/administrative/library/suic.htm

National Funeral Directors Association (NFDA). Provides resources related to funerals and funeral costs, body disposition, and bereavement support.
800-228-6332; 262-789-1880
http://www.nfda.org

National Hospice and Palliative Care Organization (NHPCO). Provides information about hospice care and supplies an online national directory of hospices listed by state and city.
703-243-5900
http://www.nhpco.org

National Institute on Aging. Provides fact sheets and brochures on aging-related topics.
http://www.nih.gov/nia

National Osteoporosis Foundation. Provides information on the causes, prevention, detection, and treatment of osteoporosis.
http://www.nof.org

Partnership for Caring. Provides information about right-to-die issues and supplies advance directives that meet specific state requirements.
800-989-9455
http://www.partnershipforcaring.org

U.S. Administration on Aging. Provides fact sheets, statistical information, and Internet links to other resources on aging.
202-619-7501
http://www.aoa.gov

The following organizations provide information about organ donation and donor cards.

National Kidney Foundation
212-889–2210
http://www.kidney.org

U.S. Department of Health and Human Services
http://www.organdonor.gov

SELECTED BIBLIOGRAPHY

Angerer, P., et al. 2001. Effect of oral postmenopausal hormone replacement on progression of atherosclerosis: A randomized, controlled trial. *Arteriosclerosis, Thrombosis, and Vascular Biology* 21(2): 262–268.

Byock, I. 2000. Palliative care. In *On Our Own Terms: Moyers on Dying,* ed. Public Affairs Television, 10–11. New York: WNET.

Centers for Disease Control and Prevention. 2000. Health-related quality of life among adults with arthritis. *Morbidity and Mortality Weekly Report* 49(17): 366–369.

Corr, C. A. 1998. Enhancing the concept of disenfranchised grief. *Omega: Journal of Death and Dying* 38: 1–20.

Ditto, P. H., et al. 2001. Advance directives as acts of communication: A randomized controlled trial. *Archives of Internal Medicine* 161(3): 421–430.

Felson, D. T., et al. 2000. Osteoarthritis: New insights Part 1: The disease and its risk factors. *Annals of Internal Medicine* 133(8): 635–646.

Folkman, S., and S. Greer. 2000. Promoting psychological well-being in the face of serious illness: When theory, research and practice inform each other. *Psycho-Oncology* 9: 11–19.

Friedland, R. P., et al. Patients with Alzheimer's disease have reduced activities in midlife compared with healthy control-group members. *Proceedings of the National Academy of Sciences* 98(6): 3440–3445.

Golin, C. E., et al. 2000. A prospective study of patient-physician communication about resuscitation. *Journal of the American Geriatrics Society* 48: S52–S60.

Health Resources and Services Administration. 2000. *Organ Donation* (http://www.organdonor.gov; retrieved September 9, 2000).

Hospice care. 2001. *Journal of the American Medical Association* 285((7): 970.

Kendall, C. E. 2000. A double dose of double effect. *Journal of Medical Ethics* 26: 204–205.

Kritz-Silverstein, D., E. Barrett-Connor, and C. Corbeau. 2001. Cross-sectional and prospective study of exercise and depressed mood in the elderly. *American Journal of Epidemiology* 153(6): 596–603.

Kübler-Ross, E. 1997. *On Death and Dying.* Reprint Edition. New York: Simon & Schuster.

Laurin, D., et al. 2001. Physical activity and risk of cognitive impairment and dementia in elderly persons. *Archives of Neurology* 58(3): 498–504.

Lynn, J. 2001. Serving patients who may die soon and their families. The role of hospice and other services. *Journal of the American Medical Association* 285(7): 925–932.

Mulnard, R. A., et al. 2000. Estrogen replacement therapy for treatment of mild to moderate Alzheimer disease: A randomized controlled trial. Alzheimer's Disease Cooperative Study. *Journal of the American Medical Association* 283(8): 1007–1015.

National Eye Institute. 2000. *Age-Related Macular Degeneration* (http://www.nei.nih.gov/publications /armd-p.htm; retrieved November 15, 2000).

National Eye Institute. 2000. *Glaucoma* (http://www.nei.nih.gov/publications/glau-pat.htm; retrieved November 15, 2000).

Nicodemus, K. K., A. R. Folsom, and K. E. Anderson. 2001. Menstrual history and risk of hip fractures in postmenopausal women in the Iowa Women's Health Study. *American Journal of Epidemiology* 153(3): 251–255.

NIH Consensus Development Panel on Osteoporosis Prevention, Diagnosis, and Therapy. 2001. Osteoporosis prevention, diagnosis, and therapy. *Journal of the American Medical Association* 285(6): 785–795.

Oregon Health Division. 2001. *Oregon's Death with Dignity Act: Three Years of Legalized Physician-Assisted Suicide* (http://www.ohd.hr.state.or.us/chs/pas/ar-smmry.htm; retrieved May 2, 2001).

Ostir, G. V., et al. 2000. Emotional well-being predicts subsequent functional independence and survival. *Journal of the American Geriatrics Society* 48(5): 473–478.

Russell, R. M., H. Rassmussen, and A. Lichenstein. 1999. Modified food guide pyramid for people over seventy years of age. *Journal of Nutrition* 129: 751–753.

Rutter, C. M., et al. 2001. Changes in breast density associated with initiation, discontinuation, and continuing use of hormone replacement therapy. *Journal of the American Medical Association* 285(2): 171–176.

Silveira, M. J., et al. 2000. Patients' knowledge of options at the end of life. *Journal of the American Medical Association* 284(19): 2483–2488.

Tierney, W. M., et al. 2001. The effect of discussions about advance directives on patients' satisfaction with primary care. *Journal of General Internal Medicine* 16(1): 32–40.

Windler, D., and N. Dickert. 2001. The consent process for cadaveric organ procurement. How does it work? How can it be improved? *Journal of the American Medical Association* 285(3): 329–333.

15

Conventional and Complementary Medicine: Skills for the Health Care Consumer

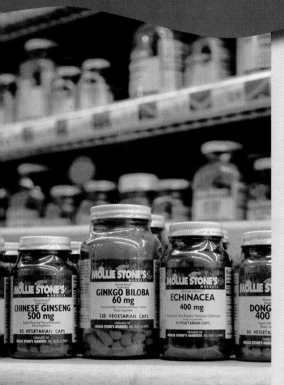

LOOKING AHEAD

After reading this chapter, you should be able to

- Explain the self-care decision-making process and discuss options for self-treatment

- Describe the basic premises, practices, and providers of conventional medicine

- Describe the basic premises, practices, and providers of complementary and alternative medicine

- Explain how to communicate effectively with a health care provider and how to evaluate different forms of treatment

- Discuss different types of health insurance plans

Today, people are becoming more confident of their ability to solve personal health problems on their own. People who manage their own health care gather information and learn skills from physicians, friends, classes, books, magazines, Web sites, or self-help groups; solicit opinions and advice; make decisions; and take action. They know how to practice safe, effective self-care, and they know how to make decisions about professional medical care, whether conventional Western medicine or complementary and alternative medicine. This chapter will help you develop the skills both to identify and manage medical problems and to make the health care system work effectively for you.

SELF-CARE: MANAGING MEDICAL PROBLEMS

Effectively managing medical problems involves developing several skills. First, you need to learn how to be a good observer of your own body and assess your symptoms. You also must be able to decide when to seek professional advice and when you can safely deal with the problem on your own. You need to know how to safely and effectively self-treat common medical problems. Finally, you need to know how to develop a partnership with physicians and other care providers and how to carry out treatment plans.

Self-Assessment

Symptoms are signals from our bodies, alerting us that something may be wrong. Many symptoms are an expression of the body's attempt to heal itself. For example, a fever may be an attempt to make the body less hospitable to infectious agents, and a cough can help clear the airways and protect the lungs. Carefully observing symptoms lets you identify those signals that suggest you need professional assistance. Begin by noting when the symptom began, how often and when it occurs, what makes it worse, what makes it better, and whether you have any associated symptoms. You can also monitor your body's vital signs, such as temperature and heart rate. For some conditions, such as urinary tract infections and diabetes, medical self-tests can help you make informed decisions about when to self-treat and when you should seek medical attention.

Decision Making: Knowing When to See a Physician

In general, you should check with a physician for symptoms with the following characteristics:

1. *Severe.* If the symptom is very severe or intense, medical assistance is advised. Examples include severe pains, major injuries, and other emergencies.

2. *Unusual.* If the symptom is peculiar and unfamiliar, it is wise to check it out with your physician. Examples include unexplained lumps, changes in a mole, problems with vision, difficulty swallowing, numbness, weakness, unexplained weight loss, and blood in sputum, urine, or stool.

3. *Persistent.* If the symptom lasts longer than expected, seek medical advice. Examples in adults include fever for more than 5 days, a cough lasting longer than 2 weeks, a sore that doesn't heal within a month, and hoarseness lasting longer than 3 weeks.

4. *Recurrent.* If a symptom tends to return again and again, medical evaluation is advised. Examples include recurrent headaches, stomach pains, and backache.

Sometimes a single symptom is not a cause for concern, but a combination of symptoms may suggest a more serious problem. For example, a fever with a stiff neck suggests meningitis.

If you decide you need professional help, you must decide how urgent the problem is. If it is a true emergency, you should go (or call someone to take you) to the nearest emergency room (ER). Emergencies would include:

- Major trauma or injury, such as head injury, suspected broken bone, deep wound, severe burn, eye injury, or animal bite
- Uncontrollable bleeding or internal bleeding, as indicated by blood in the sputum, vomit, or stool
- Intolerable and uncontrollable pain or severe chest pain
- Severe shortness of breath
- Persistent abdominal pain, especially if associated with nausea and vomiting

- Poisoning or drug overdose
- Loss of consciousness or seizure
- Stupor, drowsiness, or disorientation that cannot be explained
- Severe or worsening reaction to an insect bite or sting or to a medication, especially if breathing is difficult

If your problem is not an emergency but still requires medical attention, call your physician's office. Often you can be given medical advice over the phone without the inconvenience of a visit.

WWW. Self-Treatment: Many Options

In most cases, your body can heal itself. Patience and careful self-observation are often the best choices in self-treatment. Before reaching for medication, consider all your nondrug options, which are usually safe, easy, and highly effective. Massage, ice packs, and neck exercises may be more helpful than drugs in relieving headaches, for example. Other nondrug options include getting enough rest, increasing exercise, drinking more water, using a humidifier, making ergonomic adjustments at work, and so on. For conditions caused or aggravated by stress, relaxation exercises, meditation, and other stress-management techniques usually help.

If these strategies aren't enough, you may decide to treat yourself with nonprescription or **over-the-counter (OTC) medications.** These are medicines that the Food and Drug Administration (FDA) has determined are safe for use without a physician's prescription. There are about 100,000 OTC drugs on the market; about 60% of all medications are sold over the counter. Many OTC drugs were formerly prescription drugs: More than 600 products sold over the counter today use ingredients or dosage strengths that were available only by prescription 20 years ago.

Although many OTC products are highly effective in relieving symptoms and sometimes in curing illness, others are unnecessary or divert attention from better ways of coping. Many ingredients in OTC drugs—perhaps 70%—have not been proven to be effective, a fact the FDA does not dispute. And any drug may have risks and side effects. Follow these simple guidelines to use OTC drugs safely:

1. Always read labels, and follow directions carefully. The information on most OTC drug labels now appears in a standard format developed by the FDA (Figure 15-1);

over-the-counter (OTC) medication A medication or product that can be purchased by the consumer without a prescription.

Terms

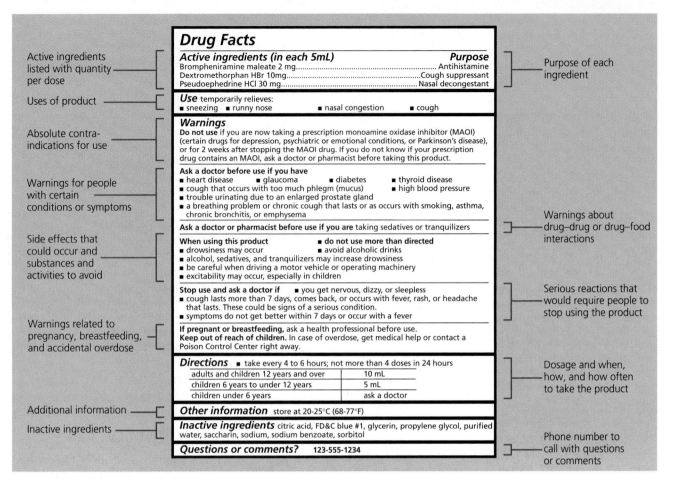

Active ingredients
listed with quantity
per dose

Uses of product

Absolute contra-
indications for use

Warnings for people
with certain
conditions or symptoms

Side effects that
could occur and
substances and
activities to avoid

Warnings related to
pregnancy, breastfeeding,
and accidental overdose

Additional information

Inactive ingredients

Drug Facts

Active ingredients (in each 5mL)   **Purpose**
Brompheniramine maleate 2 mg.. Antihistamine
Dextromethorphan HBr 10mg...Cough suppressant
Pseudoephedrine HCl 30 mg.. Nasal decongestant

Use temporarily relieves:
■ sneezing ■ runny nose   ■ nasal congestion   ■ cough

Warnings
Do not use if you are now taking a prescription monoamine oxidase inhibitor (MAOI)
(certain drugs for depression, psychiatric or emotional conditions, or Parkinson's disease),
or for 2 weeks after stopping the MAOI drug. If you do not know if your prescription
drug contains an MAOI, ask a doctor or pharmacist before taking this product.

Ask a doctor before use if you have
■ heart disease   ■ glaucoma   ■ diabetes   ■ thyroid disease
■ cough that occurs with too much phlegm (mucus)   ■ high blood pressure
■ trouble urinating due to an enlarged prostate gland
■ a breathing problem or chronic cough that lasts or as occurs with smoking, asthma,
  chronic bronchitis, or emphysema

Ask a doctor or pharmacist before use if you are taking sedatives or tranquilizers

When using this product   ■ do not use more than directed
■ drowsiness may occur   ■ avoid alcoholic drinks
■ alcohol, sedatives, and tranquilizers may increase drowsiness
■ be careful when driving a motor vehicle or operating machinery
■ excitability may occur, especially in children

Stop use and ask a doctor if   ■ you get nervous, dizzy, or sleepless
■ cough lasts more than 7 days, comes back, or occurs with fever, rash, or headache
  that lasts. These could be signs of a serious condition.
■ symptoms do not get better within 7 days or occur with a fever

If pregnant or breastfeeding, ask a health professional before use.
Keep out of reach of children. In case of overdose, get medical help or contact a
Poison Control Center right away.

Directions ■ take every 4 to 6 hours; not more than 4 doses in 24 hours

adults and children 12 years and over	10 mL
children 6 years to under 12 years	5 mL
children under 6 years	ask a doctor

Other information store at 20-25°C (68-77°F)

Inactive ingredients citric acid, FD&C blue #1, glycerin, propylene glycol, purified
water, saccharin, sodium, sodium benzoate, sorbitol

Questions or comments?   123-555-1234

Purpose of each
ingredient

Warnings about
drug–drug or drug–food
interactions

Serious reactions that
would require people to
stop using the product

Dosage and when,
how, and how often
to take the product

Phone number to
call with questions
or comments

Figure 15-1   Reading and understanding OTC drug labels.   SOURCE: Food and Drug Administration. 1999. Over-the-counter human drugs; labeling requirements; final rule. *Federal Register 64,* no. 51 (17
March): 13254–13303.

2. Do not exceed the recommended dosage or length of treatment unless you discuss this change with your physician.

3. Use caution if you are taking other medications, because OTC and prescription drugs and herbs can interact. If you have questions about drug interactions, ask your physician or pharmacist *before* you mix medicines.

4. Try to select medications with one active ingredient rather than combination ("all-in-one") products. A product with multiple ingredients is likely to include drugs for symptoms you don't have.

5. When choosing medications, try to buy **generic drugs,** which contain the same active ingredient as the brand-name product but generally at a much lower cost.

6. If you are pregnant or nursing or have a chronic condition such as kidney disease, consult your physician before self-medicating.

7. The expiration date marked on many medications is an estimate of how long the *unopened* medication is likely to be potent. Once the package is opened, the medication will probably be potent for about a year if stored properly. Mark the date on the package when you open it, and dispose of it safely after a year by taking it to a pharmacy or hospital.

8. Store your medications in a cool, dry place—not the medicine cabinet in your bathroom—that is out of the reach of children.

9. Use special caution with aspirin. Because of an association with a rare but serious problem known as Reye's syndrome, aspirin should not be used by children or adolescents who may have the flu, chicken pox, or any other viral illness.

Only a few basic medicines and supplies are really needed in your home medicine cabinet; they include such items as adhesive bandages and antibacterial ointment for minor wounds; a thermometer for taking your tempera-

Table 15-1	Use of Complementary and Alternative Therapies in the United States	
		Percent Who Used Therapy at Least Once in Past 12 Months
Relaxation techniques		16.3
Herbal medicine		12.1
Massage		11.1
Chiropractic		11.0
Spiritual healing (by others)		7.0
Megavitamins		5.5
Self-help group		4.8
Imagery		4.5
Commercial diet		4.4
Folk remedies		4.2
Lifestyle diet		4.0
Energy healing		3.8
Homeopathy		3.4
Hypnosis		1.2
Biofeedback		1.0
Acupuncture		1.0
Any therapy		42.1

SOURCE: Eisenberg, D. M., et al. 1998. Trends in alternative medicine use in the United States, 1990–1997: Results of a follow-up national survey. *Journal of the American Medical Association* 280: 1569–1575.

ture; ibuprofen, aspirin, or similar drugs for minor pain or fever; antihistamines for allergies; antacids for heartburn and indigestion; hydrocortisone cream or baking soda for skin irritations; lozenges for sore throat; needle-nosed tweezers for splinters; elastic bandages, ice packs, and heating pads for sprains and strains; cough syrup for coughs; decongestant for nasal congestion; and sunscreen to prevent sunburn. Additional items depend on the particular health problems you or your family are likely to have.

PROFESSIONAL MEDICAL AND HEALTH CARE: CHOICES AND CHANGE

When self-treatment is not appropriate or sufficient, you need to seek professional medical care, whether by going to a hospital emergency room, by scheduling an appointment with your physician, or by accessing some other part of the American medical and health care system. This system is a broad network of individuals and organizations, including independent practitioners, allied health care providers, hospitals, clinics, and public and private insurance programs.

In recent years, many Americans have also sought health care from practitioners of **complementary and alternative medicine (CAM)**, defined as those therapies and practices that do not form part of conventional, or "mainstream," health care and medical practices as taught in most U.S. medical schools and offered in most U.S. hospitals. The most commonly used CAM therapies are relaxation techniques, herbal medicine, massage, and chiropractic (Table 15-1). Consumers turn to CAM for a large variety of purposes related to health and well-being, such as boosting their immune system, lowering their cholesterol levels, losing weight, quitting smoking, or enhancing their memory. There are indications that people with chronic conditions, including cancer, asthma, autoimmune diseases, and HIV infection, are particularly likely to try CAM therapies. Despite their growing popularity, many CAM practices remain controversial, and individuals need to be critically aware of safety issues. In the next sections of this chapter, we examine the principles and providers of both **conventional medicine**—the dominant medical system in the United States and Europe, also referred to as standard Western medicine or biomedicine—and of complementary and alternative medicine, with particular attention to consumer issues.

CONVENTIONAL MEDICINE

Referring to conventional medicine as "standard Western medicine" draws attention to the fact that it differs from the various medical systems that have developed in China, Japan, India, and other parts of the world. Calling it "biomedicine" reflects the concept that conventional medicine is based on the findings of a variety of biological sciences.

Premises and Assumptions of Conventional Medicine

One of the important characteristics of Western medicine is the belief that disease is caused by identifiable physical factors. This belief can be traced back to Hippocrates, the

Terms

generic drug A drug that is not registered or protected by a trademark; a drug that does not have a brand name.

complementary and alternative medicine (CAM) Therapies or practices that are not part of conventional or mainstream health care and medical practice as taught in most U.S. medical schools and available at most U.S. health care facilities; examples of CAM practices include acupuncture, herbal remedies, and homeopathy.

conventional medicine A system of medicine based on the application of the scientific method; diseases are thought to be caused by identifiable physical factors and characterized by a representative set of symptoms; also called biomedicine or standard Western medicine.

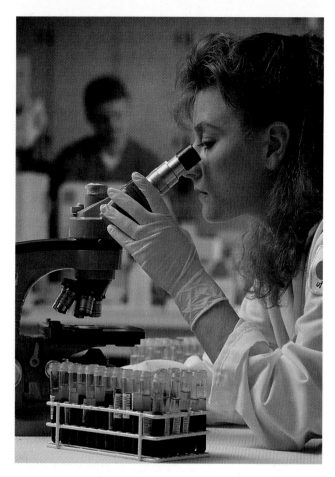

Conventional Western medicine is firmly grounded in scientific explanations resulting from the application of the scientific method to a question or problem. The identification of viruses, bacteria, and other microorganisms as a key cause of disease led to many public health measures and treatments that reduced deaths from infectious diseases in the United States.

of destroying pathogens or preventing them from causing serious infection. The public health measures of the nineteenth and twentieth centuries—chlorination of drinking water, sewage disposal, food safety regulations, vaccination programs, education about hygiene, and so on—are an outgrowth of this kind of orientation. (As described in Chapter 1, these public health measures are largely responsible for the 25-year increase in life expectancy that Americans experienced in the twentieth century.)

The implementation of public health measures is one way to control pathogens; another is the use of drugs. The discovery and development of sulfa drugs, antibiotics, and steroids in the twentieth century, along with advances in chemistry that made it possible to identify the active ingredients in common herbal remedies, paved the way for the current close identification of Western medicine with **pharmaceuticals** (medical drugs, both prescription and over-the-counter). Western medicine also relies heavily on surgery and on advanced medical technology to discover the physical causes of disease and to remove or destroy them.

Finally, Western medicine is based on scientific ways of obtaining knowledge and explaining phenomena. Scientific explanations have a blend of characteristics that set them apart from other types of explanations, such as those based on common sense, faith, or authority. Scientific explanations are

- *Empirical*—they are based on the evidence of the senses and on objective and systematic observation, often carried out under carefully controlled conditions; they must be capable of verification by others.
- *Rational*—they follow the rules of logic and are consistent with known facts.
- *Testable*—either they are verifiable through direct observation or they lead to predictions about what should occur under conditions not yet observed.
- *Parsimonious*—they explain phenomena with the fewest number of assumptions.
- *General*—they have broad explanatory power.
- *Rigorously evaluated*—they are constantly evaluated for consistency with the evidence and known principles, for parsimony, and for generality.
- *Tentative*—scientists are willing to entertain the possibility that their explanations are faulty.

Western medicine translates the scientific method into practice through the research process, a highly refined and well-established approach to exploring the causes of disease and ensuring the safety and efficacy of treatments. Research studies range from case studies—descriptions of a single patient's illness and treatment—to clinical trials conducted on large populations and carried out under carefully controlled conditions over a period of many years. The process of drug development is equally rigorous. Drugs are developed and tested through an elaborate

Greek physician of the fourth century B.C. who is credited with placing the practice of medicine on a scientific footing. In Hippocrates' time, the causes of disease were thought to include the interplay of various forces and elements; today, Western medicine identifies the causes of disease as pathogens, such as bacteria and viruses, genetic factors, and unhealthy lifestyles that result in changes at the molecular and cellular levels. In most cases, however, the focus is primarily on the physical causes of the illness rather than mental or spiritual imbalance.

Another feature that distinguishes Western biomedicine from other medical systems is the concept that every disease is defined by a certain set of symptoms and that these symptoms are similar in most patients suffering from this disease. Western medicine tends to treat illness as an isolated biological disturbance that can occur in any human being, rather than as integral in some way to the individual with the illness.

Related to the idea of illness as the result of invasion by outside factors is the strong orientation toward methods

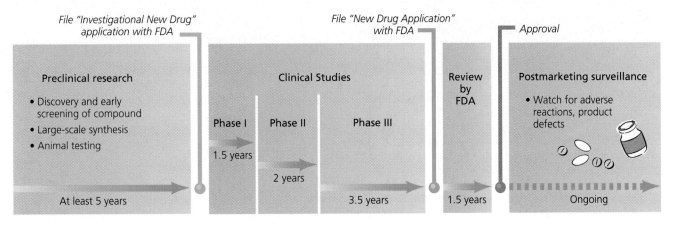

Figure 15-2   Timeline for drug development.   Once preclinical research indicates that a drug is both safe and effective, it can be tested in humans. In Phase I trials, a small group of healthy human volunteers is given the treatment to screen it for safety and to establish a maximum safe dose. In Phase II trials, a small group of patients with the condition the drug is supposed to improve is given the treatment to help screen for adverse effects and to determine appropriate dosages. In Phase III trials, a larger group of patients is given the treatment to determine if it is effective and what the common side effects are. Researchers and the FDA have made efforts to shorten the process, but thorough drug testing takes many years.   SOURCE: Timeline for drug development. 2000. *Scientific American,* April.

course that begins with preliminary research in the lab and continues through trials with human participants, review and approval by the FDA, and monitoring of the drug's effects after it is on the market (Figure 15-2).

When results of research studies are published in medical journals, a community of scientists, physicians, researchers, and scholars have the opportunity to share the findings and enter a dialogue about the subject. Publication of research often prompts further research designed to replicate and confirm the findings, challenge the conclusions, or pursue a related line of thought or experiment.

The Providers of Conventional Medicine

Conventional medicine is practiced by a wide range of health care professionals in the United States. Several kinds of professionals are permitted to practice medicine independently; these include medical doctors, osteopaths, podiatrists, optometrists, and dentists.

• **Medical doctors** are practitioners who hold a doctor of medicine (M.D.) degree from an accredited medical school. During graduate medical study, called a residency and lasting from three to eight years, M.D.s choose a specialty and obtain a medical license. Twenty-three medical specialties are currently approved by the American Board of Medical Specialties, each with its own rule-making and certifying body. Examples of specialties and their areas of interest include allergy and immunology (disorders of the immune system), anesthesiology (pain relief during medical procedures), dermatology

(disorders of the skin), emergency medicine (acute illness and injury), internal medicine (comprehensive care), neurology (disorders of the brain and nervous system), ophthalmology (disorders and injuries of the eyes), pathology (diagnosis and monitoring of disease, mainly through laboratory techniques), plastic surgery (repair of physical defects), psychiatry (mental and emotional disorders), radiology (diagnosis and treatment of disease through radiological methods, such as X ray), and urology (disorders of the reproductive and urinary systems). The larger specialties are further divided into subspecialties; for example, internal medicine includes such subspecialties as cardiology and gastroenterology.

• **Doctors of osteopathic medicine** (D.O.) are graduates of osteopathic medical schools, which place special emphasis on musculoskeletal problems and manipulative therapy. M.D.s and D.O.s are the two types of "complete" physicians in the United States, meaning they are fully trained and licensed to perform surgery and prescribe medication.

pharmaceuticals Medical drugs, both prescription and over-the-counter.

medical doctor An independent practitioner who holds a doctor of medicine degree from an accredited medical school.

doctor of osteopathic medicine A medical practitioner who has graduated from an osteopathic medical school; osteopathy incorporates the theories and practices of scientific medicine but focuses on musculoskeletal problems and manipulative therapy.

Terms

Health-related research is now described in popular newspapers and magazines rather than just medical journals, meaning that more and more people have access to the information. Greater access is certainly a plus, but news reports of research studies may oversimplify both the results and what those results mean to the average person. Researchers do not set out to mislead people, but they must often strike a balance between reporting promising preliminary findings to the public, thereby allowing people to act on them, and waiting 10–20 years until long-term studies confirm (or disprove) a particular theory.

All this can leave you in a difficult position. You cannot become an expert on all subjects, capable of effectively evaluating all the available health news. However, the following questions can help you better assess the health advice that appears in the popular media:

1. *Is the report based on research or on an anecdote?* Information or advice based on one or more carefully designed research studies has more validity than one person's experiences.

2. *What is the source of the information?* A study published in a respected peer-reviewed journal has been examined by editors and other researchers in the field, people who are in a position to evaluate the merits of a study and its results. Research presented at medical meetings should be considered very preliminary because the results have not yet undergone a thorough pre-publication review. It is also wise to ask who funded a study to determine whether there is any potential for bias. Information from government agencies and national research organizations is usually considered fairly reliable.

3. *How big was the study?* A study that involves many subjects is more likely to yield reliable results than a study involving only a few people. Another important indication that a finding is meaningful is if several different studies yield the same results.

4. *Who were the participants involved in the study?* Research findings are more likely to apply to you if you share important characteristics with the participants of the study. For example, the results of a study on men over age 50 who smoke may not be particularly meaningful for a 30-year-old nonsmoking woman. Even less applicable are studies done in test tubes or on animals. Such research should be considered very preliminary in terms of its applicability to humans. Promising results from laboratory or animal research frequently cannot be replicated in human study subjects.

5. *What kind of study was it?* Epidemiological studies involve observation or interviews in order to trace the relationship among lifestyle, physical characteristics, and diseases. While epidemiological studies can suggest links, they cannot establish cause-and-effect relationships. Clinical or interventional studies or trials involve testing the effects of different treatments on groups of people who have similar lifestyles and characteristics. They are more likely to provide conclusive evidence of a cause-and-effect relationship. The best interventional studies share the following characteristics:

- *Controlled.* A group of people who receive the treatment is compared with a matched group who do not receive the treatment.

- *Randomized.* The treatment and control groups are selected randomly.

- *Double-blind.* Researchers and participants are unaware of who is receiving the treatment.

- *Multicenter.* The experiment is performed at more than one institution.

A third type of study, meta-analysis, involves combining the results of individual studies to get an overall view of the effectiveness of a treatment.

6. *What do the statistics really say?* First, are the results described as "statistically significant"? If a study is large and well designed, its results can be deemed statistically significant, meaning there is less than a 5% chance that the findings resulted from chance. Second, are the results stated in terms of relative or absolute risk? Many findings are reported in terms of relative risk—how a particular treatment or condition affects a person's disease risk. Consider the following examples of relative risk:

- According to some estimates, taking estrogen without progesterone can increase a postmenopausal woman's risk of dying from endometrial cancer by 233%.

- Giving AZT to HIV-infected pregnant women reduces prenatal transmission of HIV by about 90%.

The first of these two findings seems far more dramatic than the second—until one also considers absolute risk, the actual risk of the illness in the population being considered. The absolute risk of endometrial cancer is 0.3%; a 233% increase based on the effects of estrogen raises it to 1%, a change of 0.7%. Without treatment, about 25% of infants born to HIV-infected women will be infected with HIV; with treatment, the absolute risk drops to about 2%, a change of 23%. Because the absolute risk of an HIV-infected mother passing the virus to her infant is so much greater than a woman's risk of developing endometrial cancer (25% compared with 0.3%), a smaller change in relative risk translates into a much greater change in absolute risk.

7. *Is new health advice being offered?* If the media report new guidelines for health behavior or medical treatment, examine the source. Government agencies and national research foundations usually consider a great deal of evidence before offering health advice. Above all, use common sense, and check with your physician before making a major change in your health habits based on news reports.

SOURCES: Medical research: Finding the best information. 2000. *Journal of the American Medical Association* 284(10): 1336. Medicine and the media. 1999. *Harvard Women's Health Watch,* February. Medical hype: How to read between the lines. 1998. *Consumer Reports on Health,* October. Making sense of health research. 1998. *Healthline,* May.

- **Podiatrists** are practitioners who specialize in the medical and surgical care of the feet; they hold a doctor of podiatric medicine (D.P.M.) degree.

- **Optometrists** are practitioners trained to examine the eyes, detect eye diseases, and treat vision problems; they hold a doctor of optometry (O.D.) degree.

- **Dentists** specialize in the care of the teeth and mouth. They are graduates of four-year dental schools and hold the doctor of dental surgery (D.D.S.) or doctor of medical dentistry (D.M.D.) degree.

In addition to these practitioners, there are millions of other trained health care professionals, known as **allied health care providers,** working in the United States. Some of them are licensed to work independently; others are permitted to work under medical supervision or medical referral. They include registered nurses (R.N.), licensed vocational nurses (L.V.N.), physical therapists, social workers, registered dietitians (R.D.), physician assistants (P.A.), nurse practitioners, and certified nurse midwives.

Choosing a Primary Care Physician

Most experts believe it is best to have a primary care physician, someone who gets to know you, who coordinates your medical care, and who refers you to specialists when you need them. Primary care physicians include those certified in family practice, internal medicine, pediatrics, and obstetrics-gynecology. These physicians are able to diagnose and treat the vast majority of common health problems; they also provide many preventive health services. The best time to look for a physician is before you are sick.

To select a physician, begin by making a list of possible choices. If your insurance limits the health care providers you can see, check the plan's list first. Ask for recommendations from family, friends, coworkers, local medical societies, and the physician referral service at a local clinic or hospital. Once you have the names of a few physicians you might want to try, call their offices to find out information such as the following:

- Is the physician covered by your health plan and accepting new patients?

- What are the office hours, and when is the physician or office staff available? What do patients do if they need urgent care or have an emergency?

- Which hospitals does the physician use?

- How many other physicians are available to "cover" when he or she isn't available, and who are they?

- How long does it usually take to get a routine appointment?

- Does the physician (or a nurse or physician assistant) give advice over the phone for common medical problems?

Finally, schedule a visit with the physician you think you would most like to use. During that first visit, you'll get a sense of how well matched you are and how well he or she might meet your medical needs. After the visit, consider whether you felt comfortable with the physician, felt listened to and respected, and understood what you were told. Although you may want to give the relationship some time to develop, you should trust your own reactions when deciding whether a particular health care provider is the right one for you.

Getting the Most out of Your Medical Care

The key to getting the most out of your medical care is good communication with your physician and other members of the health care team. Studies show that patients who are more active in interacting with physicians, who ask more questions, enjoy better health outcomes.

Developing a Partnership with Your Physician The image of the all-knowing physician and the passive patient is slowly fading. What is emerging is more of a physician-patient *partnership,* in which the physician acts more like a consultant and the patient participates more actively. You should expect your physician to be attentive, caring, able to listen, and able to clearly explain things to you. You also have to do your part. You need to be assertive in a firm but not aggressive manner. You need to express your feelings and concerns, ask questions, and, if necessary, be persistent. If your physician is unable to communicate clearly with you in spite of your best efforts, then you probably need to change physicians.

When you have an appointment with your physician, make a written list of your most important concerns and questions, along with notes about your symptoms. Present your concerns at the beginning of the visit, to set the agenda. Be specific and concise about your symptoms, and be open and honest about your concerns. Let

Terms

podiatrist A practitioner who holds a doctor of podiatric medicine degree and specializes in the medical and surgical care of the feet.

optometrist A practitioner who holds a doctor of optometry degree and is trained to examine the eyes, detect eye diseases, and prescribe corrective lenses.

dentist A practitioner who holds a doctor of medical dentistry or doctor of dental surgery degree and who specializes in the prevention and treatment of diseases and injuries of the teeth, mouth, and jaws.

allied health care providers Health care professionals who typically provide services under the supervision or control of independent practitioners.

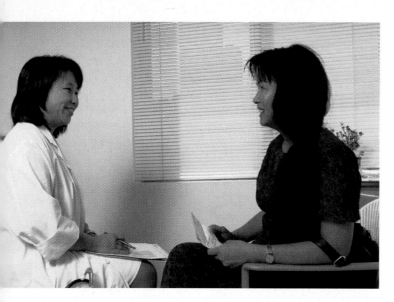

Good communication is a crucial factor in a satisfactory physician-patient partnership.

your physician know if you are taking any drugs, are allergic to any medications, are breastfeeding, or may be pregnant.

COMMUNICATE! To build a partnership with your physician, let him or her know that you want to be an active participant in your health care. One way to do that is to ask questions; another is to ask for written information or literature about your condition or sources where you can read more. Offer information about your personal or family history if you think it's relevant (or remind the physician of such information if it's part of your health record); for example, "I started using a new fabric softener about a month ago—could that be causing this rash?" Discuss your treatment plan with your physician, especially if you're not comfortable with any part of it. For example, "I had a hard time with the side effects of that medication the last time I took it. Is there anything else available?" or "I think I'm mildly depressed, but I don't really want to take an antidepressant. Are there any behavioral things that would help me, like exercise or yoga?"

WW. The Diagnostic Process An important part of your visit is the medical history, which includes your primary reason for the visit, your current symptoms, your past medical history, and your social history (job, family life, major stressors, living conditions, and health habits). Keeping up-to-date records of your medical history can help you provide your physician with key facts about your health.

The next step is the physical exam, which usually begins with a review of vital signs: blood pressure, heart rate (pulse), breathing rate, and temperature. Depending on your primary complaint, your physician may give you a complete physical, or the exam may be directed to specific areas, such as your ears, nose, and throat.

Finally, your physician may order medical tests to complete the diagnosis. Physicians can order X rays, biopsies, blood and urine tests, scans of various types, and a wide array of **endoscopies** to view, probe, or analyze almost any part of the body. If your physician orders a medical test for you, be sure you know why you need it, what the risks and benefits of the test are for you, how you should prepare for it (for example, by fasting or discontinuing medications or herbal remedies), and what the test will involve. Also ask what the test results mean, since no test is 100% accurate—**false positives** and **false negatives** do occur—and interpretation of some procedures is subjective.

At the end of the visit, briefly repeat the physician's diagnosis, prognosis, and instructions, and make sure you understand your next steps, such as making another appointment, phoning for test results, watching for new symptoms, and so on. You may also want to ask about the possibility of using e-mail for follow-up.

Prescription Medications and Surgical Treatments
Once the diagnosis is made, you and your physician can consider treatment options. Many conditions can be treated in a variety of ways; in some cases, lifestyle changes should be considered along with other options.

If lifestyle changes aren't an option, your physician may prescribe prescription medications for you. Although these powerful drugs—**antibiotics,** heart medications, insulin, and scores of others—save thousands of lives each year, they need to be treated carefully. Each year, more than 7000 deaths occur in hospitals alone from medication errors. Prescription drugs may also have side effects that didn't show up in clinical trials; consumers should be especially alert for adverse effects if they are taking a drug that is new to the market.

Another problem is that physicians may overprescribe drugs, sometimes in response to pressure by patients. Consumers are now the target of multibillion-dollar direct-to-consumer (DTC) advertising campaigns for prescription drugs, which may cause patients to press physicians to prescribe particular drugs.

A recent area of concern is the advent of online pharmacies. Although convenient, some online pharmacies may sell products or engage in practices that are illegal in the offline world. The Food and Drug Administration (FDA) recommends that consumers avoid sites that offer to prescribe drugs for the first time without a physical exam, sell prescription drugs without a prescription, or sell drugs not approved by the FDA. You should also

There are many potential benefits of e-mail communication with your physician. Both you and your physician may find it more convenient than phone calls or personal appointments because you can send messages briefly, at convenient times. It allows for clarification and advice in writing, which can remove any doubt about what your physician is recommending. Unlike telephone conversations, e-mail is self-documenting, meaning that copies of both your e-mail and those of your physician can be placed in your medical file. For information such as test results, having a written record can be very helpful.

If you like the idea, talk with your physician about the possibility of e-mail communication. If he or she already has a system set up, ask about the policies and procedures. The following guidelines can help you use e-mail with your physician effectively and safely:

- Find out what types of transactions can be carried out over e-mail. For example, can appointment scheduling and prescription refills be handled with e-mail?

- Do not use e-mail communication for emergencies and other time-sensitive issues or for confidential or sensitive information.

- Be concise—to save time for both yourself and your physician.

- Put the type of transaction and your name and medical record number in the appropriate place designated by your physician. She or he may ask that certain information be included in the subject line of your e-mail or at the top of the body of the message.

- If requested, send a reply to the physician's e-mail to acknowledge that you've received and understood the message.

- Keep copies of any e-mail that you send or receive.

- Be aware that your physician may share your e-mail with office staff or other consultants.

SOURCES: American Medical Association. 2000. *Guidelines for Physician-Patient Electronic Communications* (http://www.ama-assn.org/ama/pub/category/2386.html; retrieved December 17, 2000). Sands, D. Z. 2000. *How to Communicate with Your Doctor Using Email* (http://www.healthology.com/focus_article.asp?f=healthcare&rc=healthcare_emaildoctor; retrieved October 19, 2000).

---

avoid sites that do not provide access to a registered pharmacist to answer questions or that do not provide a U.S. address and phone number to contact if there's a problem. The National Association of Boards of Pharmacy sponsors a voluntary certification program for Internet pharmacies; to be certified, a pharmacy must have a state license in good standing and allow regular inspections.

Patients also share some responsibility for problems with prescription drugs. An estimated 30–50% of the more than 3 billion prescriptions dispensed annually in the United States are not taken correctly and thus do not produce the desired results. Consumers can increase the effectiveness of their treatment and decrease the chances of adverse effects by asking the following questions:

- *Do I really need this prescription, or are there nondrug alternatives?*

- *What is the name of the medication, and what is it supposed to do, within what period of time?*

- *How and when do I take the medication, how much do I take, and for how long? What should I do if I miss a dose?*

- *What other medications, foods, drinks, or activities should I avoid?* Other drugs, including alcohol, herbs, and OTC drugs, can interact with medications, diminishing or increasing their effect. For example, certain antibiotics, including ampicillin and tetracycline, may prevent oral contraceptives from working. Others may increase the effects of sunlight on the skin.

- *What are the side effects, and what do I do if they occur?*

- *Can I take a generic drug rather than a brand-name one?* Generic drugs contain the same ingredients as the original brand-name drug, but they may contain different inactive ingredients. They are usually substantially less expensive, but sometimes physicians have reasons for preferring a particular brand.

- *Is there written information about the medication?* There are many sources of information, including the FDA-approved inserts in drug packaging and books and pamphlets.

---

endoscopy A medical procedure in which a viewing instrument is inserted into a body cavity or opening. Specific procedures are named for the area viewed: inside joints (arthroscopy), inside airways (bronchoscopy), inside the abdominal cavity (laparoscopy), and inside the lower portion of the large intestine, or sigmoid colon (sigmoidoscopy).

false positive A test result that incorrectly detects a disease or condition in a healthy person.

false negative A test result that fails to correctly detect a disease or condition.

antibiotic A substance derived from a mold or bacterium that inhibits the growth of other microorganisms.

Terms

Another treatment option your physician may propose is surgery. Each year, more than 70 million operations and related procedures are performed in the United States. If your physician recommends surgery, make sure you know the answers to these questions:

- *Why do I need surgery at this time?* Your physician should be able to explain the reason for the surgery and what is likely to happen if you don't have it. Getting a second opinion about surgery is recommended and may be required by your health insurance plan.

- *What are the risks and complications of the surgery?* Overall risk depends on the type of operation performed, the surgeon, and your general state of health. Ask about the **mortality rate** (risk of death) and the **morbidity rate** (risk of nonlethal complications).

- *Can the operation be performed on an outpatient basis?* **Outpatient** (ambulatory) surgery has many advantages, including lower costs and fewer opportunities for hospital-associated complications.

- *What can I expect before, during, and after surgery?* Knowing what to expect can help you prepare for the surgery and speed your recovery.

COMMUNICATE! Drug manufacturers try to sell their products directly to the public through their advertising, whether for over-the-counter medications, prescription drugs, or dietary supplements. Critically examine and evaluate an ad in a magazine or on TV for a health-related product or service. What is the manufacturer communicating about the product and about health in general? What underlying premises can you discern in the way the product is presented and the promises the manufacturer makes? Does the ad contain any hidden messages? Are there any aspects of the ad you feel are misleading? Do you find it easy or difficult to resist the appeal of the ad and the product?

WW. COMPLEMENTARY AND ALTERNATIVE MEDICINE

Although conventional medicine is also taught and practiced in non-Western countries, many cultures have developed and continue to use medical systems based on philosophies and concepts very different from those of Western medicine. Today, many forms of medicine from Asia, as well as from indigenous systems of healing that developed in societies around the world, are being practiced in the United States and are becoming increasingly popular. These systems are referred to as **traditional medicine,** or, in the context of conventional Western medicine, complementary and alternative medicine.

These traditional systems and practices tend to view health more holistically, as a balance of body systems—mental, emotional, and spiritual, as well as physical. All aspects of the person are thought to be interrelated, forming an integrated system—a principle called **holism.** An imbalance or disharmony in any aspect can stress the body and lead to illness; the goal of traditional medicine is to strengthen the body's defenses and restore harmony. Thus, where conventional Western medicine tends to focus on the body, on the physical causes of disease, and on ways to eradicate pathogens in order to restore health, traditional medicine tends to focus on an integration of mind, body, and spirit and to seek ways to restore the whole person to harmony so that he or she can regain health. Where conventional medicine is based on science, traditional medicine tends to be based on accumulated experience.

With the objective of encouraging scientific research on some of the more promising alternative therapies, the National Institutes of Health created the Office of Alternative Medicine in 1992. It was soon recognized that many people were using such "alternative" approaches in addition to conventional medical treatments, rather than in their place. In other words, they wanted to complement, not replace, conventional medical practices. Thus, the term "complementary and alternative" has become accepted to describe therapies that are not currently considered mainstream health care practices in the United States. Accordingly, the Office of Alternative Medicine has been renamed the National Center for Complementary and Alternative Medicine (NCCAM).

NCCAM groups CAM practices into five domains: alternative medical systems, mind-body interventions, biological-based therapies, manipulative and body-based methods, and energy therapies (Figure 15-3). What follows is a general introduction to the types of CAM available and a brief description of some of the more widely used ones. To learn more about any of these approaches, consult the For More Information section at the end of the chapter.

Alternative Medical Systems

Many cultures elaborated complete systems of medical philosophy, theory, and practice long before the current biomedical approach was developed. The complete systems that are best known in the United States are probably traditional Chinese medicine (TCM), also known as traditional Oriental medicine, and homeopathy. Traditional medical systems have also been developed in many other regions of the world, including North, Central, and South America; the Middle East; India; Tibet; and Australia. In many countries, these medical approaches continue to be used today—frequently alongside Western medicine and quite often by physicians trained in Western medicine.

Alternative medical systems tend to have concepts in common, perhaps because of contact between the Mediterranean area, the Middle East, India, and China in

Domain	Characteristics	Examples
Alternative Medical Systems	Involve complete systems of theory and practice that have evolved independently of and often long before the conventional biomedical approach	Traditional Chinese medicine; Kampo; Ayurveda (India); Native American, Aboriginal, African, Middle-Eastern, Tibetan, Central and South American medical systems; homeopathy; naturopathy
Mind-Body Interventions	Employ a variety of techniques designed to make it possible for the mind to affect bodily function and symptoms	Meditation, certain uses of hypnosis, prayer, mental healing
Biological-Based Therapies	Include natural and biologically based practices, interventions, and products, many of which overlap with conventional medicine's use of dietary supplements	Herbal, special dietary, orthomolecular,* and individual biological therapies
Manipulative and Body-Based Methods	Include methods that are based on manipulation and/or movement of the body	Chiropractic, osteopathy, massage therapy
Energy Therapies	Focus on energy fields within the body (biofields) or from other sources (electromagnetic fields)	Qi gong, Reiki, therapeutic touch, bioelectromagnetic-based therapies

*Orthomolecular therapies are treatments of diseases with varying, but usually high, concentrations of chemicals, including minerals (e.g., magnesium), hormones (e.g., melatonin), or vitamins.

Figure 15-3   The five domains of CAM practices.

ancient times. For example, the concept of life force or energy exists in many cultures. In traditional Chinese medicine, the life force contained in all living things is called *qi* (sometimes spelled chi). In Ayurveda, the traditional medical system of India, the life force is called *prana*.

Most traditional medical systems think of disease as a disturbance or imbalance not just of physical processes but also of forces and energies within the body, the mind, and the spirit. Treatment aims at reestablishing equilibrium, balance, and harmony. Because the whole patient, rather than an isolated set of symptoms, is treated in most comprehensive alternative medical systems, it is rare that only a single treatment approach is used. Most commonly, multiple techniques and methods are employed and are continually adjusted according to the changes in the patient's health status that occur naturally or are brought about by the treatment.

Traditional Chinese Medicine (TCM)   In **traditional Chinese medicine (TCM)**, the free and harmonious flow of qi produces health—a positive feeling of well-being and vitality in body, mind, and spirit. Illness occurs when the flow of qi is blocked or disturbed. TCM works to restore and balance the flow of blocked qi; the goal is not only to treat illnesses but also to increase energy, prevent disease, and support the immune system.

Two of the primary treatment methods in TCM are herbal remedies and **acupuncture**. Chinese herbal remedies number about 5,800 and include plant products, animal parts, and minerals. The use of a single medicinal botanical is rare in Chinese herbal medicine; rather, several different plants are combined in very precise

Terms

mortality rate The number of deaths occurring in a population of a given size in a given time period.

morbidity rate The number of illnesses or injuries occurring in a population of a given size in a given time period.

outpatient A person receiving medical attention without being admitted to the hospital.

traditional medicine Medical systems that have developed in many non-Western cultures; also referred to as complementary and alternative medicine.

holism The principle that all aspects of a person are interrelated and form an integrated system.

traditional Chinese medicine (TCM) The traditional medical system of China, which views illness as the result of a disturbance in the flow of qi, the life force; therapies include acupuncture, herbal medicine, and massage.

acupuncture Insertion of long, thin needles into the skin at points along meridians, pathways through which qi is believed to flow; needles correct imbalances in qi; a practice common in traditional Chinese medicine.

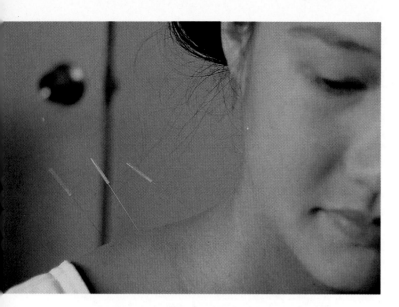

Acupuncture is one of the key treatment methods in traditional Chinese medicine. It involves the insertion of long, thin needles at appropriate points in the skin to restore balance to the flow of qi.

proportions, often to make a tea or soup. For example, a remedy might include a primary herb that targets the main symptom, a second herb that enhances the effects of the primary herb, a third that lessens side effects, and a fourth that helps deliver ingredients to a particular body site.

Acupuncture works to correct disturbances in the flow of qi through the insertion of long, thin needles at appropriate points in the skin. Qi is believed to flow through the body along several meridians, or pathways, and there are approximately 360 acupuncture points located along these meridians. The points chosen for acupuncture are highly individualized for each patient, and they change over the course of treatment as the patient's health status changes.

The World Health Organization has compiled a list of over 40 conditions in which acupuncture may be beneficial. At a conference called by the National Institutes of Health (NIH), a panel of experts found evidence that acupuncture was effective in relieving nausea and vomiting after chemotherapy and pain after surgery, including dental surgery. They added, however, that there is not yet enough evidence to show that acupuncture is effective for headaches, menstrual cramps, tennis elbow, back pain, carpal tunnel syndrome, asthma, or other conditions. Although Western researchers might acknowledge the effects of acupuncture, they typically use a different framework for understanding them. For example, they might explain pain relief not in terms of qi but in terms of stimulation of the central nervous system and release of hormones and neurotransmitters.

Although more than 1 million Americans receive acupuncture each year, there have been few adverse events (negative effects) associated with it in the United States. Nonetheless, problems can occur from the improper insertion and manipulation of needles and from the use of unsterile needles. The FDA regulates acupuncture needles like other standard medical devices and requires that they be sterile. A majority of states require some form of licensing or credentialing for practitioners of acupuncture, but the requirements for licensure vary widely.

Homeopathy   An alternative medical system of Western origin, **homeopathy** was developed about 200 years ago by the German physician Samuel Hahnemann (1755–1843) and is based on two main principles: "like cures like," and remedies become more effective with greater dilution. "Like cures like" summarizes the concept that a substance that produces the symptoms of an illness or disease in a healthy person can cure the illness when given in very minute quantities. Remedies containing very small quantities of a particular substance are obtained by repeatedly diluting the original solution. The extent of dilution varies, but the final extract is often so dilute that few, if any, of the original molecules are left in it. According to homeopathic thinking, such highly diluted extracts not only retain some form of biological activity but actually become more potent.

Over 1000 different substances (plant and animal parts, minerals, and chemicals) can be used to prepare homeopathic remedies, and each of these substances is thought to have different effects at different dilutions. That means a homeopath must not only choose the correct remedy for a particular patient but also decide on the specific dilution of that remedy in order to achieve the desired effect.

In order to assess a patient's condition, homeopaths generally spend quite a bit of time talking with a patient and assessing his or her physical, psychological, and emotional health before deciding on the correct remedy at the proper dilution. This intensive interaction between the practitioner and the patient might play an important role in the success of the therapy. Indeed, critics of homeopathy often attribute its reported effectiveness to this nonspecific "placebo effect." However, when the results of 185 homeopathic trials were analyzed recently, it was concluded that the clinical effects of homeopathy could not be completely explained by the placebo effect. At the same time, homeopathy was not found to be effective for any single clinical condition. Homeopathy remains one of the most controversial forms of CAM.

Because of the extremely dilute nature of homeopathic remedies, it is generally assumed that they are safe. To date, the FDA has not found any serious adverse events associated with the use of homeopathy, with the possible exception of situations in which a patient might have been successfully treated with standard medical approaches but chose to rely solely on homeopathy. The

A placebo is a chemically inactive substance or ineffective proce-dure that a patient believes is an effective medical therapy for his or her condition. Researchers frequently give placebos to the control group in an experiment testing the efficacy of a particu-lar treatment. By comparing the effects of the actual treatment with the effects of the placebo, researchers can judge whether or not the treatment is effective. The so-called placebo effect occurs when a patient improves after receiving a placebo. In such cases, the effect of the placebo on the patient cannot be attributed to the specific actions or properties of the drug or procedure.

Researchers have consistently found that 30–40% of all pa-tients given a placebo show improvement. This result has been observed for a wide variety of conditions or symptoms, includ-ing coughing, seasickness, depression, migraines, and angina. For some conditions, placebos have been effective in up to 70% of patients. In some cases, people given a placebo even report having the side effects associated with an actual drug.

A clear demonstration of the placebo effect occurred in a re-cent study that examined the effectiveness of a drug used to treat benign enlargement of the prostate. The men who partici-pated in the study were randomly assigned to one of two groups: One group received the medication; the other received a placebo, a look-alike dummy pill. More than half the men who got the placebo pills reported significant relief from their symptoms, including faster urine flow. This was despite the fact that men on the placebo actually experienced an *increase* in the size of their prostates. Many placebo recipients also reported side effects of the "medication." How did the men in the study experience fewer symptoms despite no improvement in their condition (prostate enlargement)? Researchers hypothesize that the patients' positive expectations of the medication's effects may have resulted in decreased nerve activity and muscle relax-ation affecting the bladder, prostate, and urethra.

The placebo effect can be exploited by unscrupulous people who sell worthless medical treatments to the scientifically unso-phisticated public. But placebo power can also be harnessed for its beneficial effects. When a skilled and compassionate medical practitioner provides a patient with a sense of confidence and hope, the positive aspects of placebo power can boost the ben-efits of standard medical treatment. Getting well, like getting sick, is a complex process. Anatomy, physiology, mind, emo-tions, and the environment are all inextricably entwined. But the placebo effect does show that belief can have both psycho-logical and physical effects.

SOURCES: Nordenberg, T. 2000. The healing power of placebos. *FDA Consumer,* January/February. The powerful placebo: An effect without a cause. 2000. *Harvard Men's Health Watch,* June. Brown, W. A. 1998. The placebo effect. *Scientific American* 278(1): 90–95.

FDA regulates homeopathic remedies, but they are subject to many fewer restrictions than prescription or over-the-counter drugs. A few states require practitioners to have special licenses, but most providers practice ho-meopathy as a specialty under another medical license, such as medical doctor or nurse practitioner.

Mind-Body Interventions

Mind-body interventions make use of the integral con-nection between mind and body and the effect each can have on the other. They include many of the stress-management techniques discussed in Chapter 2, includ-ing meditation, yoga, visualization, t'ai chi ch'van, and biofeedback. Psychotherapy, support groups, prayer, and music, art, and dance therapy can also be thought of as mind-body interventions. Obviously, there is no clear line between these forms of CAM and conventional medicine. The placebo effect is one of the most widely known examples of mind-body interdependence.

Some forms of **hypnosis** are considered to be CAM therapies, although the use of hypnotherapy for certain conditions was accepted more than 40 years ago by the American Medical Association. Hypnosis involves the in-duction of a state of deep relaxation during which the pa-tient is more suggestible (more easily influenced). While the patient is in such a hypnotic trance, the practitioner tries to help him or her change unwanted behavior or deal with pain and other symptoms. Hypnosis is some-times used in smoking cessation programs and as a non-drug approach to anxiety disorders such as phobias and chronic conditions such as irritable bowel syndrome.

Hypnosis can be used by medical professionals (M.D.s, D.O.s, D.D.S.s) but is also offered by hypnotherapists. Physicians are certified by their own associations; many states require hypnotherapists to be licensed, but the re-quirements for licensing vary substantially. There is little regulation of practitioners of other relaxation techniques, but it is very rare that adverse events result from such techniques. Many studies have shown that support groups, friendships, strong family relationships, and prayer can all have a positive impact on health.

homeopathy An alternative medical system of Western origin in which illnesses are treated by giving very small doses of drugs that in larger doses in a healthy person would produce symptoms like those of the illness.

hypnosis The process by which a practitioner induces a state of deep relaxation in which an individual is more suggestible; commonly used in cases of pain, phobia, and addiction.

Terms

Biological-Based Therapies

Biological-based therapies consist primarily of herbal therapies or remedies, botanicals, and dietary supplements. Herbal remedies are a major component of all indigenous forms of medicine; prior to the development of pharmaceuticals at the end of the nineteenth century, people everywhere in the world relied on materials from nature for pain relief, wound healing, and treatment of a variety of ailments. Herbal remedies are also a common element in most systems of traditional medicine. Much of the **pharmacopoeia** of modern scientific medicine originated in the folk medicine of native peoples, and many drugs used today are derived from plants.

A majority of botanical products are sold as dietary supplements, that is, in the form of tablets, pills, capsules, liquid extracts, or teas. Like foods, dietary supplements must carry ingredient labels (see Chapter 9 for more about dietary supplement labeling). As with food products, it is the responsibility of the manufacturers to ensure that their dietary supplements are safe and properly labeled prior to marketing. The FDA is responsible for monitoring the labeling and accompanying literature of dietary supplements and for overseeing their safety once they are on the market.

Well-designed clinical studies have been conducted on only a small number of botanicals. Among the most thoroughly tested plant extracts are St. John's wort (*Hypericum perforatum*), ginkgo (*Ginkgo biloba*), and the different coneflowers (*Echinacea purpurea, Echinacea angustifolia,* and *Echinacea pallida*). Participants in clinical trials with St. John's wort, ginkgo, and echinacea experienced only minor adverse events. However, most clinical trials of this type last only for a few weeks, so the tests did not indicate whether it is safe to take these botanicals for longer periods of time. They also didn't indicate whether higher or lower dosages would be more or less effective or cause more or fewer adverse events.

For the vast majority of other botanicals, there are almost no reliable research findings on efficacy or safety. That is extremely worrisome since, of all the CAM approaches, the consumption of botanical supplements has the greatest potential to result in serious and even life-threatening consequences.

Manipulative and Body-Based Methods

Touch and body manipulation are long-standing forms of health care. Manual healing techniques are based on the idea that misalignment or dysfunction in one part of the body can cause pain or dysfunction in another part; correcting these misalignments can bring the body back to optimal health.

Manual healing methods are an integral part of osteopathic medicine, now considered a form of conventional medicine. Other physical healing methods include massage, acupressure, Feldenkrais, Rolfing, and numerous other techniques. The most commonly accepted of the CAM manual healing methods is **chiropractic,** a method that focuses on the relationship between structure, primarily of joints and muscles, and function, primarily of the nervous system, to maintain or restore health. An important therapeutic procedure is the manipulation of joints, particularly those of the spinal column. However, chiropractors also use a variety of other techniques, including physical therapy, exercise programs, patient education and lifestyle modification, and orthotics (mechanical supports and braces) to treat patients. They do not use drugs or surgery.

Chiropractors, or doctors of chiropractic, are trained for a minimum of four full-time academic years at accredited chiropractic colleges. Chiropractic is accepted by many health care and health insurance providers to a far greater extent than the other types of CAM therapies. Promising results have been reported with the use of chiropractic techniques in acute low back pain, neck pain, and headaches. However, there are no well-controlled studies to support manipulation for asthma, gastrointestinal problems, infectious diseases, or other nonmechanical problems.

A caution is in order regarding chiropractic: Spinal manipulation performed by a person without proper chiropractic training can be extremely dangerous. There are several organizations, in particular the American Chiropractic Association, that can help you locate a licensed chiropractor near you.

Terms

biological-based therapies CAM therapies that include natural and biologically based practices, interventions, and products; examples include herbal remedies and dietary supplements.

pharmacopoeia A collection of drugs and medicinal preparations.

chiropractic A system of manual healing most frequently used to treat musculoskeletal problems; the primary treatment is manipulation of the spine and other joints. Practitioners hold a doctor of chiropractic degree and are licensed.

energy therapies Forms of CAM treatment that use energy fields originating either within the body or from outside sources to promote healing.

qigong A component of traditional Chinese medicine that combines movement, meditation, and regulation of breathing to enhance the flow of qi, improve blood circulation, and enhance immune function.

therapeutic touch A CAM practice based on the premise that healers can identify and correct energy imbalances by passing their hands over the patient's body.

Reiki A CAM practice intended to correct disturbances in the flow of life energy and enhance the body's healing powers through the use of thirteen hand positions on the patient.

In February 2000, the FDA issued an advisory warning of interactions between St. John's wort and drugs used to treat HIV infection, heart disease, and several other conditions. Because St. John's wort uses the same metabolic pathway as a number of drugs, it reduces their concentration in the blood and thus their effectiveness. For example, organ transplant patients who took St. John's wort experienced symptoms of transplant rejection because St. John's wort reduced the effectiveness of antirejection drugs. In May 2000, the FDA issued a warning about botanicals containing aristolochic acid. In 1990–1992, Chinese herbs containing aristolochic acid caused severe kidney damage and bladder cancer in patients at a weight-loss clinic in Belgium. Due to a manufacturing error, aristolochia had been inadvertently substituted for another ingredient in weight-loss pills.

These FDA warnings reflect growing safety concerns about herbal remedies, botanicals, and dietary supplements, which now represent a $15-billion-a-year industry in the United States.

Drug Interactions

As in the case of St. John's wort, the chemicals in botanicals can interact dangerously with prescription and over-the-counter drugs. Botanicals may decrease the effects of drugs, making them ineffective, or increase their effects, in some cases making them toxic. Alarmingly, a high percentage of patients fail to tell their physicians about their use of herbal substances. Botanicals can also interact with each other, and many manufacturers are offering new combinations of botanicals without scientific information about the interactions of the individual ingredients.

Lack of Standardization

A related problem is the lack of standardization in the manufacturing of herbal products in the United States. The Dietary Supplement Health and Education Act of 1994 requires that supplement labels list the name and quantity of each ingredient. However, confusion can result because different plant species —with distinct chemical compositions and effects—may have the same common name. The content of herbal preparations is also variable. A *Consumer Reports* study found that the active ingredient in widely sold ginseng products varied widely, with some pills containing twenty times as much as others. Part of the reason for such variation is the difficulty of identifying the active ingredients in botanicals and isolating and standardizing their concentrations. The chemical composition of a supplement is also affected by the growing, harvesting, processing, and storage conditions of plants.

Contamination, Adulteration, and Toxicity

A variety of Ayurvedic and traditional Chinese remedies contain heavy metals such as lead, mercury, and arsenic as part of the formula. Some Chinese herbal remedies have been found to contain pharmaceutical drugs, including tranquilizers and steroids. Others contain herbs not listed on the label, sometimes substituting herbs that have toxic effects, as in the case of the weight-loss pills used in the Belgian clinic. Furthermore, many plants are poisonous or can cause damage to the liver or kidney if taken over long periods of time. Experts have also advised against taking supplements that contain raw animal parts, particularly central nervous system tissue, out of concern that disease may be transmissible this way.

The Role of Government in Safety Issues

Some European governments assume greater responsibility in regulating botanicals than the U.S. government. In Germany, herbal medicine has a long history, but herbs are considered medicines rather than supplements; they are prescribed by physicians, although low-dose preparations are available over the counter, and manufacturing is standardized. Botanicals do not have to be proven effective to be marketed, but they do have to be proven safe.

In the United States, because herbs are considered supplements rather than food or drug products, they do not have to meet FDA food and drug standards for safety or effectiveness, nor do they currently have to meet any manufacturing standards. The manufacturer is responsible for ensuring that a supplement is safe before it is marketed; the FDA has the power to restrict a substance if it is found to pose a health risk after it is on the market. Because U.S. manufacturers can put almost anything into an herbal supplement, American consumers are at risk for buying and using products that may be not just useless but harmful as well. Part of the reasoning behind this situation is that "natural" products are considered safer than conventional medicines. As the incidents with St. John's wort and aristolochic acid demonstrate, this is not always the case.

Energy Therapies

Energy therapies are forms of treatment that use energy fields originating either within the body (biofields) or from other sources (electromagnetic fields). Biofield therapies are based on the idea that energy fields surround and penetrate the body and can be influenced by movement, touch, pressure, or the placement of hands in or through the fields. **Qigong,** a component of traditional Chinese medicine, combines movement, meditation, and regulation of breathing to enhance the flow of qi, improve blood circulation, and enhance immune function. **Therapeutic touch** is derived from the ancient technique of "laying-on of hands"; it is based on the premise that healers can identify and correct energy imbalances by passing their hands over the patient's body. **Reiki** is one form of therapeutic touch; it is intended to correct disturbances in the flow of life energy and enhance the body's healing powers through the use of thirteen specific hand positions on the patient.

According to the Federal Trade Commission, consumers waste billions of dollars on unproven, fraudulently marketed, and sometimes useless or even harmful health care products and treatments. In addition, those with serious medical problems may waste valuable time before seeking proper treatment. Health fraud is a business that sells false hope. It preys on people who are victims of diseases that have no medical cure and on people who want shortcuts to weight loss or improvements to personal appearance.

The first rule of thumb for evaluating any health claim is that if it sounds too good to be true, it probably is. Also, be on the lookout for the typical phrases and marketing techniques fraudulent promoters use to deceive consumers:

- The product is advertised as a quick and effective cure-all for a wide range of ailments.

- The promoters use words like *scientific breakthrough, miraculous cure, secret ingredient,* or *ancient remedy.* Also remember that just because a product is described as "natural" or unprocessed does not necessarily mean it's safe.

- The promoter claims the government or the medical profession has conspired to suppress the product.

- The advertisement includes undocumented case histories claiming amazing results.

- The product is advertised as available from only one source, and payment is required in advance.

- The promoter promises a no-risk "money-back guarantee." Be aware that many fly-by-night operators are not around to respond to your request for a refund.

To check out a particular product, talk to a physician or another health care professional and to family members and friends. Be wary of treatments offered by people who tell you to avoid talking to others. Check with the Better Business Bureau or local attorney general's office to see whether other consumers have lodged complaints about the product or the product's marketer. You can also check with the appropriate health professional group. For example, check with the American Diabetes Association or the National Arthritis Foundation if the products are promoted for diabetes or arthritis.

If you think you have been a victim of health fraud or if you have an adverse reaction that you think is related to a particular supplement, you can report it to the appropriate agency:

- *False advertising claims:* Contact the FTC by phone (877-FTC-HELP); by mail (Consumer Response Center, Federal Trade Commission, Washington, DC 20580); or online (http://www.ftc.gov; click on Complaint form). You can also contact your state attorney general's office, your state department of health, or the local consumer protection agency (check your local telephone directory).

- *False labeling on a product:* Contact the FDA district office consumer complaint coordinator for your area. (The FDA regulates safety, manufacturing, and product labeling.)

- *Adverse reaction to a supplement:* Call a doctor or other health care provider immediately. You may also report your adverse reaction to FDA MedWatch by calling 800-INFO-FDA or by visiting the MedWatch Web site (http://www.fda.gov/medwatch).

SOURCES: Federal Trade Commission. 1999. *Fraudulent Health Claims: Don't Be Fooled.* Washington, D.C.: Federal Trade Commission. Kurtzweil, P. 1999. How to spot health fraud. *FDA Consumer,* November/December. Food and Drug Administration. 1999. *How to Report Adverse Reactions and Other Problems with Products Regulated by FDA* (http://www.fda.gov/opacom/backgrounders/problem.html; retrieved July 19, 2000).

Bioelectromagnetics is the study of the interaction between living organisms and electromagnetic fields, both those produced by the organism itself and those produced by outside sources. The recognition that the body produces electromagnetic fields has led to the development of many diagnostic procedures in Western medicine, including electroencephalography (EEG), electrocardiography (ECG), and nuclear magnetic resonance (NMR) scans. **Bioelectromagnetic-based therapies** involve the use of electromagnetic fields to manage pain and to treat conditions such as asthma. Although promising, the available research is still very limited and does not allow firm conclusions about the efficacy of these therapies. Most scientists believe that consumer products containing small magnets have no significant effect on the human body.

Evaluating Complementary and Alternative Therapies

Because there is less information available about complementary and alternative therapies, as well as less regulation of associated products and providers, it is important for consumers to take an active role when they are thinking about using them.

Working with Your Physician   The NCCAM advises consumers not to seek complementary therapies without first visiting a conventional health care provider for an evaluation and diagnosis of their symptoms. It's usually best to discuss and try conventional treatments that have been shown to be beneficial for your condition. If you are

Terms   **bioelectromagnetic-based therapies** CAM therapies based on the notion that electromagnetic fields can be used to promote healing and manage pain.

The act of writing down feelings and thoughts about stressful life events has been shown to help people with chronic conditions improve their health. In one recent study, people with asthma or rheumatoid arthritis were asked to write down their feelings about the most stressful event in their lives; they wrote for 20 minutes a day over a three-day period. In follow-up exams four months later, nearly half of the patients who engaged in expressive writing experienced positive changes in their condition such as improved lung function or reduced joint pain. Only about a quarter of the control group, who wrote about their daily plans, experienced a positive change in health.

Investigators remain unsure why writing about one's feelings has beneficial effects. It is possible that expressing feelings about a traumatic event helps people work through the event and put it behind them. The resulting sense of release and control may reduce stress levels and have positive physical effects such as reduced heart rate and blood pressure and improved immune function. Alternatively, expressive writing may change the way people think about previous stressful events in their lives and help them cope with new stressors. Whatever the cause, it's clear that expressive writing can be a safe, inexpensive, and effective supplement to standard treatment of certain chronic illnesses.

What about the effects of expressive writing on otherwise healthy individuals? Other studies have, in fact, found such a benefit: People who wrote about traumatic experiences reported fewer symptoms, fewer days off work, fewer visits to the doctor, improved mood, and a more positive outlook.

If you'd like to try expressive writing to help you deal with a traumatic event, set aside a special time—15 minutes a day for four consecutive days, for example, or one day a week for four weeks. Write in a place where you won't be interrupted or distracted. Explore your very deepest thoughts and feelings and why you feel the way you do. Don't worry about grammar or coherence or about what someone else might think about what you're writing; you are writing just for yourself. You may find the writing exercise to be distressing in the short term—sadness and depression are common when dealing with feelings about a stressful event—but most people report relief and contentment soon after writing for several days.

SOURCES: Smyth, J. M., et al. 1999. Effects of writing about stressful experiences on symptom reduction in patients with asthma or rheumatoid arthritis: A randomized trial. *Journal of the American Medical Association* 281(14): 1304–1309. Spiegel, D. 1999. Healing words: Emotional expression and disease outcome. *Journal of the American Medical Association* 281(14): 1328–1329. Pennebaker, J. 1997. *Opening Up: The Healthy Power of Expressing Emotions.* New York: Guilford Press.

thinking of trying any alternative therapies, it is critically important to tell your physician in order to avoid any dangerous interactions with conventional treatments you are receiving. Areas to discuss with your physician include the following:

- *Safety:* Is there something unsafe about the treatment in general or for you specifically? Are there safety issues you should be aware of, such as the use of disposable needles in acupuncture?
- *Effectiveness:* Is there any research about the use of the therapy for your condition?
- *Timing:* Is the immediate use of a conventional treatment indicated?
- *Cost:* Is the therapy likely to be very expensive, especially in light of the potential benefit?

If appropriate, schedule a follow-up visit with your physician to assess your condition and your progress after a certain amount of time using a complementary therapy. Keep a symptom diary to more accurately track your symptoms and gauge your progress. (Symptoms such as pain and fatigue are very difficult to recall with accuracy, so an ongoing symptom diary is an important tool.) If you plan to pursue a therapy against your physician's advice, you need to tell him or her.

For dietary supplements, particularly botanicals, pharmacists can also be an excellent source of information, especially if they are familiar with other medications you are taking.

Questioning the CAM Practitioner   You can also get information from individual practitioners and from schools, professional organizations, and state licensing boards. Ask about education, training, licensing, and certification. If appropriate, check with local or state regulatory agencies or the consumer affairs department to determine if any complaints have been lodged against the practitioner. When talking with a CAM practitioner, ask for a full description of the therapy and any potential side effects, how long the therapy should continue before it can be determined if it is beneficial, and how much it will cost. Tell the practitioner about any conventional treatments you are receiving. If anything an alternative practitioner says or recommends directly conflicts with advice from your physician, discuss it with your physician before making any major changes in any current treatment regimen or in your lifestyle.

Doing Your Own Research   You can investigate CAM therapies on your own by going to the library or doing research online, although caution is in order when using Web sites for the various forms of CAM. A good place to start is the Web sites of government agencies like the FDA or NCCAM and of universities and similar organizations that conduct government-sponsored research on CAM approaches (see For More Information at the end of the chapter).

If possible, also talk to people with the same condition you have who have received the same treatment. Remember, though, that patient testimonials shouldn't be used as the sole criterion for choosing a therapy or assessing its safety and efficacy. Controlled scientific trials usually provide the best information and should be consulted whenever possible. Perhaps more so than for any other consumer products and services, the use of complementary and alternative medicine calls for consumer skills, critical thinking, and caution.

COMMUNICATE! It makes sense to talk with your physician if you are thinking about trying a complementary therapy, such as acupuncture or chiropractic, and it is critically important to talk with him or her about any dietary supplements you are taking or thinking about taking. As mentioned in the text, you have a right to expect your physician to be able to discuss complementary and alternative therapies with you. To get started, you might say something like, "A friend of mine tried acupuncture for tendinitis and he said it helped. What do you think about my trying it for my elbow?" or "I've read that St. John's wort can help with mild depression. Do you think I should try it? Is there any reason I shouldn't?"

Why Do Consumers Use Complementary Medicine?

Why are American consumers attracted to complementary and alternative medicine? Numerous reasons have been proposed. CAM often offers hope to people who have been disappointed by conventional medical therapies or who have chronic conditions that are incurable with conventional medical treatments. People with cancer, AIDS, and arthritis are among the heaviest users of CAM. Those most likely to use CAM are elderly people, approximately 80% of whom have at least one chronic health problem, and teenagers, who are concerned about their appearance and respond to a variety of appeals. Both these groups may be particularly susceptible to fraudulent claims for products promising new, quick, or easy ways to stay thin, strong, or attractive. A major source of CAM's appeal is that CAM practitioners often spend much more time listening and touching their patients than conventional physicians. Patients may find CAM practitioners to be warmer, more empathetic, and less rushed than their conventional counterparts.

Some experts speculate that the persuasive appeal of complementary and alternative medicine may come from the power of its underlying beliefs and cultural assumptions, which offer patients an experience they are missing in conventional medicine. People using CAM may feel they are connecting to nature or a more natural version of society; they may also feel a connection to vital energy or a life force, such as qi. They may view CAM as operating from a more holistic, person-centered body of knowledge than Western science, and they may find their quest for health imbued with an almost sacred quality. According to this view, CAM is attractive because of what it offers people when their sense of intactness and connection with the world is threatened by illness: empowerment, participation, authenticity, connection to nature and the universe, a renewed sense of purpose and meaning, and a new set of behavioral options. The assumptions of CAM can redefine the experience of illness in ways that inspire and empower the individual.

Despite many profound and irreconcilable philosophical differences between conventional medicine and CAM, there are abundant opportunities for learning, collaborating, and providing parallel care. Within each is an enormous amount of time-tested information that has its own logic and use. In the future, greater understanding and collaboration across boundaries will certainly benefit the patient-consumer.

PAYING FOR HEALTH CARE

Whether you choose conventional medicine or complementary and alternative medicine, you or your insurance company, or both, will have to pay for your health care. The American health care system is one of the most advanced and comprehensive in the world, but it is also the most expensive. In 1999, the nation spent more than $1 trillion on health care, or $4300 per person (Figure 15-4). Health care is currently financed by a combination of private and public insurance plans, patient out-of-pocket payments, and government assistance. Most nonelderly Americans receive their health insurance through their employers.

Despite high spending, not everyone is included in this financing system. More than 48 million people (17% of the population), the vast majority of them employed, have no health care insurance at all. The uninsured include almost 11 million children—15% of all American children—most in working, low-income families. Lack of insurance affects both access to care and quality of care.

Health care costs soared in the 1980s and then were contained to some extent in the 1990s by a large-scale switch from private insurance to managed care (discussed below), which is designed to achieve cost economies. But the savings from this switch were likely a one-time phenomenon, since more than 80% of working Americans are now covered by managed-care plans. Experts predict that health costs will increase drastically in the near future, with much of the increase borne by private insurers and individuals.

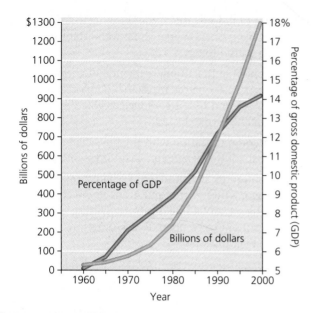

Figure 15-4 U.S. health care expenditures. SOURCE: Health Care Financing Administration (http://www.hcfa.gov).

Health Insurance

Health insurance enables people to receive health care they might not otherwise be able to afford. Health insurance plans are either fee-for-service (or indemnity) or managed care. With both types the individual or the employer pays a basic premium, usually on a monthly basis; there are often other payments as well.

In a fee-for-service or indemnity plan, you can use any medical provider (such as a physician or a hospital) you choose. You or the provider sends the bill to your insurance company, which pays part of it. Usually you have to pay a "deductible" amount each year, ranging from $100 up to several hundred dollars, before the insurer starts covering your expenses. Once you meet the deductible, most plans pay a percentage—often 80%—of what they consider the "usual and customary" charge for covered services.

Managed-care plans have agreements with certain physicians, hospitals, and health care providers to give a range of services to plan members at reduced cost. In general, you have lower out-of-pocket costs and less paperwork with a managed-care plan than with an indemnity plan, but you also have less freedom in choosing health care providers. Most Americans with job-based insurance are covered by managed care plans, which may follow several different models:

• **Health maintenance organizations (HMOs)** offer members a range of services for a set monthly fee.

You choose a primary care physician who manages your care and refers you to specialists if you need them.

• **Preferred provider organizations (PPOs)** are plans that have arrangements with physicians and other providers who have agreed to accept lower fees.

• **Point-of-service (POS) plans** are options offered by many HMOs, in which you can see a physician outside the plan and still be partially covered.

Americans who are 65 or older and younger people with certain disabilities can be covered by **Medicare,** a federal health insurance program that helps pay for both hospitalization and physician services. **Medicaid** is a joint federal-state health insurance program that covers some low-income people, especially children, pregnant women, and people with certain disabilities.

Choosing a Policy

Choosing health insurance can be complicated; it's important to evaluate the coverage provided by different plans and decide which one is best for you. Consider these questions:

• Do you want to have a wide choice of providers (in which case a fee-for-service plan would be preferable), or is a more limited choice acceptable in exchange for the lower cost of a managed-care plan?

• Does the plan include the physicians and hospitals you want?

• Does the plan provide the benefits you and your family need? (Consider such services as diagnostic tests and X rays, prescription medications, hospital costs, physical therapy, well baby care, eye care, mental health services, preventive care, complementary therapies such as acupuncture, home health care, and so on.)

managed-care plan A health care program that integrates the financing and delivery of services by using designated providers, utilization review, and financial incentives for following the plan's policies.

health maintenance organization (HMO) A prepaid health insurance plan in which patients receive health care from designated providers.

preferred provider organization (PPO) A prepaid health insurance plan in which providers agree to deliver services for discounted fees; patients can go to any provider, but using nonparticipating providers results in higher costs to the patient.

point-of-service (POS) plan A managed-care plan that covers treatment by an HMO physician but permits patients to seek treatment elsewhere with a higher copayment.

Medicare A federal health insurance program for people 65 or older and for younger people with certain disabilities.

Medicaid A federally subsidized state-run plan of health care for people of low income.

Terms

- Does the plan fit your budget? (Include monthly premiums, annual deductibles, copayments for physician visits and drugs, and the cost of going outside the plan for special services.)

Colleges typically provide medical services through a student health center; some require students to purchase additional insurance if they are not covered by family policies. It's usually economical to remain on a family policy as long as possible. After college, most people secure group coverage through their employer or through membership in an organization. Whatever your options, be sure to consider the plans carefully and use your critical thinking skills to find the one that best suits your needs.

Tips for Today

Most of the time, you can take care of yourself without consulting a health care provider. When you do need professional care, you can continue to take responsibility for yourself by making informed, reasoned decisions about the care you obtain, whether conventional or complementary and alternative.

Right now you can

- Make sure you have basic first aid supplies at home and prepare or buy a small first aid kit for your car or office.

- Make sure you have enough on hand of any prescription medication that you take and that your prescription is up to date.

- Research any alternative or complementary practice or product you are using, either at the library or online, to find out if it is considered safe.

- Sit back in your chair and practice relaxation through breathing: Inhale slowly and deeply, imagining warm air flowing to all parts of your body; exhale from your abdomen, imagining tension flowing out of your body; continue for five or ten minutes or until you feel relaxed.

SUMMARY

- Informed self-care requires knowing how to evaluate symptoms. It's necessary to see a physician if symptoms are severe, unusual, persistent, or recurrent.

- Self-treatment doesn't necessarily require medication, but OTC drugs can be a helpful part of self-care.

- Conventional medicine is characterized by a focus on the external, physical causes of disease; the identification of a set of symptoms for different diseases; the development of public health measures to prevent disease and drugs and surgery to treat them;

the use of rational, scientific thinking to understand and explain phenomena; and a well-established research methodology.

- Conventional practitioners include medical doctors, doctors of osteopathic medicine, podiatrists, optometrists, and dentists, as well as allied health care providers.

- Good communication with the physician and other members of the health care team is essential.

- Preparation for a visit to a physician should include making a written list of questions or concerns and bringing a list of all medications. During the visit, it's important to be open, to ask questions, and to request clarification.

- The diagnostic process involves a medical history, a physical exam, and medical tests.

- Safe use of prescription drugs requires knowledge of what the medication is supposed to do, how and when to take it, and what the side effects are.

- All surgical procedures carry risk; patients should ask about alternatives and get a second opinion.

- Complementary and alternative medicine (CAM) is defined as those therapies and practices that do not form part of conventional or "mainstream" health care and medical practice as taught in most U.S. medical schools and offered in most U.S. hospitals.

- CAM is characterized by a view of health as a balance and integration of body, mind, and spirit; a focus on ways to restore the individual to harmony so that he or she can fight disease and regain health; and a body of knowledge based on accumulated experience and observations of patient reactions.

- Alternative medical systems are complete systems of medical philosophy, theory, and practice. Traditional Chinese medicine and homeopathy are two of the best known in the United States.

- Mind-body interventions include meditation, yoga, breathwork, group support, hypnosis, and prayer.

- Biological-based therapies consist of herbal remedies, botanicals, and dietary supplements.

- Manipulative and body-based methods include massage and other physical healing techniques; the most commonly accepted is chiropractic.

- Energy therapies are designed to influence the flow of energy in and around the body.

- Because there is less information available about CAM and less regulation of its practices and providers, consumers must use critical thinking skills and exercise caution.

- In general, CAM may be attractive to consumers because it allows people to redefine the experience of illness in ways that empower the individual.

- Health insurance plans are usually described as either fee-for-service (indemnity) or managed-care plans. Indemnity plans allow consumers more choice in medical providers, but managed-care plans are less expensive.

- Government programs include Medicaid, for the poor, and Medicare, for those who are 65 and over or chronically disabled.

JOURNAL ENTRY

1. Interactions among over-the-counter and prescription drugs and herbal remedies are potentially serious. Make a list of every drug and herbal remedy you've used in the past three months. How many did you use? Do you know for certain that you haven't risked a dangerous interaction? Check the labels on all the products you used for warnings; if you are unsure about any interactions, take your list to your pharmacist or health care practitioner for advice.

2. Critical Thinking Examine a news report on a research study. From the report, try to determine key acts about the research (see the box on p. 352 in the chapter): source of the information, size and type of the study, characteristics of the participants, findings, and conclusions. How much information is actually included in the media report? Is there enough information for you to critically evaluate the findings? If possible, compare the media report to the actual study findings. (Abstracts of most medical studies can be found on the Library of Medicine's PubMed Web site: http://www.ncbi.nlm.nih.gov/entrez.) Write a short essay about your findings.

FOR MORE INFORMATION

Books and Articles

American Medical Women Association. 2001. *Complete Family Health Book.* New York: Golden Books. *A comprehensive guide to family health.*

Brody, H. 2000. *The Placebo Response.* New York: Cliff Street Books. *Describes the placebo effect and how it may be used to benefit health.*

Howard Hughes Medical Institute, ed. 2000. *Exploring the Biomedical Revolution.* Baltimore: Johns Hopkins University Press. *Explores biomedical research and its impact on the fight against human disease.*

Medical Economics Staff, ed. 2001. *PDR for Nonprescription Drugs and Dietary Supplements,* 22nd ed. Montvale, N.J.: Medical Economics. *A clinical reference covering food and drug interactions, side effects, contraindications, costs, and other information. Medical Economics also publishes volumes covering prescription drugs and herbal medicines.*

Micozzi, M. S. 2001. *Fundamentals of Complementary and Alternative Medicine,* 2nd ed. St. Louis: Mosby. *Provides information on the development and key ideas and approaches of alternative and complementary systems and therapies.*

Organizations, Hotlines, and Web Sites

Agency for Healthcare Research and Quality (AHRQ). Provides practical, evidence-based information on health care treatments and outcomes for consumers and practitioners.
  800-358-9295
  http://www.ahrq.gov

American Academy of Medical Acupuncture (AAMA). Provides information about acupuncture and a searchable directory of medical doctors who have been certified by the American Board of Medical Acupuncture.
  323-937-5514
  http://www.medicalacupuncture.org

American Board of Medical Specialties. Provides information on board certification, including information on specific physicians.
  866-275-2267
  http://www.abms.org

American Chiropractic Association. Provides information on chiropractic care, consumer tips, and a searchable directory of certified chiropractors.
  http://www.amerchiro.org

American Medical Association (AMA). Provides information about physicians, including their training, licensure, and board certification.
  http://www.ama-assn.org

American Osteopathic Association. Provides information on osteopathic physicians, including board certification.
  800-621-1773
  http://www.aoa-net.org

Government gateways to health information. The following government sites have links to a wealth of information on health promotion, diseases and disorders, prescription and OTC drugs, and many other topics.

CDC Health Information A to Z
  http://www.cdc.gov/health/diseases.htm

FDA Information for Consumers
  http://www.fda.gov/opacom/morecons.html

Healthfinder
  http://www.healthfinder.gov

National Library of Medicine: MedlinePlus
   http://www.nlm.nih.gov/medlineplus
NIH Health Information Index
   http://www.nih.gov/health
U.S. Consumer Gateway: Health
   http://www.consumer.gov/health.htm
National Center for Complementary and Alternative Medicine (NCCAM). Provides general information packets, answers to frequently asked questions about CAM, consumer advice for safer use of CAM, research abstracts, and bibliographies.
   888-644-6226
   http://nccam.nih.gov
National Center for Homeopathy. Provides information about homeopathy and a directory of member practitioners.
   http://www.homeopathic.org
National Certification Commission for Acupuncture and Oriental Medicine (NCCAOM). Promotes nationally recognized standards of competency and safety in acupuncture, Chinese herbology, and Oriental bodywork therapy; includes a searchable directory of certified practitioners.
   703-548-9004
   http://www.nccaom.org
National Council Against Health Fraud. Provides news and information about health fraud and quackery and links to related sites.
   http://www.ncahf.org
Quackwatch. Provides information on health fraud, quackery, and health decision making.
   http://www.quackwatch.com

See also the listings for Chapters 2 and 9; the section on dietary supplements in Chapter 9 (p. 206) suggests books and Web sites with more information on supplements.

SELECTED BIBLIOGRAPHY

Ayanian, J. Z., et al. 2000. Unmet health needs of uninsured adults in the United States. *Journal of the American Medical Association* 284(16): 2061–2069.

Bell, R. A., R. L. Kravitz, and M. S. Wilkes. 2000. Direct-to-consumer prescription drug advertising, 1989–1998. A content analysis of conditions, targets, inducements, and appeals. *Journal of Family Practice* 49(4): 329–335.

Bell, R. A., M. S. Wilkes, and R. L. Kravitz. 2000. The educational value of consumer-targeted prescription drug print advertising. *Journal of Family Practice* 49(12): 1092–1098.

Blumenthal, D. 2001. Controlling health care expenditures. *New England Journal of Medicine* 344(10): 766–769.

Bordens, K. S., and B. B. Abbott. 2002. *Research Design and Methods: A Process Approach.* 5th ed. New York: McGraw-Hill.

Burak, L. J., and A. Damico. 1999. Effects of direct-to-consumer advertising of pharmaceutical products on college students. *Health Marketing Quarterly* 17(2): 19–29.

Eisenberg, D. M. 1997. Advising patients who seek alternative medical therapies. *Annals of Internal Medicine* 127: 61–69.

Eisenberg, D. M., et al. 1998. Trends in alternative medicine use in the United States, 1990–1997: Results of a follow-up national survey. *Journal of the American Medical Association* 280(18): 1569–1575.

Ernst, E. 2001. A primer of complementary and alternative medicine commonly used by cancer patients. *Medical Journal of Australia* 174(2): 88–92.

Foster, D. F., et al. 2000. Alternative medicine use in older Americans. *Journal of the American Geriatric Society* 48(12): 1560–1565.

Gardiner, P., and W. Wornham. 2000. Recent review of complementary and alternative medicine used by adolescents. *Current Opinion in Pediatrics* 12(4): 298–302.

Health Care Financing Administration. 2001. *National Health Expenditures Aggregate and per Capita Amounts, Percent Distribution, and Average Annual Percent Growth, by Sources of Funds: Selected Calendar Years 1960–1999.* (http://www.hcfa.gov/stats/nhe-oact/tables/t1.htm; retrieved May 2, 2001).

Health Care Financing Administration. 2001. *National Health Expenditures and Selected Economic Indicators, Levels and Average Annual Percent Change: Selected Calendar Years 1980–2010* (http://www.hcfa.gov/stats/NHE-Proj/proj2000/tables/table1.htm; retrieved May 2, 2001).

Henkel, J. 2000. Buying drugs online: It's convenient and private, but beware of "rogue sites." *FDA Consumer,* January–February.

Institute of Medicine Committee on Quality of Health Care in America. 2001. *Crossing the Quality Chasm: A New Health System for the 21st Century.* Washington, D.C.: National Academy Press.

Kaptchuk, T. J., and D. M. Eisenberg. 1998. The persuasive appeal of alternative medicine. *Annals of Internal Medicine* 129(12): 1061–1065.

Leape, L. L. 2000. Institute of Medicine medical error figures are not exaggerated. *Journal of the American Medical Association* 284(1): 95–97.

Linde, K., et al. 1998. Are the clinical effects of homeopathy placebo effects? A meta-analysis of placebo-controlled trials. *Lancet* 350(9081): 834–843.

Mechanic, D., D. D. McAlpine, and M. Rosenthal. 2001. Are patients' office visits with physicians getting shorter? *New England Journal of Medicine* 344(3): 198–204.

Murphy, D. R. 2000. Chiropractic rehabilitation of the cervical spine. *Journal of Manipulative and Physiological Therapeutics* 23(6): 404–408.

National Center for Complementary and Alternative Medicine. (2001. *Considering Complementary and Alternative Therapies?* (http://nccam.nih.gov/nccam/fcp/faq/considercam.html; retrieved May 2, 2001).

National Center for Complementary and Alternative Medicine. 2000. Major domains of complementary and alternative medicine. (http://nccam. nih.gov/nccam/fcp/classify; retrieved December 20, 2000).

National Institutes of Health. 1997. *Acupuncture: NIH Consensus Statement* (http://odp.od.nih.gov/consensus/cons/107/107statement.htm; retrieved December 29, 2000).

Nortier, J. L., et al. 2000. Urothelial carcinoma associated with the use of a Chinese herb (*Aristolochia fangchi*). *The New England Journal of Medicine* 342(23): 1686–1692.

Participating in medical research studies. 2001. *Journal of the American Medical Association* 285(5): 686.

Piscitelli, S. C., et al. 2000. Indinavir concentrations and St. John's wort. *Lancet* 355(9203): 547–548.

Prescription for trouble. 2001. *Consumer Reports,* February.

Ruschitzka, R., et al. 2000. Acute heart transplant rejection due to Saint John's wort. *Lancet* 355(9203): 548–549.

Schroeder, S. A. 2001. Prospects for expanding health insurance coverage. *New England Journal of Medicine* 344(11): 847–852.

Soon, S. L., and R. I. Crawford. 2001. Recurrent erythema nodosum associated with Echinacea herbal therapy. *Journal of the American Academy of Dermatology* 44(2): 298–299.

Personal Safety: Protecting Yourself from Unintentional Injuries and Violence

16

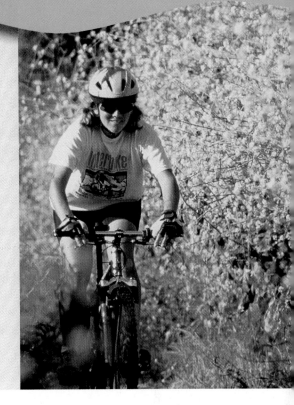

LOOKING AHEAD

After reading this chapter, you should be able to

- List the most common types of unintentional injuries and strategies for preventing them

- Describe factors that contribute to violence and intentional injuries

- Discuss different forms of violence and how to protect yourself from intentional injuries

- List strategies for helping others in an emergency situation

Each year, about 150,000 Americans die from injuries, and many more are temporarily or permanently disabled. Injuries can be intentional or unintentional. An **intentional injury** is one that is purposely inflicted, by either oneself or another person; examples are homicide, suicide, and assault. If an injury occurs when no harm is intended, it is considered an **unintentional injury.** Motor vehicle crashes, falls, and fires often result in unintentional injuries. (The word *accidents* was formerly used to describe unintentional injuries, but it is now considered inaccurate because it suggests events beyond human control. *Injuries* are predictable outcomes of factors that can be controlled or prevented.) Although Americans tend to express more concern about intentional injuries, unintentional injuries are actually more common. On an average day in the United States, there are 58 homicides, 85 suicides, 265 deaths from unintentional injuries, 3200 suicide attempts, 20,400 interper-

sonal assaults, and 100,000 unintentional injury–related emergency room visits.

Unintentional injuries are the fifth leading cause of death among all Americans and the leading cause of death and disability among children and young adults. Heart disease, cancer, and stroke are responsible for more deaths each year than injuries, but because unintentional injuries are so common among people, they account for more **years of potential life lost** than any other cause of

intentional injury An injury that is purposely inflicted, by either oneself or another person.

unintentional injury An injury that occurs without harm being intended.

years of potential life lost The difference between an individual's life expectancy and his or her age at death.

Terms

369

Table 16-1	Unintentional Injuries in the United States	
	Deaths	Disabling Injuries
Motor vehicle	41,300	2,200,000
Home	28,800	6,900,000
Leisure	24,100	8,000,000
Work	5,100	3,800,000
All classes*	96,900	20,800,000

*Deaths and injuries for the four separate classes total more than the "All classes" figures because of rounding and because some deaths and injuries are included in more than one class.

SOURCE: National Safety Council. 2000. *Injury Facts.* Itasca, Ill.: National Safety Council.

death. Suicide and homicide rank eighth and thirteenth respectively on the list of leading causes of death among Americans; because they often affect young people, they also account for many years of potential life lost. Injuries affect all segments of the population, but they are particularly common among men, minorities, and people with low incomes, primarily due to social, environmental, and economic factors.

UNINTENTIONAL INJURIES

Injury situations are generally categorized into four general classes, based on where they occur: motor vehicle injuries, home injuries, leisure injuries, and work injuries (Table 16-1). In all of these arenas, the action you take can mean the difference between injury or death and no injury at all.

Motor Vehicle Injuries

Motor vehicle crashes are the leading cause of death for Americans between the ages of 1 and 29. **Motor vehicle injuries** also result in the majority of cases of paralysis due to spinal injuries, and they are the leading cause of severe brain injury in the United States.

Factors Contributing to Motor Vehicle Injuries Common causes of motor vehicle injuries are speeding, aggressive driving, fatigue, cell phones and other distractions, the use of alcohol and other drugs, and the incorrect use of safety belts and other safety devices.

SPEEDING   Nearly two-thirds of all motor vehicle crashes are caused by bad driving, especially speeding. As speed

increases, momentum and the force of impact increase, and the time allowed for the driver to react (reaction time) decreases. Speed limits are posted to establish the safest maximum speed limit for a given area under ideal conditions; if visibility is limited or the road is wet, the safe maximum speed may be considerably lower.

AGGRESSIVE DRIVING   Speeding is also a hallmark of aggressive drivers—those who operate a motor vehicle in an unsafe and hostile manner. Other characteristics of aggressive driving include frequent, erratic, and abrupt lane changes; tailgating; running red lights or stop signs; passing on the shoulder; and blocking other cars trying to change lanes or pass. Aggressive drivers increase the risk of crashes for themselves and others; injuries may also occur if drivers stop their vehicles and confront each other following an incident. One in four U.S. drivers admits to driving aggressively at least some of the time.

FATIGUE AND SLEEPINESS   Driving requires mental alertness and attentiveness. Studies have shown that sleepiness causes slower reaction time, reduced vigilance, and delayed information processing. Research shows that even mild sleep deprivation causes a deterioration in driving ability comparable to that caused by a 0.05% blood alcohol concentration—a level considered hazardous when driving.

CELL PHONES AND OTHER DISTRACTIONS   Anything that distracts a driver—a bad mood, pets or children in the car—can increase the risk of a motor vehicle injury. Several common causes of crashes, including failing to yield and disregarding traffic signals and stop signs have been linked to driver distraction, and it is estimated that distraction is a contributing factor in 25–50% of all crashes. As the use of cell phones has spread, their potential to distract drivers has been recognized. Studies have documented a higher rate of crashes among cell phone users compared to nonusers.

ALCOHOL AND OTHER DRUGS   Alcohol is involved in about half of all fatal crashes. Alcohol-impaired driving is illegal in all states; the legal blood alcohol concentration (BAC) varies by state from 0.08% to 0.10%, but people are impaired at much lower BACs. The combination of fatigue and alcohol use increases the risk even further. Because alcohol affects reason and judgment as well as the ability to make fast, accurate, and coordinated movements, a person who has been drinking will be less likely to recognize that he or she is impaired. Use of many over-the-counter and all psychoactive drugs is also potentially dangerous if you plan to drive.

SAFETY BELTS, AIR BAGS, AND CHILD SAFETY SEATS   Only 68% of motor vehicle occupants use safety belts, even though you are twice as likely to be injured in a crash if you do not wear one. Of drivers not wearing a safety belt

On January 1, 2001, a law banning the use of handheld cellular phones while driving went into effect in Suffolk County, New York. Officials in New York City have proposed a similar ban that would require drivers to use headsets, earpieces, or voice-activated devices or face fines of up to $150. If the ban is passed, New York will join Suffolk County and cities including Brooklyn Heights, Ohio, and Brookline, Massachusetts, in prohibiting the use of a phone while driving unless both hands are on the steering wheel.

Although research findings have been mixed, the available evidence suggests that use of a cell phone while driving can, indeed, increase the risk of motor vehicle crashes. One study found that motorists who talk on the phone face a fourfold increase in their risk of a collision; the risk of a fatal crash is also higher. It is unclear, however, if bans such as those in Suffolk County will help reduce the risk: Studies have not found much benefit in the use of headsets, perhaps because it is the mental distraction of talking that is a factor in crashes rather than one hand holding the phone.

The safest strategy is not to use your phone while driving. For people who live in areas where cell phone use is legal while driving and who choose to use a phone, the following strategies may help increase safety:

- Be very familiar with your phone and its functions, especially speed dial and redial.

- Store frequently called numbers on speed dial so you can place calls without looking at the phone.

- Use a hands-free device so that you can keep both hands on the steering wheel.

- Let the person you are speaking to know you are driving and be prepared to end the call at any time.

- Don't place or answer calls in heavy traffic and hazardous weather conditions.

- Don't take notes or look up phone numbers while driving.

- Time calls so that you can place them when you are at a stop.

- Never engage in stressful or emotional conversations while on the road. If you are discussing a complicated or emotional matter, pull over to the side of the road or into a parking lot to complete your conversation.

Remember, as a driver, your primary obligation is to pay attention to the road—for your own safety and the safety of others.

SOURCES: Lueck, T. J. 2000. Giuliani and Vallone call for limits on use of cell phones by drivers. *New York Times*, December 20. World of Wireless Communications. 2000. *Consumer Resources: Driving Safety Tips* (http://www.wow-com/consumer/driving/safetyold.cfm; retrieved December 16, 2000). Redelmeier, D. A., and R. J. Tibshirani. 1997. Association between cellular-telephone calls and motor vehicle collisions. *New England Journal of Medicine* 336(7): 453–458.

---

who have been killed in automobile crashes, an estimated 60–70% would have survived if they had been wearing one. If you wear a combination lap and shoulder belt, your chances of surviving a crash are three to four times better than those of a person who doesn't wear one.

Some people think that if they are involved in a crash, they are better off being thrown free of their vehicle. In fact, the chances of being killed are 25 times greater if you are thrown from a vehicle. Safety belts also provide protection from the "second collision." If a car is traveling at 65 mph and hits another vehicle, the car stops first; then the occupants stop because they are traveling at the same speed. The second collision occurs when the occupants of the car hit something inside the car, such as the steering column or windshield. The safety belt stops the second collision from occurring and spreads the stopping force of the collision over the body.

Since 1998, all new cars have been equipped with dual air bags—one for the driver and one for the front passenger. Although air bags provide supplementary protection in the event of a collision, most are useful only in head-on collisions. They also deflate immediately after inflating and therefore do not provide protection in collisions involving multiple impacts.

Air bags deploy forcefully and can injure a child or short adult who is improperly restrained or sitting too close to the dashboard. To ensure that air bags work safely, always follow these basic guidelines: Place infants in rear-facing infant seats in the back seat; transport children age 12 and under in the back seat; always use safety belts or appropriate safety seats; and keep 10 inches between the air bag cover and the breastbone of the driver or passenger. If necessary, adjust the steering wheel or use seat cushions to ensure that an inflating air bag will hit a person in the chest and not in the face. Children who have outgrown child safety seats but are still too small for adult safety belts alone (usually ages 4 to 8) should be

motor vehicle injuries Unintentional injuries and deaths involving motor vehicles in motion, both on and off the highway or street; incidents causing motor vehicle injuries include collisions between vehicles and collisions with objects or pedestrians.

Terms

secured using booster seats that ensure that the safety belt is positioned low across their waist.

In the rare event that a person cannot comply with air bag guidelines, permission to install an on-off switch that temporarily disables the air bag can be applied for from the National Highway Traffic Safety Administration (NHTSA). Air bags currently prevent far more injuries than they cause and are expected to save at least 3200 lives each year once they are installed in all vehicles.

Preventing Motor Vehicle Injuries About 75% of all motor vehicle collisions occur within 25 miles of home and at speeds lower than 40 mph. Strategies for preventing motor vehicle injuries include the following:

- Obey the speed limit. If you have to speed to get there on time, you're not allowing enough time.

- Always wear a safety belt. Fasten the lap belt, even if the vehicle has automatic shoulder belts. The shoulder strap should cross the collarbone and the lap belt should fit low and snug across the hips and pelvic area. Pregnant women should position the lap belt as low as possible on the pelvic area.

- Never drive under the influence of alcohol or other drugs. Never ride with a driver who has been drinking or using drugs.

- Keep your car in good working order. Regularly inspect the tires, oil and fluid levels, windshield wipers, spare tire, and so on.

- Always allow enough following distance. Use the "3-second rule": When the vehicle ahead passes a reference point, count out 3 seconds. If you pass the reference point before you finish counting, drop back and allow more following distance.

- Always increase your following distance and slow down if weather or road conditions are poor.

- Choose interstate highways rather than rural roads. Highways are much safer because of better visibility, wider lanes, fewer surprises, and other factors.

- Always signal when turning or changing lanes.

- Stop completely at stop signs. Follow all traffic laws.

- Take special care at intersections. Always look left, right, and then left again. Make sure you have plenty of time to complete your maneuver in the intersection.

- Don't pass on two-lane roads unless you're in a designated passing area and have a clear view ahead.

- Children under the age of 12 should ride in the back seat of a motor vehicle. Young children and infants should ride in approved child safety seats appropriate for their age and size.

Motorcycles and Mopeds About one out of every ten traffic fatalities among people age 15–34 involves someone riding a motorcycle. Injuries from motorcycle collisions are generally more severe than those involving automobiles because motorcycles provide little, if any, protection. Moped riders face additional challenges. Mopeds usually have a maximum speed of 30–35 mph and have less power for maneuverability, especially in an emergency. Strategies for preventing motorcycle and moped injuries include the following:

- Maximize your visibility by wearing light-colored clothing, driving with your headlights on, and correctly positioning yourself in traffic.

- Develop the necessary skills. Lack of skill, especially when evasive action is needed to avoid a collision, is a major factor in motorcycle and moped injuries. Skidding from improper braking is the most common cause of loss of control.

- Wear a helmet. Helmets should be marked with the symbol DOT, certifying that they conform to federal safety standards established by the Department of Transportation.

- Protect your eyes with goggles, a face shield, or a windshield.

- Drive defensively, particularly when changing lanes at intersections, and never assume that you've been seen by other drivers.

Bicycles Injuries to bicyclists and pedestrians are considered motor vehicle–related because they are usually caused by motor vehicles. Bicycle injuries result primarily from riders not knowing or understanding the rules of the road, failing to follow traffic laws, not having sufficient skill or experience to handle traffic conditions, or being intoxicated. Bicycles are considered vehicles; bicyclists must obey all traffic laws that apply to automobile drivers, including stopping at traffic lights and stop signs.

Head injuries are involved in about two-thirds of all bicycle-related deaths. Wearing a helmet reduces the risk of head injury by 85%, but fewer than 50% of cyclists wear helmets. Safe cycling strategies include the following:

- Wear safety equipment, including a helmet, eye protection, gloves, and proper footwear. Secure the bottom of your pant legs with clips, and secure your shoelaces so they don't get tangled in the chain.

- Maximize your visibility by wearing light-colored, reflective clothing. Equip your bike with reflectors, and use lights, especially at night or when riding in wooded or other dark areas.

- Ride with the flow of traffic, not against it, and follow all traffic laws. Use bike paths when they are available.

- Ride defensively; never assume that drivers have seen you. Be especially careful when turning or crossing at corners and intersections. Watch for cars turning right.

Wearing a bicycle helmet can help you avoid serious head injury, brain damage, or even death in the event of a collision or fall. Helmets have a layer of stiff foam, which absorbs shock and cushions a blow to your head, covered by a thin plastic shell that will "skid" along the ground. When you shop for a helmet, remember the four S's: size, strap, straight, and sticker.

• *Size:* Try on several different sizes before making your selection; it may take several tries before you find the most comfortable fit. The helmet should be very snug but not overly tight on your head. Pads are usually provided to help adjust the fit. A good salesperson can also help you get the right fit. When the helmet is strapped onto your head, it should not move more than an inch in any direction, and you should not be able to pull or twist it off no matter how hard you try.

• *Strap:* Be sure that the chin strap fits snugly under your chin and that the V in the strap meets under your ear. Avoid thin straps, which can be uncomfortable. Check to be sure that the buckle is strong and won't pop open and that the straps are sturdy.

• *Straight:* The helmet should sit straight on your head, not tilted back or forward (see the figure). A rule of thumb is that the rim should be about two finger widths above your eyebrows (depending on the height of your forehead).

• *Sticker:* Since March 1999, helmets sold in the United States must meet uniform safety standards established by the U.S. Consumer Product Safety Commission (CPSC). Look for a sticker or label that says the helmet meets the CPSC standard. If a helmet does not have one, it does not meet federal safety standards and should not be used.

You are more likely to wear your helmet if it is comfortable, so be sure that vents on the helmet provide airflow to promote cooling and sweat control. You will be safer with a brightly col-ored helmet that makes you more visible to drivers, especially in rainy, foggy, or dark conditions. Reflective tape will also increase your visibility. Finally, a helmet is a good place to put emergency information (your name, address, and phone number, plus any emergency medical conditions and an emergency contact). Tape change inside the helmet for a phone call.

If you are involved in a crash, replace your helmet. Even if the helmet doesn't have any visible signs of damage, its ability to protect your head may be compromised. As the Bicycle Helmet Safety Institute says, "No one ever complains about the cost of their second bike helmet."

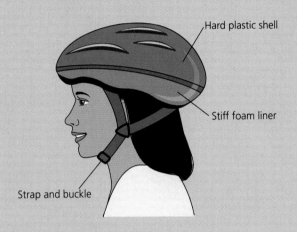

Hard plastic shell

Stiff foam liner

Strap and buckle

SOURCES: Bicycle Helmet Safety Institute. 2000. *A Consumer's Guide to Bicycle Helmets* (http://www.helmets.org/webdocs/guide.htm; retrieved July 26, 2000). National Safety Council. 2000. *Choose the Right Helmet for Your Favorite Summer Sport* (http://www.nsc.org/pubs/fsh/archive/summr00/helmet.htm; retrieved July 26, 2000).

• Stop at all traffic lights and stop signs. Know and use hand signals.

• Continue pedaling at all times when moving (no coasting) to help keep the bike stable and to maintain your balance.

• Keep your bike in good working condition.

Home Injuries

A person's place of residence, whether it be a house, an apartment, a trailer, or a dormitory, is considered home. People spend a great deal of time at home and feel that they are safe and secure there. However, home can be a dangerous place. The most common fatal **home injuries** are falls, fires, poisoning, suffocation, and unintentional firearm injuries.

Falls Most deaths occurring from falls involve falling on stairs or steps or from one level to another. Falls also occur on the same level, from tripping, slipping, or stumbling. Alcohol is a contributing factor in many falls. Strategies for preventing falls include the following:

• Install handrails and nonslip applications in the shower and bathtub.

home injuries Unintentional injuries and deaths that occur in the home and on home premises to occupants, guests, domestic servants, and trespassers; falls, burns, poisonings, suffocations, unintentional shootings, drownings, and electrical shocks are examples.

Terms

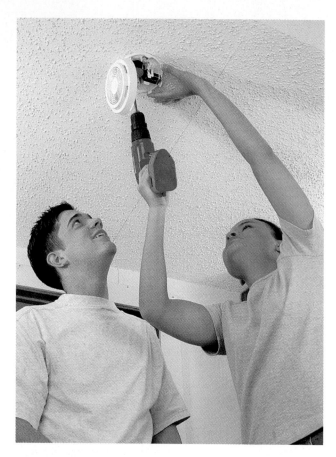

The risk of dying in a fire is reduced by half if you use a smoke detector. Install detectors on every floor, check them monthly, and replace the batteries at least once a year.

- Keep floors, stairs, and outside areas clear of objects or conditions that could cause slipping or tripping, such as ice, snow, electrical cords, and toys.

- Put a light switch by the door of every room so no one has to walk across a room to turn on a light. Use night lights in bedrooms, halls, stairs, and bathrooms.

- When climbing a ladder, use both hands. Never stand higher than the third step from the top. When using a stepladder, make sure the spreader brace is in the locked position. With straight ladders, set the base out 1 foot for every 4 feet of height. Don't use chairs to reach things.

- If there are small children in the home, place gates at the top and bottom of stairs. Never leave a baby unattended on a bed or table. Install window guards to prevent children from falling out of windows.

Fires   A death caused by a residential fire occurs every 2 hours. Cooking is now the leading cause of home fire injuries; careless smoking is the leading cause of fire deaths, followed by problems with heating equipment and arson. To prevent fires, it's important to dispose of all cigarettes in ashtrays and to never smoke in bed. Other

strategies include proper maintenance of fireplaces, furnaces, heaters, chimneys, and electrical outlets, cords, and appliances. If you use a portable heater, keep it at least 3 feet away from curtains, bedding, or anything else that might catch fire. Never leave heaters on unattended.

It's important to be adequately prepared to handle fire-related situations. Plan at least two escape routes out of each room, and designate a location outside the home as a meeting place. For practice, stage a home fire drill; do it at night, since that's when most deadly fires occur.

Install smoke detectors on every level of your home. Your risk of dying in a fire is almost twice as high if you do not use them. Clean them and check the batteries once a month, and replace the batteries at least once a year. More than 90% of U.S. homes have at least one smoke alarm, but about half are no longer functioning a year after installation, usually because batteries need to be replaced or dust needs to be cleaned out of the unit.

If a fire does occur, following these strategies can help prevent injuries:

- Get out as quickly as possible, and go to the designated meeting place. Don't stop for a keepsake or a pet. Never hide in a closet or under a bed. Once outside, count heads to see if everyone is out. If you think someone is still inside, tell the firefighters; never go back inside a burning building.

- If you're trapped in a room, feel the door. If it is hot, or if smoke is coming in through the cracks, don't open it; use the alternative escape route. If you can't get out of a room, go to the window and shout or wave for help.

- Smoke inhalation is the largest cause of death and injury in fires. To avoid inhaling smoke, crawl along the floor away from the heat and smoke. Cover your mouth and nose, ideally with a wet cloth, and take short, shallow breaths.

- If your clothes catch fire, don't run. Drop to the ground, cover your face, and roll back and forth to smother the flames. Remember: stop-drop-roll.

Poisoning   More than 2 million poisonings and over 9000 poison-related deaths occur every year in the United States. Poisons come in many forms, some of which are not typically considered poisons. For example, medications are safe when used as prescribed, but overdosing and incorrectly combining medications with another substance may result in poisoning. Other poisonous substances in the home include cleaning agents, petroleum-based products, insecticides and herbicides, cosmetics, nail polish and remover, and many houseplants. All potentially poisonous substances should be used only as directed and stored carefully, out of the reach of children.

The most common type of poisoning by gases is carbon monoxide poisoning. Carbon monoxide gas is emitted by motor vehicle exhaust and some types of heating equipment. The effects of exposure to this colorless, odorless gas include headache, blurred vision, and shortness of breath, followed by dizziness, vomiting, and unconsciousness. Carbon monoxide detectors similar to smoke detectors are available for home use. To prevent poisoning by gases, never operate a vehicle in an enclosed space, have your furnace inspected yearly, and use caution with any substance that can produce toxic fumes.

A key strategy for preventing serious poisoning injuries is to look up the phone number for the nearest Poison Control Center and post it in a convenient location. It is also a good idea to keep syrup of ipecac on hand. This nonprescription plant extract can be used to induce vomiting, but *it should be used only on the advice of the Poison Control Center or your physician.* If a poisoning does occur, it's important that you act quickly. Remove the poison from contact with the victim's eyes, skin, or mouth, or move the victim away from contact with poisonous gases. Call the Poison Control Center immediately for instructions; do not follow the emergency instructions on product labels because they may be incorrect. Depending on the situation, you may be instructed to give the victim water to drink, to flood affected parts of the skin or eyes with water, or to induce vomiting. If you are advised to go to an emergency room, take the poisonous substance or container with you.

Suffocation and Choking Suffocation accounts for nearly 4000 deaths annually in the United States. Young children account for nearly half of these deaths. Children can suffocate if they put small items in their mouths, get tangled in their crib bedding, or get trapped in airtight appliances like old refrigerators. Keep small objects out of reach of children under age 3, and don't give them raw carrots, hot dogs, popcorn, or hard candy. Examine toys carefully for small parts that could come loose; don't give plastic bags or balloons to small children.

Many choking victims can be saved with the **Heimlich maneuver** (Figure 16-1). The American Red Cross recommends the Heimlich maneuver (also called "abdominal thrusts") as the easiest and safest thing to do when an adult is choking. Back blows administered in conjunction with abdominal thrusts are an acceptable procedure for dislodging an object from the throat of an infant.

Firearms More than half of all unintended firearm deaths occur to people age 10–29. People who use firearms should remember the following:

- Never point a loaded gun at something you do not intend to shoot.
- Store unloaded firearms under lock and key, in a place separate from the ammunition.
- Always inspect firearms carefully before handling.
- Behave in the safe and responsible manner advocated in firearms safety courses.

Proper storage is critical. Do not assume that young children cannot fire a gun: About 25% of 3–4-year-olds and 70% of 5–6-year-olds have enough finger strength to pull a trigger. Every year, about 120 Americans are unintentionally shot to death by children under 6. An estimated 8.3 million children live in households with unlocked guns, including 2.6 million who live in households where guns are stored loaded or with ammunition nearby.

Probably the best advice for anyone who picks up a gun is to assume it is loaded. Too many deaths and injuries occur when someone unintentionally shoots a friend while under the impression that the gun he or she is handling is not loaded. In addition, if you plan to handle a gun, you should avoid the use of alcohol and drugs, which may affect your judgment and coordination. (Firearms and intentional injuries are discussed later in the chapter.)

Leisure Injuries

Leisure activities encompass a large part of our free time, so it is not surprising that **leisure injuries** are a significant health-related problem in the United States. Specific safety strategies for activities associated with leisure injuries include the following:

- Don't swim alone, in unsupervised places, under the influence of alcohol, or for an unusual length of time; use caution when swimming in unfamiliar surroundings or in water colder than 70°F. Check the depth of water before diving. Make sure residential pools are fenced and that children are never allowed to swim unsupervised.
- Always use a **personal flotation device** (life jacket) when on a boat.
- For all sports and recreational activities, make sure facilities are safe, follow the rules, and practice good sportsmanship. Develop adequate skill in the activity, and use proper safety equipment.
- If using equipment such as skateboards, mountain bikes, or all-terrain vehicles, wear a helmet and other safety equipment, and avoid excessive speeds and unsafe stunts.

Terms

Heimlich maneuver A maneuver developed by Henry J. Heimlich, M.D., to help force an obstruction from the airway.

leisure injuries Unintentional injuries and deaths that occur in public places or places used in a public way, not involving motor vehicles; includes most sports and recreation deaths and injuries; falls, drownings, burns, and heat and cold stress are examples.

personal flotation device A device designed to save a person from drowning by buoying up the body while in the water; also called a *life jacket*.

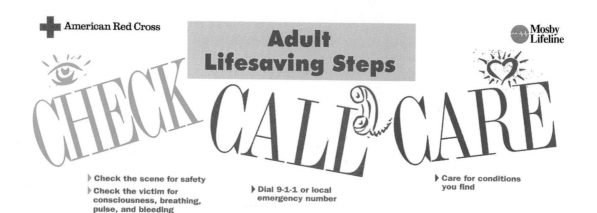

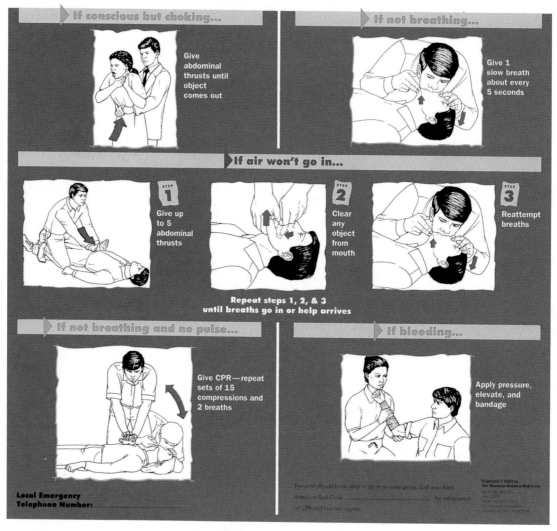

American Red Cross

Mosby Lifeline

Adult Lifesaving Steps

CHECK CALL CARE

▸ Check the scene for safety
▸ Check the victim for consciousness, breathing, pulse, and bleeding

▸ Dial 9-1-1 or local emergency number

▸ Care for conditions you find

If conscious but choking...

Give abdominal thrusts until object comes out

If not breathing...

Give 1 slow breath about every 5 seconds

If air won't go in...

STEP 1 Give up to 5 abdominal thrusts

STEP 2 Clear any object from mouth

STEP 3 Reattempt breaths

Repeat steps 1, 2, & 3 until breaths go in or help arrives

If not breathing and no pulse...

Give CPR—repeat sets of 15 compressions and 2 breaths

If bleeding...

Apply pressure, elevate, and bandage

Local Emergency Telephone Number: _____

Figure 16-1 Rescue breathing, first aid for choking, and ways to control bleeding; procedures recommended by the American Red Cross. SOURCE: Courtesy of the American Red Cross. All rights reserved in all countries.

- If you are active in excessively hot and humid weather, drink plenty of fluids, rest frequently in the shade, and slow down or stop if you feel uncomfortable. Danger signals of heat stress include excessive perspiration, dizziness, headache, muscle cramps, nausea, weakness, rapid pulse, and disorientation.
- Do not use alcohol or other drugs during recreational activities—such activities require coordina-

tion and sound judgment. Don't chew gum or eat while active to avoid choking.

In-Line Skating Injuries   More than 26 million Americans use in-line skates, and more than 250,000 are injured badly enough each year to wind up in an emergency room. Injuries to the wrist and head are most common. To reduce your risk of being injured while rollerblading, wear a helmet, elbow and knee pads, wrist guards, a long-sleeved shirt, and long pants; don't mix skating and drinking.

Scooter Injuries   The most common injuries associated with scooters are arm or hand fractures and dislocations, cuts and bruises, and sprains; 85% of injuries have involved children under the age of 15. Viewing scooters as toys more than transportation may lead riders to ignore important safety precautions:

- Wear a helmet that meets bicycle helmet standards, along with knee and elbow pads.
- Be sure that handlebars, the steering column, and all nuts and bolts are securely fastened.
- Ride on smooth, paved surfaces away from motor vehicle traffic. Avoid streets and surfaces with water, sand, gravel, or dirt.
- Don't ride after dark.
- Closely supervise young children.

COMMUNICATE!   It takes extra time and effort to be safe, and sometimes people don't want to be bothered with taking necessary precautions. If you have a friend or family member who resists safety measures—whether it's wearing a safety belt in a car, a helmet on a bike, a personal flotation device on a boat, or safety equipment while in-line skating, skateboarding, or riding a scooter—you can do him or her a favor by insisting that the safety measures be taken. You may make some impression on the person by quoting the kind of statistics mentioned in this chapter, but your best argument may simply be, "I care about you and I don't want you to get hurt."

Work Injuries

The highest risk of **work injuries** occurs among laborers. Although laborers make up less than half of the workforce, they account for more than 75% of all work-related injuries and illnesses. Most fatal occupational injuries involve crushing injuries, severe lacerations, burns, and electrocutions; among women, the leading cause of workplace injury deaths is homicide.

Back problems account for more than 20% of work injuries; many of these could be prevented through proper lifting technique (Figure 16-2):

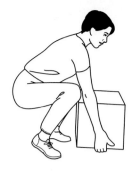

Figure 16-2   Correct lifting technique.   Stay upright, bending at the knees and hips.

- Avoid bending at the waist. Remain in an upright position and crouch down if you need to lower yourself to grasp the object. Bend at the knees and hips.
- Place feet securely about shoulder-width apart; grip the object firmly.
- Lift gradually, with straight arms. Avoid quick, jerky motions. Lift by standing up or pushing with your leg muscles. Keep the object close to your body.
- If you have to turn, change the position of your feet. Twisting is a common and dangerous cause of injury. Plan ahead so that your pathway is clear and turning can be minimized.
- Put the object down gently, reversing the rules for lifting.

Musculoskeletal injuries and disorders in the workplace include **repetitive strain injuries (RSIs)**. RSIs are caused by repeated strain on a particular part of the body. Twisting, vibrations, awkward postures, and other stressors may contribute to RSIs. **Carpal tunnel syndrome** is one type of RSI that has increased in recent years due to increased use of computers, both at work and in the home. Whatever the working conditions, employees should make a conscious effort to avoid hazardous situations.

work injuries Unintentional injuries and deaths that arise out of and in the course of gainful work, such as falls, electrical shocks, exposure to radiation and toxic chemicals, burns, cuts, back sprains, and loss of fingers or other body parts in machines.

repetitive strain injury (RSI) A musculoskeletal injury or disorder caused by repeated strain to the hand, arm, wrist, or other part of the body; also called cumulative trauma disorder (CTD).

carpal tunnel syndrome Compression of the median nerve in the wrist, often caused by repetitive use of the hands, such as in computer use; characterized by numbness, tingling, and pain in the hands and fingers; can cause nerve damage.

Terms

Carpal tunnel syndrome (CTS) is a repetitive strain injury characterized by pressure on the median nerve in the wrist. The median nerve travels from the forearm to the hand through a tunnel in the wrist formed by the wrist bones (carpals) and associated tendons and covered by a ligament. The median nerve can become compressed for a variety of reasons, including swelling of the surrounding tendons caused by pregnancy, diabetes, arthritis, or repetitive wrist motions during activities such as typing, cutting, or carpentry work. Symptoms of CTS include numbness, tingling, burning, and/or aching in the hand, particularly in the thumb and the first three fingers. The pain may worsen at night and may shoot up from the hand as far as the shoulder.

Many cases of carpal tunnel syndrome clear up on their own or with minimal treatment. Modification of the movement that is causing the problem is critically important. For example, adjusting the height of a computer keyboard so that the wrists can be held straight during typing can help relieve pressure on the wrists. CTS is often first treated by immobilizing the wrist with a splint during the night. People may also be given anti-inflammatory drugs or injections of cortisone in the wrist to reduce swelling. In a small percentage of severe cases, surgery to cut the ligament and reduce the pressure on the nerve may be recommended.

If you engage in activities like typing or cutting that involve repetitive motions, there are some strategies you can try to reduce your risk of developing carpal tunnel syndrome. Begin by modifying your work environment to reduce the stress on your wrists. Alternate activities to avoid spending long stretches of time engaged in the same motion. Warm up your wrists before you begin any repetitive motion activity, and take frequent breaks to stretch and flex your wrists and hands:

- Extend your arms out in front of you and stretch your wrists by pointing your fingers to the ceiling; hold for a count of five. Then straighten your wrists and relax your fingers for a count of five.

- With arms extended, make a tight fist with both hands and then bend your wrists so your knuckles are pointed toward the floor; hold for a count of five. Then straighten your wrists and relax your fingers for a count of five.

Repeat these stretches several times, and finish by letting your arms hang loosely at your sides and shaking them gently for several seconds.

SOURCE: American Academy of Orthopaedic Surgeons. 2000. *Exercises to Do at Work to Prevent Carpal Tunnel Syndrome* (http://orthoinfo.aaos.org/fact/thr_report.cfm?Thread_ID=15&topcategory=Hand; retrieved March 11, 2001). National Institute of Neurological Disorders and Stroke. 2000. *Carpal Tunnel Syndrome* (http://www.ninds.nih.gov/health_and_medical/disorders/carpal_doc.htm; retrieved March 11, 2001). Detecting carpal tunnel syndrome. 1999. *Journal of the American Medical Association* 282(2): 206.

VIOLENCE AND INTENTIONAL INJURIES

Violence—the use of physical force with the intent to inflict harm, injury, or death upon oneself or another—is a major public health concern in the United States. More than 2 million Americans are victims of violent injury each year; about three violent crimes occur every minute. In general, the overall violent crime rate increased between the 1950s and 1970s and then leveled off until the mid1980s, when it again began to rise. Since 1993, however, the rate of violent crime has declined by over 20%; the homicide rate in 1999 was at its lowest level since 1966. In comparison to other industrialized countries, U.S. rates of of violence are abnormally high in only two areas—homicide and firearm-related deaths. The U.S. homicide death rate is four to ten times that of similar countries, and the firearm death rate in the United States exceeds that of other developed countries eightfold.

Factors Contributing to Violence

Most intentional injuries and deaths are associated with an argument or the committing of another crime. However, there are a great many forms of violence, and no single factor can explain all of them.

Social Factors   Rates of violence are not the same throughout society; they vary by geographic region, neighborhood, socioeconomic level, and many other factors. In the United States, violence is highest in the West, followed by the South, and among those who are disadvantaged in some way. Neighborhoods that are disadvantaged in status, power, and economic resources are typically the ones with the most violence. Rates of violence are highest among young people and minorities, groups that have relatively little power. People under age 25 account for nearly half the arrests for violent crimes in the United States and about 40% of the arrests for homicide.

Violence in the Media   The mass media play a major role in exposing audiences of all ages to violence as an acceptable and effective means of solving problems. Children may view as many as 10,000 violent acts on television and in movies each year. The consequences of violence, on both perpetrator and victim, are shown much less frequently.

The role of media violence on violent behavior is an area of controversy. However, it makes sense for parents to be aware of the potential influence of the media on their children. A child may not clearly understand the distinctions between the fantasy world portrayed in the

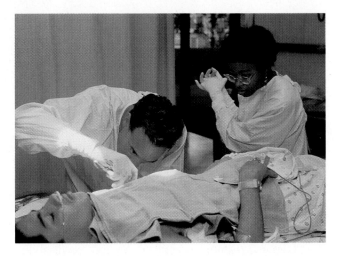

For every violent death that occurs in the United States, there are at least 100 nonfatal injuries caused by violence. The victims of most types of violence are statistically likely to be young (under 25 years), poor, in a minority, urban, and—except for rape and domestic violence—male.

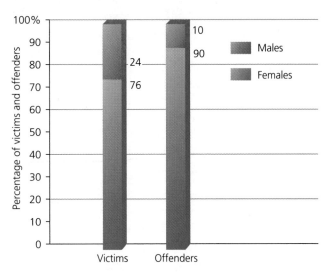

(a) Homicide victims and offenders by sex

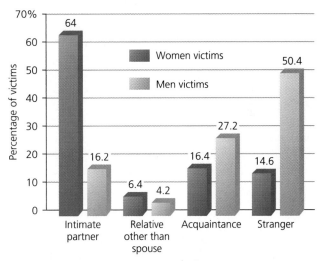

(b) Adult victims of violence by victim-offender relationship and sex of victim

Www. VITAL STATISTICS

Figure 16-3 Facts about violence in the United States.
SOURCES: Federal Bureau of Investigation. 2000. *Crime in the United States. Uniform Crime Reports, 1999.* Washington, D.C.: U.S. Department of Justice. Tjaden, P., and N. Thoennes. 2000. *Full Report of the Prevalence, Incidence, and Consequences of Violence Against Women.* Washington, D.C.: U.S. Department of Justice.

media and the complexities of the real world. Watching programs with children gives parents the opportunity to talk to children about violence and its consequences, to explain that violence is not the best way to resolve conflicts or solve problems, and to point out examples of positive behaviors such as kindness and cooperation.

Gender In most cases, violence is committed by men (Figure 16-3). Males are more than nine times more likely than females to commit murder, and three times more likely than females to be murdered. Some researchers have suggested that the male hormone testosterone is in some way linked to aggressive behavior. Others point to prevailing cultural attitudes about male roles (men as dominant and controlling) as an explanation for the high rate of violence among men. However, these theories do not explain just why it is that violent men are more likely to live in the West, belong to minorities, be poor, and be young.

Women do commit acts of violence, including a small but substantial proportion of murders of spouses. This fact has been used to argue that women have the same capacity to commit violence as men, but most researchers feel that there are substantial differences. Men often kill their wives as the culmination of years of violence or after stalking them; they may kill the entire family and themselves at the same time. Women virtually never kill in these circumstances; rather, they kill their husbands after repeated victimization or while being beaten.

Interpersonal Factors Although most people fear attack from strangers, the majority of victims are acquainted with their attacker (see Figure 16-3). Approximately 60% of murders of women and 80% of sexual assaults are committed by someone the woman knows. In many cases, the people we need to fear the most live in our own household. Crime victims and violent criminals tend to share many characteristics—that is, they are likely to be young, male, in a minority, and poor.

Alcohol and Other Drugs Substance abuse and dependence are consistently associated with interpersonal violence and suicide. Intoxication affects judgment and may increase aggression in some people, causing a small argument to escalate into a serious physical confrontation. On college campuses, alcohol is involved in about 95% of all violent crimes.

Firearms Many criminologists feel that the high rate of homicide in the United States is directly related to the fact that we are the only industrialized country in which handguns are widespread and easily available. Simply put, most victims of assaults with other weapons don't die, but the death rate from assault by handgun is extremely high. The possession of a handgun can change a suicide attempt to a completed suicide and a violent assault to a murder. Every hour, guns are used to kill four people in the United States.

Over 100,000 deaths and injuries occur in the United States each year as a result of the use of firearms. Firearms are used in more than two-thirds of homicides, and studies reveal a strong correlation between the incidence of gun ownership and homicide rates for a given area of the country. Over half of all suicides involve a firearm, and people living in households in which guns are kept have a risk of suicide that is five or more times greater than that of people living in households without guns.

Assault

Assault is the use of physical force by a person or persons to inflict injury or death on another; homicide, aggravated assault, and robbery are examples of assault. The victims of assaultive injuries and their perpetrators tend to resemble one another in terms of ethnicity, educational background, psychological profile, and reliance on weapons. In many cases, the victim actually magnifies the confrontation through the use of a weapon.

Homicide

Men, teenagers, young adults, and members of minority groups, particularly African Americans and Latinos, are most likely to be murder victims. Poverty and unemployment have been identified as key factors in homicide, and this may account for the high rates of homicide among blacks and other minority groups. Most homicides are committed with a firearm, occur during an argument, and occur among people who know one another. Intrafamilial homicide, where the perpetrator and victim are related, accounts for about one out of every eight homicides. About 40% of family homicides are committed by spouses, usually following a history of physical and emotional abuse directed at the woman. Wives are more likely to be murdered than husbands, and when a wife kills her husband, it is usually in self-defense.

Gang-Related Violence

Gangs are most frequently associated with large cities, but gang activity also extends to the suburbs and even to rural areas. It is estimated that more than 800,000 Americans belong to gangs; the average age for joining a gang is 14. Most gangs control a particular territory and will oppose other gangs, as well as police and community efforts to eliminate them. Gangs may be involved in illegal drug trade, extortion, and "protection" schemes. Violence may result from conflicts over territory or illegal activities.

Gangs are more common in areas that are poor and suffer from high unemployment, population density, and crime. In these areas, an individual may feel that his or her chance of legitimate success in life is out of reach and know that involvement in the drug market makes some gang members rich. Often, gangs also serve as a mechanism for companionship, self-esteem, support, and security; indeed, in some areas, gang membership may be viewed as the only possible means of survival.

Hate Crimes

When bias against another person's race or ethnicity, national origin, religion, sexual orientation, or disability motivates a criminal act, the offense is classified as a hate crime. Hate crimes may be committed against people or property; those against people may include intimidation, assault, and even rape or murder. Crimes against property most frequently involve graffiti, the desecration of churches or synagogues, cross burnings, and other acts of vandalism or property damage.

About 10,000 hate crimes are reported every year; many more go unreported. Crimes against people make up about 70% of all incidents; intimidation and assault are the most common offenses. Racial or ethnic bias was cited as the motivating bias in 55% of the hate crimes reported in 1999; religion was cited in 18% of the cases, sexual orientation in 17%, and national origin in 11%.

Hate crimes may be extremely brutal acts perpetrated at random on total strangers by multiple offenders. Research indicates that a substantial number of hate crimes are committed by males under age 20. Hate crimes are frequently, but not always, associated with fringe groups that have extremist ideologies, such as the Ku Klux Klan and neo-Nazi groups. The Southern Poverty Law Center tracks more than 450 hate groups and group chapters currently active in the United States; the rapid growth of hate sites on the Internet is another area of concern.

To combat hate crimes, individuals and communities must foster tolerance, understanding, and an appreciation of differences among people.

School Violence

According to the National School Safety Center, more than 275 school-associated violent deaths of students, faculty, and administrators have occurred since 1992. A majority of these deaths occurred in urban areas and involved use of a firearm; as with other types of violence, both victims and offenders were predominantly young men. Homicide and suicide are the most serious and least common types of violence in schools; an estimated 400,000 less serious incidents of violence and crime occur each year, including theft, vandalism, and fights not involving weapons.

Children are actually much safer at school than away from it. Less than 1% of all homicides among youths age 5–19 occur at school, and 90% of schools report no incidents of serious violence. Children and adolescents are far more likely to be killed by an adult in their own home or away from school than they are to die as a result of school-associated violence. According to the CDC, the overall number of violent incidents has decreased steadily since 1992; however, the number of multiple-victim events may have increased.

Characteristics associated with youths who have caused school-associated violent deaths include a history of uncontrollable angry outbursts, violent and abusive language and behavior, isolation from peers, depression and irritability, access to and preoccupation with weapons, and lack of support and supervision from adults. Recommendations for reducing school violence include offering classroom training in anger management and improved self-control, providing mental health and social services for students in need, developing after-school programs that help students build self-esteem and make friends, and keeping guns out of the hands of children and out of schools.

Family and Intimate Violence

Family violence generally refers to any rough and illegitimate use of physical force, aggression, or verbal abuse by one family member toward another. Such abuse may be physical and/or psychological in nature. Based upon reported cases each year, an estimated 5–7 million women and children are abused in the United States.

Battering   Studies reveal than 95% of domestic violence victims are women. Violence against wives/intimate partners, or battering, occurs at every level of society but is more common at lower socioeconomic levels. It occurs more frequently in relationships with a high degree of conflict—an apparent inability to resolve arguments through negotiation and compromise. About 25% of women report having been physically assaulted or raped by an intimate partner.

At the root of much of this abusive behavior is the need to control another person: Abusive partners are controlling partners. They not only want to have power over another person, but also believe they are entitled to it, no matter what the cost to the other person. Abuse includes behavior that physically harms, arouses fear, prevents a person from doing what she wants, or compels her to behave in ways she does not freely choose.

In abusive relationships, the abuser (in most cases a man) usually has a history of violent behavior, traditional beliefs about gender roles, and problems with alcohol abuse. He has low self-esteem and seeks to raise it by dominating and imposing his will on another person. Research has revealed a three-phase cycle of battering, con-

sisting of a period of increasing tension, a violent explosion and loss of control, and a period of contriteness, in which the man begs forgiveness and promises it will never happen again. The batterer is drawn back to this cycle over and over again, but he never succeeds in changing his feelings about himself.

Battered women often stay in violent relationships for years. They may be economically dependent on their partners, believe their children need a father, or have low self-esteem themselves. They may love or pity their husbands, or they may believe they'll eventually be able to stop the violence. They usually leave the relationship only when they become determined that the violence must end. Battered women's shelters offer physical protection, counseling, support, and other types of assistance.

Stalking and Cyberstalking   Battering is closely associated with **stalking**, characterized by harassing behaviors such as following or spying on a person and making verbal, written, or implied threats. In the United States, it is estimated that 1 million women and 400,000 men are stalked each year; about 87% of stalkers are men. About half of female victims are stalked by current or former intimate partners; of these, 80% had been physically or sexually assaulted by that partner during the relationship. A stalker's goal may be to control or scare the victim or to keep her or him in a relationship. Most stalking episodes last a year or less, but victims may experience social and psychological effects long after the stalking ends.

The use of the Internet, e-mail, chat rooms, and other electronic communications devices to stalk another person is known as **cyberstalking.** As with offline stalking, the majority of stalkers are men, and the majority of victims are women, although there have been same-sex cyberstalking incidents. Cyberstalkers may send harassing or threatening e-mails or chat room messages to the victim, or they may encourage others to harass the victim—for example, by impersonating the victim and posting inflammatory messages and personal information on bulletin boards or in chat rooms. Guidelines for staying safe online include the following:

- Never use your real name as an e-mail username or chat room nickname. Select an age- and gender-neutral identity.

---

stalking Repeatedly harassing or threatening a person through behaviors such as following a person, appearing at a person's residence or workplace, leaving written messages or objects, making harassing phone calls, or vandalizing property; frequently directed at a former intimate partner.

cyberstalking The use of e-mail, chat rooms, bulletin boards, or other electronic communications devices to stalk another person.

Terms

There are no sure ways to tell whether someone will become abusive or violent toward an intimate partner, but there are warning signs that you can look for. (Remember that, although most abusive relationships involve male violence directed at a woman, women can also be abusive, as can partners in a same-sex relationship. Because most abusers are male, the following material refers to the abuser as "he.") If you are concerned that a person you are involved with has the potential for violence, observe his or her behavior, and ask yourself these questions:

- What is this person's attitude toward women? How does he treat his mother and his sister? How does he work with female students, female colleagues, or a female boss? How does he treat your women friends?

- What is his attitude toward your autonomy? Does he respect the work you do and the way you do it? Or does he put it down, or tell you how to do it better, or encourage you to give it up? Does he tell you he'll take care of you?

- How self-centered is he? Does he want to spend leisure time on your interests or his? Does he listen to you? Does he remember what you say?

- Is he possessive or jealous? Does he want to spend every minute with you? Does he cross-examine you about things you do when you're not with him?

- What happens when things don't go the way he wants them to? Does he blow up? Does he always have to get his way?

- Is he moody, mocking, critical, or bossy? Do you feel as if you're "walking on eggshells" when you're with him?

- Do you feel you have to avoid arguing with him?

- Does he drink too much or use drugs?

- Does he refuse to use condoms or take other precautions for safer sex?

Listen to your own uneasiness, and stay away from any man who disrespects women, who wants or needs you intensely and exclusively, and who has a knack for getting his own way almost all the time.

If you are in a serious relationship with a controlling person, you may already have experienced abuse. Consider the questions on the following list:

- Does your partner constantly criticize you, blame you for things that are not your fault, or verbally degrade you?

- Does he humiliate you in front of others?

- Is he suspicious or jealous? Does he accuse you of being unfaithful or monitor your mail or phone calls?

- Does he "track" all your time? Does he discourage you from seeing friends and family?

- Does he prevent you from getting or keeping a job or attending school? Does he control your shared resources or restrict your access to money?

- Has he ever pushed, slapped, hit, kicked, bitten, or restrained you? Thrown an object at you? Used a weapon on you?

- Has he ever destroyed or damaged your personal property or sentimental items?

- Has he ever forced you to have sex or to do something sexually you didn't want to do?

- Does he anger easily when drinking or taking drugs?

- Has he ever threatened to harm you or your children, friends, pets, or property?

- Has he ever threatened to blackmail you if you leave?

If you answered yes to one or more of these questions, you may be experiencing domestic abuse. If you believe you or your children are in imminent danger, look in your local telephone directory for a women's shelter, or call 9-1-1. If you want information, referrals to a program in your area, or assistance, contact one of the organizations listed in For More Information at the end of the chapter.

SOURCES: Family Violence Prevention Fund. 1996. *Take Action Against Domestic Violence.* San Francisco, Calif.: Family Violence Prevention Fund. How to tell if you're in an abusive situation. 1994. *San Francisco Chronicle,* 24 June. Jones, A. 1994. *Next Time She'll Be Dead.* Boston: Beacon Press.

- Avoid filling out profiles for accounts related to e-mail use or chat room activities with information that could be used to identify you.

- Do not share personal information in public spaces anywhere online or give it to strangers.

- Learn how to filter unwanted e-mail messages.

- If you do experience harassment online, do not respond to the harasser. Log off or surf elsewhere.

If you receive unwanted online contact, make it clear to that person that you want all contact to stop. If harassment continues, contact the harasser's Internet service provider (ISP) by identifying the domain of the stalker's account (after the "@" sign); most ISPs have an e-mail address for complaints. Often, an ISP can try to stop the conduct by direct contact with the harasser or by closing his or her account. Save all communications for evidence, and contact your ISP and your local police department.

Violence Against Children   At least 1 million American children are physically abused by their parents every year. Parental violence is one of the five leading causes of death for children age 1–18. Parents who abuse children tend to have low self-esteem, to believe in physical punishment, to have a poor marital relationship, and to have been abused themselves (although many people who were abused as children do not grow up to abuse their own children). Poverty, unemployment, and social isolation are characteristics of families in which children are abused. Single parents, both men and women, are at especially high risk for abusing their children. Very often one child, whom the parents consider different in some way, is singled out for violent treatment.

Elder Abuse   Each year, at least 500,000 older persons are abused; only one in six incidents is reported. Most abusers are family members who are serving as caregivers. Elder abuse can take different forms: physical, sexual, or emotional abuse, financial exploitation, neglect, or abandonment. Neglect is the most common form of abuse, accounting for about 55% of reported cases; physical abuse accounts for about 15% of reported cases and financial exploitation for about 13%. Abuse often occurs when caring for a dependent adult becomes too stressful for the caregiver, especially if the elder is incontinent, has suffered mental deterioration, or is violent. Abuse may become an outlet for frustration. Many believe that the solution to elder abuse is support in the form of greater social and financial assistance, such as adult day-care centers and education and public care programs.

> **COMMUNICATE!**   It's normal to feel angry when someone you love or trust lets you down, but don't let your anger hurt you or anyone else. Learn to talk about your feelings and to express yourself calmly, describing your disappointment, frustration, anger, or displeasure without losing your temper. For example, you might say, "I am so disappointed and angry that you repeated what I told you in confidence." Learn to listen to others without getting upset if they give you negative feedback; try to see the situation from the other person's point of view. Look for creative ways to negotiate difficult problems and find compromises. Anger is part of life, but it shouldn't control you or your relationships.

Sexual Violence

The use of force and coercion in sexual relationships is one of the most serious problems in human interactions. The most extreme manifestation of sexual coercion—forcing a person to submit to another's sexual desires—is rape, but sexual coercion occurs in many more subtle forms, including sexual harassment.

Sexual Assault: Rape   Sexual coercion that relies on the threat and use of physical force or takes advantage of circumstances that render a person incapable of giving consent (such as when drunk) constitutes **sexual assault** or **rape.** When the victim is younger than the legally defined "age of consent," the act constitutes **statutory rape,** whether or not coercion is involved. Coerced sexual activity in which the victim knows or is dating the rapist is often referred to as **date rape** (or acquaintance rape).

Any woman—or man—can be a rape victim. It is conservatively estimated that at least 3.5 million females are raped annually in the United States. Some men are raped by other men, perhaps 10,000 annually; the majority of male victims are not in prison and most know their assailant.

WHO COMMITS RAPE?   Men who commit rape may be any age and come from any socioeconomic group. Some rapists are exploiters in the sense that they rape on the spur of the moment and mainly want immediate gratification. Some attempt to compensate for feelings of sexual inadequacy and an inability to obtain satisfaction otherwise. Others are more hostile and sadistic and are primarily interested not in sex but in hurting and humiliating a particular woman or women in general.

Most women are in much less danger of being raped by a stranger than of being sexually assaulted by a man they know or date. Surveys suggest that as many as 25% of women have had experiences in which the men they were dating persisted in trying to force sex despite pleading, crying, screaming, or resisting. Surveys have also found that more than 60% of all rape victims were raped by a current or former spouse, boyfriend, or date; and as many as 60% of battered women may have been raped by their husbands.

Most cases of date rape are never reported to the police, partly because of the subtlety of the crime. Usually no weapons are involved, and direct verbal threats may not have been made. Rather than being terrorized, the victim usually is attracted to the man at first. Victims of date rape tend to shoulder much of the responsibility for the incident, questioning their own judgment and behavior rather than blaming the aggressor.

FACTORS CONTRIBUTING TO DATE RAPE   One factor in date rape appears to be the double standard about appropriate sexual behavior for men and women. Although the general status of women in society has improved, it is still a commonly held cultural belief that nice women don't say yes to sex (even when they want to) and that real men don't take no for an answer.

There are also widespread differences between men and women in how they perceive romantic encounters and signals. In one study, researchers found that men tend to interpret women's actions on dates, such as smiling or talk-

> **sexual assault** or **rape**   The use of force to have sex with someone against that person's will.
>
> **statutory rape**   Sexual interaction with someone under the legal age of consent.
>
> **date rape**   Sexual assault by someone the victim knows or is dating; also called *acquaintance rape*.

Guidelines for Women

- Believe in your right to control what you do. Set limits, and communicate these limits clearly, firmly, and early. Say "no" when you mean "no."

- Be assertive with someone who is sexually pressuring you. Men often interpret passivity as permission.

- If you are unsure of a new acquaintance, go on a group or double date. If possible, provide your own transportation.

- Remember that some men assume sexy dress and a flirtatious manner mean a desire for sex.

- Remember that alcohol and drugs interfere with clear communication about sex.

- Use the statement that has proven most effective in stopping date rape: "This is rape, and I'm calling the police."

Guidelines for Men

- Be aware of social pressure. It's OK not to "score."

- Understand that "no" means "no." Don't continue making advances when your date resists or tells you she wants to stop. Remember that she has the right to refuse sex.

- Don't assume sexy dress and a flirtatious manner are invitations to sex, that previous permission for sex applies to the current situation, or that your date's relationships with other men constitute sexual permission for you.

- Remember that alcohol and drugs interfere with clear communication about sex.

ing in a low voice, as indicating an interest in having sex, while the women interpreted the same actions as just being "friendly." Men's thinking about forceful sex also tends to be unclear. One psychologist reports that men find "forcing a woman to have sex against her will" more acceptable than "raping a woman," even though the former description is the definition of rape.

DATE-RAPE DRUGS   Recently there has been an increase in the reported use of "date-rape drugs" besides alcohol. Drugs used in date-rape situations include flunitrazepam (Rohypnol), gamma hydroxybutyrate (GHB), and ketamine hydrochloride ("Special K"). As described in Chapter 7, these drugs have a variety of effects, including sedation anterograde amnesia, meaning victims have little memory of what happens while they are under the influence of the drug. The Drug-Induced Rape Prevention and Punishment Act of 1996 adds up to 20 years to the prison sentence of any rapist who uses a drug to incapacitate a victim. Strategies such as the following can help ensure that your drink is not tampered with at a bar or party:

- Check with campus or local police to find out if drug-facilitated sexual assault has occurred in your area and, if so, where.

- Drink moderately and responsibly. Avoid group drinking and drinking games.

- Be wary of opened beverages—alcoholic or nonalcoholic—offered by strangers. When at an unfamiliar bar, watch the bartender pour your drink.

- Let your date be the first to drink from the punchbowl at a bar, club, or rave.

- If an opened beverage tastes, looks, or smells strange, do not drink it. If you leave your drink

unattended, such as when you dance or use the restroom, obtain a fresh drink when you return to your table.

- If you go to a party, club, or bar, go with friends. Have a prearranged plan for checking on each other visually and verbally. If you feel giddy or lightheaded, get assistance.

DEALING WITH A SEXUAL ASSAULT   Experts disagree about whether a woman who is faced with a rapist should fight back or give in quietly to avoid being injured or gain time in the hope of escaping. Some rapists say that if a woman had screamed or resisted loudly, they would have run; others report they would have injured or killed her. (If a rapist is carrying a weapon, most experts advise against fighting unless absolutely necessary.) A woman who is raped by a stranger is more likely to be physically injured than a woman raped by someone she knows. Each situation is unique, and a woman should respond in whatever way she thinks best. If a woman chooses not to resist, it does not mean that she has not been raped.

If you are threatened by a rapist and decide to fight back, here is what Women Organized Against Rape (WOAR) recommends:

- Trust your gut feeling. If you feel you are in danger, don't hesitate to run and scream. It is better to feel foolish than to be raped.

- Yell—and keep yelling. It will clear your head and start your adrenaline going; it may scare your attacker and also bring help. Don't forget that a rapist is also afraid of pain and afraid of getting caught.

- If an attacker grabs you from behind, use your elbows for striking the neck, his sides, or his stomach.

- Try kicking. Your legs are the strongest part of your body, and your kick is longer than his reach. Kick with your rear foot and with the toe of your shoe. Aim low to avoid losing your balance.

- His most vulnerable spot is his knee; it's low, difficult to protect, and easily knocked out of place. Don't try to kick a rapist in the crotch; he has been protecting this area all his life and will have better protective reflexes there than at his knees.

- Once you start fighting, keep it up. Your objective is to get away as soon as you can.

- Remember that ordinary rules of behavior don't apply. It's OK to vomit, act "crazy," or claim to have a sexually transmitted disease.

If you are raped, tell what happened to the first friendly person you meet. Call the police, tell them you were raped, and give your location. Write down a description of your attacker as soon as possible. Don't wash or change your clothes, or you may destroy important evidence. The police will take you to a hospital for a complete exam; show the physician any injuries. Tell the police simply, but exactly, what happened. Be honest, and stick to your story.

If you decide that you don't want to report the rape to the police, be sure to see a physician as soon as possible. You need to be checked for pregnancy and STDs.

THE EFFECTS OF RAPE   Rape victims suffer both physical and psychological injury. For most, physical wounds heal within a few weeks. Psychological pain may endure and be substantial. Even the most physically and mentally strong are likely to experience shock, anxiety, depression, shame, and a host of psychosomatic symptoms after being victimized. These psychological reactions following rape are called rape trauma syndrome, which is characterized by fear, nightmares, fatigue, crying spells, and digestive upset. (Rape trauma syndrome is a form of post-traumatic stress disorder; see Chapter 3.) Self-blame is very likely; society has contributed to this tendency by perpetuating the myths that woman can actually defend themselves and that no one can be raped if she doesn't want to be. Fortunately, these false beliefs are dissolving in the face of evidence to the contrary.

Many organizations offer counseling and support to rape victims. Look in the telephone directory under Rape or Rape Crisis Center for a hotline number to call. Your campus may have counseling services or a support group.

Child Sexual Abuse   Child sexual abuse is a sexual act imposed on a minor. Adults and older adolescents are able to coerce children into sexual activity because of their authority and power over them. Threats, force, or the promise of friendship or material rewards may be used to manipulate a child. Sexual contacts are typically brief and consist of genital manipulation; genital inter-

course is much less common. One highly traumatic form of sexual abuse is **incest,** sexual activity between people too closely related to legally marry.

Sexual abusers are usually male, heterosexual, and known to the victim. The abuser may be a relative, a friend, a neighbor, or another trusted adult acquaintance. Child abusers are often pedophiles, people who are sexually attracted to children. With other adults, they may have poor interpersonal and sexual relationships and feel socially inadequate and inferior.

Sexual abuse is often unreported. Surveys suggest that as many as 27% of women and 16% of men were sexually abused as children. An estimated 150,000–200,000 new cases of child sexual abuse occur each year. It can leave lasting scars, and adults who were abused as children are more likely to suffer from low self-esteem, depression, anxiety, eating disorders, self-destructive tendencies, sexual problems, and difficulties in intimate relationships.

If you were a victim of sexual abuse as a child and feel it may be interfering with your functioning today, you may want to address the problem. A variety of approaches may help, such as joining a support group of people who have had similar experiences, confiding in a partner or friend, or seeking professional help.

Sexual Harassment   Unwelcome sexual advances, requests for sexual favors, and other verbal, visual, or physical conduct of a sexual nature constitute **sexual harassment** if such conduct explicitly or implicitly affects academic or employment decisions or evaluations; interferes with an individual's academic or work performance; or creates an intimidating, hostile, or offensive academic, work, or student living environment.

Extreme cases of sexual harassment occur when a manager, professor, or other person in authority uses his or her ability to control or influence jobs or grades to coerce people into having sex or to punish them if they refuse. A hostile environment can be created by such conduct as sexual gestures, displaying of sexually suggestive objects or pictures, derogatory comments and jokes, sexual remarks about clothing or appearance, obscene letters, and unnecessary touching or pinching.

If you have been the victim of sexual harassment, you can take action to stop it. Be assertive with anyone who uses language or actions you find inappropriate. If possible, confront your harasser either in writing, over the

Terms

incest Sexual activity between close relatives, such as siblings or parents and their children.

sexual harassment Unwelcome sexual advances, requests for sexual favors, and other conduct of a sexual nature that affects academic or employment decisions or evaluations; interferes with an individual's academic or work performance, or creates an intimidating, hostile, or offensive academic, work, or student living environment.

often, the threat of a lawsuit or other legal action is enough to stop the harasser.

What You Can Do About Violence

It is obvious that violence in our society is not disappearing and that it is a serious threat to our collective health and well-being. This is especially true on college campuses, which in a sense are communities in themselves but which sometimes lack the authority or guidance to tackle the issue of violence directly. Although government and law enforcement agencies are working to address the problem of violence, individuals must take on a greater responsibility to bring about change.

Reducing gun-related injuries may require changes in the availability, possession, and lethality of the 12 million firearms sold in the United States each year. As part of the Brady gun control law, computerized instant background checks are performed for most gun sales to prevent purchases by convicted felons, people with a history of mental instability, and certain other groups. In some states, waiting periods are required in addition to the background checks. Some groups advocate a complete and universal federal ban on the sale of all handguns.

Safety experts also advocate the adoption of consumer safety standards for guns, including features such as childproofing and indicators to show if a gun is loaded. Technologies such as fingerprint reading are now available to personalize handguns to help prevent unauthorized use. Education about proper storage is also important: Surveys indicate that in about 23% of gun-owning households, the weapon is stored loaded, and in 28% the gun is kept hidden but not locked. To be effective, any approach to firearm injury prevention must have the support of law enforcement and the community as a whole.

PROVIDING EMERGENCY CARE

A course in **first aid** can help you respond appropriately when someone is injured. One important benefit of first aid training is learning what _not_ to do in certain situations. For example, a person with a suspected neck or back injury should not be moved unless other life-threatening conditions exist. An emergency first aid guide is provided inside the back cover of this book.

Emergency rescue techniques can save the lives of people who are choking, who have stopped breathing, or whose hearts have stopped beating. As described earlier, the Heimlich maneuver is used when a victim is choking. Pulmonary resuscitation (also known as rescue breathing, artificial respiration, or mouth-to-mouth resuscitation) is used when a person is not breathing (see Figure 16-1). **Cardiopulmonary resuscitation (CPR)** is used when a pulse cannot be found. Training is required before a person can perform CPR; courses are offered by the American Red Cross and the American Heart Association.

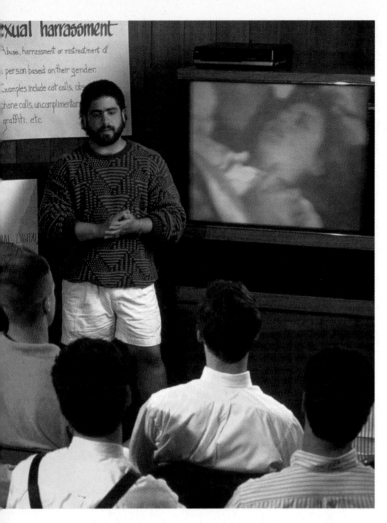

Date rape and sexual harassment are important issues for college students. The goals of this college workshop are to raise men's awareness of the double standard about appropriate sexual behavior for men and women and to examine the differences in how men and women may perceive each other's comments and actions.

telephone, or in person, informing him or her that the situation is unacceptable to you and you want the harassment to stop. Be clear: "Do not _ever_ make sexual remarks to me" is an unequivocal statement. Assemble a file or log documenting the harassment, noting the details of each incident and information about any witnesses who may be able to support your claims. You may discover others who have been harassed by the same person, which will strengthen your case. Then file a grievance with the harasser's supervisor or employer.

If your attempts to deal with the harassment internally are not successful, you can file an official complaint with your city or state Human Rights Commission or Fair Employment Practices Agency, or with the federal Equal Employment Opportunity Commission. You may also wish to pursue legal action under the Civil Rights Act or under local laws prohibiting employment discrimination. Very

College campuses can be the site of criminal activity and violence just as any other environment or living situation can be—and so they require the same level of caution and awareness that you would use in other situations. Two key points to remember: 80% of campus crimes are committed by a student against a fellow student, and alcohol or drug use is involved in 90% of campus felonies. Drinking or drug use can affect judgment and lower inhibitions, so be aware if you or another person is under the influence. Here are some suggestions for keeping yourself safe on campus:

- Don't travel alone after dark. Many campuses have shuttle buses that run from spots on campus such as the library and the dining hall to residence halls and other locations. Escorts are often available to walk with you at night.

- Be familiar with well-lit and frequently traveled routes around campus if you do need to walk alone.

- If you have a car, follow the usual precautions about parking in well-lit areas, keeping the doors locked while you are driving, and never picking up hitchhikers.

- Always have your keys ready as you approach your residence hall, room, and car. Don't lend your keys to others.

- Let friends and family members know your schedule of classes and activities to create a sort of buddy system.

- Be sure the doors and windows of your dorm room have sturdy locks, and use them.

- Don't prop open doors or hold doors open for nonstudents or nonresidents trying to enter your dorm. Be aware of nonresidents around your dorm. If someone says that he or she is meeting a friend inside, that person should be able to call the friend from outside the building.

- Keep valuables and anything containing personal information—credit cards, wallets, jewelry, and so on—hidden. Secure expensive computer and stereo equipment with cables so that it can't be easily stolen. Use a quality U-shaped lock whenever you leave a bicycle unattended.

- Be alert when using an ATM and don't display large amounts of cash.

- Stay alert and trust your instincts. Don't hesitate to call the police or campus security if something doesn't seem or feel right.

The Jeanne Clery Disclosure of Campus Security Policy and Campus Crime Statistics Act, named for a Lehigh University student who was murdered in her residence hall in 1986, requires colleges and universities to collect and report campus crime statistics. You can now review this information online at the Crime Statistics Web site of the U.S. Department of Education's Office of Postsecondary Education (http://ope.ed.gov/security/Search.asp).

SOURCES: U.S. Department of Education, Office of Postsecondary Education. 2000. *Campus Security* (http://www.ed.gov/offices/OPE/PPI/security.html; retrieved December 16, 2000). Security on Campus, Inc. 2000. *Campus Safety: Tips and Evaluation Brochure* (http://www.soconline.org/information/tips/index.html; retrieved December 16, 2000).

As a person providing assistance to someone, you are the first link in the **emergency medical services (EMS) system.** Your responsibility may be to render first aid as needed, provide emotional support for the victim, or just call for help. The basic pattern for providing emergency care is check-call-care:

- *Check the situation:* Before administering aid, make sure the scene is safe for both you and the injured person.

- *Check the victim:* Conduct a quick head-to-toe examination. Assess the victim's signs and symptoms, such as level of responsiveness, pulse, and breathing rate. Look for bleeding and any indications of broken bones or paralysis.

- *Call for help:* Call 9-1-1 or a local emergency number. Identify yourself and give as much information as you can about the condition of the victim and what happened.

- *Care for the victim:* If the situation requires immediate action (no pulse, shock, etc.), provide first aid if you are trained to do so (see Figure 16-1).

Like other kinds of behavior, preventing injuries and acting safely involve choices you make every day. You can motivate yourself to act in the safest way possible by increasing your knowledge and level of awareness, by examining your attitudes to see if they're realistic, by knowing your capacities and limitations, by adjusting your responses when environmental hazards exist, and, in general, by taking responsibility for your actions. You can't eliminate all risks and dangers from your life—no one can do that—but you can improve your chances of avoiding injuries and living to a healthy, ripe old age.

Terms

first aid Emergency care given to an ill or injured person until medical care can be obtained.

cardiopulmonary resuscitation (CPR) An emergency first aid procedure that combines artificial respiration and artificial circulation; used in first aid emergencies where breathing and blood circulation have stopped.

emergency medical services (EMS) system A system designed to network community resources for providing emergency care.

Although people worry about violence, unintentional injuries—such as those resulting from car crashes, falls, and fires—are much more common. In fact, unintentional injuries are the leading cause of death for people under the age of 35. To protect yourself from both unintentional and intentional injuries, learn to incorporate sensible safety precautions into your daily life.

Right now you can

- Pick up anything on the floor of your home that could cause tripping or slipping.

- Make sure the electrical outlets in your home are not overloaded and that extension cords do not run under rugs or where people walk.

- Test the batteries in the smoke detectors in your home and replace them if they aren't working.

- Check your bike helmet to make sure it fits properly and meets the requirements described in the box "Choosing a Bicycle Helmet." Wear it the next time you go for a bike ride.

SUMMARY

- Key factors in motor vehicle injuries include aggressive driving, speeding, a failure to wear safety belts, alcohol intoxication, fatigue, and distraction.

- Motorcycle, moped, and bicycle injuries can be prevented by developing appropriate skills, driving, or riding defensively, and wearing proper safety equipment, especially a helmet.

- Most fall-related injuries are a result of falls at floor level, but stairs, chairs, and ladders are also involved in a significant number of falls.

- Careless smoking and problems with cooking or heating equipment are common causes of fires. Being prepared for fire emergencies means planning escape routes and installing smoke detectors.

- The home can contain many poisonous substances, including medications, cleaning agents, plants, and fumes from cars and appliances.

- Performing the Heimlich maneuver can prevent someone from dying from choking.

- The proper storage and handling of firearms can help prevent injuries; assume that a gun is loaded.

- Many injuries during leisure activities result from the misuse of equipment, lack of experience, use of alcohol, and a failure to wear proper safety equipment.

- Most work-related injuries involve manual laborers. Back problems are most common; newer problems include repetitive strain injuries.

- Types of violence include assault, homicide, gang-related violence, hate crimes, school violence, workplace violence, battering, and child abuse.

- Most rape victims are women, and most know their attackers. Factors in date rape include different standards of appropriate sexual behavior for men and women and different perceptions of actions.

- Sexual harassment is unwelcome sexual advances or other conduct of a sexual nature that affects academic or employment performance or evaluations or that creates an intimidating, hostile, or offensive academic, work, or student living environment.

- Steps in giving emergency care include making sure the scene is safe for you and the injured person, conducting a quick examination of the victim, calling for help, and providing emergency first aid.

TAKE ACTION

1. Contact the American Red Cross or American Heart Association in your area, and ask about first aid and CPR classes. These courses are usually given frequently and at a variety of times and locations. They can be invaluable in saving lives. Consider taking one or both of the courses.

2. Find out what resources are available on your campus or in your community for victims of rape, hate crimes, or other types of violence. Does your campus sponsor any violence prevention programs or activities? If so, consider participating in one.

3. Contact your local fire department and obtain a checklist for fire safety procedures. What would you do if a fire started in your home? What types of evacuation procedures would be necessary? Do a practice fire drill at home to see what problems might arise in a real emergency.

4. Look up the nearest Poison Control Center in your telephone book, and post the number near your telephone. Contact the center, and ask them to send you information on poisonings. Read it carefully so you know what to do in case of poisoning.

For the next 7–10 days, keep track of any mishaps you are involved in or injuries you receive, recording them on a daily behavior record like the one shown in Chapter 1. Count each time you cut, burn, or injure yourself, fall down, run into someone, or have any other potentially injury-causing mishap, no matter how trivial. Also record any risk-taking behaviors, such as failing to wear your safety belt or bicycle helmet, drinking and driving, exceeding the speed limit, putting off home or bicycle repairs, and so on. For each entry (injury or incidence of unsafe behavior), record the date, time, what you were doing, who else was there and how you were influenced by him or her, what your motivations were, and what you were thinking and feeling at the time.

At the end of the monitoring period, examine your data. For each incident, determine both the human factors and the environmental factors that contributed to the injury or unsafe behavior. Were you tired? Distracted? Did you not realize this situation was dangerous? Did you take a chance? Did you think this incident couldn't happen to you? Was visibility poor? Were you using defective equipment? Then consider each contributing factor carefully, determining why it existed and how it could have been avoided or changed. Finally, consider what preventive actions you could take to avoid such incidents or change your behaviors in the future.

As an example, let's say that you usually don't use a safety belt when you run local errands in your car and that several factors contribute to this behavior: You don't really think you could be involved in a crash so close to home, you only go on short trips, you just never think to use it, and so on. One of the contributing factors to your unsafe behavior is inadequate knowledge. You can change this factor by obtaining accurate information about auto crashes (and their usual proximity to a victim's home) from this chapter and from library or Internet research. Just acquiring information about auto crashes and safety belt use may lead you to examine your beliefs and attitudes about safety belts and motivate you to change your behavior.

Once you're committed, you can use behavior change techniques described in Chapter 1, such as completing a contract, asking family and friends for support, and so on, to build a new habit. Put a note or picture reminding you to buckle up in your car where you can see it clearly. Recruit a friend to run errands with you and to remind you about using your safety belt. Once your habit is established, you may influence other people—especially people who ride in your car—to use safety belts all the time. By changing this behavior, you have reduced the chances that you or your passengers will suffer a serious injury or even die in a vehicle crash.

JOURNAL ENTRY

1. In your health journal, list the positive behaviors that help you avoid injuries and keep you safe. What can you do to reinforce and support these behaviors? Then list the behaviors that keep you from following safety guidelines or that put you at risk for being injured. How can you change one or more of them?

2. *Critical Thinking* Federal, state, and local governments have passed many regulations and laws to enforce a certain level of safety among citizens, such as laws regulating safety belts, helmets, and firearms. Some people believe that government should not be involved in issues of individual safety and injury prevention; others feel the government has a right to demand certain behaviors for the public good. How do you feel about this issue? Write a brief essay outlining your opinion; be sure to explain your reasoning.

FOR MORE INFORMATION

Books

Henderson, H., ed. 2001. *Domestic Violence and Child Abuse Sourcebook*. Detroit, Mich.: Omnigraphics. *Provides comprehensive, up-to-date information about domestic violence, including community and national sources of assistance.*

James, L., and D. Nahl. 2000. *Road Rage and Aggressive Driving: Steering Clear of Highway Warfare*. Amherst, N.Y.: Prometheus Books. *How to control your temper behind the wheel or understand the rage of a loved one. Also looks at other dangerous driving habits such as cell phone use.*

Kelly, K., and R. C. Duncan. 2000. *Living Safe in an Unsafe World: The Complete Guide to Family Preparedness*. New York: New American Library. *Simple advice on being prepared for emergencies, from fires to safe traveling.*

Lindquist, S. 2000. *The Date Rape Prevention Book: The Essential Guide for Girls and Women*. Naperville, Ill.: Sourcebooks. *How to avoid problem situations and what to do when confronted with danger.*

Organizations, Hotlines, and Web Sites

American Automobile Association Foundation for Traffic Safety. Pro1vides consumer information about all aspects of traffic safety; Web site has online quizzes and extensive links.

800-305-SAFE

http://www.aaafts.org

American Bar Association: Domestic Violence. Provides information on statistics, research, and laws relating to domestic violence.

http://www.abanet.org/domviol/home.html

Consumer Product Safety Commission. Provides information and advice about safety issues relating to consumer products.

http://www.cpsc.gov

CyberAngels. Provides information on online safety and help and advice for victims of cyberstalking.

http://www.cyberangels.org

National Center for Injury Prevention and Control. Provides consumer-oriented information about preventing unintentional injuries and violence.

770-488-1506

http://www.cdc.gov/ncipc

http://www.cdc.gov/safeusa

National Highway Traffic Safety Administration. Supplies materials about reducing deaths, injuries, and economic losses from motor vehicle crashes.

800-424-9393

http://www.nhtsa.dot.gov

National Safety Council. Provides information and statistics about preventing unintentional injuries.

630-285-1121

http://www.nsc.org

National Violence Hotlines. Provide information, referral services, and crisis intervention.

800-799-SAFE (domestic violence); 800-422-4453 (child abuse); 800-656-HOPE (sexual assault)

Prevent Child Abuse America. Provides statistics, information, and publications relating to child abuse, including parenting tips.

312-663-3520

http://www.preventchildabuse.org

Sexual Assault Information Page. Provides information on a wide variety of topics relating to sexual violence.

http://www.cs.utk.edu/~bartley/saInfoPage.html

The following sites provides statistics and background information on violence and crime in the United States:

Bureau of Justice Statistics

http://www.ojp.usdoj.gov/bjs

Federal Bureau of Investigation

http://www.fbi.gov

Justice Information Center

http://www.ncjrs.org

SELECTED BIBLIOGRAPHY

Brent, D. A., et al. 2000. Compliance with recommendations to remove firearms in families participating in a clinical trial for adolescent depression. *Journal of the American Academy of Child and Adolescent Psychiatry* 39(10): 1220–1226.

Burt, C. W., and M. D. Overpeck. 2001. Emergency visits for sports-related injuries. *Annals of Emergency Medicine* 37(3): 301–308.

Centers for Disease Control and Prevention. 2000. Alcohol involvement in fatal motor-vehicle crashes—United States, 1998–1999. *Morbidity and Mortality Weekly Report* 49(47): 1071–1072.

Centers for Disease Control and Prevention. 2000. Intimate partner violence among men and women. *Morbidity and Mortality Weekly Report* 49(30): 691–694.

Centers for Disease Control and Prevention. 2000. Prevalence and health consequences of stalking. *Morbidity and Mortality Weekly Report* 49(29): 653–655.

Centers for Disease Control and Prevention. 2000. Unpowered scooter-related injuries—United States, 1998–2000. *Morbidity and Mortality Weekly Report* 49(49): 1108–1110.

Centers for Disease Control and Prevention. 2001. Surveillance for fatal and nonfatal firearm-related injuries. *CDC Surveillance Summaries* 50(SS-2).

Cole, T. B. 2001. Complementary strategies to prevent firearm injury. *Journal of the American Medical Association* 285(8): 1071–1072.

Federal Bureau of Investigation. 2000. *Crime in the United States. Uniform Crime Reports,* 1999. Washington, D.C.: U.S. Department of Justice.

Li, G., et al. 2001. Use of alcohol as a risk factor for bicycling injury. *Journal of the American Medical Association* 285(7): 893–896.

Marenco, J. P., et al. 2001. Improving survival from sudden cardiac arrest. The role of the automatic external defibrillator. *Journal of the American Medical Association* 285(9): 1193–1200.

National Highway Traffic Safety Administration, Expert Panel on Driver Fatigue and Sleepiness. 2000. *Drowsy Driving and Automobile Crashes* (http://www.nhtsa.dot.gov/people/injury/drowsy_driving1/drowsy.html; retrieved December 16, 2000).

National Safety Council. 2000. *Injury Facts.* Itasca, Ill.: National Safety Council.

National School Safety Center. 2001. *Report on School Associated Violent Deaths* (http://nssc1.org/savd/savd.pdf; retrieved March 11, 2001).

Philip, P., et al. 2001. Fatigue, alcohol, and serious road crashes in France. *British Medical Journal* 322(7290): 829–830.

Rivara, F. P., et al. 2000. Effectiveness of automatic shoulder belt systems in motor vehicle crashes. *Journal of the American Medical Association* 283(21): 2826–2828.

Robinson, T. N., 2001. et al. Effects of reducing children's television and video game use on aggressive behavior: A randomized controlled trial. *Archives of Pediatrics and Adolescent Medicine* 155(1): 17–23.

Schuster, M. A., et al. 2000. Firearm storage patterns in U.S. homes with children. *American Journal of Public Health* 90(4): 588–594.

Southern Poverty Law Center. 1999. *The Year in Hate: Hate Group Count Tops 500, Internet Sites Soar* (http://www.splcenter.org/intelligenceproject/ip-4i1.html; retrieved February 24, 1999).

U.S. Department of Justice. 1999. *1999 Report on Cyberstalking: A New Challenge for Law Enforcement and Industry* (http://www.usdoj.gov:80/criminal/cybercrime/cyberstalking.htm; retrieved December 27, 2000).

Violence in the media. 2000. *Journal of the American Medical Association* 283(20): 2748.

Williamson, A. M., and A. M. Feyer. 2000. Moderate sleep deprivation produces impairments in cognitive and motor performance equivalent to legally prescribed levels of alcohol intoxication. *Occupational and Environmental Medicine* 57(10): 649–655.

Yokota, F., and K. M. Thompson. 2000. Violence in G-rated animated films. *Journal of the American Medical Association* 283(20): 2716–2720.

Environmental Health

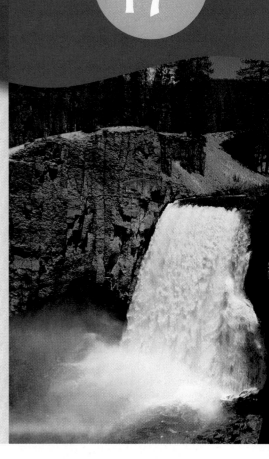

LOOKING AHEAD

After reading this chapter, you should be able to

- Describe the methods used to deal with the classic environmental concerns of clean water and waste disposal

- Discuss the effects of rapid increases in human population and list factors that may limit or slow world population growth

- Describe the short- and long-term effects of air, chemical, and noise pollution and exposure to radiation

- Outline strategies that individuals, communities, and nations can take to preserve and restore the environment

E nvironmental health has historically focused on preventing infectious diseases spread by water, waste, food, rodents, and insects. Although these problems still exist, the focus of environmental health has expanded and become more complex, for several reasons. First, we now recognize that environmental pollutants contribute not only to infectious diseases but to many chronic diseases as well. In addition, technological advances have increased our ability to affect and damage the environment. And finally, rapid population growth, which has resulted partly from past environmental improvements, means that far more people are consuming and competing for resources than ever before, magnifying the effect of humans on the environment.

Environmental health is therefore seen as encompassing all the interactions of humans with their environment and the health consequences of these interactions. Al-

though many environmental problems are complex and seem beyond the control of the individual, there are ways that people can make a difference in the future of the planet.

CLASSIC ENVIRONMENTAL HEALTH CONCERNS

Every time we venture beyond the boundaries of our everyday world, whether traveling to a less-developed

environmental health The collective interactions of humans with the environment and the short-term and long-term health consequences of those interactions.

Terms

391

In this excerpt from her book *The Sense of Wonder*, noted scientist and author Rachel Carson affirms the nurturing power of the natural world and urges us to appreciate the deep relationship between nature and the human spirit.

What is the value of preserving and strengthening this sense of awe and wonder, this recognition of something beyond the boundaries of human existence? Is the exploration of the natural world just a pleasant way to pass the golden hours of childhood or is there something deeper?

I am sure there is something much deeper, something lasting and significant. Those who dwell, as scientists or laymen, among the beauties and mysteries of the earth are never alone or weary of life. Whatever the vexations or concerns of their personal lives, their thoughts can find paths that lead to inner contentment and to renewed excitement in living. Those who contemplate the beauty of the earth find reserves of strength that will endure as long as life lasts. There is symbolic as well as actual beauty in the migration of the birds, the ebb and flow of the tides, the folded bud ready for spring. There is something infinitely healing in the repeated refrains of nature—the assurance that dawn comes after night, and spring after the winter.

SOURCE: Carson, R. 1956. *The Sense of Wonder*. New York: Harper & Row. Copyright © 1956 by Rachel Carson. Copyright © renewed 1984 by Roger Christie.

country or camping in a wilderness area, we are reminded of the importance of the basic elements of a healthy environment: clean water, sanitary waste disposal, safe food, and insect and rodent control.

Clean Water

Few things are as important to human health as adequate quantities of safe, clean drinking water. Many cities rely at least in part on wells that tap local groundwater, but often it is necessary to find lakes and rivers to supplement wells. Because such surface water is more likely to be contaminated with both organic matter and pathogenic microorganisms, it is purified in water-treatment plants before being piped into the community.

In most areas of the United States, water systems have adequate, dependable supplies, are able to control waterborne disease, and provide water without unacceptable color, odor, or taste. However, problems do occur, and the Centers for Disease Control and Prevention (CDC) estimate that 1 million Americans become ill and 900–1000 die each year from microbial illnesses from drinking water. Other concerns include pollution by hazardous chemicals from manufacturing, agriculture, and household wastes and water shortages. Some parts of the United States are experiencing rapid population growth that outstrips the ability of local systems to provide adequate water to all.

To protect the water supply, follow these guidelines:

- Take showers, not baths, to minimize your water consumption. Don't let water run when you're not actively using it while brushing your teeth, shaving, or hand-washing clothes. Don't run a dishwasher or washing machine until you have a full load.

- Install sink faucet aerators and water-efficient shower heads, which use two to five times less water with no noticeable decrease in performance.

- Purchase a water-saver toilet, or put a displacement device in your toilet tank to reduce the amount of water used with each flush.

- Fix any leaky faucets in your house. Leaks can waste thousands of gallons of water per year.

- Use organic rather than chemical fertilizers, and don't overfertilize your lawn or garden; the extra could end up in the groundwater.

- Don't pour toxic materials such as cleaning solvents, bleach, or motor oil down the drain. Store them until you can take them to a hazardous waste collection center.

Waste Disposal

Humans generate large amounts of waste, which must be handled in an appropriate manner if the environment is to be safe and sanitary.

Sewage   Most cities have sewage-treatment systems that separate fecal matter from water in huge tanks and ponds and stabilize it so that it cannot transmit infectious dis-

Terms

heavy metal A metal with a high specific gravity, such as lead, copper, or tin.

polychlorinated biphenyl (PCB) An industrial chemical used as an insulator in electrical transformers and linked to certain human cancers.

sanitary landfill A disposal site where solid wastes are buried.

eases. Once treated and biologically safe, the water is released back into the environment. The sludge that remains behind may be spread on fields as fertilizer if it is
free from **heavy metal** contamination, or it may be
burned or buried. Many cities have now begun expanded
sewage-treatment measures to remove heavy metals and
other hazardous chemicals. This action has resulted from
many studies linking exposure to such chemicals as mercury, lead, and **polychlorinated biphenyls (PCBs)** with
long-term health consequences, including cancer and
damage to the central nervous system.

Solid Waste   The bulk of the organic food garbage produced in American kitchens is now dumped in the
sewage system by way of the mechanical garbage disposal. The garbage that remains is not very hazardous
from the standpoint of infectious disease because there is
very little food waste in it, but it does represent an enormous disposal and contamination problem.

The biggest single component of household trash
(38.2% by weight) is paper products, including junk mail,
glossy mail-order catalogs, and computer printouts. Yard
waste is the next biggest source by weight (12.6% before
recycling). Plastics make up 10.2% of all trash by weight
but take up about 18% of landfill space. Most of this plastic waste is in the form of packaging, which accounts for
about one-third of the 6 million tons of plastics produced
each year in the United States. Other significant sources of
trash include metals (7.6% by weight), glass (5.7%), and
wood (5.4%). About 1% of household waste is toxic. Manufacturing, mining, and other industries all produce large
amounts of potentially dangerous materials.

Since the 1960s, much solid waste has been buried in
sanitary landfill disposal sites. Layers of solid waste are
covered with thin layers of dirt until the site is filled.
Some communities then plant grass and trees and convert
the site into a park. Landfill is relatively stable; almost no
decomposition occurs in the solidly packed waste. Bury-
ing solid waste in sanitary landfills has several disadvantages. Much of this waste contains chemicals, ranging
from leftover pesticides to nail polish remover, which
should not be released indiscriminately into the environment. Despite precautions, contaminants do leak into the
soil and groundwater. Burial is also expensive and requires huge amounts of space.

Industrial toxic waste poses an even greater disposal
problem. In 1980, Congress enacted the Superfund program to clean up inactive hazardous waste sites that are a
threat to human health and the environment. Because
many such sites are in areas with high population density,
60 million Americans live within 4 miles of a priority Superfund site. By 2000, cleanup was complete at 50% of
priority sites, but further action was still needed at about
750 priority sites and nearly 10,000 other sites.

Because of the expense and potential chemical hazards
of any form of solid waste disposal, many communities to-

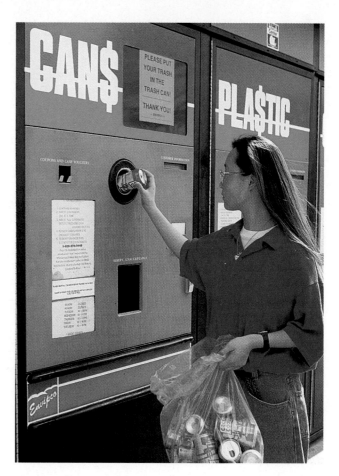

Recycling paper, cans, bottles, and plastics conserves resources, saves
energy, and keeps large amounts of solid wastes out of landfills. Some
communities have curbside pickup recycling, while others have drop-off
sites. Manufacturers and researchers are looking at new ways to use
recycled materials.

day encourage individuals and businesses to recycle their
trash. Some cities offer curbside pickup of recyclables;
others have recycling centers to which people can bring
their waste. Recycling programs have been successful in
reducing the proportion of solid waste sent to landfills: in
1980, 81% went to landfills; in 2000, about 55%.

To reduce garbage, follow these guidelines:

- Buy products with the least amount of packaging
  you can, or buy products in bulk. Buy products
  packaged in glass, paper, or metal containers; avoid
  plastic and aluminum (unless it's recycled). Reuse
  glass containers to store products bought in bulk or
  other household items.

- Buy recycled or recyclable products. Avoid dispos-
  ables; instead, use long-lasting or reusable products
  such as refillable pens and rechargeable batteries.

- Avoid using foam or paper cups and plastic stirrers
  by bringing your own china coffee mug and metal
  spoon to work or wherever you drink coffee or tea.
  Pack your lunch in reusable containers, and use a
  cloth or plastic lunch sack or a lunch box.

You can quickly and easily develop habits that direct your consumer dollar toward environmentally friendly products.

- Remember the three Rs of green consumerism:
  Reduce the amount of trash and pollution you generate by consuming and throwing away less.
  Reuse as many products as possible—either yourself or by selling them or donating them to charity.
  Recycle all appropriate materials and buy recycled products whenever possible.

- Choose products packaged in refillable, recycled, reusable containers or in readily recyclable materials, such as paper, cardboard, aluminum, or glass. Don't buy products that are excessively packaged or wrapped.

- Look for products made with the highest possible content of recycled paper, metal, glass, plastic, and other materials.

- Choose simple products containing the lowest amounts of bleaches, dyes, and fragrances. Look for organically grown foods and clothes made from organically grown cotton or Fox Fibre or another naturally colored type of cotton.

- Buy high-quality appliances that have an Energy Star seal from the EPA or some other type of certification indicating that they are energy- and water-efficient.

- Get a reusable cloth shopping bag. If you forget to bring your bag to the store, it doesn't matter much if you use a paper or plastic bag to carry your purchases home. What's important is that you reuse whatever bag you get.

- Don't buy what you don't need—borrow, rent, or share. Take good care of the things you own, repair items when they break, and replace them with used rather than new items, whenever possible. Sell or donate used items rather than throwing them out.

- Walk or bike to the store. If you must drive, do several errands at once to save energy and cut down on pollution.

- Look beyond the products to the companies that make them. Support those with good environmental records. If some of your favorite products are overpackaged or contain harmful ingredients, write to the manufacturer.

- Keep in mind that doing something is better than doing nothing. Even if you can't be a perfectly green consumer, doing your best on any purchase *will* make a difference.

SOURCES: U.S. Environmental Protection Agency. 2000. *Reduce, Reuse, and Recycle* (http://www.epa.gov/epaoswer/non-hw/muncpl/reduce.htm; retrieved January 11, 2001). Makower, J., J. Elkington, and J. Hailes. 1993. *The Green Consumer.* New York: Penguin Books. Madigan, C. O., and A. Elwood. 1995. *Life's Big Instruction Book.* New York: Warner Books.

- To store food, use glass jars and reusable plastic containers rather than foil and plastic wrap.

- Recycle your newspapers, glass, cans, paper, and other recyclables.

- Start a compost pile for your organic garbage (non-animal food and yard waste) if you have a yard.

- You can stop the delivery of junk mail by sending a request to Mail Preference Service, Direct Marketing Association, P.O. Box 9008, Farmingdale, NY 11735.

COMMUNICATE!   You can use the information and ideas in this chapter not only to make changes in your own behavior but also to help others do the same. For example, you might say, "Even though our curbside recycling program takes only newspapers and cans, I found out that the county recycling center takes all kinds of other things—cardboard, paper, plastic, magazines. I've been going every month or so. Do you want to join me next month?"

Food Inspection

Many agencies inspect food at various points in production. On the federal level, the U.S. Department of Agriculture (USDA) inspects grains and meats, and the U.S. Food and Drug Administration (FDA) is responsible for ensuring the wholesomeness of foods and regulating the chemicals that can be used in foods, drugs, and cosmetics. On the state level, public health departments inspect dairy herds, milking barns, storage tanks, tankers that transport milk, and processing plants. Local health departments inspect and license restaurants. Overall, the food distribution system in the United States is safe and efficient, but cases of foodborne illness do occur. Many cases of foodborne illness can be prevented through the proper storage and preparation of food.

Insect and Rodent Control

A great number of illnesses can be transmitted to humans by animal and insect vectors. In recent years, we have seen outbreaks of Lyme disease and Rocky Mountain spotted fever from ticks; bubonic plague from fleas on wild mammals; and West Nile virus transmitted by mosquitoes. Rodents carry forms of hantavirus, tapeworms, and *Salmonella*. Disability and death from these diseases

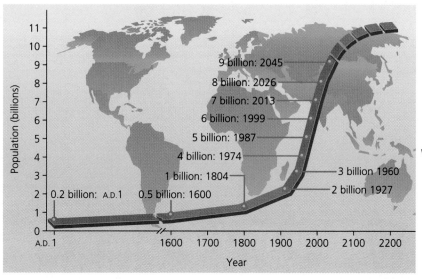

 VITAL STATISTICS

Figure 17-1 World population growth.
The United Nations estimates that the world's population will continue to increase dramatically until it stabilizes at about 11 billion people in 2200.   SOURCE: United Nations Population Division. 2001 *World Population Prospects: The 2000 Revision.* New York: United Nations.

can be prevented by spraying insecticides when necessary, wearing protective clothing, and exercising reasonable caution in infested areas.

POPULATION GROWTH

Throughout most of history, humans have been a minor pressure on the planet. About 200 million people were alive in the year A.D. 1; by the time Europeans were settling in the United States 1600 years later, the world population had increased gradually to 500 million. But then it began rising exponentially—zooming to 1 billion by about 1830, more than doubling by 1950, and then doubling again in just 40 years (Figure 17-1).

The world's population, currently about 6.1 billion, is increasing at a rate of about 78 million per year—150 people every minute. The United Nations projects that world population will exceed 9 billion by 2050 and will continue to increase until it levels off at about 11 billion in 2200. Nearly all of this increase will take place in less-developed regions. No one knows how many people the world can support, but most scientists agree that there is a limit. The primary factors that may eventually put a cap on human population are the limits of the earth's resources—land, water, energy, and food.

Although it is apparent that population growth must be controlled, population trends are difficult to influence and manage. To be successful, population management must change the condition of people's lives, especially poverty, to remove the pressures for having large families. Research indicates that the combination of improved health, better education, and increased literacy and employment opportunities for women works together with family planning to decrease fertility rates. Unfortunately,

the needs of a rapidly increasing population often use up financial resources that might otherwise be used to improve lives and ultimately slow population growth.

Ww. POLLUTION

The term *pollution* refers to any unwanted contaminant in the environment that may pose a health risk.

Ww. Air Pollution

Air pollution is not a human invention or even a new problem. The air is "polluted" naturally with every forest fire, pollen bloom, and dust storm, as well as with countless other natural pollutants. To these natural sources, humans contribute the by-products of their activities.

Air Quality and Smog   Air pollution can cause illness and death if pollutant levels are high; young children, older adults, and people with chronic health conditions are particularly at risk. The EPA uses a measure called the **Air Quality Index (AQI)** to indicate whether air pollution levels pose a health concern. AQI values run from 0 to 500; the higher the AQI, the greater the level of pollution and associated health danger. The AQI is applied to five major air pollutants: carbon monoxide, sulfur dioxide,

> **Air Quality Index (AQI)** A measure of local air quality and what it means for health. Concentrations of five major pollutants are measured and assigned index values between 0 and 500, with values above 100 considered unhealthy; the highest of the five values becomes the overall AQI for the day. Health warnings and recommendations may be issued when AQI values exceed 100.
>
> Terms

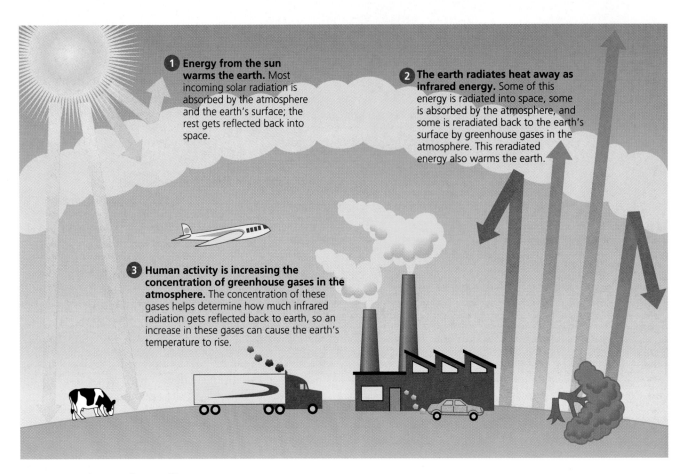

Figure 17-2   The greenhouse effect.

① **Energy from the sun warms the earth.** Most incoming solar radiation is absorbed by the atmosphere and the earth's surface; the rest gets reflected back into space.

② **The earth radiates heat away as infrared energy.** Some of this energy is radiated into space, some is absorbed by the atmosphere, and some is reradiated back to the earth's surface by greenhouse gases in the atmosphere. This reradiated energy also warms the earth.

③ **Human activity is increasing the concentration of greenhouse gases in the atmosphere.** The concentration of these gases helps determine how much infrared radiation gets reflected back to earth, so an increase in these gases can cause the earth's temperature to rise.

nitrogen dioxide, particulate matter, and ground-level ozone. A major source of these pollutants is the burning of **fossil fuels** by vehicles and power plants. Information on local AQI values is often available in newspapers, on television and radio, on the Internet, and from state and local telephone hotlines.

The term **smog** was first used in the early 1900s in London to describe the combination of smoke and fog. What we typically call smog today is a mixture of pollutants, with ground-level ozone being the key ingredient. Major smog occurrences are linked to the combination of several factors. Heavy motor vehicle traffic, high temperatures, and sunny weather can increase the production of ozone. Pollutants are also more likely to build up in areas with little wind and/or where a topographic feature such as a mountain range or valley prevents the wind from pushing out stagnant air.

A weather event called a **temperature inversion** also contributes to smog buildup. A temperature inversion occurs when there is little or no wind and a layer of warm air traps a layer of cold air next to the ground. Normally, the sun heats the earth, making the air closest to the ground warmer than that just above it. Warm air rises and is replaced by cooler air, which in turn is warmed and

rises, thereby producing a natural circulation. This circulation, combined with horizontal winds, prevents pollutants from reaching dangerous levels of concentration. When there is a temperature inversion, this replacement and cleansing action cannot occur. The effect is like covering an area with a dome that traps all the pollutants and prevents vertical dispersion. If this condition persists for several days, the buildup of pollutants may reach dangerous levels and threaten people's health.

The Greenhouse Effect and Global Warming   The temperature of the earth's atmosphere depends on the balance between the amount of energy the planet absorbs from the sun (mainly as high-energy ultraviolet radiation) and the amount of energy radiated back into space as lower-energy infrared radiation. Key components of temperature regulation are carbon dioxide, water vapor, methane, and other "greenhouse gases"—so named because, like a pane of glass in a greenhouse, they let through visible light from the sun but trap some of the resulting infrared radiation and reradiate it back to the earth's surface. This reradiation causes a buildup of heat that raises the temperature of the lower atmosphere, a natural process known as the **greenhouse effect** (Figure

17–2). Without it, the atmosphere would be far cooler and much more hostile to life.

Human activity may be tipping this balance toward **global warming.** The concentration of greenhouse gases is increasing because of human activity, especially the combustion of fossil fuels. Carbon dioxide levels in the atmosphere have increased rapidly since the onset of the Industrial Revolution, and current levels are higher than at any time in the past 160,000 years. Deforestation, often by burning, also sends carbon dioxide into the atmosphere and reduces the number of trees available to convert carbon dioxide into oxygen. But energy use in the developed world is the primary cause of increases in the concentrations of greenhouse gases. The United States alone is responsible for one-third of the world's total emissions of carbon dioxide.

According to a 2001 report from the United Nations–sponsored Intergovernmental Panel on Climate Change, the average global temperature will likely increase by about 2.5–10.4°F (1.4–5.8°C) by 2100, with a corresponding significant rise in sea level. Although the full implications of climate change are unknown, possible consequences include increased rainfall and flooding in some regions and increased drought in others; increased mortality from heat stress, severe weather events, urban air polution, and tropical diseases (due to the spread of disease-carrying organisms like mosquitoes); and a poleward shift of about 50–350 miles (150–550 km) in the location of vegetation zones, affecting crop yields, irrigation demands, and forest productivity.

Since record-keeping began in the mid-1800s, 8 of the 10 hottest years have occurred since 1990. Data from tree rings and other sources suggest that recent temperatures are the warmest in 1000 years. What can be done? The Kyoto Protocol to the UN Convention on Climate Change calls for industrialized countries to cut greenhouse gas emissions to about 5.2% below 1990 levels by 2008–2012; U.S. emissions, however, have actually increased by more than 10% since 1990.

Thinning of the Ozone Layer   A second air pollution problem is the thinning of the **ozone layer** of the atmosphere, a fragile, invisible layer about 10–30 miles above the earth's surface, shielding the planet from the sun's hazardous ultraviolet (UV) rays. Since the mid-1980s, scientists have observed the seasonal appearance and growth of a "hole" in the ozone layer over Antarctica. More recently, thinning over other areas—including Canada, Scandinavia, the northern United States, Russia, Australia, and New Zealand—has been noted.

The ozone layer is being destroyed primarily by **chlorofluorocarbons (CFCs),** industrial chemicals used as coolants in refrigerators and in home and automobile air conditioners; as foaming agents in some rigid foam products, including insulation; as propellants in some kinds of aerosol sprays (most such sprays were banned in 1978);

and as solvents. When CFCs rise into the atmosphere, winds carry them toward the polar regions and chemical reactions occur that destroy ozone.

Since 1979, about 15% of Antarctic ozone has been destroyed, although locally and seasonally up to 95% of the ozone disappears (forming the "hole"). The hole above Antarctica in late 2000 was larger and deeper than any previous ozone hole, and it extended over populated areas of South America, where residents were advised to stay indoors and take other measures to avoid UV exposure. (UV radiation levels under the hole were high enough to cause sunburn within 7 minutes.) In the Northern Hemisphere, ozone levels have declined by about 10% since 1980, and certain areas may be temporarily depleted in late winter and early spring by as much as 40%.

The loss of ozone is of concern because without the ozone layer to absorb the sun's UV radiation, life on earth would be impossible. The potential effects of increased long-term exposure to UV light for humans include skin cancer, wrinkling and aging of the skin, cataracts and blindness, and reduced immune response. UV light may interfere with photosynthesis and cause lower crop yields; it may also kill phytoplankton and krill, the basis of the ocean food chain.

Worldwide production and use of CFCs has declined rapidly since the danger to the ozone layer was recognized. However, future ozone losses are inevitable because CFCs persist in the atmosphere for 50–150 years.

Terms

fossil fuels Buried deposits of decayed animals and plants that are converted into carbon-rich fuels by exposure to heat and pressure over millions of years; oil, coal, and natural gas are fossil fuels.

smog Hazy atmospheric conditions resulting from increased concentrations of ground-level ozone and other pollutants. Smog most commonly occurs when oxides of nitrogen and hydrocarbons, primarily from motor vehicle exhaust, react in the presence of sunlight; also known as *photochemical smog*. (The term was first used to describe the combination of smoke and fog in early-twentieth-century London.)

temperature inversion A weather condition in which a cold layer of air is trapped by a warm layer so that pollutants cannot be dispersed.

greenhouse effect A warming of the earth due to a buildup of carbon dioxide and certain other gases.

global warming An increase in the earth's atmospheric temperature when averaged across seasons and geographical regions.

ozone layer A layer of ozone molecules (O_3) in the upper atmosphere that screens out UV rays from the sun.

chlorofluorocarbons (CFCs) Chemicals used as spray-can propellants, refrigerants, and industrial solvents, implicated in the destruction of the ozone layer.

Recent years have seen both progress and setbacks on environmental issues, and new problems continue to be recognized. The following are just a few issues of current concern.

More and More Consumers

Birth rates are dropping worldwide, from an average of 3.7 children per woman in 1980 to 3.2 in 1990 and 2.7 in 2000. Despite this trend, world population continues to skyrocket, increasing by about 9000 people every hour. It's estimated that world population will grow by more than a billion people between 2000 and 2013. A larger population puts an even greater strain on the earth's resources. Although much of this increase is occurring in the developing countries, people in industrialized countries consume the bulk of the energy and resources. The World Wildlife Fund estimates that if people in the developing world consumed as much as those living in the richest countries, humans would need another two planets to cope.

Waiting for the Ozone Layer to Heal

Since the chemicals responsible for the thinning of the ozone layer were identified, the production and use of most of these compounds have greatly declined. Unfortunately, the thinning of the ozone layer is likely to continue for some time because CFCs and other ozone-destroying agents persist in the atmosphere for decades. The "hole" in the ozone layer over Antarctica has continued to grow, both in size and depth, and now extends over populated areas during part of the year. Thinning in the ozone layer over the Arctic, northern Europe, and North America has also been noted. People in many parts of the world may soon be subject to periodic UV alerts, with people advised to stay indoors or wear complete sun protection.

Rising Temperatures and Severe Weather

Scientists continue to debate the extent of global warming and degree to which human activities are contributing to it. Another area of debate, one in which the public has a great deal of interest, is whether global warming could be responsible for the apparent recent increase in severe weather events—hurricanes, droughts, floods, tornadoes, and other catastrophes. In the past 20 years, the United States has been hit with $170 billion worth of weather-related damage; to date, 1998 was both the hottest year on record in the United States and the year with the greatest number of severe weather events. Worldwide, the number of natural disasters has increased more than fourfold since the 1950s. Researchers cannot conclusively link global warming to extreme weather at this time, but answers may begin to emerge as more data are collected and better computer models are created. Recent data does suggest that global warming is increasing the frequency and severity of El Niño, a periodic disruption of the ocean-atmosphere system in the tropical Pacific that has important consequences for weather around the world.

Transportation: SUVs and HEVs

Despite recent increases in gas prices in the United States, more than 70% of American commuters drive alone to work, and low-fuel-economy sport utility vehicles (SUVs) remain popular. Every gallon of gas burned puts about 20 pounds of carbon dioxide into the atmosphere, contributing to global warming; motor vehicles are also key sources of ozone and other pollutants. Some SUVs average fewer than 10 miles per gallon, and the largest SUVs increase greenhouse gas emissions by 6 or more tons per year compared to an average car.

On the bright side, 2000 saw the introduction of a new class of car, the hybrid electric vehicle (HEV). HEVs combine a conventional internal combustion engine with an electric motor, resulting in about twice the fuel economy of conventional vehicles. The combination allows for the extended range and rapid refueling that consumers are accustomed to from conventional cars. The HEVs currently for sale are priced competitively and can travel 500–700 miles on a single tank of gas. Researchers hope that hybrid technology can be extended to all classes of vehicles and that Americans can be convinced to use more-fuel-efficient vehicles and to travel more frequently on public transportation, in carpools, or on foot.

Acid Precipitation   A by-product of many industrial processes, **acid precipitation** occurs when atmospheric pollutants combine with moisture in the air and fall to earth as highly acidic rain, snow, sleet, or hail. It occurs especially when coal containing large amounts of sulfur is burned and chemicals are released into the atmosphere. Acidification of lakes and streams due to acid precipitation has completely eradicated fish and other aquatic species in some areas. Trees are also affected because acid precipitation damages leaves, strips the soil of key nutrients, and releases toxic substances such as heavy metals from the soil. Acid precipitation also corrodes metals and damages stone and paint on buildings, monuments, and cars. The areas currently most affected are Canada, Scandinavia, parts of central Europe, and, in the United States, the Adirondacks, the mid-Appalachian highlands, the upper Midwest, and high elevations in the West.

Energy Use and Air Pollution   Americans are the biggest energy consumers in the world. About 75% of the energy we use comes from fossil fuels—oil, coal, and natural gas; the remainder comes from nuclear power and renewable energy sources (such as hydroelectric, wind, and solar power). Energy consumption is at the root of many environmental problems, especially those relating to air pollution. Automobile exhaust and the burning of oil and coal by industry and by electricity-generating plants are primary causes of smog, acid precipitation, and the greenhouse effect. The mining of coal and the extraction and transportation of oil cause pollution on land and in the water; coal miners often suffer from serious health problems related to their jobs. Nuclear power generation creates hazardous wastes and carries the risk of dangerous releases of radiation. Two key strategies for controlling energy use are conservation and the development of nonpolluting, renewable sources of energy.

Indoor Air Pollution Potentially dangerous pollutants also occur in the home. Some of these compounds trigger allergic responses, and others have been linked to cancer. Common indoor pollutants include environmental tobacco smoke (ETS); carbon monoxide and other combustion by-products from wood stoves, fireplaces, kerosene heaters and lamps, and gas ranges; formaldehyde gas from resins used in particle board, plywood paneling, and some carpeting and upholstery; and biological pollutants, including bacteria, dust mites, mold, and animal dander.

To help prevent air pollution—both outdoors and indoors—try the following strategies:

- Cut back on driving. Ride your bike, walk, use public transportation, or carpool.

- Keep your car tuned up and well maintained. Use only unleaded gas, and keep your tires inflated at recommended pressures. To save energy when driving, avoid quick starts, stay within the speed limit, limit the use of air conditioning, and don't let your car idle unless absolutely necessary. Have your car's air conditioner checked and serviced by a station that uses environmentally friendly refrigerants.

- Buy energy-efficient appliances, and use them only when necessary. Run the washing machine, dryer, and dishwasher only when you have full loads, and do laundry in warm or cold water instead of hot; don't overdry your clothes. Clean refrigerator coils and clothes dryer lint screens frequently. Towel or air-dry your hair rather than using an electric dryer.

- Replace incandescent bulbs with compact fluorescent bulbs (not fluorescent tubes). Although they cost more initially, they'll save you money over the life of the bulb.

- Make sure your home is well-insulated with ozone-safe agents; use insulating shades and curtains to keep heat in during winter and out during summer. Seal any openings that produce drafts. In cold weather, put on a sweater and turn down the thermostat. In hot weather, wear lightweight clothing and, whenever possible, use a fan instead of an air conditioner to cool yourself.

- Plant trees in your yard and neighborhood. Because they recycle carbon dioxide, trees work against global warming. They also provide shade and cool the air, so less air conditioning is needed.

- Before discarding a refrigerator, air conditioner, or humidifier, check with the waste hauler or your local government to ensure that ozone-depleting refrigerants will be removed prior to disposal. If you use a metered-dose inhaler, ask your physician if an ozone-safe inhaler is available for your medication.

- To prevent indoor air pollution, keep your house adequately ventilated, and buy some houseplants; they have a natural ability to rid the air of harmful pollutants.

- Keep paints, cleaning agents, and other chemical products in their original, tightly sealed containers.

- Don't smoke, and don't allow others to smoke in your room, apartment, or home. If these rules are too strict for your situation, limit smoking to a single, well-ventilated room.

- Clean and inspect chimneys, furnaces, and other appliances regularly. Install carbon monoxide detectors.

COMMUNICATE! Many people resist the idea of carpooling, even though it's an excellent way to lower the number of cars on the road and thus reduce the amount of motor vehicle exhaust entering the air. If you find you have classmates or colleagues traveling to school or work at about the same time as you, see if you can set up a carpool with them. You might say, "I notice that we come to work from the same neighborhood every day. Would you be interested in carpooling? We'd be able to use the carpool lane on the highway, so we'd avoid some of the traffic slowdowns, and we'd both save on gas and mileage—to say nothing of helping the environment a little."

Chemical Pollution

Chemical pollution is by no means a new problem, but today, new chemical substances are constantly being created and introduced into the environment—as pesticides, herbicides, solvents, cleaning fluids, flame retardants, and hundreds of other products. We have many more chemicals, in more concentrated forms and in wider use, and larger numbers of people are exposed and potentially exposed to them than ever before. The following are brief descriptions of just a few current problems.

acid precipitation Rain, snow, sleet, or hail with a low pH (acid), caused by atmospheric moisture combining with products of industrial combustion to form acids such as sulfur dioxide; harmful to forests and lakes, which cannot tolerate changes in acidity/alkalinity.

Terms

Residents of poor and minority communities are often exposed to more environmental toxins than residents of wealthier communities, and they are more likely to suffer from health problems caused or aggravated by pollutants. Poor neighborhoods are often located near highways and industrial areas that have high levels of air pollution; they are also common sites for hazardous waste production and disposal. Residents of substandard housing are more likely to come into contact with lead, asbestos, carbon monoxide, pesticides, and other hazardous pollutants associated with peeling paint, old plumbing, poorly maintained insulation and heating equipment, and attempts to control high levels of pests such as cockroaches and rodents. Poor people are more likely to have jobs that expose them to asbestos, silica dust, and pesticides, and they are more likely to catch and consume fish contaminated with PCBs, mercury, and other toxins.

The most thoroughly researched and documented link among poverty, the environment, and health is lead poisoning in children. Many studies have shown that children of low-income black families are much more likely to have elevated levels of lead in their blood than white children. One survey found that two-thirds of urban African American children from families earning less than $6000 a year had elevated lead levels. The CDC and the American Academy of Pediatrics recommend annual testing of blood lead levels for all children under age 6, with more frequent testing for children at special risk.

Asthma is another health threat that appears to be linked with both environmental and socioeconomic factors. The number of Americans with asthma has grown dramatically in the past 20 years; most of the increase has occurred in children, with African Americans and the poor hardest hit. Researchers are not sure what accounts for this increase, but suspects include household pollutants, pesticides, air pollution, cigarette smoke, and allergens like cockroaches. These risk factors are likely to cluster in poor urban areas where inadequate health care may worsen asthma's effects.

A new push for research on the health effects of exposure to toxins on low-income communities is being called for by the environmental justice movement. New studies are investigating the links between environmental factors and respiratory problems, skin diseases, and cancer. While health researchers seek to quantify the health impacts, neighborhood activists continue to fight against the "dumping" of pollution in poor communities.

Asbestos   A mineral-based compound, asbestos was widely used for fire protection and insulation in buildings until the late 1960s. Microscopic asbestos fibers can be released into the air when this material is applied or when it later deteriorates or is damaged. These fibers can lodge in the lungs, causing **asbestosis,** lung cancer, and other serious lung diseases. Similar conditions are risks in the coal mining industry, from exposure to coal and silica dust (black lung disease), and in the textile industry, from exposure to cotton fibers (brown lung disease).

Lead   Lead poisoning continues to be a serious problem, particularly among children living in older buildings and adults who are exposed to lead in the workplace. When lead is ingested or inhaled, it can damage the central nervous system, cause mental impairment, hinder oxygen transport in the blood, and create digestive problems. Severe lead poisoning may cause coma or even death. Young children can easily ingest lead from their environment by picking up dust and dirt on their hands and then putting their fingers in their mouth. Lead-based paints are believed to be the chief culprit in lead poisoning of children. They were banned from residential use in 1978, but as many as 57 million American homes still contain lead paint. The use of lead in plumbing is now also banned, but some old pipes and faucets contain lead that can leach into drinking water.

Lead gets into the air from industrial and vehicle emissions, from tobacco smoke and paint dust, and from the burning of solid wastes that contain lead. Levels of lead in the air have dropped sharply as leaded gas use has declined, but many vehicles still use leaded fuel. Other sources of lead are foods stored or served in lead-glazed pottery or lead crystal and processed foods sold in lead-soldered cans.

Pesticides   **Pesticides** are used primarily for two purposes: to prevent the spread of insect-borne diseases and to maximize food production by killing insects that eat crops. Both uses have risks as well as benefits. Most pesticide hazards to date have been a result of overuse, but there are concerns about the health effects of long-term exposure to small amounts of pesticide residues in foods, especially for children.

Mercury   A naturally occurring metal, mercury is a toxin that affects the nervous system and may damage the brain, kidneys, and gastrointestinal tract; increase blood pressure and heart rate; and cause cancer. Mercury slows fetal and child development and causes irreversible deficits in brain function. Coal-fired power plants are the largest producers of mercury; other sources include mining and smelting operations and the disposal of consumer products containing mercury.

Mercury persists in the environment, and large, long-lived fish may carry high levels of mercury. The FDA recommends that pregnant women, women of childbearing age who may become pregnant, women who are breast-

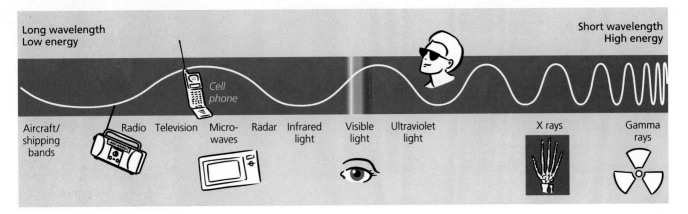

Long wavelength
Low energy

Short wavelength
High energy

Aircraft/ shipping bands Radio Television Micro- waves Radar Infrared light Visible light Ultraviolet light X rays Gamma rays

Cell phone

Figure 17-3 Electromagnetic radiation. Electromagnetic radiation takes the form of waves that travel through space. The length of the wave determines the type of radiation: The shortest waves are high-energy gamma rays; the longest are radio waves and extremely low frequency waves used for communication between aircraft, ships, and submarines. Different types of electromagnetic radiation have different effects on health.

feeding, and young children not consume shark, swordfish, king mackerel, and tilefish. Because of health concerns, some cities and stores have banned the sale of mercury fever thermometers.

To the preceding list of real and potential chemical pollution problems, we can add recent concern about arsenic in drinking water, formaldehyde in synthetic building materials, and other by-products of our industrial age. Hazardous wastes are also found in the home, including automotive supplies, paint supplies, art and hobby supplies, insecticides, batteries, computer and electronic components, and household cleaners containing sodium hydroxide (lye) or ammonia. Many cities provide guidelines about approved disposal methods and have hazardous waste collection days. Look in the government pages of your phone book under Environmental Health or Hazardous Waste.

To prevent chemical pollution, follow these guidelines:

- When buying products, read the labels, and try to buy the least toxic ones available. Choose nontoxic nonpetrochemical cleansers, disinfectants, polishes, and other personal and household products.

- Dispose of your household hazardous wastes properly. If you have questions, contact your local environmental health office or health department. Don't burn trash.

- Buy organic produce or produce that has been grown locally. Wash, scrub, and, if appropriate, peel fruits and vegetables. Consider eating less meat; animal products require more pesticides, fertilizer, water, and energy to produce.

- If you must use pesticides or toxic household products, store them in a locked place where children

and pets can't get to them. Don't measure chemicals with food-preparation utensils, and wear gloves whenever handling them.

- If you have your house fumigated for pest control, be sure to hire a licensed exterminator. Keep everyone, including pets, out of the house while the crew works and, if possible, for a few days after.

Radiation

Radiation can come in different forms, such as ultraviolet rays, microwaves, or X rays, and from different sources, such as the sun, uranium, and nuclear weapons (Figure 17-3). Of most concern to health are gamma rays produced by radioactive sources such as nuclear weapons, nuclear energy plants, and radon gas; these high-energy waves are powerful enough to penetrate objects and break molecular bonds. Although gamma radiation cannot be seen or felt, its effects at high doses can include **radiation sickness** and death; at lower doses, chromosome damage, sterility, tissue damage, cataracts, and cancer can occur. Other types of radiation can also affect health; for

asbestosis A lung condition caused by inhalation of microscopic asbestos fibers, which inflame the lung and can lead to lung cancer.

pesticides Chemicals used to prevent the spread of diseases transmitted by insects and to maximize food production by killing insects that eat crops.

radiation Energy transmitted in the form of rays, waves, or particles.

radiation sickness An illness caused by excess radiation exposure, marked by low white blood cell counts and nausea; possibly fatal.

Terms

It takes only a few minutes to write to an elected official, but it can make a difference on an issue you care about. To give your letter the greatest possible impact, use these guidelines:

- Use your own words and your own stationery.

- Be clear and concise. Keep your letter to one or two paragraphs, never more than one page.

- Focus on only one subject in each letter, and identify it clearly. Refer to legislation by its name or number.

- Request a specific action—vote a particular way on a piece of legislation, request hearings, cosponsor a bill—and state your reasons for your position.

- If you live or work in the legislator's district, say so.

- Don't be insulting or unnecessarily critical.

Your phone book has addresses of all state and local representatives. You can write to the president or vice president at the White House:

President (Vice President) _____
White House
Washington, D.C. 20500
president@whitehouse.gov
vice.president@whitehouse.gov

United States senators and representatives can be reached at the following addresses:

The Honorable _____   The Honorable _____
U.S. Senate   U.S. House of Representatives
Washington, D.C. 20510   Washington, D.C. 20515

Members of Congress also have e-mail addresses and many have Web sites; you can find a directory of this information at http://lcweb.loc.gov/global/legislative/email.html.

example, exposure to UV radiation from the sun or from tanning salons can increase the risk of skin cancer.

Nuclear weapons pose a health risk of the most serious kind to all species. Reducing weapon stockpiles is a challenge and a goal for the twenty-first century. Power-generating plants that use nuclear fuel also pose health problems. When **nuclear power** was first developed as an alternative to oil and coal, it was promoted as clean, efficient, inexpensive, and safe. In general, this has proven to be the case. However, despite all the built-in safeguards and regulating agencies, accidents in nuclear power plants do happen, and the consequences of such accidents are far more serious than similar accidents in other types of power-generating plants. An additional, enormous problem is disposing of the radioactive wastes these plants generate. To date, no storage method has been devised that can provide infallible, infinitely durable shielding for nuclear waste.

Another area of concern is the use of radiation in medicine, primarily the X ray. From a personal health point of view, individuals should never have a "routine" X ray examination; each such exam should have a definite purpose, and its benefits and risks should be carefully weighed. Recently, there has also been concern about electromagnetic radiation associated with such common modern devices as microwave ovens, computer monitors, cellular telephones, and even high-voltage power lines. These forms of radiation do have effects on health, but research results are inconclusive.

Another area of concern is **radon,** a naturally occurring radioactive gas found in certain soils, rocks, and building materials. When the breakdown products of radon are inhaled, they cling to lungs and bombard sensitive tissue with radioactivity. Radon can enter a home by rising though the soil into the basement through dirt floors, cracks, and other openings. Research into whether exposure to low levels of radon significantly increases the risk of lung cancer has yielded mixed results. However, the EPA recommends that people test their homes for radon and take appropriate actions to bring elevated levels down.

To avoid radiation, follow these guidelines:

- If your physician orders an X ray, ask why it is necessary. Only get X rays that you really need, and keep a record of every X ray exam.

- Check with your local or state health department to find out if there are radon problems in your area. If there are, consider buying a home radon testing kit.

- Find out if there are radioactive sites in your area. If you live or work near such a site, form or join a community action group to get the site cleaned up.

Terms

nuclear power The use of controlled nuclear reactions to produce steam, which in turn drives turbines to produce electricity.

radon A naturally occurring radioactive gas emitted from rocks and natural building materials that can become concentrated in insulated homes, causing lung cancer.

decibel A unit for expressing the relative intensity of sounds on a scale from 0 for the average least perceptible sound to about 120 for the average pain threshold.

tinnitus Ringing in the ears, a condition that can be caused by excessive noise exposure.

Noise Pollution

The potential health effects of loud or persistent noise in the environment include hearing loss and stress. Prolonged exposure to sounds above 80–85 **decibels** (a measure of the intensity of a sound wave) can cause permanent hearing loss. Whispering has an intensity of about 30 decibels; normal conversation, 50–60 decibels; heavy traffic, 90 decibels; a rock concert, 120 decibels; and a jet engine, 150 decibels. The Occupational Safety and Health Administration (OSHA) sets legal standards for noise in the workplace, but no laws exist regulating noise levels at rock concerts, which often exceed OSHA standards for the workplace.

Most hearing loss occurs in the first 2 hours of exposure, and hearing usually recovers within 2 hours after the noise stops. But if exposure continues or is repeated frequently, hearing loss may be permanent. The employees of a club where rock music is played loudly are at much greater risk than the patrons of the club, who might be exposed for only 2 hours at a time. Another possible effect of exposure to excessive noise is **tinnitus,** a condition of more or less continuous ringing or buzzing in the ears. Excessive noise is also an environmental stressor, producing the typical stress response described in Chapter 2. A chronic and prolonged stress response can have serious effects on health.

To avoid noise pollution, follow these guidelines:

- Wear ear protectors when working around noisy machinery.
- When listening to music on a headset with a volume range of 1–10, keep the volume no louder than 4; your headset is too loud if you can't hear people around you speaking in a normal tone of voice.
- Avoid loud music. Don't sit or stand near speakers or amplifiers at a rock concert, and don't play a car radio or stereo so high that you can't hear the traffic.
- Avoid any exposure to painfully loud sounds, and avoid repeated exposure to any sounds above 80 decibels.

HEALING THE ENVIRONMENT

Faced with a vast array of confusing and complex environmental issues, you may feel overwhelmed and conclude that there isn't anything you can do about global problems. But this is not true. If everyone made individual changes in his or her life, the impact would be tremendous. At the same time, it is important to recognize that large corporations and manufacturers are the ones primarily responsible for environmental degradation. To influence them, people have to become educated, demand changes in production methods, and elect people to office who consider environmental concerns along with sound business incentives.

Large-scale changes and individual actions complement each other. What you do every day *does* count. Following the suggestions throughout this chapter will help you make a difference in the environment. In addition, you can become a part of larger community actions to work for a healthier world by educating friends, supporting environmental causes, and contacting your elected representatives.

Tips for Today

Environmental health involves protecting ourselves from environmental dangers and protecting the environment from the dangers we ourselves create. The two are intimately connected, and both require that we take responsibility for our actions every day.

Right now you can

- Turn the lights off in any unoccupied rooms.
- Plan to buy compact fluorescent light bulbs to replace your incandescent ones.
- Turn the heat down a few degrees and put on a sweater, or turn the air conditioner off and change into shorts.
- Make an appointment to have your car checked if it's not running well or needs a tune-up.
- Check your trash can for recyclable items—soda cans, plastic water bottles, white paper, magazines—and put aside any you find for recycling or take them to your recycling bins.

SUMMARY

- Environmental health encompasses all the interactions of humans with their environment and the health consequences of those interactions.
- Concerns with water quality focus on pathogenic organisms and hazardous chemicals from industry and households, as well as on water shortages.
- Sewage treatment prevents pathogens from contaminating drinking water; it must also often deal with heavy metals and hazardous chemicals.
- The amount of garbage is growing all the time; paper is the biggest component. Recycling can help solid waste disposal problems.
- The world's population is increasing rapidly, especially in the developing world.
- Increased amounts of air pollutants are especially dangerous for children, older adults, and people with chronic health problems.
- Factors contributing to the development of smog include heavy motor vehicle traffic, hot weather, stagnant air, and temperature inversion.

- Carbon dioxide and other natural gases act as a "greenhouse" around the earth, increasing the temperature of the atmosphere. Levels of these gases are rising through human activity.
- The ozone layer that shields the earth's surface from the sun's UV rays has thinned and developed holes in certain regions.
- Acid precipitation occurs when certain atmospheric pollutants combine with moisture in the air.
- Indoor pollutants can trigger allergies and illness in the short term and cancer in the long term.
- Potentially hazardous chemical pollutants include asbestos, lead, pesticides, and mercury. Proper handling and disposal are critical.
- Radiation can cause radiation sickness, chromosome damage, and cancer, among other health problems.
- Loud or persistent noise can lead to hearing loss and/or stress.
- The impact of personal changes made by every concerned individual could be tremendous.

TAKE ACTION

1. Prepare an inventory to find out what hazardous chemicals you have in your household. Read the labels for disposal instructions. If there aren't any instructions, call your local health department and ask how to dispose of specific chemicals. Also ask if there are hazardous waste disposal sites in your community or special pickup days. If possible, get rid of some or all of the hazardous wastes in your home.

2. Investigate the recycling facilities in your community. Find out how materials are recycled and what they are used for in their recycled state. If recycling isn't available in your community, contact your local city hall to find out how a recycling program can be started.

JOURNAL ENTRY

1. In your health journal, list the positive behaviors that help you protect the environment. What can you do to reinforce and support these behaviors? Then list the behaviors that may harm the environment. How can you change one or more of them?

2. *Critical Thinking* Some developing nations want to "catch up" with the West in terms of economic development and standard of living by using the same kinds of industrial practices that developed nations have used to get where they are. They are cutting down forests to raise cattle for beef, using pesticides that have been banned in the developed nations, and polluting their water and air with industrial and agricultural wastes. Do you think it's fair to expect them to be environmentally conscious when the developed nations were not? Do they have a right to the same standard of living that Americans have, no matter what the environmental costs? Write a short essay that makes a case for or against their continuing use of these practices.

FOR MORE INFORMATION

Books

Getis, J. 1999. *You Can Make a Difference: Be Environmentally Responsible*, 2nd ed. New York: McGraw-Hill. *Describes environmental problems and suggestions for individual action.*

Nadakavukaren, A. 2000. *Our Global Environment: A Health Perspective*, 5th ed. Prospect Heights, Ill.: Waveland Press. *A broad survey of major environmental issues and their effects on personal and community health.*

Stevens, W. K. 2001. *The Change in the Weather: People, Weather, and the Science of Climate*. New York: Delacorte. *Describes the scientific debate about global warming and severe weather events and what might be done to reverse current trends.*

Yassi, A. 2001. *Basic Environmental Health*. New York: Oxford University Press. *A comprehensive introduction to environmental health concerns.*

Useful annual or biennial publications include the following:

Brown, L., et al. 2001. *State of the World 2001*. New York: Norton.

National Wildlife Federation. 2001. *2001 Conservation Directory*. Washington D.C.: National Wildlife Federation.

World Resources Institute. 2000. *World Resources 2000–2001*. New York: Oxford University Press.

Organizations, Hotlines, and Web Sites

The Earth Times. An international online newspaper devoted to global environmental issues.

http://www.earthtimes.org

Energy Efficiency and Renewable Energy Network (EREN). U.S. Department of Energy. Provides information about alternative fuels and tips for saving energy at home and in your car.

http://www.eren.doe.gov

Environmental News Network. Provides daily environmental news and special reports in print, audio, and video.

http://www.enn.com

Fuel Economy. Provides information on the fuel economy of cars made since 1985 and tips on improving gas mileage.

http://www.fueleconomy.gov

Garbage. Provides information and links about ways to reduce solid and hazardous waste.

http://www.learner.org/exhibits/garbage

Indoor Air Quality Information Hotline. Answers questions, provides publications, and makes referrals.

800-438-4318

National Lead Information Center. Provides information packets and specialist advice.

800-LEAD-FYI

National Safety Council Environmental Health Center. Provides information on lead, radon, indoor air quality, hazardous chemicals, and other environmental issues.

800-55-RADON (Radon Hotline)

http://www.nsc.org/ehc.htm

Ozone Hole Tour. An illustrated look at the science behind the Antarctic ozone hole.

http://www.atm.ch.cam.ac.uk/tour

Student Environmental Action Coalition (SEAC). A coalition of student and youth environmental groups; Web site has contact information for local groups.

215-222-4711

http://www.seac.org

United Nations. Several UN programs are devoted to environmental problems on a global scale; the Web sites provide information on current and projected trends and on international treaties developed to deal with environmental issues.

http://www.undp.org/popin (Population Division)

http://www.unep.org (Environment Programme)

U.S. Environmental Protection Agency (EPA). Provides information about EPA activities and many consumer-oriented materials.

http://www.epa.gov

Worldwatch Institute. A public policy research organization focusing on emerging global environmental problems and the links between the world economy and the environment.

http://www.worldwatch.org

There are many national and international organizations working on environmental health problems. A few of the largest and best known are listed below:

Greenpeace: 800-326-0959; http://www.greenpeace.org

National Audubon Society: 212-979-3000; http://www.audubon.org

National Wildlife Federation: 202-797-6800; http://www.nwf.org

Nature Conservancy: 703-841-5300; http://www.tnc.org

Sierra Club: 415-977-5500; http://www.sierraclub.org

SELECTED BIBLIOGRAPHY

American Council for an Energy-Efficient Economy. 2000. *Green Book: Market Trends* (http://www.greenercars.org/gctext.html; retrieved January 13, 2001).

Brown, L., et al. 2001. *State of the World 2001.* New York: Norton.

Centers for Disease Control and Prevention. 2000. Recommendations for blood lead screening of young children enrolled in Medicaid: Targeting a group at high risk. *MMWR Recommendations and Reports* 49(RR14): 1–13.

Centers for Disease Control and Prevention. 2001. Blood and hair mercury levels in young children and women of childbearing age—United States, 1999. *Morbidity and Mortality Weekly Report* 50(8): 140–143.

D'Agnese, J. 2000. Why has our weather gone wild? *Discover,* June, 72.

Epstein, P. R. 2000. Is global warming harmful to health? *Scientific American,* August, 50–57.

Friedrich, M. J. 2000. Poor children subject to "environmental injustice." *Journal of the American Medical Association* 283(23): 3057–3058.

Gleick, P. H. 2001. Safeguarding our water: Making every drop count. *Scientific American,* February.

Intergovernmental Panel on Climate Change. 2001. *Climate Change 2001: Impacts, Adaptation and Vulnerability.* Geneva: Intergovernmental Panel on Climate Change.

International Center for Technology Assessment. 1998. *The Real Price of Gas* (http://www.icta.org/projects/trans/rlprexsm.htm; retrieved March 3, 1999).

National Oceanic and Atmospheric Administration. 2000. *2000 Southern Hemisphere Ozone Hole Area* (http://www.cpc.ncep.noaa.gov/products/stratosphere/sbuv2to/ozone_hole_plot.gif; retrieved January 12, 2001).

National Research Council. 2000. *Toxicological Effects of Methylmercury.* Washington, D.C.: National Academy Press.

Sala, O. E., et al. 2000. Global biodiversity scenarios for the year 2100. *Science* 287(5459): 1770–1774.

Samet, J. M., et al. 2000. Fine particulate air pollution and mortality in 20 U.S. cities, 1987–1994. *New England Journal of Medicine* 343(24): 1742–1749.

United Nations Population Division. 2001. *World Population Prospects: The 2000 Revision.* New York: United Nations.

U.S. Department of Energy, Hybrid Electric Vehicle Program. 2000. *What Is an HEV?* (http://www.ott.doe.gov/hev/what.html; retrieved January 13, 2001).

U.S. Environmental Protection Agency. 2000. *Air Quality Index: A Guide to Air Quality and Your Health.* Pub. no. EPA-454/R-00-005.

U.S. Environmental Protection Agency. 2000. *Municipal Solid Waste Generation, Recycling, and Disposal in the United States.* Pub. no. EPA-530/F-00-024.

U.S. Environmental Protection Agency. 2001. *America's Children and the Environment.* Washington, D.C.: U.S. Environmental Protection Agency.

U.S. Environmental Protection Agency, Superfund Program. 2000. *Superfund Cleanup Figures* (http://www.epa.gov/superfund/actin/process/mgmtrpt.htm; retrieved January 11, 2001).

U.S. Global Change Research Project. 2000. *Climate Change Impacts on the United States.* Washington, D.C.: U.S. Global Change Research Project.

Nutritional Content of Popular Items from Fast-Food Restaurants

Arby's

	Serving size	Calories	Protein	Total fat	Saturated fat	Total carbohydrate	Sugars	Fiber	Cholesterol	Sodium	Vitamin A	Vitamin C	Calcium	Iron	% calories from fat
	g		g	g	g	g	g	g	mg	mg	% Daily Value				
Regular roast beef	154	388	23	19	7	33	N/A	3	43	1009	N/A	N/A	N/A	N/A	44
Super roast beef	247	523	25	27	9	50	N/A	5	43	1189	N/A	N/A	N/A	N/A	46
French dip	195	475	30	22	8	40	N/A	3	55	1411	N/A	N/A	N/A	N/A	41
Junior roast beef	126	324	17	14	5	35	N/A	2	30	779	N/A	N/A	N/A	N/A	39
Roast chicken Caesar sandwich	300	660	41	24	5	70	N/A	N/A	80	1900	N/A	N/A	N/A	N/A	33
Roast turkey & swiss	327	630	42	30	8	52	N/A	N/A	80	1670	N/A	N/A	N/A	N/A	43
Breaded chicken fillet	240	623	28	28	5	46	N/A	5	45	1016	N/A	N/A	N/A	N/A	40
Han 'n cheese	169	359	24	14	5	34	N/A	2	53	1283	N/A	N/A	N/A	N/A	35
Jalapeño bites	110	330	7	21	9	29	N/A	2	40	670	N/A	N/A	N/A	N/A	57
Cheddar curly fries	120	333	5	18	4	40	N/A	0	3	1016	N/A	N/A	N/A	N/A	49
Potato cakes	85	204	2	12	2	20	N/A	0	0	397	N/A	N/A	N/A	N/A	53
Red ranch dressing	14	75	0	6	1	5	N/A	0	0	115	N/A	N/A	N/A	N/A	72
French-toastix	124	430	10	21	5	52	N/A	3	0	550	N/A	N/A	N/A	N/A	44
Jamocha shake	340	384	15	10	3	62	N/A	0	36	262	N/A	N/A	N/A	N/A	23

N/A: not available.

SOURCE: Triare Restaurant Group, 1998–2000, http://www.arbysrestaurant.com. Permission pending.

Burger King

	Serving size	Calories	Protein	Total fat	Saturated fat	Total carbohydrate	Sugars	Fiber	Cholesterol	Sodium	Vitamin A	Vitamin C	Calcium	Iron	% calories from fat
	g		g	g	g	g	g	g	mg	mg	% Daily Value				
Whopper®	278	680	29	39	12	53	9	4	80	940	10	15	10	30	52
Whopper Jr.®	172	420	20	24	8	32	6	2	55	520	4	8	8	20	51
Double Whopper® w/cheese	387	1020	53	65	25	55	9	4	170	1460	15	15	30	40	57
BK Big Fish™ sandwich	263	710	24	38	14	67	4	4	50	1200	2	0	8	20	48
BK Broiler® chicken sandwich	258	550	30	25	5	52	5	3	105	1110	6	10	6	20	41
Chicken Tenders® (8 pieces)	123	340	22	19	5	20	0	<1	50	840	0	0	0	4	50
Ranch dipping sauce	28	120	1	13	2	1	N/A	N/A	5	85	N/A	N/A	N/A	N/A	98
Barbecue dipping sauce	28	35	0	0	0	9	N/A	N/A	0	400	N/A	N/A	N/A	N/A	0
French fries, medium	116	370	4	17	5	49	0	4	0	760	0	2	0	6	41
Onion rings, medium	94	330	5	16	4	41	5	3	0	470	0	0	10	0	44
Chocolate shake, medium	397	440	12	10	6	75	67	4	30	330	8	0	30	15	21
Croissan'wich® w/sausage, egg & cheese	153	500	19	36	13	26	5	1	190	1020	8	0	15	15	65
French toast sticks	112	390	6	20	4.5	46	11	2	0	440	0	0	6	10	46
Dutch apple pie	113	340	2	14	3	15	23	1	0	470	2	0	0	8	37
Chicken club sandwich	242	620	30	32	8	54	6	4	75	1460	6	10	8	20	47

N/A: not available.

SOURCE: Burger King Corporation, 2001, http://www.burgerking.com. Burger King® trademarks, trade name, and Nutritional Guide are reproduced with permission from Burger King Brands, Inc.

Domino's Pizza

(1 serving = 2 of 8 slices or ¼ of 14-inch pizza; 2 of 8 slices or ¼ of 12-inch pizza; 1 6-inch pizza)

	Serving size	Calories	Protein	Total fat	Saturated fat	Total carbohydrate	Sugars	Fiber	Cholesterol	Sodium	Vitamin A	Vitamin C	Calcium	Iron	% calories from fat
	g		g	g	g	g	g	g	mg	mg	% Daily Value				
14-inch lg. hand-tossed cheese	219	516	21	15	7	75	6	4	32	1080	18	0	26	23	26
14-inch lg. thin crust cheese	148	382	17	17	7	43	6	2	32	1172	18	0	32	8	40
14-inch lg. deep dish cheese	257	677	26	30	11	80	9	5	41	1575	21	<1	33	31	40
12-inch med. hand-tossed cheese	159	375	15	11	5	55	5	3	23	776	13	0	19	17	26
12-inch med. thin crust cheese	106	273	12	12	5	31	4	2	23	835	13	0	23	5	40
12-inch med. deep dish cheese	181	482	19	22	8	56	6	3	30	1123	15	<1	24	22	41
6-inch deep dish cheese	216	598	23	28	10	68	7	4	36	1341	17	<1	30	30	42
Toppings: pepperoni	*	98	5	9	3	<1	<1	<1	20	364	†	†	†	†	83
ham	*	31	5	2	<1	<1	<1	<1	12	292	†	†	†	†	58
Italian sausage	*	110	5	9	3	3	<1	<1	22	342	†	†	†	†	74
bacon	*	153	8	13	4	<1	<1	<1	22	424	†	†	†	†	77
beef	*	111	6	10	4	<1	<1	<1	21	309	†	†	†	†	81
anchovies	*	45	9	2	<1	<1	<1	<1	18	791	†	†	5	6	40
extra cheese	*	68	7	6	3	<1	<1	<1	15	228	11	†	12	†	79
cheddar cheese	*	71	5	6	3	<1	<1	<1	18	110	4	†	13	†	76
Barbeque buffalo wings	25	50	5	2	<1	2	1	<1	26	175	†	†	†	†	36
Breadsticks (1 piece)	37	116	3	4	<1	16	<1	<1	0	152	†	†	†	†	31
Double cheesy bread	43	142	4	6	2	18	<1	<1	6	183	†	†	†	†	38

* Topping information is based on minimal portioning requirements for one serving of a 14-inch large pizza; add the values for toppings to the values for a cheese pizza. The following toppings supply fewer than 15 calories per serving: green and yellow peppers, onion, olives, mushrooms, pineapple.

† Contains less than 2% of the Daily Value of these nutrients.

SOURCE: Domino's Pizza, 2001, http://www.dominos.com. Reproduced with permission from Domino's Pizza LLC.

Jack in the Box

	Serving size	Calories	Protein	Total fat	Saturated fat	Total carbohydrate	Sugars	Fiber	Cholesterol	Sodium	Vitamin A	Vitamin C	Calcium	Iron	% calories from fat
	g		g	g	g	g	g	g	mg	mg	% Daily Value				
Breakfast Jack®	126	280	17	12	5	28	3	1	190	750	8	6	15	20	39
Supreme croissant	164	530	21	34	10	37	6	0	225	1060	8	6	10	10	58
Hamburger	104	250	12	9	3.5	30	5	2	30	610	0	0	10	20	32
Jumbo Jack®	271	550	27	30	10	43	12	2	75	880	10	15	15	25	49
Sourdough Jack®	233	690	34	45	15	37	3	2	105	1180	15	15	20	25	59
Chicken fajita pita	230	320	24	10	4.5	34	6	3	55	850	20	25	20	15	28
Grilled chicken fillet	242	480	27	24	6	39	6	4	65	1110	8	15	20	25	45
Chicken supreme	305	830	33	49	7	66	5	3	65	2140	10	15	20	20	53
Jack Spicy Chicken®	252	570	24	29	2.5	52	9	2	50	1020	8	15	15	10	46
Garden chicken salad	253	200	23	9	4	8	4	3	65	420	70	20	20	4	41
Blue cheese dressing	57	210	1	15	2.5	11	4	0	25	750	0	0	2	0	64
Chicken teriyaki bowl	502	670	26	4	1	128	27	3	15	1730	130	40	10	25	5
Monster taco	138	270	12	17	6	19	2	4	30	630	10	4	20	8	57
Egg rolls (3 pieces)	170	440	15	24	6	40	5	4	30	1020	15	20	8	25	49
Chicken breast pieces (5)	150	360	27	17	3	24	0	1	80	970	4	2	2	10	43
Stuffed jalapeños (7 pieces)	168	530	16	31	12	46	5	4	60	1730	20	35	30	8	53
Barbeque dipping sauce	28	45	1	0	0	11	7	0	0	310	0	4	0	0	0
Seasoned curly fries	125	410	6	23	5	45	0	4	0	1010	6	0	4	10	51
Onion rings	120	450	7	25	5	50	3	3	0	780	4	30	4	15	50
Cappuccino classic ice cream shake	16 oz	630	11	29	17	80	58	0	90	320	15	0	35	0	41

SOURCE: Jack's Nutrition Facts, Rev. 2000. The following trademarks are owned by Jack in the Box, Inc.: Breakfast Jack,® Jumbo Jack,® Sourdough Jack,® Jack in the Box.® Reproduced with permission from Jack in the Box Inc.

KFC

	Serving size	Calories	Protein	Total fat	Saturated fat	Total carbohydrate	Sugars	Fiber	Cholesterol	Sodium	Vitamin A	Vitamin C	Calcium	Iron	% calories from fat
	g		g	g	g	g	g	g	mg	mg	% Daily Value				
Original Recipe® breast	153	400	29	24	6	16	0	1	135	1116	*	*	4	6	54
Original Recipe® thigh	91	250	16	18	4.5	6	0	1	95	747	*	*	2	4	65
Extra crispy chicken breast	168	470	39	28	8	17	0	<1	160	874	*	*	2	6	54
Extra crispy chicken thigh	118	380	21	27	7	14	0	<1	118	625	*	*	2	6	64
Hot & spicy breast	180	505	38	29	8	23	9	1	162	1170	*	*	6	6	52
Hot & spicy thigh	107	355	19	26	7	13	0	1	126	630	*	*	2	4	66
Tender Roast sandwich w/sauce	211	350	32	15	3	26	1	1	75	880	4	*	4	10	39
Tender Roast sandwich w/o sauce	177	270	31	5	1.5	23	<1	1	65	690	*	*	4	10	17
Hot wings (6 pieces)	135	471	27	33	8	18	0	2	150	1230	*	*	4	8	63
Colonel's Crispy Strips™ (3)	115	300	26	16	4	18	1	1	56	1165	2	*	*	6	48
Chunky chicken pot pie	368	770	29	42	13	69	8	5	70	2160	80	2	10	10	49
Corn on the cob	162	150	5	1.5	0	35	8	2	0	20	2	6	*	*	9
Mashed potatoes w/gravy	136	120	1	6	1	17	0	2	,1	440	*	*	*	2	45
BBQ baked beans	156	190	6	3	1	33	13	6	5	760	8	*	8	10	14
Cole slaw	142	232	2	13.5	2	26	20	3	8	284	9	58	3	*	52
Biscuit (1)	56	180	4	10	2.5	20	2	<1	0	560	*	*	2	6	50
Potato salad	160	230	4	14	2	23	9	3	15	540	10	*	2	15	55

*Contains less than 2% of the Daily Value of these nutrients.

SOURCE: KFC Corporation, 2001, http://www.kfc.com. Reproduced with permission from Kentucky Fried Chicken Corporation.

Taco Bell

	Serving size	Calories	Protein	Total fat	Saturated fat	Total carbohydrate	Sugars	Fiber	Cholesterol	Sodium	Vitamin A	Vitamin C	Calcium	Iron	% calories from fat
	g		g	g	g	g	g	g	mg	mg	% Daily Value				
Taco	86	170	9	10	4	12	<1	3	30	330	8	0	8	4	53
Taco Supreme®	124	210	9	14	6	14	2	3	40	350	8	6	10	6	60
Double Decker Taco Supreme®	109	380	15	18	7	39	3	9	40	760	8	6	15	10	43
Beef soft taco	109	210	11	10	4	20	1	3	30	570	8	0	8	6	43
Chicken soft taco	109	190	13	7	2.5	19	1	2	35	480	4	2	8	4	33
Chicken Burrito Supreme	117	410	20	16	6	49	4	8	45	1120	45	8	15	10	35
Beef Double Burrito Supreme	319	510	23	23	9	52	4	11	60	1500	50	8	15	15	41
Chili cheese burrito	156	330	13	13	5	40	2	4	25	900	20	0	15	6	35
Bean burrito	218	370	13	12	3.5	54	3	12	10	1080	45	0	15	15	29
Nachos Supreme	218	440	14	24	7	44	3	9	35	800	0	6	15	15	49
Nachos BellGrande®	342	760	20	39	11	83	4	17	35	1300	10	8	20	20	46
Pintos 'n cheese	140	180	9	8	4	18	1	10	15	640	45	0	15	10	40
Mexican rice	148	190	5	9	3.5	23	,1	,1	15	750	100	2	15	8	43
Beef Fiesto Burrito	202	370	14	15	5	49	3	4	30	1110	30	0	10	10	36
Meximelt®	148	290	15	15	7	22	2	4	45	830	8	0	20	6	47
Chalupa Supreme,® beef	171	380	14	23	8	29	3	3	40	580	6	8	15	10	55
Chalupa nacho cheese, chicken	171	350	16	19	4.5	29	3	2	25	640	6	8	8	10	49
Gordita Supreme,® beef	171	300	17	14	5	27	4	3	35	550	2	6	15	10	42
Gordita Santa Fe,® chicken	171	370	17	20	4	30	3	3	40	610	4	6	15	10	49

SOURCE: Taco Bell Corporation, 2001, http;://www.tacobell.com. Reproduced with permission from the Taco Bell Corporation.

Wendy's

	Serving size	Calories	Protein	Total fat	Saturated fat	Total carbohydrate	Sugars	Fiber	Cholesterol	Sodium	Vitamin A	Vitamin C	Calcium	Iron	% calories from fat
	g		g	g	g	g	g	g	mg	mg		% Daily Value			
Single w/everything	219	420	25	20	7	37	8	3	70	930	6	10	15	25	43
Big Bacon Classic	282	580	33	31	12	45	11	3	95	1500	15	20	25	30	48
Jr. hamburger	118	280	15	10	3.5	34	7	2	30	610	2	2	10	20	32
Jr. bacon cheeseburger	166	390	20	20	8	34	7	2	55	870	8	10	15	20	46
Grilled chicken sandwich	189	300	24	8	1.5	36	8	2	55	730	4	10	10	15	24
Caesar side salad (no dressing)	92	110	9	6	2.5	6	1	1	15	600	35	25	15	6	49
Grilled chicken salad (no dressing)	338	190	22	8	1.5	10	5	4	45	680	120	60	20	10	38
Taco salad (no dressing)	468	380	26	19	10	28	8	8	65	1040	45	45	35	25	45
Blue cheese dressing (2T)	28	180	1	19	3.5	0	0	0	15	170	0	0	2	0	95
Ranch dressing, reduced fat, calories (2T)	28	60	1	5	1	2	1	0	10	240	0	0	2	0	75
Soft breadstick	44	130	4	3	.5	23	N/A	1	5	250	0	0	4	9	21
Biggie fries	159	470	7	23	3.5	61	0	6	0	150	0	15	3	7	44
Baked potato w/broccoli & cheese	411	470	9	14	2.5	80	6	9	5	470	35	120	20	25	27
Baked potato w/chili & cheese	439	620	20	24	9	83	7	9	40	780	20	60	35	30	35
Chili, small, plain	227	210	15	7	2.5	21	5	5	30	800	8	6	8	6	30
Chili, large w/cheese & crackers	363	405	28	16.5	7	37	8	7	60	1380	14	10	22	26	37
Chicken nuggets (5)	75	230	11	16	3	11	0	0	30	470	0	2	2	2	63
Barbeque sauce	28	45	1	0	0	10	7	0	0	160	0	0	0	4	0
Frosty dairy dessert, medium	298	440	11	11	7	73	56	0	50	260	20	0	41	8	23
Chicken club sandwich	216	480	30	21	5	44	6	2	65	1000	4	10	10	15	39

N/A: not available.

SOURCE: Wendy's International, Inf., 2001, http://www.wendys.com. Reproduced with permission from Wendy's International, Inc.

Information on additional foods and restaurants is available online:

Arby's: http://www.arbysrestaurant.com

Burger King: http://www.burgerking.com

Domino's Pizza: http://www.dominos.com

Hardees: http://www.hardees.com

Jack in the Box: http://www.jackinthebox.com

KFC: http://www.kfc.com

McDonald's: http://www.mcdonalds.com

Subway: http://www.subway.com

Taco Bell: http://www.tacobell.com

Wendy's: http://www.wendys.com

White Castle: http://www.whitecastle.com

Index

Page references in boldface refer to pages on which terms are defined. Page references followed by a "t" refer to tables.

cigarette smoking. *See* smoking; tobacco
cigarette tar, **169**
cigars, 172–173
cilia, 171, 295
circumcision, 78–**79**
cirrhosis, 7, 160–**161**, 164, 303
civil unions, 68
clarity (MDMA), 141, 145
clear cell cancer, 280
climate change, 304, 396–398
clinical breast exam (CBE), 286t
clinical death, **334**–335
clinical psychologists, 54
clitoris, **77**, 84
clonazepam, 140
clonidine, 178
cloning, 90
clove cigarettes, 173–174
club drugs, 141
cluster headaches, 28
CMV (cytomegalovirus), 265
coagulation disorder, 310
coarctation of the aorta, 271
cocaine, 131t, 135t, 137, 140–142
codeine, 135t, 139
codependency, **148**–149, 166–167
coffee, 143. *See also* caffeine
cognitive distortions, 46–**47**
cohabitation, 67
coitus interruptus (withdrawal), 107t, 116, 119
cola drinks, 143
colds, 302
cold sores, 303, 315–316
college students
    binge drinking, 162–164, 163t
    drug-treatment programs, 148
    nonmedical drug use statistics, 131t
    smoking, 172
    stress, 28–29
colon cancer, 276–277, 284, 286t
colonoscopy, 286
colostrum, **91**, 99
commitment, 61–62, 69–70, 73
communication
    conflict and conflict resolution, 65
    contraception, 88, 120
    effective, 64
    families, 73
    feedback, 64
    nonverbal, 63–64
complementary and alternative medicine (CAM)
    biological-based therapies, 357, **360**–361
    definition, **349**
    energy therapies, 357, **360**–362
    evaluation of, 362–364
    five domains of, 356–357
    homeopathy, 349t, 358–**359**
    hypnosis, 349t, **359**
    manipulative and body-based methods, 357, 360
    mind-body interventions, 357, 359
    organizations and Web sites, 367–368
    reasons for using, 364
    traditional Chinese medicine, 356–358, **357**, 361
    use statistics, 349t
compulsions, **50**, 131
compulsive gambling, 132–133
compulsive overeaters, 253–254
compulsive shopping, 133
computed tomography (CT), 268, **270**, 287
conception, **88**–89
condoms
    female, 111–112, 117t, 118t
    male, **108**–112, 117t, 118t
    prevalence of use, 119
    STD prevention, 109–110, 312–313, 315, 319–320
conflict and conflict resolution, 65
congenital heart disease, **270**–271
congenital malformations, 94–**95**
congenital syphilis, 318
congestive heart failure, **270**–271
consumer guidelines
    adoption, 125

alcohol advertising, 154
bicycle helmets, 373
birth plan, 97
common cold treatments, 302
complementary and alternative medicine, 618–619
contraceptives, 111
dietary supplements, 81, 206, 237
diet pills and aids, 250
end-of-life care, 336–338
exercise instructors, equipment, and facilities, 230
fat and sugar substitutes, 245
functional foods, 237
funerals, 339
green (environmentally-friendly) consumerism, 394
HIV tests, 311
mental health professionals, 55
over-the-counter medications, 348
tobacco cessation products, 178
weight loss products and strategies, 410–414
See also advertising; media
Consumer Product Safety Commission (CPSC), 373
contagion, 297, 302
contagious diseases, 302–**303**. *See also* infectious diseases
continuation rates, **105**
contraception, 104–129
    barrier methods, 104, 109–115, 117t
    choice of methods, 118–120
    contraceptive implants, 106–108
    effectiveness, 105, 118t
    emergency, 108
    hormonal methods, 104–109, 117t
    injectable contraceptives, 108
    natural methods, 104–105, **114**–116, 117t
    principles, 104–105
    risks of, 107t
    surgical methods, 105, 116–117
    See also oral contraceptives
contraceptive behavior, 104–**105**
contraceptive failure rates, **105**
contraceptive implants, 106–108, 119
contraceptive sponges, 111, **114**, 117t
contractions, **96**–98
conventional medicine, **349**–356
    choosing a primary care physician, 353
    definition, 349
    diagnostic process, 354
    medications and surgical treatments, 354–356
    partnership with physician, 353–354
    premises and assumptions, 350–351
    providers, 351–353
coping strategies, 24, 36, 247, 340–341
Copper T-380A, 109, 118t
coronary angiograms, 268
coronary arteries, 259
coronary bypass surgery, 268
coronary heart disease (CHD), 161, 170–**171**, 264, **267**, 272. *See also* cardiovascular disease
coronary stents, 268
coronary thrombosis, **267**
corpus luteum, **80**–81
corpus spongiosum, 78
Corr, Charles, 340
corticosteroids, 298
cortisol, **22**, 26
costs of health care, 364–365
cough medicines, 302
court shoes, 230
Cowper's glands, 78
CPR (cardiopulmonary resuscitation), 268–**269**
crabs (lice), 318
crack cocaine, 135t, 137, 140, 142
C-reactive protein, 265
creatine monohydrate, 227
creativity, 43, 54
cremation, 340
Creutzfeldt-Jakob disease (CJD), 300, 304–305
Crime Statistic Web site, 387
cross-training, 232
cruciferous vegetables, 289

Cruzan, Nancy Beth, 336
crystal (amphetamines), 135t, 137, 142
CTS (carpal tunnel syndrome), 377–378
culture
    abortion and, 122
    attitudes toward aging, 332
    attitudes toward death, 334
    body image and, 251
    circumcision and, 78
    role in health, 4–7
    stress and, 25
    See also ethnicity
cumulative trauma disorder (CTD), **377**
cunnilingus, **86**
CVD. *See* cardiovascular disease
CVS (chorionic villi sampling), **93**
cybersex, 87
cyberstalking, **381**–382
cytokines, 296–297
cytomegalovirus (CMV), 265, 303

Dalkon Shields, 108–109
DASH diet, 272
date rape, 141, **383**–384
date-rape drugs, 141, 384
dating, 66–67. *See also* intimate relationships
Day of the Dead, 334
death
    advance directives, 338–**339**, 344
    coming to terms with, 343
    coping with dying, 340–341
    coping with loss, 341–343
    definitions of, 334–335
    from injuries, 370t
    leading causes, 4–5, 5t
    wills, **334**–336
Death with Dignity Act of 1994, 337
decibels, **402**–403
decongestants, 302
deep breathing, 34–35
DEET, 281, 301
defense mechanisms, **45**–46
defense of marriage acts (DOMAs), 68
deforestation, 397
dehydration, 229
dehydroepiandrosterone (DHEA), 227
delirium tremens (DTs), 140, **162**–163
delusions, 52
dementia, **330**–332
demoralization, 44–45
dentists, 353
Department of Health and Human Services, 344–345
depersonalization, **144**
Depo-Provera, 108, 118t
depressants, **140**
depression
    aging, 326, 331
    alcohol use, 161
    cardiovascular disease, 262
    exercise and, 220
    lifetime prevalence, 48t
    postpartum, 99
    symptoms, **50**
    treatment, 51–52
    warning signs of suicide, 50
DES (diethylstilbestrol), 89, 280, 282
desert herb, 250
designated drivers, 159
dexfenfluamine (Redux), 251
DHEA (dehydroepiandrosterone), 227
diabetes
    alcohol use, 161
    cardiovascular heart disease, 262
    exercise and, 220
    glycemic index, **264**–265
    symptoms, 240
    treatment, 241
    warning signs and testing, 241
Dia de los Muertos, 334
Diagnostic and Statistical Manual of Mental Disorders, 133
diaphragmatic breathing, 35
diaphragms, **112**–113, 117t, 119

CHAPTER 1
Taking Charge of Your Health

Multiple Choice

1. An out-of-date definition of health is:
   a. fulfillment of personal potential.
   b. personal wellness.
   c. absence of disease.
   d. multidimensional.

2. All of the following are dimensions of wellness described in the book EXCEPT:
   a. planetary wellness.
   b. emotional wellness.
   c. interpersonal wellness.
   d. socioeconomic wellness.

3. Self-acceptance is most representative of:
   a. physical wellness.
   b. emotional wellness.
   c. intellectual wellness.
   d. spiritual wellness.

4. The leading cause of death among Americans is:
   a. heart disease.
   b. infection.
   c. cancer.
   d. stroke.

5. The *Healthy People 2010* report includes all of the following EXCEPT:
   a. a goal of increasing quality and years of healthy life.
   b. a goal of eliminating health disparities among Americans.
   c. specific objectives in different focus areas related to wellness.
   d. specific budget goals for all federally funded health programs.

6. The most important contributor to wellness for most people is:
   a. health behavior.
   b. health care.
   c. heredity.
   d. environment.

7. Which of the following behaviors is linked with the greatest number of the leading causes of death in the United States?
   a. overconsumption of alcohol
   b. poor diet
   c. cigarette smoking
   d. physical inactivity

8. A target behavior may best be described as:
   a. a risky behavior of a loved one that you would like to see changed.
   b. a risky behavior of your own that you would like to change.
   c. the thing you do that is most risky.
   d. a risky behavior of yours that your family or physician tries to get you to change.

9. Probably the LEAST effective health behavior change strategy is:
   a. changing several behaviors at once.
   b. charting health behaviors.
   c. setting up short-term reward systems.
   d. selecting the easiest-to-change behavior as the first target for change.

10. Parts of a plan of action for making a behavior change include all of the following EXCEPT:
    a. modifying your environment.
    b. designing a health journal.
    c. setting up a system of rewards.
    d. involving the people around you.

True or False

T F 1. Wellness requires learning about and protecting yourself from environmental hazards.

T F 2. Personal wellness is defined primarily by a high level of cardiovascular fitness.

T F 3. A major *Healthy People 2010* objective is to increase longevity among Americans.

T F 4. A healthy person has learned how to manage stress effectively.

T F 5. Focusing on several target behaviors at once increases your chances of succeeding in changing the behaviors.

T F 6. Most people are likely to be motivated by long-term goals such as avoiding disease 20 or 30 years from now.

T F 7. Some health behaviors are difficult or impossible to change without outside assistance.

T F 8. A good role model is a person who has reached the goal you are striving for.

T F 9. You are more likely to succeed if you pursue your behavior change program without telling friends or family members

T F 10. Personal health contracts tend to set people up for failure by creating expectations that cannot be filled.

ANSWERS: Multiple Choice: 1. c (p. 1); 2. d (p. 2); 3. b (p. 2); 4. a (p. 5, Table 1-1); 5. d (p.3); 6. a (p. 9); 7. c (p. 5, Table 1-1); 8. b (p. 10); 9. a (p. 10); 10. b (p. 5). True or False: 1. T (p. 2); 2. F (p. 1); 3. F (p. 3); 4. T (p. 9); 5. F (p. 10); 6. F (p. 11); 7. T (p. 12); 8. T (p. 12); 9. F (p. 15); 10. F (p. 15).

Name _____ Section _____ Date _____

WELLNESS WORKSHEET I

Evaluate Your Lifestyle

All of us want optimal health. But many of us do not know how to achieve it. Taking this quiz, adapted from one created by the U.S. Public Health Service, is a good place to start. The behaviors covered in the test are recommended for most Americans. (Some of them may not apply to people with certain diseases or disabilities or to pregnant women, who may require special advice from their physicians.) After you take the quiz, add up your score for each section.

	Almost always	Sometimes	Never
Tobacco Use			
If you never use tobacco, enter a score of 10 for this section and go to the next section.			
1. I avoid using tobacco.	2	1	0
2. I smoke only low-tar-and-nicotine cigarettes *or* I smoke a pipe or cigar *or* I use smokeless tobacco.	2	1	0
Tobacco Score: _____			
Alcohol and Other Drugs			
1. I avoid alcohol *or* I drink no more than 1 (women) or 2 (men) drinks a day.	4	1	0
2. I avoid using alcohol or other drugs as a way of handling stressful situations or problems in my life.	2	1	0
3. I am careful not to drink alcohol when taking medications, such as for colds or allergies, or when pregnant.	2	1	0
4. I read and follow the label directions when using prescribed and over-the-counter drugs.	2	1	0
Alcohol and Other Drugs Score: _____			
Nutrition			
1. I eat a variety of foods each day, including five or more servings of fruits and vegetables.	3	1	0
2. I limit the amount of fat and saturated fat in my diet.	3	1	0
3. I avoid skipping meals.	2	1	0
4. I limit the amount of salt and sugar I eat.	2	1	0
Nutrition Score: _____			
Exercise/Fitness			
1. I engage in moderate exercise for 20–60 minutes, 3–5 times a week.	4	1	0
2. I maintain a healthy weight, avoiding overweight or underweight.	2	1	0
3. I do exercises to develop muscular strength and endurance at least twice a week.	2	1	0
4. I spend some of my leisure time participating in physical activities such as gardening, bowling, golf, or baseball.	2	1	0
Exercise/Fitness Score: _____			

(over)

	Almost always	Sometimes	Never
Emotional Health			
1. I enjoy being a student, and I have a job or do other work that I like.	2	1	0
2. I find it easy to relax and express my feelings freely.	2	1	0
3. I manage stress well.	2	1	0
4. I have close friends, relatives, or others I can talk to about personal matters and call on for help.	2	1	0
5. I participate in group activities (such as church and community organizations) or hobbies that I enjoy.	2	1	0

Emotional Health Score: _____

	Almost always	Sometimes	Never
Safety			
1. I wear a safety belt while riding in a car.	2	1	0
2. I avoid driving while under the influence of alcohol or other drugs.	2	1	0
3. I obey traffic rules and the speed limit when driving.	2	1	0
4. I read and follow instructions on the labels of potentially harmful products or substances, such as household cleaners, poisons, and electrical appliances.	2	1	0
5. I avoid smoking in bed.	2	1	0

Safety Score: _____

	Almost always	Sometimes	Never
Disease Prevention			
1. I know the warning signs of cancer, diabetes, heart attack, and stroke.	2	1	0
2. I avoid overexposure to the sun and use sunscreens.	2	1	0
3. I get recommended medical screening tests (such as blood pressure checks and Pap tests), immunization, and booster shots.	2	1	0
4. I practice monthly breast/testicle self-exams.	2	1	0
5. I am not sexually active *or* I have sex with only one mutually faithful, uninfected partner *or* I always engage in safer sex (using condoms) *and* I do not share needles to inject drugs.	2	1	0

Disease Prevention Score: _____

What Your Scores Mean

Scores of 9 and 10 Excellent! Your answers show that you are aware of the importance of this area to wellness. More important, you are putting your knowledge to work for you by practicing good health habits. As long as you continue to do so, this area should not pose a serious health risk. It's likely that you are setting an example for your family and friends to follow. Since you earned a very high test score on this part of the test, you may want to focus on other areas where your scores indicate room for improvement.

Scores of 6–8 Your health practices in this area are good, but there is room for improvement. Look again at the items you answered with a "Sometimes" or "Never." What changes can you make to improve your score? Even a small change can often help you achieve better health.

Scores of 3–5 Your health risks are showing! You may need more information about the risks you are facing and about why it is important for you to change these behaviors. Perhaps you need help in deciding how to successfully make the changes you desire.

Scores of 0–2 Your answers show that you may be taking serious and unnecessary risks with your health. Perhaps you are not aware of the risks and what to do about them. You can easily get the information and help you need to improve, if you wish. The next step is up to you.

CHAPTER 2
Stress: The Constant Challenge

Multiple Choice

1. The division of our nervous system that triggers the stress response is the
   _____ division.
   a. autonomic
   b. parasympathetic
   c. sympathetic
   d. somatic

2. The fight-or-flight reaction produces:
   a. bronchial constriction.
   b. blood sugar reduction.
   c. increased digestion.
   d. increased blood cell production.

3. Which of the following is a brain chemical that helps to relieve pain?
   a. cortisol
   b. epinephrine
   c. norepinephrine
   d. endorphin

4. Our behavioral responses to stressors are managed by our:
   a. autonomic nervous system.
   b. parasympathetic nervous system.
   c. sympathetic nervous system.
   d. somatic nervous system.

5. Which of the following characteristics is most closely associated with the Type A
   personality?
   a. tolerance
   b. cynicism
   c. sense of inner purpose
   d. optimism

6. Eustress might be triggered by:
   a. getting a bad grade.
   b. winning the lottery.
   c. being physically attacked.
   d. experiencing homeostasis.

7. Which of the following is one of the stages of the general adaptation syndrome?
   a. alarm
   b. ambivalence
   c. anger
   d. anxiety

8. All of the following are effective techniques for managing stress EXCEPT:
   a. exercising regularly.
   b. meditating.
   c. drinking caffeine.
   d. prioritizing tasks.

9. All of the following are strategies for overcoming insomnia EXCEPT:
   a. keeping to a regular schedule.
   b. avoiding alcohol before bedtime.
   c. exercising just before bedtime.
   d. having a snack just before bedtime.

10. Another term for imagery is:
   a. progressive relaxation.
   b. visualization.
   c. meditation.
   d. biofeedback.

True or False

T F 1. Stressors are events or situations that trigger the stress response.

T F 2. The two body systems that control the physical responses to stressors are the nervous system and the endocrine system.

T F 3. The parasympathetic division of the nervous system triggers the fight-or-flight reaction.

T F 4. The fight-or-flight reaction occurs only when physical action is required to deal with a stressor.

T F 5. A person with a Type A personality who tends to be hostile and cynical has an increased risk of heart disease.

T F 6. A high level of stress can impair the immune system, thereby increasing one's risk for colds and allergy attacks.

T F 7. Exercise can help you manage stress only if performed at least four times a week.

T F 8. Blood pressure and heart rate increase during the relaxation response.

T F 9. Progressive relaxation involves focusing on a single word and taking deep breaths.

T F 10. Keeping a stress journal will help you identify and cope with daily stressors.

ANSWERS: Multiple Choice: 1. c (p. 22); 2. d (p. 23); 3. d (p. 23); 4. d (p. 24); 5. b
(p. 24); 6. b (p. 25); 7. a (p. 25); 8. c (p. 31); 9. c (p. 31); 10. b (p. 34). True or False:
1. T (p. 22); 2. T (p. 22); 3. F (p. 22); 4. F (p. 24); 5. T (p. 24); 6. T (p. 27); 7. F (p. 30);
8. F (pp. 33–34); 9. F (p. 34); 10. T (p. 36).

Name _____ Section _____ Date _____

 WELLNESS WORKSHEET 2

Identify Your Stress Level and Your Key Stressors

How High Is Your Stress Level?

Many symptoms of excess stress are easy to self-diagnose. To help determine how much stress you experience on a daily basis, answer the following questions.

Yes No

____ 1. How many of the symptoms of excess stress listed below do you experience frequently? Circle the appropriate symptoms.

Yes No

____ ____ 2. Are you easily startled or irritated?

____ ____ 3. Are you increasingly forgetful?

____ ____ 4. Do you have trouble falling or staying asleep?

____ ____ 5. Do you continually worry about events in your future?

____ ____ 6. Do you feel as if you are constantly under pressure to produce?

____ ____ 7. Do you frequently use tobacco, alcohol, or other drugs to help you relax?

____ ____ 8. Do you often feel as if you have less energy than you need to finish the day?

____ ____ 9. Do you have recurrent stomachaches or headaches?

____ ____ 10. Is it difficult for you to find satisfaction in simple life pleasures?

____ ____ 11. Are you often disappointed in yourself and others?

____ ____ 12. Are you overly concerned with being liked or accepted by others?

____ ____ 13. Have you lost interest in intimacy or sex?

____ ____ 14. Are you concerned that you do not have enough money?

Experiencing some of the stress-related symptoms or answering "yes" to a few questions is normal. However, if you experience a large number of stress symptoms or you answered "yes" to a majority of the questions, you are likely experiencing a high level of stress. Take time out to develop effective stress-managemnent techniques. Many coping strategies that can aid you in dealing with your college stressors are described in this chapter. Additionally, your school's counseling center can provide valuable support.

Symptoms of Excess Stress

Physical Symptoms	**Emotional Symptoms**	**Behavioral Symptoms**
Dry mouth	Anxiety or edginess	Crying
Excessive perspiration	Depression	Disrupted eating habits
Frequent illnesses	Fatigue	Disrupted sleeping habits
Gastrointestinal problems	Hypervigilance	Harsh treatment of others
Grinding of teeth	Impulsiveness	Increased use of tobacco, alcohol, or other drugs
Headaches	Inability to concentrate	Problems communicating
High blood pressure	Irritability	Sexual problems
Pounding heart	Trouble remembering things	Social isolation
Stiff neck or aching lower back		

Insel/Roth, *Core Concepts in Health*, Brief Ninth Edition. © 2002 The McGraw-Hill Companies, Inc.

(over)

STUDY GUIDE

Weekly Stress Log

Now that you are familiar with the signals of stress, complete the weekly stress log to map patterns in your stress levels and identify sources of stress. Enter a score for each hour of each day according to the ratings listed below.

	A.M.							P.M.												Average
	6	7	8	9	10	11	12	1	2	3	4	5	6	7	8	9	10	11	12	*Average*
Monday																				
Tuesday																				
Wednesday																				
Thursday																				
Friday																				
Saturday																				
Sunday																				
Average																				

Ratings

1 = No anxiety; general feeling of well-being
2 = Mild anxiety; no interference with activity
3 = Moderate anxiety; specific signal(s) of stress present
4 = High anxiety; interference with activity
5 = Very high anxiety and panic reactions; general inability to engage in activity

To identify daily or weekly patterns in your stress level, average your stress rating for each hour and each day. For example, if your scores for 6:00 A.M. are 3, 3, 4, 3, and 4, with blanks for Saturday and Sunday, your 6:00 A.M. rating would be 17 ÷ 5, or 3.4 (moderate to high anxiety). Finally, calculate an average weekly stress score by averaging your daily average stress scores. Your weekly average will give you a sense of your overall level of stress.

Identifying Sources of Stress

External stressors: List several people, places, or events that caused you a significant amount of discomfort this week. _____

_____

_____

_____

Internal stressors: List any recurring thoughts or worries that produced feelings of discomfort this week.

_____

_____

_____

_____

CHAPTER 3
Psychological Health

Multiple Choice

1. Which of the following best describes psychological health?
   a. being psychologically normal
   b. having no symptoms of mental disorders
   c. achieving self-actualization
   d. conforming to social demands

2. Self-actualized people are:
   a. critical.
   b. verbal.
   c. realistic.
   d. self-absorbed.

3. Unlike realistic self-talk, positive thinking involves:
   a. substituting a positive thought for a negative one.
   b. making your thoughts as logical and accurate as possible.
   c. acknowledging only one's successes.
   d. developing a lasting positive self-concept.

4. Achieving healthy self-esteem involves all of the following EXCEPT:
   a. developing a positive self-concept.
   b. meeting challenges to self-esteem.
   c. developing defense mechanisms.
   d. learning to deal with anger.

5. An example of negative self-talk is:
   a. I overdid it last night. Next time I'll make different choices.
   b. It may not be the best speech I'll ever give, but it was good enough to earn a grade of "B."
   c. I wonder why my boss wants to see me? I'll just have to wait and see.
   d. I got a bad grade on this paper because I'm incompetent at everything.

6. Shyness is:
   a. social anxiety.
   b. relatively uncommon.
   c. not inherited.
   d. seldom outgrown.

7. A phobia is:
   a. a persistent fear of a specific thing.
   b. a heart attack symptom.
   c. a common response to stress.
   d. a mood disorder.

8. A key symptom of post-traumatic stress disorder is:
   a. reexperiencing a trauma in dreams.
   b. having recurrent, unwanted thoughts.
   c. experiencing sudden surges in anxiety.
   d. hearing voices when no one is present.

9. Which of the following may be symptomatic of depression?
   a. poor appetite
   b. insomnia
   c. restlessness
   d. all of the above

10. Characteristics of schizophrenia include all of the following EXCEPT:
    a. disorganized thoughts.
    b. increased social activity.
    c. delusions.
    d. auditory hallucinations.

True or False

T F 1. Normality is a key component of psychological health.

T F 2. Self-acceptance is a prerequisite for positive psychological health.

T F 3. Developing an adult identity is easier in a culture where many roles are possible.

T F 4. Participating in organized religion, spending time in nature, and volunteering in one's community are all possible paths to spiritual wellness.

T F 5. A pessimistic outlook is typically learned during childhood.

T F 6. Psychologically healthy people always express their anger rather than suppressing it.

T F 7. Fear of public speaking is an example of a social phobia.

T F 8. There is a strong association between severe depression and suicide.

T F 9. Manic behavior is characterized by lethargy.

T F 10. Keeping a journal promotes emotional and physical wellness.

ANSWERS: Multiple Choice: 1. c (p. 42); 2. c (p. 42); 3. a (p. 45); 4. c (pp. 44, 47);
5. d (p. 46); 6. a (p. 48); 7. a (p. 48); 8. a (p. 50); 9. d (p. 50); 10. b (p. 52).
True or False: 1. F (p. 41); 2. T (p. 42); 3. F (p. 44); 4. T (p. 45); 5. T (p. 46);
6. F (p. 47); 7. T (p. 48); 8. T (p. 50); 9. F (p. 51); 10. T (p. 53).

WELLNESS WORKSHEET 3

Recognizing Signs of Mood and Anxiety Disorders

Part I. Depression and Bipolar Disorder

You should get evaluated by a professional if you've had five or more of the following symptoms for more than 2 weeks or if any of these symptoms cause such a big change that you can't keep up your usual routine.

When You're Depressed:

_____ You feel sad or cry a lot, and it doesn't go away.

_____ You feel guilty for no reason; you feel you're no good; you've lost your confidence.

_____ Life seems meaningless, or you think nothing good is ever going to happen again.

_____ You have a negative attitude a lot of the time, or it seems as if you have no feelings.

_____ You don't feel like doing a lot of the things you used to like—music, sports, being with friends, going out, and so on—and you want to be left alone most of the time.

_____ It's hard to make up your mind. You forget lots of things, and it's hard to concentrate.

_____ You get irritated often. Little things make you lose your temper; you overract.

_____ Your sleep pattern changes: You start sleeping a lot more or you have trouble falling asleep at night; or you wake up really early most mornings and can't get back to sleep.

_____ Your eating pattern changes: You've lost your appetite or you eat a lot more.

_____ You feel restless and tired most of the time.

_____ You think about death or feel as if you're dying or have thoughts about committing suicide.

When You're Manic:

_____ You feel high as a kite . . . like you're on top of the world.

_____ You get unrealistic ideas about the great things you can do . . . things that you really can't do.

_____ Thoughts go racing through your head, you jump from one subject to another, and you talk a lot.

_____ You're a nonstop party, constantly running around.

_____ You do too many wild or risky things—with driving, with spending money, with sex, and so on.

_____ You're so "up" that you don't need much sleep.

_____ You're rebellious or irritable and can't get along at home or school or with your friends.

If you are concerned about depression in yourself or a friend, or if you are thinking about hurting or killing yourself, talk to someone about it and get help immediately. There are many sources of help: a good friend; an academic or resident advisor; the staff at the student health or counseling center; a professor, coach, or advisor; a local suicide or emergency hotline (get the phone number from the operator or directory) or the 911 operator; or a hospital emergency room.

Part II. Are You Overly Anxious?

The self-test below was developed to help screen for common anxiety disorders. Answere "yes" or "no" for each question based on your experiences *during the past month*.

Yes   No

Panic disorder

_____   _____   1.   Did you experience a sudden unexplained attack of intense fear, anxiety, or panic for no apparent reason? (If "yes," continue with questions a–c; if "no," go to question 2.)

_____   _____   a.   Were you afraid you might have more of these attacks?

_____   _____   b.   Were you worried that these attacks could mean you were losing control, having a heart attack, or "going crazy"?

_____   _____   c.   Did these attacks cause changes or avoidance patterns in your behavior?

(over)

STUDY GUIDE

Yes	No		
____	____	2.	Have you been afraid of not being able to get help or not being able to escape in certain situations, such as being on a bridge, in a crowded store, or in similar situations?
____	____	3.	Have you been afraid or unable to travel alone?

Generalized anxiety disorder

Yes	No		
____	____	4.	Have you persistently worried about several different things, such as work, school, family, and money?
____	____	5.	Did you find it difficult to control your worrying?
____	____	6.	Did persistent worrying or nervousness cause problems with your work or your dealings with people?

Obsessive-compulsive disorder

Yes	No		
____	____	7.	Did you have persistent, senseless thoughts you could not get out of your head, such as thoughts of death, illnesses, aggression, sexual urges, contamination, or others?
____	____	8.	Did you spend more time than necessary doing things over and over again, such as washing your hands, checking things, or counting things?
____	____	9.	Did you spend more than one hour a day involved in your senseless thoughts or your needless checking, washing, or counting?

Social phobia

Yes	No		
____	____	10.	Were you afraid to do things in front of people, such as public speaking, eating, performing, or teaching?
____	____	11.	Did you avoid or feel very uncomfortable in situations involving people, such as parties, weddings, dating, dances, and other social events?

Post-traumatic stress disorder

Yes	No		
____	____	12.	Have you ever had an extremely frightening, traumatic, or horrible experience—such as being the victim of a violent crime, being seriously injured in a car crash, being sexually assaulted, seeing someone seriously injured or killed, or being the victim of a natural disaster? (If "yes," continue with questions a–e.)
____	____	a.	Did you relive the experience through recurrent dreams, preoccupations, or flashbacks?
____	____	b.	Did you seem less interested in important things, not "with it," or unable to experience or express emotions?
____	____	c.	Did you have problems sleeping, concentrating, or keeping your temper?
____	____	d.	Did you avoid anything that reminded you of the original horrible event?
____	____	e.	Did you have some of the above problems for more than one month?

Consider seeking professional assistance if your daily functioning is impaired or if you are significantly troubled by any of the areas in which you answered "yes."

SOURCES: Part I from National Institute of Mental Health. 1999. *Let's Talk About Depression* (http://www.nimh.nih.gov/publicat/letstalk.cfm; retrieved August 31, 2000). Part II adapted with permission from Freedom from Fear. 1998. *Anxiety Disorders Screening Day Questionnaire.* New York: Freedom from Fear.

CHAPTER 4
Intimate Relationships and Communication

Multiple Choice

1. Our gender role is defined for us by our:
   a. genes.
   b. culture.
   c. decisions.
   d. sexual experiences.

2. All of the following are associated with long-term love relationships EXCEPT:
   a. loyalty.
   b. idealization of the other person.
   c. respect.
   d. interest in the other person.

3. Jealousy:
   a. proves the existence of commitment in a relationship.
   b. is associated with high self-esteem.
   c. is more closely related to insecurity than to love.
   d. secures a relationship by putting strict controls on the partners.

4. The most destructive way of dealing with anger is probably to:
   a. suppress it.
   b. talk about your feelings.
   c. give yourself some space until your anger subsides.
   d. negotiate and explore alternatives.

5. First attraction is usually based on:
   a. easily observable characteristics.
   b. personality traits.
   c. basic values.
   d. future aspirations.

6. The factor that most separates people who cohabit from those who don't is:
   a. age.
   b. ethnicity.
   c. religiousness.
   d. socioeconomic status.

7. The adoption of "best friend" roles in a relationship is a common characteristic of:
   a. long-term marriages.
   b. cohabitating couples.
   c. relationships that have just begun.
   d. gay and lesbian relationships.

8. Which one of the following statements about marriage is TRUE?
   a. About 25% of marriages in the United States end in divorce.
   b. The primary functions and benefits of marriage are very different from other types of personal relationships.
   c. People are marrying at younger ages than in the past.
   d. Today, people tend to marry for personal, emotional reasons rather than for practical or economic reasons.

9. About _____ of all children under 18 live with only one parent.
   a. 4%
   b. 16%
   c. 28%
   d. 42%

10. Which of the following tends to be TRUE about strong families?
   a. They are without problems.
   b. They seek counseling about any difficult problems that arise.
   c. They avoid talking about disagreements.
   d. They know they care for one another without having to show it.

True or False

T F 1. Successful intimate relationships are more likely for people who have high self-esteem.

T F 2. Intimate partnerships tend to last longer and be more stable than friendships.

T F 3. For most people, love sustains a relationship and sex intensifies a relationship.

T F 4. Nonverbal communication is only a small part of the overall communication that occurs between two people.

T F 5. Men and women approach communication and conversation differently.

T F 6. Most young people today find partners through dating.

T F 7. About 50–55% of all American marriages end in divorce.

T F 8. Social stigma is the primary problem for single mothers.

T F 9. Marital satisfaction usually declines after children have left home.

T F 10. Healthy stepfamilies are less cohesive and more adaptable than healthy primary families.

ANSWERS: Multiple Choice: 1. b (p. 60); 2. b (p. 61); 3. c (p. 63); 4. a (p. 65); 5. a (p. 66); 6. c (p. 67); 7. d (p. 67); 8. d (p. 67); 9. c (p. 72); 10. b (p. 73). True or False: 1. T (p. 59); 2. F (p. 61); 3. T (p. 61); 4. F (p. 63); 5. T (pp. 64–65); 6. F (p. 66); 7. T (p. 70); 8. F (p. 72); 9. F (pp. 71–72); 10. T (p. 72).

WELLNESS WORKSHEET 4

Intimate Relationships

Part I. Love Maps Questionnaire

Emotionally intelligent couples have richly detailed "love maps"—they know about each other's history, major goals and beliefs, and day-to-day struggles. To assess the quality of your current love maps, answer each of the following questions with "true" or "false."

T   F   1. I can name my partner's best friends.

T   F   2. I can tell you what stresses my partner is currently facing.

T   F   3. I know the names of some of the people who have been irritating my partner lately.

T   F   4. I can tell you some of my partner's life dreams.

T   F   5. I am very familiar with my partner's religious beliefs and ideas.

T   F   6. I can tell you about my partner's basic philosophy of life.

T   F   7. I can list the relatives my partner likes the least.

T   F   8. I know my partner's favorite music.

T   F   9. I can list my partner's three favorite movies.

T   F   10. My partner is familiar with my current stresses.

T   F   11. I know the three most special times in my partner's life.

T   F   12. I can tell you the most stressful thing that happened to my partner as a child.

T   F   13. I can list my partner's major aspirations and hopes in life.

T   F   14. I know my partner's major current worries.

T   F   15. My partner knows who my friends are.

T   F   16. I know what my partner would want to do if he or she suddenly won the lottery.

T   F   17. I can tell you in detail my first impressions of my partner.

T   F   18. Periodically, I ask my partner about his or her world right now.

T   F   19. I feel that my partner knows me pretty well.

T   F   20. My partner is familiar with my hopes and aspirations.

Scoring: Give yourself one point fror each "true" answer.

10 or above: This is an area of strength in your relationship. You have a fairly detailed map of your partner's everyday life, hopes, fears, and dreams. If you maintain this level of knowledge and understanding of each other, you'll be well equipped to handle any problem areas that crop up in your relationship.

Below 10: Your relationship could stand some improvement in this area. By taking the time to learn more about your partner now, you'll find your relationship becomes stronger.

(over)

Part II. Rate Your Family's Strengths

This Family Strengths Inventory was developed by researchers who studied the strengths of over 3000 families. To assess your family (either the family you grew up in or the family you have formed as an adult), circle the number that best reflects how your family rates on each strength. A number 1 represents the lowest rating and a number 5 represents the highest.

	Low				High
1. Spending time together and doing things with each other	1	2	3	4	5
2. Commitment to each other	1	2	3	4	5
3. Good communication (talking with each other often, listening well, sharing feelings with each other)	1	2	3	4	5
4. Dealing with crises in a positive manner	1	2	3	4	5
5. Expressing appreciation to each other	1	2	3	4	5
6. Spiritual wellness	1	2	3	4	5
7. Closeness of relationship between spouses	1	2	3	4	5
8. Closeness of relationship between parents and children	1	2	3	4	5
9. Happiness of relationship between spouses	1	2	3	4	5
10. Happiness of relationship between parents and children	1	2	3	4	5
11. Extent to which spouses make each other feel good about themselves (self-confident, worthy, competent, and happy)	1	2	3	4	5
12. Extent to which parents help children feel good about themselves	1	2	3	4	5

Scoring: Add the numbers you have circled. A score below 39 indicates below-average family strengths. Scores between 39 and 52 are in the average range. Scores above 53 indicate a strong family. Low scores on individual items identify areas that families can profitably spend time on. High scores are worthy of celebration but shouldn't lead to complacency. Like gardens, families need loving care to remain strong.

What do you think is your family's major strength? What do you like best about your family?

What about your family would you most like to change?

SOURCE: Part I from Gottman, J. M., and N. Silver. 1999. *The Seven Principles for Making Marriage Work.* New York: Three Rivers Press. Used by permission of Crown Publishers, a division of Random House. Part II from Stinnett, N., and J. DeFrain. 1986. *Secrets of Strong Families.* Copyright © 1985 by Nick Stinnett and John Defrain. By permission of Little, Brown and Company.

CHAPTER 5
Sexuality, Pregnancy, and Childbirth

Multiple Choice

1. The male germ cell(s) is (are) the:
   a. sperm.
   b. penis.
   c. testes.
   d. scrotum.

2. Puberty is first marked by:
   a. the development of differentiated genitalia.
   b. achievement of emotional maturity.
   c. an ability to reproduce.
   d. the development of secondary sex characteristics.

3. A strategy for relieving symptoms of premenstrual syndrome is:
   a. limit salt intake to minimize bloating.
   b. use alcohol for muscle relaxation.
   c. avoid exercise to minimize fatigue.
   d. increase intake of red meat to increase levels of iron.

4. The phase of the sexual response cycle unique to men is:
   a. resolution.
   b. plateau.
   c. refractory period.
   d. excitement.

5. If the egg is not fertilized, it lasts about _____ hours and then disintegrates.
   a. 2
   b. 12
   c. 24
   d. 48

6. In which of the following techniques for overcoming infertility are eggs and sperm surgically placed into the oviducts prior to fertilization?
   a. in vitro fertilization
   b. gamete intrafallopian transfer
   c. nuclear transfer
   d. zygote intrafallopian transfer

7. Pregnancy tests seek to detect the presence of:
   a. human chorionic gonadotropin.
   b. prostaglandins.
   c. estrogen.
   d. progesterone.

8. Which method of prenatal testing analyzes hormone levels to determine the probability of fetal abnormalities?
   a. ultrasonography
   b. amniocentesis
   c. chorionic villus sampling
   d. triple screen marker

9. All of the following are characteristic of fetal alcohol syndrome EXCEPT:
   a. unusual facial characteristics.
   b. mental impairments.
   c. heart defects.
   d. spina bifida.

10. During the second stage of labor:
    a. the amniotic sac ruptures.
    b. contractions become more intense during transition.
    c. the baby moves through the birth canal.
    d. the placenta is expelled.

True or False

T F 1. The function of the scrotum is to keep the testes at a lower temperature than the rest of the body.

T F 2. Worldwide, most male infants are circumcised.

T F 3. The final phase of the sexual response cycle is the orgasmic phase.

T F 4. Most forms of sexual dysfunction are treatable.

T F 5. Complications from sexually transmitted diseases are a primary cause of female infertility.

T F 6. Women of normal weight gain an average of 18–25% of their initial weight during pregnancy.

T F 7. The triple marker screen is used to determine the sex of the fetus.

T F 8. Ectopic pregnancy is the leading cause of pregnancy-related death in the United States.

T F 9. Putting babies on their backs to sleep lowers their risk for sudden infant death syndrome (SIDS).

T F 10. About 1 in 10 babies born in the United States is delivered by cesarean section.

ANSWERS: Multiple Choice: 1. a (p. 76); 2. d (p. 79); 3. a (p. 82); 4. c (pp. 83–84); 5. c (p. 88); 6. b (p. 89); 7. a (p. 90); 8. d (p. 93); 9. d (p. 94); 10. c (p. 98).
True or False: 1. T (p. 77); 2. F (p. 78); 3. F (p. 83); 4. T (p. 84); 5. T (p. 89); 6. T (p. 91); 7. F (p. 93); 8. T (p. 96); 9. T (p. 96); 10. F (p. 99).

Name _____ Section _____ Date _____

WELLNESS WORKSHEET 5

Creating a Family Health Tree

Knowing that a specific disease runs in your family allows you to watch closely for the early warning signs and get appropriate screening tests. It can also help you target important health habits to adopt. You can put together a simple family health tree by compiling key facts on your primary relatives; siblings, parents, aunts and uncles, and grandparents. If possible, have your primary relatives fill out a family health history record like the one below.

Family Health History

Name: _____ Ethnicity: _____ Date of birth: _____

Blood and Rh type: _____ Occupation: _____

Please note any serious or chronic diseases you have experienced, with special attention to the following:

_____ Alcoholism

_____ Allergies

_____ Arthritis

_____ Asthma

_____ Blood diseases (hemophilia, sickle-cell disease, thalassemia, hemochromatosis)

_____ Cancer (breast, colon, ovarian, skin, stomach, etc.)

_____ Cystic fibrosis

_____ Diabetes

_____ Epilepsy

_____ Familial high blood cholesterol levels

_____ Hearing defects

_____ Heart defects

_____ Huntington's disease

_____ Hypertension (high blood pressure)

_____ Learning disabilities (dyslexia, attention-deficit/hyperactivity disorder, autism)

_____ Liver disease (particularly hepatitis)

_____ Lupus

_____ Mental illness (bipolar disorder, schizophrenia)

_____ Mental impairment (Down syndrome, fragile X, etc.)

_____ Migraine headaches

_____ Miscarriages or neonatal deaths

_____ Multiple sclerosis

_____ Muscular dystrophy

_____ Myasthenia gravis

_____ Obesity

_____ Phenylketonuria (PKU)

_____ Respiratory disease (emphysema, bacterial pneumonia)

_____ Rh disease

_____ Skin disorders (particularly psoriasis)

_____ Thyroid disorders

_____ Tay-Sachs disease

_____ Tuberculosis

_____ Visual disorders (dyslexia, glaucoma, retinitis pigmentosa)

_____ Other (please list):

(over)

List any important health-related behaviors (including tobacco use, dietary and exercise habits, and alcohol use):

Please note names of your relatives below, along with indications of any illnesses, such as those listed on the previous page, which affected them. If they are deceased, list age and cause. Also make note of their lifestyle habits such as smoking.

Father: _____

_____

_____

Mother:_____

_____

_____

Brothers and sisters:_____

_____

_____

Children of brothers and sisters: _____

_____

_____

If you don't have enough information on past generations, you can get clues by requesting death certificates from state health departments or medical records from relatives' physicians or hospitals where they died. Once you've collected the information you want, plug it into a tree format and look for patterns. In general, the more relatives you have with a particular condition and the closer they are to you, the greater your risk. Nongenetic factors such as health habits also play a role. Signs of a strong hereditary influence include appearance of a disease largely on one side of the family, developing the disease despite good health habits, and early onset of the disease. If you note clear patterns, you may want to discuss your health tree with your physician or a genetic counselor.

SOURCE: Adapted from March of Dimes Birth Defects Foundation. 1992. *Genetic Counseling*. Copyright © 1992 March of Dimes Birth Defects Foundation. Used with permission.

CHAPTER 6
Contraception and Abortion

Multiple Choice

1. Oral contraceptives prevent pregnancy by:
   a. acting as a sperm barrier.
   b. causing spontaneous abortion.
   c. preventing ovulation.
   d. killing sperm.

2. Which of the following methods of contraception is most effective at preventing pregnancy?
   a. male condom
   b. oral contraceptives
   c. intrauterine device
   d. Norplant implants

3. Depo-Provera is administered:
   a. by skin patch.
   b. by injection.
   c. by implantation.
   d. orally.

4. Which of the following does NOT damage latex when used as a lubricant with condoms?
   a. Vaseline
   b. baby oil
   c. K-Y jelly
   d. hand lotion

5. Which of the following methods of contraception provides the most protection against HIV infection?
   a. latex male condom
   b. Depo-Provera injections
   c. diaphragm with spermicide
   d. oral contraceptives

6. Which of the following is NOT an advantage of diaphragm use?
   a. Its use is limited to times of sexual activity.
   b. It has few side effects.
   c. It decreases risk for toxic shock syndrome.
   d. It decreases risk for human papillomavirus infection.

7. The fertility awareness method is NOT recommended for any woman:
   a. for whom pregnancy would be a serious problem.
   b. who has very irregular menstrual cycles.
   c. who needs protection against STDs.
   d. all of the above.

8. The *Roe v. Wade* decision:
   a. made abortion legal during the first trimester of pregnancy but illegal during the second and third trimesters.
   b. made abortion legal during the first two trimesters but gave states the right to regulate certain factors.
   c. gave states the right to regulate abortion as long as they do not impose an undue burden on women seeking the procedure.
   d. required physicians to test a fetus for viability if the fetus is estimated to be 20 weeks or older.

9. Approximately what percentage of abortions that are done after the 12th week of gestation are performed on teenagers?
   a. 5%
   b. 15%
   c. 25%
   d. 35%

10. The abortion method used in about 90% of all U.S. abortions is:
   a. suction curettage.
   b. dilation and evacuation.
   c. manual vacuum aspiration.
   d. mifepristone.

True or False

T F 1. The active ingredients in oral contraceptives are progesterone and testosterone.

T F 2. Pap tests are recommended for women who begin taking oral contraceptives because OCs may temporarily increase a woman's susceptibility to some STDs.

T F 3. Norplant is the most effective reversible contraceptive currently available.

T F 4. Emergency contraception works by inhibiting or delaying ovulation.

T F 5. Spontaneous expulsion of the IUD occurs in about 40% of users.

T F 6. It's okay to keep condoms in a pocket or wallet.

T F 7. The surgical risks associated with female and male sterilization are about equal.

T F 8. The case of *Webster v. Reproductive Health Services* legalized abortion.

T F 9. The number of abortions performed in the United States has increased steadily since the *Roe v. Wade* decision.

T F 10. Medical abortion can be administered up to 49 days after the last menstrual period.

ANSWERS: Multiple Choice: 1. c (p. 104); 2. d (p. 107); 3. b (p. 108); 4. c (p. 110); 5. a (p. 109); 6. c (p. 113); 7. d (p. 116); 8. b (pp. 120–121); 9. d (p. 122); 10. a (p. 123). True or False: 1. F (p. 105); 2. T (p. 106); 3. T (p. 107); 4. T (p. 108); 5. F (p. 109); 6. F (p. 110); 7. F (p. 116); 8. F (p. 121); 9. F (p. 122): 10. T (p. 124).

Name _____ Section _____ Date _____

WELLNESS WORKSHEET 6

Contraception and Abortion

Part I. Which Contraceptive Method Is Right for You and Your Partner?

If you are sexually active, you need to use the contraceptive method that will work best for you. A number of factors may be involved in your decision. The following questions will help you sort out these factors and choose an appropriate method. Answer yes (Y) or no (N) for each statement as it applies to you and, if appropriate, your partner.

Y or N

_____ 1. I like sexual spontaneity and don't want to be bothered with contraception at the time of sexual intercourse.

_____ 2. I need a contraceptive immediately.

_____ 3. It is very important that I do not become pregnant now.

_____ 4. I want a contraceptive method that will protect me and my partner against STDs.

_____ 5. I prefer a contraceptive method that requires the cooperation and involvement of both partners.

_____ 6. I have sexual intercourse frequently.

_____ 7. I have sexual intercourse infrequently.

_____ 8. I am forgetful or have a variable daily routine.

_____ 9. I have more than one sexual partner.

_____ 10. I have heavy periods with cramps.

_____ 11. I prefer a method that requires little or no action or bother on my part.

_____ 12. I am a nursing mother.

_____ 13. I want the option of conceiving immediately after discontinuing contraception.

_____ 14. I want a contraceptive method with few or no side effects.

If you answered "yes" to the numbers of statements listed on the left, the method on the right might be a good choice for you:

1, 3, 6, 10, 11	Oral contraceptives
1, 3, 6, 8, 10, 11	Contraceptive implants
1, 3, 6, 8, 10, 11, 12	Contraceptive injections
1, 3, 6, 8, 11, 12, 13	IUD
2, 4, 5, 7, 8, 9, 12, 13, 14	Condoms (male and female)
5, 7, 12, 13, 14	Diaphragm with spermicide and cervical cap
2, 5, 7, 8, 12, 13, 14	Vaginal spermicides and sponge
5, 7, 13, 14	FAM and withdrawal

Your answers may indicate that more than one method would be appropriate for you. To help narrow your choices, circle the numbers of the statements that are *most* important for you. Before you make a final choice, talk with your partner(s) and your physician. Consider your own lifestyle and preferences as well as characteristics of each method (effectiveness, side effects, costs, and so on). For maximum protection against pregnancy and STDs, you might want to consider combining two methods.

(over)

Insel/Roth, *Core Concepts in Health*, Brief Ninth Edition. © 2002 The McGraw-Hill Companies, Inc.

Part II. Your Position on the Legality and Morality of Abortion

To help define your own position on abortion, answer the following series of questions.

	Agree	Disagree
1. The fertilized egg is a human being from the moment of conception.	_____	_____
2. The rights of the fetus at any stage take precedence over any decision a woman might want to make regarding her pregnancy.	_____	_____
3. The rights of the fetus depend upon its gestational age: further along in the pregnancy, the fetus has more rights.	_____	_____
4. Each individual woman should have final say over decisions regarding her health and body; politicians should not be allowed to decide.	_____	_____
5. In cases of teenagers seeking an abortion, parental consent should be required.	_____	_____
6. In cases of married women seeking an abortion, spousal consent should be required.	_____	_____
7. In cases of late abortion, tests should be done to determine the viability of the fetus.	_____	_____
8. The federal government should provide public funding for abortion to ensure equal access to abortion for all women.	_____	_____
9. The federal government should not allow states to pass their own abortion laws; there should be uniform laws for the entire country.	_____	_____

10. Does a woman's right to choose whether or not to have an abortion depend upon the circumstances surrounding conception or the situation of the mother? In which of the following situations, if any, would you support a woman's right to choose to have an abortion (check where appropriate)?

_____ An abortion is necessary to maintain the woman's life or health.

_____ The pregnancy is a result of rape or incest.

_____ A serious birth defect has been detected in the fetus.

_____ The pregnancy is a result of the failure of a contraceptive method or device.

_____ The pregnancy occurred when no contraceptive method was in use.

_____ A single mother, pregnant for the fifth time, wants an abortion because she feels she cannot support another child.

_____ A pregnant 15-year-old high school student feels having a child would be too great a disruption in her life and keep her from reaching her goals for the future.

_____ A pregnant 19-year-old college student does not want to interrupt her education.

_____ The father of the child has stated he will provide no support and is not interested in helping raise the child.

_____ Parents of two boys wish to terminate the mother's pregnancy because the fetus is male rather than female.

STUDY GUIDE

CHAPTER 7
The Use and Abuse of Psychoactive Drugs

Multiple Choice

1. Which of the following characteristics is commonly associated with addictive behaviors?
    a. strong compulsion
    b. loss of control
    c. escalating use
    d. all of the above

2. Which of the following is most closely associated with physical dependence on a drug?
    a. poor performance at work or school
    b. withdrawal symptoms
    c. escalating use of a drug
    d. expressing a desire to cut down on drug use

3. The method of drug use that significantly increases the user's risk for hepatitis and HIV infection is:
    a. inhalation.
    b. ingestion.
    c. injection.
    d. absorption through the skin.

4. If a person responds to an inert substance as if it were an active drug, he or she is experiencing:
    a. a placebo effect.
    b. state dependence.
    c. synesthesia.
    d. altered states of consciousness.

5. Opioids:
    a. relieve pain.
    b. stimulate activity.
    c. induce alertness.
    d. cause hallucinations.

6. Which of the following is a central nervous system depressant?
    a. alcohol
    b. heroin
    c. marijuana
    d. LSD

7. The most likely physical reaction to amphetamine ingestion is:
    a. sedation.
    b. fatigue.
    c. delirium.
    d. alertness.

8. The most widely used illegal drug in the United States is:
   a. alcohol.
   b. crack cocaine.
   c. heroin.
   d. marijuana.

9. The active ingredient in marijuana is:
   a. ephedrine.
   b. psilocybin.
   c. tetrahydrocannabinol.
   d. benzodiazepine.

10. Significant physical withdrawal symptoms can occur in users of all of the following EXCEPT:
    a. amphetamines.
    b. alcohol.
    c. caffeine.
    d. LSD.

True or False

T F   1. Addictive behaviors are associated exclusively with psychoactive drugs.

T F   2. Two symptoms of drug dependence are tolerance and withdrawal.

T F   3. Access to drugs increases most dramatically in high school.

T F   4. Heroin and other injectable drugs are responsible for many cases of HIV infection in the United States.

T F   5. Cocaine is a central nervous system stimulant.

T F   6. Ephedrine is a safe, natural stimulant.

T F   7. Substances in marijuana have some potential medical uses.

T F   8. Inhalants are present in many legal, seemingly harmless products.

T F   9. People whose jobs do not involve hazards cannot legally be tested for drugs.

T F 10. Drug substitution treatment programs are losing favor because of their relatively high cost.

ANSWERS: Multiple Choice: 1. d (p. 131); 2. b (p. 134); 3. c (p. 136); 4. a (p. 138);
5. a (p. 139); 6. a (p. 140); 7. d (p. 142); 8. d (p. 143); 9. c (p. 143); 10. d (p. 144).
True or False: 1. F (p. 130); 2. T (p. 134); 3. F (p. 135); 4. T (p. 136); 5. T (p. 140);
6. F (p. 142); 7. T (p. 144); 8. T (p. 145); 9. F (p. 147); 10. F (p. 147).

Name _____ Section _____ Date _____

WELLNESS WORKSHEET 7
Addictive Behaviors

Part I. General Addictive Behavior Checklist
Choose an activity or a behavior in your life that you feel may be developing into an addiction. Ask yourself the following questions about it, and answer yes (Y) or no (N).

Activity/behavior: _____

_____ 1. Do you engage in the activity on a regular basis?

_____ 2. Have you engaged in the activity over a long period of time?

_____ 3. Do you currently engage in this activity more than you used to?

_____ 4. Do you find it difficult to stop or to avoid the activity?

_____ 5. Have you tried and failed to cut down on the amount of time you spend on the activity?

_____ 6. Do you turn down or skip social/recreational events in order to engage in the activity?

_____ 7. Does your participation in the activity interfere with your attendance and/or performance at school and/or work?

_____ 8. Have friends or family members spoken to you about the activity and indicated they think you have a problem?

_____ 9. Has your participation in the activity affected your reputation?

_____ 10. Have you lied to friends or family members about the amount of time, money, and other resources that you put into the activity?

_____ 11. Do you feel guilty about the resources that you put into the activity?

_____ 12. Do you engage in the activity when you are worried, frustrated, or stressed or when you have other painful feelings?

_____ 13. Do you feel better when you engage in the activity?

_____ 14. Do you often spend more time engaged in the activity than you plan to?

_____ 15. Do you have a strong urge to participate in the activity when you are away from it?

_____ 16. Do you spend a lot of time planning for your next opportunities to engage in the activity?

_____ 17. Are you often irritable and restless when you are away from the activity?

_____ 18. Do you use the activity as a reward for all other accomplishments?

(over)

Insel/Roth, *Core Concepts in Health*, Brief Ninth Edition. © 2002 The McGraw-Hill Companies, Inc.

Part II. Checklist for Drug Dependency

If you wonder whether you are becoming dependent on a drug, ask yourself the following questions. Answer yes (Y) or no (N).

_____ 1. Do you take the drug regularly?

_____ 2. Have you been taking the drug for a long time?

_____ 3. Do you always take the drug in certain situations or when you're with certain people?

_____ 4. Do you find it difficult to stop using the drug? Do you feel powerless to quit?

_____ 5. Have you tried repeatedly to cut down or control your use of the drug?

_____ 6. Do you need to take a larger dose of the drug in order to get the same high you're used to?

_____ 7. Do you feel specific symptoms if you cut back or stop using the drug?

_____ 8. Do you frequently take another psychoactive substance to relieve withdrawal symptoms?

_____ 9. Do you take the drug to feel "normal"?

_____ 10. Do you go to extreme lengths or put yourself in dangerous situations to get the drug?

_____ 11. Do you hide your drug use from others? Have you ever lied about what you're using or how much you use?

_____ 12. Do people close to you ask you about your drug use?

_____ 13. Are you spending more and more time with people who use the same drug as you?

_____ 14. Do you think about the drug when you're not high, figuring out ways to get it?

_____ 15. If you stop taking the drug, do you feel bad until you can take it again?

_____ 16. Does the drug interfere with your ability to study, work, or socialize?

_____ 17. Do you skip important school, work, social, or recreational activities in order to obtain or use the drug?

_____ 18. Do you continue to use the drug despite a physical or mental disorder or despite a significant problem that you know is worsened by drug use?

_____ 19. Have you developed a mental or physical condition or disorder because of prolonged drug use?

_____ 20. Have you done something dangerous or that you regret while under the influence of the drug?

Evaluation

On each of these checklists, the more times you answer yes, the more likely it is that you are developing an addiction. If your answers suggest abuse or dependency, talk to someone at your school health clinic or to your physician about taking care of the problem before it gets worse.

STUDY GUIDE

CHAPTER 8
Alcohol and Tobacco

Multiple Choice

1. If a beverage is 100 proof, it contains _____ alcohol.
   a. 10%
   b. 25%
   c. 50%
   d. 100%

2. Which of the following is NOT a symptom of flushing syndrome?
   a. increased heart rate
   b. headache
   c. hives
   d. disorientation

3. Women generally have higher BACs than men after consuming the same amount of alcohol because they:
   a. drink more.
   b. are less experienced drinkers.
   c. have a higher percentage of body fat.
   d. don't eat when they drink.

4. The "holiday heart" syndrome is caused by:
   a. long-term alcohol use.
   b. binge drinking.
   c. alcohol combined with marijuana.
   d. alcohol withdrawal.

5. Which of the following statements comparing college students who binge drink with non–binge drinkers is FALSE?
   a. Binge drinkers are more likely to drink and drive.
   b. Binge drinkers are more likely to consider themselves problem drinkers.
   c. Binge drinkers are more likely to engage in unplanned, unprotected sex.
   d. Binge drinkers are less likely to keep up with their schoolwork.

6. The addictive drug in cigarettes is:
   a. benzo(a)pyrene.
   b. formaldehyde.
   c. tar.
   d. nicotine.

7. The immediate effects of smoking a cigarette include which of the following?
   a. increased blood pressure
   b. improved sense of taste
   c. decreased heart rate
   d. increased appetite

8. The most widespread cause of death among cigarette smokers is:
   a. coronary heart disease.
   b. lung cancer.
   c. pancreatic cancer.
   d. emphysema.

9. Smoking causes a condition called _____, in which air sacs in the lungs are gradually destroyed.
   a. asthma
   b. aortic aneurysm
   c. chronic bronchitis
   d. emphysema

10. Compared to cigarettes, cigar smoke contains up to 30 times more of which ingredient?
    a. nicotine
    b. benzo(a)pyrene
    c. carbon monoxide
    d. ammonia

True or False

T F   1. Alcohol is the leading cause of death among people between 15 and 24.

T F   2. The rate of alcohol metabolism cannot be accelerated.

T F   3. People can usually drive safely with a BAC of up to 0.20%.

T F   4. The consumption of alcohol in any amount has beneficial effects on the cardiovascular system.

T F   5. Children with fetal alcohol syndrome are born impaired, but they usually catch up with their peers both physically and mentally by age 5.

T F   6. Most alcoholics need professional help to stop drinking.

T F   7. About a dozen chemicals in tobacco smoke are linked to the development of cancer.

T F   8. Due to increased rates of smoking among women, lung cancer has surpassed breast cancer as the leading cause of cancer death among women.

T F   9. Spit tobacco products deliver a dose of nicotine comparable to that provided by cigarettes.

T F   10. Clove cigarettes are a safe alternative to regular cigarettes.

ANSWERS: Multiple Choice: 1. c (p. 154); 2. d (p. 156); 3. c (p. 156); 4. b (p. 160); 5. b (p. 162); 6. d (p. 167); 7. a (p. 167); 8. a (p. 170); 9. d (p. 171); 10. c (p. 173). True or False: 1. T (p. 154); 2. T (p. 156); 3. F (p. 156, table 8-1); 4. F (p. 160); 5. F (p. 161); 6. T (p. 165); 7. F (p. 169); 8. T (p. 171); 9. T (p. 173); 10. F (p. 173).

Name _____ Section _____ Date _____

WELLNESS WORKSHEET 8

Alcohol and Tobacco

Part I. Do You Have a Problem with Alcohol?

To determine if you may have a drinking problem, complete the following two screening tests.

A. CAGE Screening Test

Answer yes or no to the following questions:

Have you ever felt you should ..... Cut down on your drinking?
Have people .... Annoyed you by criticizing your drinking?
Have you ever felt bad or .... Guilty about your drinking?
Have you ever had an .... Eye-opener (a drink first thing in the morning to steady
your nerves or get rid of a hangover)?

One "yes" response suggests a possible alcohol problem. If you answered yes to more than one question, it is highly likely that a problem exists. In either case, it is important that you see your physician or other health care provider right away to discuss your responses to these questions.

B. AUDIT Screening Test

For each question, choose the answer that best describes your behavior. Then total your scores.

Questions	Points					Your Score
	0	1	2	3	4	
1. How often do you have a drink containing alcohol?	Never	Monthly or less	2–4 times a month	2–3 times a week	4 or more times a week	_____
2. How many drinks containing alcohol do you have on a typical day when you are drinking?	1 or 2	3 or 4	5 or 6	7 to 9	10 or more	_____
3. How often do you have six or more drinks on one occasion?	Never	Less than monthly	Monthly	Weekly	Daily or almost daily	_____
4. How often during the last year have you found that you were not able to stop drinking once you had started?	Never	Less than monthly	Monthly	Weekly	Daily or almost daily	_____
5. How often during the last year have you failed to do what was normally expected because of drinking?	Never	Less than monthly	Monthly	Weekly	Daily or almost daily	_____
6. How often during the last year have you needed a first drink in the morning to get yourself going after a heavy drinking session?	Never	Less than monthly	Monthly	Weekly	Daily or almost daily	_____
7. How often during the last year have you had a feeling of guilt or remorse after drinking?	Never	Less than monthly	Monthly	Weekly	Daily or almost daily	_____
8. How often during the last year have you been unable to remember what happened the night before because you had been drinking?	Never	Less than monthly	Monthly	Weekly	Daily or almost daily	_____
9. Have you or has someone else been injured as a result of your drinking?	No	Yes, but not in the last year (2 points)		Yes, during the last year (4 points)		_____
10. Has a relative, friend, doctor, or other health worker been concerned about your drinking or suggested you cut down?	No	Yes, but not in the last year (2 points)		Yes, during the last year (4 points)		_____

Total _____

A total score of 8 or more indicates a strong likelihood of hazardous or harmful alcohol consumption.

Even if you answered no to all four items in the CAGE screening test and scored below 8 on the AUDIT screening test, if you are encountering drinking-related problems with your academic performance, job, relationships, or health, or with the law, you should consider seeking help.

(over)

Part II. Nicotine Dependence: Are You Hooked?

Answer each question in the list below, giving yourself the appropriate points.

_____ 1. How soon after yhou wake up do you have your first cigarette?

    a. within 5 minutes (3)

    b. 6–30 minutes (2)

    c. 31–60 minutes (1)

    d. After 60 minutes (0)

_____ 2. Do you find it difficult to refrain from smoking in places where it is forbidden, such as the library, a theater, or a doctor's office?

    a. yes (1)

    b. no (0)

_____ 3. Which cigarette would you most hate to give up?

    a. the first one in the morning (1)

    b. any other (0)

_____ 4. How many cigarettes a day do you smoke?

    a. 10 or less (0)

    b. 11–20 (1)

    c. 21–30 (2)

    d. 31 or more (3)

_____ 5. Do you smoke more frequently during the first hours after waking than during the rest of the day?

    a. yes (1)

    b. no (0)

_____ 6. Do you smoke if you are so ill that you are in bed most of the day?

    a. yes (1)

    b. no (o)

_____ TOTAL

A total score of 7 or greater indicates that you are very dependent on nicotine and are likely to experience withdrawal symptoms when you stop smoking. A score of 6 or less indicates low to moderate dependence.

SOURCES: CAGE test: National Institute on Alcohol Abuse and Alcoholism. 1996. *Alcoholism: Getting the Facts*. NIH Publication No. 96-4153. AUDIT test: Saunders, J. B., et al. 1993. Development of the Alcohol Use Disorders Identification Test (AUDIT): WHO collaborative project on early detection of persons with harmful alcohol consumption—II. *Addiction*. 88: 791–804, June. Reprinted with permission from Carfax Publishing, a division of Taylor & Francis Ltd. http://www.tandf.co.uk. Nicotine dependence test: Heatherton, T. F., et al. 1991. The Fagerstrom Test for Nicotine Dependence: A revision of the Fagerstrom Tolerance Questionnaire. *British Journal of Addictions* 86(9): 1119–1127.

CHAPTER 9
Nutrition Basics

Multiple Choice

1. On average, adults need to consume about ____ calories per day.
   a. 1200
   b. 1500
   c. 2000
   d. 2500

2. The building blocks of protein are called:
   a. soluble fiber.
   b. complex carbohydrates.
   c. amino acids.
   d. fatty acids.

3. If you consume more protein than you need, the excess will be:
   a. excreted in urine.
   b. expired during respiration.
   c. stored as fat.
   d. stored as muscle.

4. Which of the following contains trans fat?
   a. partially hydrogenated oil
   b. olive oil
   c. safflower oil
   d. fish oil

5. A good source of omega-3 fatty acids is:
   a. bread.
   b. rice.
   c. vegetables.
   d. fish.

6. Health experts recommend that we reduce our fat intake to _____ of total calories.
   a. 10% or less
   b. 30% or less
   c. 50% or less
   d. 70% or less

7. Increasing intake of which of the following would be a beneficial dietary change for most Americans?
   a. refined carbohydrates
   b. protein
   c. vitamin supplements
   d. dietary fiber

(over)

8. For which food group in the Food Guide Pyramid is the largest number of daily servings recommended?
   a. bread, cereals, rice, and pasta
   b. vegetables
   c. fruit
   d. milk, yogurt, and cheese

9. How many daily servings of vegetables are recommended by the Food Guide Pyramid?
   a. 1–2
   b. 2–3
   c. 3–5
   d. 6–11

10. For dietary supplements, which of the following is regulated by the FDA?
    a. potency
    b. effectiveness
    c. purity
    d. labels on packaging

True or False

T F 1. A gram of carbohydrate supplies more calories than a gram of fat.

T F 2. Meat and fish are examples of incomplete proteins.

T F 3. When unsaturated oils are hydrogenated, trans fatty acids are produced.

T F 4. Hydrogenation is a process that makes fats healthy for consumption.

T F 5. A high-fiber diet can help manage diabetes.

T F 6. Vitamins are needed by the body to initiate or regulate chemical reactions.

T F 7. Free radicals prevent the damage caused to the body by antioxidants.

T F 8. One serving of meat or chicken (3 ounces) is about the same size as a small paperback book.

T F 9. The recommended daily limit for sodium consumption is equivalent to 1 tablespoon of salt.

T F 10. Women need to consume nutrient-dense foods because they have higher calorie needs than men.

ANSWERS: Multiple Choice: 1. c (p. 184); 2. c (p. 185); 3. c (p. 185); 4. a (p. 186); 5. d (p. 186); 6. b (p. 187); 7. d (p. 190); 8. a (p. 196); 9. c (p. 197); 10. d (p. 206). True or False: 1. F (p. 184); 2. F (p. 185); 3. T (p. 186); 4. F (p. 186); 5. T (p. 190); 6. T (p. 190); 7. F (p. 192); 8. F (p. 197); 9. F (p. 200); 10. F (p. 202).

Name _____ Section _____ Date _____

WELLNESS WORKSHEET 9

Your Daily Diet Versus the Food Guide Pyramid

1. **Keep a food record:** Keep a record of everything you eat on a typical day.

2. **Compare your servings to the Food Guide Pyramid.** Complete the chart below using your food record. Your portion sizes may have been smaller or larger than the serving sizes given in the Pyramid; be sure to translate your intake into actual Pyramid servings as you complete the chart. For example, if you consumed 1½ cups of spaghetti, you would count it as three servings from the grain group. To determine the recommended number of servings for your calorie intake, refer to the following table.

Food Guide Pyramid Recommendations: Number of Servings at Three Calorie Levels

	1600 calories per day (sedentary women, older adults)	2200 calories per day (children, teenage girls, active women, sedentary men)	2800 calories per day (teenage boys, active men, very active women)
Grain group (servings)	6	9	11
Vegetable group (servings)	3	4	5
Fruit group (servings)	2	3	4
Dairy group (servings)[a]	2–3	2–3	2–3
Meat group (ounces)[b]	5	6	7

[a] Women who are pregnant or lactating, teenagers, and young adults to age 24 need 3 servings.
[b] The Pyramid recommends 2–3 servings per day, the equivalent of 5–7 ounces of cooked lean meat, poultry, or fish.

Food Group	Pyramid Serving Sizes	Recommended Servings	Actual Servings
Bread, Cereal, Rice, and Pasta	• 1 slice bread • 1 oz ready-to-eat cereal • ½ cup cooked cereal, rice, or pasta		
Vegetable	• 1 cup raw leafy vegetables • ½ cup other cooked or raw vegetables • ¾ cup vegetable juice		
Fruit	• 1 medium apple, banana, or orange • ½ cup fresh, chopped, cooked, or canned fruit • ¾ cup fruit juice		
Milk, Yogurt, and Cheese	• 1 cup milk or yogurt • 1½ oz natural cheese • 2 oz processed cheese		
Meat, Poultry, Fish, Dry Beans, Eggs, and Nuts	• 2–3 oz cooked lean meat, poultry, or fish • 1 oz meat = ½ cup cooked dry beans, 1 egg, 2 tablespoons peanut butter, or ⅓ cup nuts		

Below, list the foods you consumed that don't fit into the major food groups (fats such as mayonnaise, butter, margarine, salad dressings, and sour cream; added sugars such as candy, jam, and regular soda; and alcoholic beverages).

_____   _____   _____

_____   _____   _____

_____   _____   _____

(over)

STUDY GUIDE

3. **Evaluate your food choices within the groups:** Some choices within each food group are particularly healthy, while others should be eaten only in moderation. To further evaluate your current diet, indicate the number of servings you consumed of the following foods.

Foods to emphasize:
____ whole grains
____ dark-green leafy vegetables
____ orange fruits and vegetables
____ legumes
____ citrus, melon, berries
____ cruciferous vegetables
____ low-fat or nonfat dairy products
____ fish (baked, broiled, or steamed)

Food to limit:
____ processed, sweetened grains
____ high-fat meats, poultry skin
____ deep-fried foods
____ full-fat dairy products
____ regular soda, sweetened tea, fruit drink/punch
____ foods from the Pyramid tip (fats, added sugars)
____ alcoholic beverages

4. **Make healthy changes:** Bring your diet in line with the Pyramid by adding servings of food groups for which you fall short of the recommendations. To maintain a healthy weight, you may need to balance these additions with reductions in other areas—by eliminating some of the fats, oils, sweets, and alcohol you consume, by cutting extra servings from food groups for which your intake is more than adequate; or by making healthier choices within the foods groups. Make a list of foods to add and a list of foods to limit or eliminate:

Foods to add:

_____

_____

_____

_____

Foods to limit or eliminate:

_____

_____

_____

_____

CHAPTER 10
Exercise for Health and Fitness

Multiple Choice

1. Which of the following is NOT an element of health-related fitness?
    a. body composition
    b. muscular strength
    c. cardiorespiratory endurance
    d. speed

2. Flexibility is best described as:
    a. the ability to move without pain during exercise.
    b. the ability to move the joints through their full range of motion.
    c. sustained motion without resistance.
    d. the ability to move rapidly during exercise.

3. Healthy body composition is characterized by a:
    a. high proportion of fat tissue and a low proportion of fat-free mass.
    b. low proportion of fat tissue and a low proportion of fat-free mass.
    c. low proportion of fat tissue and a high proportion of fat-free mass.
    d. high proportion of fat tissue and a high proportion of fat-free mass.

4. Regular exercise does all the following EXCEPT:
    a. raises metabolic rate
    b. decreases levels of high-density lipoproteins
    c. builds bone density
    d. protects cells from free radicals

5. Which of the following is LEAST beneficial for developing cardiorespiratory endurance?
    a. jogging
    b. cycling
    c. weight lifting
    d. swimming

6. Cardiorespiratory endurance exercise intensity is measured according to the:
    a. duration of a workout.
    b. heart rate.
    c. distance traveled.
    d. number of exercise sessions per week.

7. In order to improve cardiorespiratory endurance, a person should perform a minimum of _____ minutes of continuous or intermittent aerobic activity, 3–5 days per week.
    a. 10
    b. 20
    c. 45
    d. 60

8. Muscular strength and endurance are developed best by activities that:
   a. involve continuous rhythmic movements of large-muscle groups.
   b. gently extend joints beyond their normal range of motion.
   c. involve working with weights or against another type of resistance.
   d. decrease body fat.

9. Which kind of stretching achieves the greatest range of motion?
   a. static
   b. ballistic
   c. active
   d. passive

10. Which strategy will contribute to the success of your fitness program?
    a. Be sure to have water or commercial sports drinks on hand.
    b. Buy one pair of shoes that you can use for all of your fitness activities.
    c. If joining a health club, sign a long-term contract.
    d. Add protein supplements to your diet.

True or False

T F   1. Approximately 25% of Americans are not regularly active.

T F   2. Exercise increases the efficiency of the body's metabolism.

T F   3. Weight-bearing exercise can help prevent osteoporosis.

T F   4. Regular exercise can improve mood, lessen depression, and boost creativity.

T F   5. To improve cardiorespiratory endurance, it is best to exercise at your maximum heart rate.

T F   6. Isometric exercise involves applying muscular force with movement.

T F   7. In a weight training program, use of a light weight and a high number of repetitions develops endurance more than strength.

T F   8. Most women develop large, bulky muscles from a regular, moderate program of resistance exercise.

T F   9. Ballistic stretching develops a high degree of flexibility with little risk of injury.

T F 10. The proper treatment for a strained muscle includes resting the affected area, applying ice until the swelling subsides, compressing the area with an elastic bandage, and elevating the affected body part.

ANSWERS: Multiple Choice: 1. d (p. 217); 2. b (p. 218); 3. c (p. 218); 4. b (p. 219);
5. c (p. 223); 6. b (p. 223); 7. b (p. 224); 8. c (p. 225); 9. d (p. 228); 10. a (p. 229).
True or False: 1. F (p. 217); 2. T (p. 218); 3. T (p. 219); 4. T (p. 220); 5. F (p. 223);
6. F (p. 225); 7. T (p. 226); 8. F (p. 227); 9. F (p. 228); 10. T (p. 231).

Name _____ Section _____ Date _____

WELLNESS WORKSHEET 10

Assessing and Developing Physical Fitness

Once you've decided whether you should obtain medical clearance before making a change in your exercise program, the next step is to assess your current level of physical fitness. The test presented here will allow you to make a relatively simple assessment of cardiorespiratory endurance.

Part I. Assessing Cardiorespiratory Endurance

1.5-Mile Run-Walk Test

Don't attempt this test unless you have completed at least 6 weeks of some type of conditioning activity. You may want to practice pacing yourself prior to taking the test to avoid going too fast at the start and becoming fatigued before you finish. Allow yourself a day or two to recover from your practice run before taking the test. Before beginning this test, warm up with some walking, easy jogging, and stretching exercises.

1. Ask someone with a stopwatch, clock, or watch with a second hand to time you.

2. Take the test on a running track or course that is flat and provides measurements of up to 1.5 miles. Cover the distance as fast as possible, at a pace that is comfortable for you. You can run or walk the entire distance or use some combination of running and walking.

3. Note the time it takes you to complete the 1.5-mile distance.

    Your time: ____ : ____ (minutes:seconds)

4. Cool down by walking or jogging slowly for about 5 minutes.

5. Determine the rating for your score by consulting the table below. If you are unable to complete the entire 1.5 miles, consider yourself very poor in CRE.

Standards for the 1.5-Mile Run-Walk Test (minutes:seconds)

Women	Superior	Excellent	Good	Fair	Poor	Very Poor
Age: 18–29	11:00 or less	11:15–12:45	13:00–14:15	14:30–15:45	16:00–17:30	17:45 or more
30–39	11:45 or less	12:00–13:30	13:45–15:15	15:30–16:30	16:45–18:45	19:00 or more
40–49	12:45 or less	13:00–14:30	14:45–16:30	16:45–18:30	18:45–20:45	21:00 or more
50–59	14:15 or less	14:30–16:30	16:45–18:30	18:45–20:30	20:45–23:00	23:15 or more
60 and over	14:00 or less	14:15–17:15	17:30–20:15	20:30–22:45	23:00–24:45	25:00 or more

Men						
Age: 18–29	9:15 or less	9:30–10:30	10:45–11:45	12:00–12:45	13:00–14:00	14:15 or more
30–39	9:45 or less	10:00–11:00	11:15–12:15	12:30–13:30	13:45–14:45	15:00 or more
40–49	10:00 or less	10:15–11:45	12:00–13:00	13:15–14:15	14:30–16:00	16:25 or more
50–59	10:45 or less	11:00–12:45	13:00–14:15	14:30–15:45	16:00–17:45	18:00 or more
60 and over	11:15 or less	11:30–13:45	14:00–15:45	16:00–17:45	18:00–20:45	21:00 or more

SOURCES: Formula for maximal oxygen consumption taken from McArdle, W. D., F. I. Katch, and V. L. Katch. 1991. *Exercise Physiology: Energy, Nutrition, and Human Performance.* Philadelphia: Lea & Febiger, pp. 225–226. Ratings based on norms from the Cooper Institute for Aerobics Research, Dallas, Texas, *The Physical Fitness Specialist Manual,* revised 1993. Used with permission.

(over)

STUDY GUIDE

Part II. Personal Fitness Program Plan and Contract

A. I, _____, am contracting with myself to follow a physical fitness
(name)

program to work toward the following goals:

1. _____

2. _____

3. _____

B. My program plan is as follows:

Activities	Components (Check ✔)					Intensity	Duration	Frequency (Check ✔)						
	CRE	MS	ME	F	BC			M	Tu	W	Th	F	Sa	Su

C. My program will begin on _____. My program includes the following schedule of
(date)

   minigoals. For each step in my program, I will give myself the reward listed.

_____   _____   _____
(minigoal 1)   (date)   (reward)

_____   _____   _____
(minigoal 2)   (date)   (reward)

_____   _____   _____
(minigoal 3)   (date)   (reward)

D. I will use the following tools to monitor my program and my progress toward my goals:

_____
(list any charts, graphs, or journals you plan to use)

_____

I sign this contract as an indication of my personal commitment to reach my goal.

_____   _____
(your signature)   (date)

I have recruited a helper who will witness my contract and _____

_____
(list any way your helper will participate in your program)

_____   _____
(witness's signature)   (date)

CHAPTER 11
Weight Management

Multiple Choice

1. The most important factor in assessing a person's body composition is:
   a. total body weight.
   b. body weight relative to age.
   c. proportion of body weight that is fat.
   d. body weight relative to height.

2. Which of the following elements in the energy-balance equation is under an individual's control?
   a. energy for food digestion
   b. energy for resting metabolism
   c. energy for basic body functions
   d. energy intake from food

3. People are at greater risk for coronary heart disease if they tend to gain weight in the:
   a. thighs.
   b. hips.
   c. abdomen.
   d. buttocks.

4. Body image is determined by:
   a. one's own thinking.
   b. hydrostatic weighing.
   c. height-weight charts.
   d. calculation of body mass index.

5. Resting metabolic rate is:
   a. the energy required to maintain basic body functions.
   b. the sum of all the processes by which food energy is used by the body.
   c. the body's total daily energy expenditure.
   d. the energy required to digest food.

6. If you were trying to control your weight, you should increase your consumption of which of the following?
   a. protein
   b. complex carbohydrates
   c. sugar
   d. fat

7. Strength training can assist with weight loss because it:
   a. can target specific areas of the body where you want to lose fat.
   b. reduces appetite.
   c. burns more calories than cardiorespiratory exercise.
   d. increases fat-free mass, which raises the metabolic rate.

8. All of the following are good strategies for managing weight EXCEPT:
   a. measuring portion sizes with a food scale.
   b. eating more quickly.
   c. planning your meals and snacks.
   d. serving food in small bowls or plates.

9. Weight loss usually declines after the first phase of a diet because:
   a. dieters generally start cheating after a few weeks.
   b. metabolism starts to slow to compensate for weight changes.
   c. most weight loss at the beginning is due to loss of body water.
   d. most diets do not account for underlying problems, such as food combining or allergies.

10. Bulimia nervosa is characterized by:
    a. refusal to eat enough food to maintain normal, healthy body weight.
    b. high fat intake and low level of physical activity.
    c. alternating binging and purging.
    d. normal food consumption interrupted by episodes of binge eating.

True or False

T F 1. The range for healthy percent body fat is lower for women than for men.

T F 2. Obesity is a risk factor for cancer.

T F 3. Height-weight charts directly measure body fat.

T F 4. Excess body fat is a major risk factor for diabetes mellitus.

T F 5. Fat stored in the hips is less of a health risk than fat stored in the abdomen.

T F 6. Regular exercise reduces resting metabolic rate.

T F 7. Obesity is more common among men of high socioeconomic status.

T F 8. To maintain weight loss, a person must maintain the behaviors that helped him or her lose the weight in the first place.

T F 9. Prescription drugs for weight loss are a good choice for people who need to lose less than 15 pounds.

T F 10. For an obese person, losing small amounts of weight can significantly improve physical and emotional health.

ANSWERS: Multiple Choice: 1. c (p. 237); 2. d (p. 238); 3. c (p. 241); 4. a (pp. 241–242);
5. a (p. 242); 6. b (p. 245); 7. d (p. 246); 8. b (p. 248); 9. c (p. 247); 10. c (p. 253).
True or False: 1. F (pp. 236–237); 2. T (p. 240); 3. F (p. 238); 4. T (p. 240); 5. T (p. 241); 6. F
(p. 243); 7. T (p. 244); 8. T (p. 244); 9. F (p. 251); 10. T (p. 252).

Name _____ Section _____ Date _____

WELLNESS WORKSHEET 11

What Triggers Your Eating?

This test is designed to provide you with a score for five factors that describe many people's eating. This information will put you in a better position to manage your eating behavior and control your weight. Circle the number that indicates to what degree each situation is likely to make you start eating.

Social

	Very Unlikely								**Very Likely**
1. Arguing or having a conflict with someone	1	2	3	4	5	6	7	8	9	10
2. Being with others when they are eating	1	2	3	4	5	6	7	8	9	10
3. Being urged to eat by someone else	1	2	3	4	5	6	7	8	9	10
4. Feeling inadequate around others	1	2	3	4	5	6	7	8	9	10

Emotional

5. Feeling bad, such as being anxious or depressed	1	2	3	4	5	6	7	8	9	10
6. Feeling good, happy, or relaxed	1	2	3	4	5	6	7	8	9	10
7. Feeling bored or having time on my hands	1	2	3	4	5	6	7	8	9	10
8. Feeling stressed or excited	1	2	3	4	5	6	7	8	9	10

Situational

9. Seeing an advertisement for food or eating	1	2	3	4	5	6	7	8	9	10
10. Passing by a bakery, cookie shop, or other enticement to eat	1	2	3	4	5	6	7	8	9	10
11. Being involved in a party, celebration, or special occasion	1	2	3	4	5	6	7	8	9	10
12. Eating out	1	2	3	4	5	6	7	8	9	10

Thinking

13. Making excuses to myself about why it's OK to eat	1	2	3	4	5	6	7	8	9	10
14. Berating myself for being so fat or unable to control my eating	1	2	3	4	5	6	7	8	9	10
15. Worrying about others or about difficulties I am having	1	2	3	4	5	6	7	8	9	10
16. Thinking about how things should or shouldn't be	1	2	3	4	5	6	7	8	9	10

Physiological

17. Experiencing pain or physical discomfort	1	2	3	4	5	6	7	8	9	10
18. Experiencing trembling, headache, or light-headedness associated with not eating or having too much caffeine	1	2	3	4	5	6	7	8	9	10
19. Experiencing fatigue or feeling overtired	1	2	3	4	5	6	7	8	9	10
20. Experiencing hunger pangs or urges to eat, even though I've eaten recently	1	2	3	4	5	6	7	8	9	10

(over)

Insel/Roth, *Core Concepts in Health,* Brief Ninth Edition. © 2002 The McGraw-Hill Companies, Inc.

STUDY GUIDE

Scoring

Total your scores for each category, and enter them below. Then rank the scores by marking the highest score 1, next highest score 2, and so on. Focus on the highest ranked categories first, but any score above 24 is high and indicates that you need to work on that category.

Category	Total Score	Rank Order
Social (Items 1–4)	_____	_____
Emotional (Items 5–8)	_____	_____
Situational (Items 9–12)	_____	_____
Thinking (Items 13–16)	_____	_____
Physiological (Items 17–20)	_____	_____

What Your Score Means

Social A high score here means you are very susceptible to the influence of others. Work on better ways to communicate more assertively, handle conflict, and manage anger. Challenge your beliefs about the need to be polite and the obligations you feel you must fulfill.

Emotional A high score here means you need to develop effective ways to cope with emotions. Work on developing skills in stress management, time management, and communication. Practicing positive but realistic self-talk can help you handle small daily upsets.

Situational A high score here means you are especially susceptible to external influences. Try to avoid external cues to eat and respond differently to those you cannot avoid. Control your environment by changing the way you buy, store, cook, and serve food. Anticipate potential problems, and have a plan for handling them.

Thinking A high score here means that the way you think—how you talk to yourself, the beliefs you hold, your memories, and your expectations—have a powerful influence on your eating habits. Try to be less self-critical, less perfectionistic, and more flexible in your ideas about the way things ought to be. Recognize when you're making excuses or rationalizations that allow you to eat.

Physiological A high score here means that the way you eat, what you eat, or medications you are taking may be affecting your eating behavior. You may be eating to reduce physical arousal or deal with physical discomfort. Try eating three meals a day, supplemented with regular snacks if needed. Avoid too much caffeine. If any medication you're taking produces adverse physical reactions, switch to an alternative, if possible. If your medications may be affecting your hormone levels, discuss possible alternatives with your physician.

SOURCE: Adapted from Nash, J. D. 1997. *The New Maximize Your Body Potential*. Palo Alto, Calif.: Bull Publishing. Reprinted with permission from Bull Publishing Company.

CHAPTER 12
Cardiovascular Disease and Cancer

Multiple Choice

1. The type of blood vessel that delivers nutrients to the tissues and picks up waste-carrying blood is the:
    a. artery.
    b. capillary.
    c. ventricle.
    d. vein.

2. Smoking affects the cardiorespiratory system in which one of the following ways?
    a. It decreases blood pressure.
    b. It increases the amount of oxygen available to the heart.
    c. It reduces levels of HDL in the bloodstream.
    d. It reduces blood clotting.

3. Which of the following diastolic blood pressure readings would be typical for a healthy adult?
    a. 50
    b. 80
    c. 120
    d. 150

4. A type of chest pain that may be a sign of heart disease is:
    a. arrhythmia.
    b. thrombosis.
    c. aneurysm.
    d. angina.

5. Dietary changes that can protect against cardiovascular diseases include all of the following EXCEPT:
    a. decreasing fiber intake.
    b. decreasing fat intake.
    c. replacing animal proteins with soy proteins.
    d. increasing fish and seafood consumption.

6. Metastasis occurs when:
    a. cancer cells break off and invade other parts of the body.
    b. cancer cells begin to divide rapidly within an organ.
    c. a tumor grows big enough to interfere with body functions.
    d. a nonmalignant group of cells grows slowly.

7. Cancers of the blood-forming cells are:
    a. carcinomas.
    b. leukemias.
    c. lymphomas.
    d. sarcomas.

8. The most common cause of cancer death in the United States is:
   a. breast cancer.
   b. prostate cancer.
   c. lung cancer.
   d. colon cancer.

9. Which of the following types of cancer is linked to a sexually transmitted disease?
   a. ovarian cancer
   b. testicular cancer
   c. prostate cancer
   d. cervical cancer

10. Using a sunscreen with an SPF rating of 15 means that you:
    a. can stay in the sun for 15 minutes without getting burned.
    b. can stay in the sun 15 times longer without getting burned than if you didn't use it.
    c. are protected against the full range of ultraviolet radiation.
    d. can remain in the sun as long as the UV index is below 15.

True or False

T F   1. Moderate physical activity reduces the risk of heart disease.

T F   2. Chronic hostility and anger increase one's risk of heart attack.

T F   3. At age 60, women are at greater risk for heart attack than are men.

T F   4. Hypertension usually has no symptoms.

T F   5. It is not necessary to report a transient ischemic attack to a physician.

T F   6. The primary risk factor for lung cancer is tobacco smoke.

T F   7. Age is a key risk factor for both colon and prostate cancer.

T F   8. One woman in 20 will develop breast cancer.

T F   9. Oral cancers can be linked to the use of spit tobacco and alcohol.

T F 10. Estrogen is a cancer promoter.

ANSWERS: Multiple Choice: 1. b (p. 259); 2. c (p. 260); 3. b (p. 266); 4. d (p. 267); 5. a (p. 271); 6. a (p. 274); 7. b (p. 275); 8. c (p. 276); 9. d (p. 279); 10. b (p. 281). True or False: 1. T (p. 262); 2. T (p. 262); 3. F (p. 263); 4. T (p. 266); 5. F (p. 270); 6. T (p. 276); 7. T (pp. 276, 278); 8. F (p. 277); 9. T (p. 282); 10. T (p. 284).

Name _____ Section _____ Date _____

 WELLNESS WORKSHEET 12

Cardiovascular Disease and Cancer

Part I. Are You at Risk for Cardiovascular Disease?

Your risk for CVD depends on a variety of factors, many of which are under your control. To help identify your risk factors, circle the response for each risk category that best describes you.

1. Gender and Age
   - 0 Female age 55 or younger; male age 45 or younger
   - 2 Female over age 50 or male over age 45

2. Heredity
   - 0 Neither parent suffered a heart attack or stroke before age 60.
   - 3 One parent suffered a heart attack or stroke before age 60.
   - 7 Both parents suffered a heart attack or stroke before age 60.

3. Smoking
   - 0 Never smoked
   - 3 Quit more than 2 years ago and lifetime smoking is less than 5 pack-years*
   - 6 Quit less than 2 years ago and/or lifetime smoking is greater than 5 pack-years*
   - 8 Smoke less than 1/2 pack per day
   - 13 Smoke more than 1/2 pack per day
   - 15 Smoke more than 1 pack per day

4. Environmental Tobacco Smoke
   - 0 Do not live or work with smokers
   - 2 Exposed to ETS at work
   - 3 Live with smoker
   - 4 Both live and work with smokers

5. Blood Pressure
   The average of the last three readings:
   - 0 130/80 or below
   - 1 131/81 to 140/85
   - 5 141/86 to 150/90
   - 9 151/91 to 170/100
   - 13 Above 170/100

6. Total Cholesterol
   The average of the last three readings:
   - 0 Lower than 190
   - 1 190 to 210
   - 2 Don't know
   - 3 211 to 240
   - 4 241 to 270
   - 5 271 to 300
   - 6 Over 300

7. HDL Cholesterol
   The average of the last three readings:
   - 0 Over 65 mg/dl
   - 1 55 to 65
   - 2 Don't know HDL
   - 3 45 to 54
   - 5 35 to 44
   - 7 25 to 34
   - 12 Lower than 25

8. Exercise
   - 0 Exercise three times a week
   - 1 Exercise once or twice a week
   - 2 Occasional exercise less than once a week
   - 7 Rarely exercise

9. Diabetes
   - 0 No personal or family history
   - 2 One parent with diabetes
   - 6 Two parents with diabetes
   - 9 Type 1 diabetes
   - 13 Type 2 diabetes

10. Weight
    - 0 Near ideal weight
    - 1 6 pounds or less above ideal weight
    - 3 7 to 19 pounds above ideal weight
    - 5 20 to 40 pounds above ideal weight
    - 7 More than 40 pounds above ideal weight

11. Stress
    - 0 Relaxed most of the time
    - 1 Occasional stress and anger
    - 2 Frequently stressed and angry
    - 3 Usually stressed and angry

*Pack-years can be calculated by multiplying the number of packs you smoked per day by the number of years you smoked. For example, if you smoked a pack and a half a day for 5 years, you would have smoked the equivalent of 1.5 × 5 = 7.5 pack-years.

Total Score	Estimated Risk of Early Heart Attack or Stroke
Less than 20	Low risk
20–29	Moderate risk
30–45	High risk
Over 45	Extremely high risk

(over)

Insel/Roth, *Core Concepts in Health*, Brief Ninth Edition. © 2002 The McGraw-Hill Companies, Inc.

Part II. Skin Cancer Risk Assessment

Skin cancer is the most common cancer of all when cases of the highly curable forms are included in the count. Your risk of skin cancer from the ultraviolet radiation in sunlight depends on several factors. Take the quiz below to see how sensitive you are. The higher your UV-risk score, the greater your risk of skin cancer—and the greater your need to take precautions against too much sun. Score 1 point for each true statement:

_____ 1. I have blond or red hair.

_____ 2. I have light-colored eyes (blue, gray, green).

_____ 3. I freckle easily.

_____ 4. I have many moles.

_____ 5. I had two or more blistering sunburns as a child.

_____ 6. I spent lots of time in a tropical climate as a child.

_____ 7. I have a family history of skin cancer.

_____ 8. I work outdoors.

_____ 9. I spend a lot of time in outdoor activities.

_____ 10. I like to spend as much time in the sun as I can.

_____ 11. I sometimes go to a tanning parlor or use a sunlamp.

_____ **Total score**

Score	Risk of skin cancer from UV radiation
0	Low
1–3	Moderate
4–7	High
8–11	Very high

Part III. Do You Eat Enough Cancer Fighters?

Track your diet for 3 days, putting a mark ("1" for day 1, "2" for day 2, "3" for day 3) next to any food you eat:

_____ Orange and yellow vegetables and (some) fruits, including apricots, cantaloupe, carrots, corn, papaya, pumpkin, red and yellow peppers, sweet potatoes, and winter squash

_____ Dark-green leafy vegetables, including chard; kale; romaine and other dark lettuces; spinach; and beet, collard, dandelion, mustard, and turnip greens

_____ Cruciferous vegetables, including bok choy, broccoli, brussels sprouts, cabbage, cauliflower, and turnips

_____ Citrus fruits, including grapefruit, lemon, lime, orange, and tangerine

_____ Whole grains, including whole-grain bread, cereal, and pasta and brown rice

_____ Legumes, including peas; lentils; and fava, navy, kidney, pinto, black, and lima beans

_____ Berries, including strawberries, raspberries, blackberries, blueberries

_____ Garlic and other allium vegetables, including onions, leeks, chives, scallions, and shallots

_____ Soy products, including tofu, tempeh, soy milk, miso, and soybeans

_____ Other cancer-fighting fruits: apples, cherries, grapes, kiwifruit, plums, prunes, raisins, watermelon

_____ Other cancer-fighting vegetables: asparagus, beets, chili peppers, green peppers, radishes, tomatoes

Total average daily servings: _____ (day 1) + _____ (day 2) + _____ (day 3) = _____ ÷ 3 = _____

Try to eat at least five servings of cancer-fighting foods a day; the more servings, the better (as long as you maintain a healthy weight). (*Note:* Research is ongoing, and this list of cancer fighters is not comprehensive. Remember, nearly all fruits, vegetables, and grains are healthy, disease-fighting dietary choices.)

SOURCE: Part II skin cancer risk assessment adapted from Shear, N. 1996. What's your UV-risk score? Copyright © 1996 by the Consumers Union of the United States, Inc., Yonkers, NY 10703-1057, a nonprofit organization. Reprinted with permission from the June 1996 issue of *Consumer Reports on Health* for educational purposes only. No commercial use of photocopying permitted. To subscribe, call 1-800-234-1645 or visit us at www.ConsumerReport.org.

CHAPTER 13
Immunity and Infection

Multiple Choice

1. An organism that causes disease is a(an):
    a. allergen.
    b. pathogen.
    c. viral agent.
    d. parasite.

2. The release of histamines causes:
    a. infection.
    b. illness.
    c. contamination.
    d. inflammation.

3. A reaction by the body's immune system to a harmless substance such as dust is:
    a. acquired immunity.
    b. an antigen.
    c. an allergy.
    d. a vector.

4. Antibiotics are most effective against:
    a. bacteria.
    b. parasites.
    c. viruses.
    d. colds.

5. The most common forms of contagious disease are caused by:
    a. bacteria.
    b. protozoa.
    c. T cells.
    d. viruses.

6. In untreated HIV infection, the average amount of time between the initial infection and the onset of symptoms is:
    a. 1 year.
    b. 6 years.
    c. 11 years.
    d. 16 years.

7. Which of the following STDs is often asymptomatic among women?
    a. chlamydia
    b. gonorrhea
    c. hepatitis B
    d. all of the above

8. Which antibiotic is recommended to treat gonorrhea?
    a. penicillin
    b. tetracycline
    c. new, expensive antibiotics
    d. all of the above

9. The leading cause of infertility among young women is:
   a. human papillomavirus.
   b. HIV infection.
   c. syphilis.
   d. pelvic inflammatory disease.

10. Unlike HIV, hepatitis B is often transmitted through:
    a. sexual intercourse.
    b. nonsexual close contact.
    c. injection drug use.
    d. contact during childbirth.

True or False

T F 1. Lymphocytes travel in both the bloodstream and the lymphatic system.

T F 2. Acquired immunity is the ability of lymphocytes to "remember" previous infections.

T F 3. The immune system is active only when you are sick.

T F 4. Viruses cause only mild, short-term illness.

T F 5. Hand washing can prevent the transmission of pathogens.

T F 6. A woman with HIV infection is more likely to transmit the infection to a male sexual partner during intercourse than vice versa.

T F 7. HIV is not spread through casual contact.

T F 8. The customary treatment for pelvic inflammatory disease is over-the-counter medication.

T F 9. Genital warts have been linked with cervical cancer.

T F 10. The number of new cases of syphilis steadily increased in the 1990s.

ANSWERS: Multiple Choice: 1. b (p. 293); 2. d (p. 295); 3. c (p. 298); 4. a (p. 301); 5. d (p. 302); 6. c (p. 308); 7. d (pp. 313, 314, 317); 8. c (p. 314); 9. d (p. 314); 10. b (p. 317). True or False: 1. T (p. 295); 2. T (p. 297); 3. F (p. 297); 4. F (pp. 302–303); 5. T (p. 306); 6. F (p. 309); 7. T (p. 309); 8. F (p. 315); 9. T (p. 315); 10. F (p. 317).

WELLNESS WORKSHEET 13

Checklist for Avoiding Infection

The best thing you can do to prevent an infection is to limit your exposure to pathogens. The next best thing is to keep your immune system as strong as possible. Read through the following list of statements and check whether each is mostly true or mostly false for you.

True   **False**

Exposure to Pathogens

____   ____   I receive drinking water from a clean supply.

____   ____   The area in which I live has adequate sewage treatment.

____   ____   I frequently wash my hands with soap and warm water for at least 10–20 seconds.

____   ____   I avoid close contact with people who are infectious with diseases transmitted via the respiratory route (e.g., influenza, chickenpox, and tuberculosis).

____   ____   I do not inject drugs.

When Outdoors

____   ____   When hiking or camping, I do not drink water from streams, rivers, or lakes without first purifying it.

____   ____   I avoid contact with ticks, rodents, bats, and other disease carriers.

____   ____   When hiking in the woods or playing in a yard in an area where Lyme disease or other tickborne infections have been reported, I take appropriate precautions:

       ____   Wear light-colored clothing: long pants, a long-sleeved shirt, and closed shoes.

       ____   Tuck my pants into my socks, shoes, or boots.

       ____   Tuck my shirt into my pants.

       ____   Wear light-colored, tightly woven fabrics.

       ____   Wear a hat.

       ____   Stay near the center of trails.

       ____   Check myself daily for ticks.

       ____   Shower and shampoo after each outing.

       ____   Wash clothes and check equipment after each outing

       ____   Use an insect repellent containing DEET on my skin and/or a spray containing permethrin on my clothing.

____   ____   If I discover a tick attached to my skin, I remove it immediately in an appropriate

manner (fill in): _____

_____

_____

_____

(over)

Insel/Roth, *Core Concepts in Health,* Brief Ninth Edition. © 2002 The McGraw-Hill Companies, Inc.

STUDY GUIDE

True   False

In a Sexual Relationship

_____   _____   I am in a monogamous relationship with a mutually faithful, uninfected partner.

_____   _____   I use condoms.

_____   _____   I discuss STDs and prevention with new partners.

_____   _____   I avoid engaging in high-risk behaviors with any person who might carry HIV.

In the Kitchen

_____   _____   I wash my hands thoroughly with warm soapy water before and after handling food.

_____   _____   I don't let groceries sit in a warm car.

_____   _____   I avoid buying food in containers that leak, bulge, or are severely dented.

_____   _____   I use separate cutting boards for meat and for foods that will be eaten raw.

_____   _____   I thoroughly clean all equipment (cutting boards, counters, utensils) before and after use.

_____   _____   I rinse and scrub fresh fruits and vegetables carefully to remove all dirt.

_____   _____   I cook all foods thoroughly, especially beef, poultry, fish, pork, and eggs.

_____   _____   I verify that hamburgers are cooked to 160°F (71°C) with a food thermometer.

_____   _____   I store foods below 40°F (5°C).

_____   _____   I do not leave cooked or refrigerated foods at room temperature for more than 2 hours.

_____   _____   I thaw foods in the refrigerator or microwave.

_____   _____   I use only pasteurized milk and juice.

_____   _____   I avoid coughing or sneezing over foods, even when I'm healthy.

_____   _____   I cover any cuts on my hands when handling food.

To Keep Your Immune System Healthy

_____   _____   I eat a balanced diet, following the guidelines presented in the Food Guide Pyramid and the Dietary Guidelines for Americans.

_____   _____   I maintain a healthy weight.

_____   _____   I get enough sleep, 6–8 hours per night.

_____   _____   I exercise regularly.

_____   _____   I don't smoke, and I drink alcohol only in moderation.

_____   _____   I wash my hands frequently.

_____   _____   I have effective ways of coping with stress.

_____   _____   I get all recommended immunizations and booster shots.

False answers indicate areas where you could change your behavior to help avoid infectious diseases. Consider creating a behavior change strategy for any statement you checked false.

CHAPTER 14
The Challenge of Aging

Multiple Choice

1. Which of the following remains most stable as you age?
   a. intelligence
   b. hearing
   c. eyesight
   d. flexibility

2. Which of the following statements about aging is TRUE?
   a. Requirements for vitamins and minerals are significantly lower for people over age 65.
   b. Glaucoma always leads to blindness.
   c. The ability to hear high-pitched sounds increases with age.
   d. Alcohol and drug dependence are common problems among the elderly.

3. The decline in the ability to focus on close objects that occurs in many people beginning in their forties is called:
   a. cataracts.
   b. glaucoma.
   c. presbyopia.
   d. dendrite.

4. As birth rates drop, the percentage of elderly people will:
   a. increase.
   b. decrease.
   c. stay the same.
   d. fluctuate.

5. Most older Americans live:
   a. alone.
   b. with a relative.
   c. with a nonrelative.
   d. in a nursing home.

6. Which of the following is NOT a characteristic of brain death?
   a. unresponsivity
   b. incoherence
   c. flat EEG
   d. no movements or breathing

7. The testator of a will is the:
   a. attorney.
   b. person making the will.
   c. closest living relative.
   d. beneficiary of the will.

8. In 1990 in the case of Nancy Beth Cruzan, the Supreme Court ruled that:
   a. life support can only be removed from a vegetative patient if he or she has completed a living will making such a request.
   b. the right to refuse unwarranted treatment is constitutionally protected.
   c. physician-assisted suicide is illegal.
   d. there is no medical or ethical difference between withholding and withdrawing a treatment.

9. A legal document that allows one person to act as the agent of another in making medical decisions is a:
   a. living will.
   b. Uniform Donor Card.
   c. will.
   d. health care proxy.

10. All of the following are stages in Elisabeth Kübler-Ross's stages of dying theory EXCEPT:
    a. denial.
    b. adjusting.
    c. depression.
    d. bargaining.

True or False

T F   1. Older women are more likely to live in poverty than older men.

T F   2. Hormone replacement therapy protects women against all forms of cancer.

T F   3. Alzheimer's disease is an incurable form of dementia.

T F   4. Males born in the year 2000 have a longer life expectancy than females born in the same year.

T F   5. Most older Americans live in a nursing home at some point in their lives.

T F   6. Our attitudes toward death are formed in childhood and do not change much as we grow older.

T F   7. About one third of Americans die without leaving a will.

T F   8. Palliative care focuses on relieving pain in a patient not expected to recover.

T F   9. Increasing a patient's pain medication to the point where, in addition to controlling pain, it also hastens death is considered physician-assisted suicide.

T F   10. Acceptance is the final stage in Kübler-Ross's model of the psychological stages that a dying person experiences.

ANSWERS: Multiple Choice: 1. a (p. 325); 2. d (p. 326); 3. c (p. 328); 4. a (p. 332); 5. b (p. 333); 6. b (p. 334); 7. b (p. 335); 8. b (p. 336); 9. d (p. 338); 10. b (p. 340). True or False: 1. T (p. 327); 2. F (p. 329); 3. T (p. 331); 4. F (p. 332); 5. F (p. 333); 6. F (p. 335); 7. F (p. 335); 8. T (p. 336); 9. F (p. 338); 10. T (p. 340).

Name _____ Section _____ Date _____

✍ WELLNESS WORKSHEET 14

Are You Prepared for Aging?

Assess Your Current Behaviors

Are you doing everything you can now to enhance the quality of your life as you age? Read through the following list of statements and check the answer that best describes your current behavior.

Yes   **No**

_____   _____   I exercise regularly.

_____   _____   I eat wisely.

        _____   I eat meals low in fat and high in complex carbohydrates (fresh fruits and vegetables, whole-grain cereals and breads, brown rice, pasta).

        _____   I limit saturated and trans fats and get protein from fish and skinless poultry.

        _____   I use nonfat or low-fat dairy products.

        _____   I consume the recommended amount of calcium and vitamin B-12.

        _____   I limit the amount of sodium I consume.

_____   _____   My weight is in the recommended range.

_____   _____   I drink alcohol in moderation, if at all.

_____   _____   I don't use tobacco in any form.

_____   _____   I recognize the stressors in my life and take appropriate steps to control and deal with stress.

_____   _____   I perform appropriate self-examinations.

_____   _____   I have regular physical examinations that include appropriate screening tests.

_____   _____   I participate in activities that keep my mind sharp and active.

Thinking About Aging

Have you thought seriously about the changes that aging can bring? To help you begin thinking now about your life as you grow older, answer the following questions.

1. What things come to mind when you think of an older person? Can you imagine those things applying to you? What do you think you will be like when you are 70 years old?

2. What do you most look forward to as you grow older?

(over)

Insel/Roth, *Core Concepts in Health,* Brief Ninth Edition. © 2002 The McGraw-Hill Companies, Inc.

STUDY GUIDE

3. What do you most fear as you grow older?

4. How long would you like to keep working? What would you like to do after you retire? What hobbies or volunteer opportunities would you pursue?

5. Have you considered the loss of income that retirement often brings? What can you do now to help meet your economic needs in the future?

6. Older people often find themselves alone more frequently (due to the death of a spouse and/or close friends). Can you think of activities you enjoy doing alone?

7. If when you are older you are no longer able to care for yourself, what living and care arrangements would you prefer?

8. What would you do if your parents were no longer able to care for themselves?

9. List five positive and five negative things about aging.

CHAPTER 15
Conventional and Complementary Medicine:
Skills for the Health Care Consumer

Multiple Choice

1. All of the following symptoms or conditions require emergency medical care EXCEPT:
   a. loss of consciousness.
   b. recurrent stomach pain.
   c. severe shortness of breath.
   d. steadily worsening reaction to an insect bite.

2. If you have a cough that lasts longer than 2 weeks, you should:
   a. go to a hospital emergency room.
   b. call your primary physician to see if you should schedule an appointment.
   c. monitor your condition for another 1–2 weeks before contacting your physician.
   d. ask your pharmacist to recommend an over-the-counter or prescription medication.

3. The best choice in self-treatment is often:
   a. contacting your physician to see what medications you should be taking.
   b. using prescription medications from the last time you had something similar.
   c. waiting for your body to heal itself.
   d. using a medical self-test kit to determine how serious your condition is.

4. Conventional Western medicine might identify all of the following as factors contributing to or causing illness or disease EXCEPT:
   a. a streptococcal infection.
   b. a genetic tendency to obesity.
   c. a spiritual imbalance.
   d. a diet high in saturated fats and cholesterol.

5. Primary care physicians routinely do all of the following EXCEPT:
   a. provide psychiatric care.
   b. provide pediatric care.
   c. provide preventive health services, such as immunizations and cancer screening tests.
   d. provide gynecological and obstetrical care.

6. The most successful patient-physician relationship appears to be one in which:
   a. the patient relies exclusively on the physician's medical knowledge and expertise.
   b. the physician protects his or her time by discouraging or dismissing questions.
   c. the patient participates actively in decisions and the physician acts as a consultant.
   d. the physician protects the patient from confusing or distressing information and makes the important decisions about the patient's care.

7. A principle of homeopathy is:
   a. a substance that causes a disease can cure the disease in small amounts.
   b. illnesses are caused by disturbances in the flow of qi.
   c. energy fields surrounding the body can be influenced by touch and movement.
   d. mind and body are connected and changing one can change the other.

8. The manipulation of joints in the spinal column is an important procedure in:
   a. homeopathy.
   b. chiropractic.
   c. acupuncture.
   d. qigong.

9. If you are thinking of trying a complementary and alternative treatment for a medical condition, you should first discuss it with your conventional health care provider for all of the following reasons EXCEPT:
   a. the treatment might interact dangerously with a conventional treatment you are receiving.
   b. there may be a beneficial conventional treatment for your condition.
   c. you may need a conventional treatment immediately.
   d. conventional treatments are the only effective treatments.

10. An advantage of fee-for-service insurance plans over managed-care plans is:
    a. it is less expensive.
    b. it allows consumers more choice in health care providers.
    c. it is provided by the government.
    d. it is easier to get into a plan.

True or False

T F 1. The FDA guarantees the safety and effectiveness of all medications on the market, both over-the-counter and prescription.

T F 2. Generic drugs have the same active ingredient as brand-name drugs.

T F 3. For a cold, the best medication is an all-in-one product that will treat many symptoms simultaneously.

T F 4. In conventional Western medicine, each person with a particular set of symptoms is treated in a basically similar way.

T F 5. In the United States the two types of physicians fully trained and licensed to perform surgery and prescribe medication are osteopaths and homeopaths.

T F 6. The goal of complementary and alternative medicine is to rid the body of disease-causing pathogens.

T F 7. Acupuncture has been found to be effective in relieving pain after surgery.

T F 8. Hypnosis can be performed only by a licensed medical doctor.

T F 9. Because herbal remedies and botanicals are derived from plants and other naturally occurring materials, they can be assumed to be very safe.

T F 10. In a health maintenance organization, you choose a primary care physician who manages your health care and refers you to specialists if you need them.

ANSWERS: Multiple Choice: 1. b (p. 347); 2. b (p. 347); 3. c (p. 347); 4. c (p. 350); 5. a (p. 353); 6. c (p. 353); 7. a (p. 358); 8. b (p. 360); 9. d (p. 363); 10. b (p. 365). True or False: 1. F (pp. 347–348); 2. T (p. 348); 3. F (p. 348); 4. T (p. 350); 5. F (p. 353); 6. F (p. 356); 7. T (p. 358); 8. F (p. 359); 9. F (p. 361); 10. T (p. 365).

Name _____ Section _____ Date _____

✎ WELLNESS WORKSHEET 15

Your Personal Health Profile

Complete as much as possible of this personal health profile and keep it up to date.

General Information

Age: _____

Height: _____

Weight: _____

Are you currently trying to _____ gain or

_____ lose weight? (check if appropriate)

Blood pressure: _____ / _____

Blood lipid levels:

    Total cholesterol: _____

    HDL: _____

    LDL: _____

    Triglycerides: _____

Blood glucose level: _____

Medical Conditions

Check any of the following that apply to you and add other conditions that might affect your health and well-being.

_____ heart disease

_____ lung disease

_____ diabetes

_____ allergies

_____ asthma

_____ back pain

_____ arthritis

_____ other injury or joint problem

_____ substance abuse problem

_____ depression, anxiety, or another psychological disorder

_____ eating disorder

_____ other: _____

_____ other: _____

List any conditions or diseases that are common in your family and/or ethnic group.

_____

_____

_____

_____

_____

_____

Medications/Treatments

List any medications or supplements you are taking or any medical treatments you are undergoing. Include the name of the substance or treatment and its purpose. Include both prescription and over-the-counter drugs and any vitamin, mineral, or other dietary supplement you are taking.

Medication/treatment

_____

_____

_____

_____

_____

_____

Condition/purpose

_____

_____

_____

_____

_____

_____

(over)

Screening Tests and Vaccinations

To ensure that you are getting the most out of your medical care, keep a record of your screening tests and vaccinations; see Chapters 12–13 for more information on these. Fill in any additional tests and vaccinations that are appropriate for your age, gender, and medical history.

Screening test/immunization	Date last performed
Blood pressure check	
STD screening	
Cholesterol measurement	
Vision test	
Dental exam	
Pelvic exam and Pap test (women only)	
Clinical breast exam (women only)	
Other:	
Other:	
Other:	
Other:	
Tetanus/diphtheria vaccination	
Influenza vaccination	
Other:	
Other:	

Health Care Providers

Primary care physician: name _____ phone _____

Specialist physician: name _____ phone _____

    Condition treated: _____

Other health care provider: name _____ phone _____

    Condition treated: _____

Pharmacy: name _____ phone _____

Dentist: name _____ phone _____

Optometrist/ophthalmologist: name _____ phone _____

Health insurance provider: name _____ phone _____

    Policy number: _____

Dental insurance provider: name _____ phone _____

    Policy number: _____

Vision care insurance provider: name _____ phone _____

    Policy number: _____

CHAPTER 16
Personal Safety: Protecting Yourself from
Unintentional Injuries and Violence

Multiple Choice

1. The leading cause of motor vehicle injuries is:
   a. fatigue from long drives.
   b. cell phones.
   c. bad driving, especially speeding.
   d. poor vehicle maintenance.

2. Which of the following statements about the safe use of air bags is TRUE?
   a. Children younger than 12 should ride in the front seat.
   b. Riders should sit as close as possible to the passenger-side dashboard.
   c. If a car has air bags, wearing safety belts isn't necessary.
   d. The seat and steering wheel should be adjusted so that the air bag will deploy in front of the driver's chest rather than face.

3. All of the following are strategies for preventing bicycle injuries EXCEPT:
   a. riding against the flow of traffic.
   b. wearing light-colored clothing.
   c. stopping at all traffic lights.
   d. using bicycle paths.

4. Wearing a bike helmet reduces the risk of head injury by:
   a. 25%.
   b. 45%.
   c. 65%.
   d. 85%.

5. Smoke detector batteries should be checked every:
   a. week.
   b. month.
   c. 6 months.
   d. year.

6. The Heimlich maneuver is used in cases of:
   a. poisoning.
   b. choking.
   c. burns.
   d. heart attack.

7. Carpal tunnel syndrome affects the:
   a. eyes.
   b. wrists.
   c. back.
   d. skin.

8. In comparison to rates in other industrialized countries, U.S. rates of violence are abnormally high in which two areas?
   a. aggravated assault and homicide
   b. rape and robbery
   c. homicide and firearm-related deaths
   d. battering and rape

9. Which is TRUE regarding school violence?
   a. Students are less safe in school than away from school.
   b. Murder is the most common type of school violence.
   c. Victims of school violence are predominantly female.
   d. The majority of acts of school violence occur in urban areas.

10. Which of the following statements about date rape is FALSE?
    a. The double standard about appropriate sexual behavior for men and women is a factor in date rape.
    b. As many as 25% of women have had experiences in which a date tried to force sex.
    c. Most cases of date rape are reported to the police.
    d. Victims of date rape often feel responsible for the incident.

True or False

T F 1. Suicide is an example of an unintentional injury.

T F 2. A person who wears a safety belt is less than half as likely to be killed in a car crash as a person who does not.

T F 3. Automobile air bags cause more injuries than they prevent.

T F 4. More than 75% of bicyclists wear helmets.

T F 5. Most fall-related deaths occur as a result of falls on stairs or steps rather than from a height.

T F 6. About half of work injuries occur among laborers.

T F 7. Rates of violent crime are highest among people under age 25.

T F 8. Men and women are about equally likely to be victims of homicide.

T F 9. Violence against children by parents is one of the five leading causes of death for children age 1–18.

T F 10. Making sexual jokes or displaying sexually suggestive pictures can be considered sexual harassment.

ANSWERS: Multiple Choice 1. c (p. 370); 2. d (p. 371); 3. a (p. 372); 4. d (p. 372);
5. b (p. 374); 6 b (p. 375); 7. b (p. 378); 8. c (p. 378); 9. d (p. 380); 10. c (p. 383).
True or False: 1. F (p. 369); 2. T (pp. 370–371); 3. F (p. 371); 4. F (p. 372);
5. T (p. 373); 6. F (p. 377); 7. T (p. 378); 8. F (p. 379); 9. T (p. 382); 10. T (p. 385).

Name _____ Section _____ Date _____

WELLNESS WORKSHEET 16

Personal Safety Checklist

Are you doing all you can to protect yourself from violence and injuries? The following list of statements relate to intentional injury incidents that can occur in a variety of settings. Put a check next to those statements that are true for you.

At Home

_____ My home has good lighting.

_____ Doors are secured with effective locks (deadbolts).

_____ All unused doors and windows are securely locked.

_____ I always lock all windows and doors when I go out.

_____ I have a dog and/or post "Beware of Dog" signs.

_____ Landscaping around the home doesn't provide opportunities for concealment.

_____ Keys are hidden in a secure, nonobvious place.

_____ I do not give anyone the opportunity to duplicate my keys.

_____ The front door has a peephole.

_____ I do not open my door to strangers or allow them into my home or yard.

_____ I ask to see ID or call to verify that repair and utility workers are legitimate.

_____ I use my initials in phone directory listings.

_____ My answering machine message does not imply that I live alone or am not home.

_____ Everyone in the household knows how to call for help.

_____ My neighbors and I have a system for alerting one another in case of an emergency.

_____ I participate in a neighborhood watch program.

On the Street

_____ I avoid walking alone, especially at night or in less-populous areas.

_____ I dress in clothing that allows freedom of movement.

_____ I walk purposefully, in an alert and confident manner.

_____ I walk on the outside of the sidewalk, facing traffic.

_____ I check routes to my destination before leaving so as not to appear lost.

_____ I never hitchhike.

_____ I carry valuables in a secure or concealed location and take special care at ATMs.

_____ I have my keys ready when I approach my vehicle or home.

_____ I carry change for a telephone call, fare for public transportation, and a whistle to blow if I am attacked or harassed.

_____ I keep alert for suspicious behavior, and I keep at least two arm lengths between myself and strangers.

(over)

STUDY GUIDE

In My Car

_____ My car is in good working condition.

_____ I carry emergency supplies in my car.

_____ I keep my gas tank at least half full.

_____ When driving, I keep doors locked and windows rolled up at least three-quarters of the way.

_____ I park my car in well-lighted areas or parking garages.

_____ I lock my car when I leave it.

_____ I check the interior of my car before unlocking it and getting in.

_____ I don't pick up strangers.

_____ I note the location of emergency call boxes, or I have a cellular phone in my car.

_____ I use caution if my car breaks down or if I am involved in a minor crash or bumped intentionally.

_____ When I stop at a light or stop sign, I stop far enough behind the car in front to allow room to maneuver in case of emergency.

_____ I do not get into arguments with drivers of other vehicles.

On Public Transportation

_____ I wait in populated, well-lighted areas.

_____ I sit near the driver or conductor.

_____ I sit in a single seat or an outside seat.

_____ I check routes and times in advance, and confirm before boarding that the bus, subway, or train is bound for my destination.

On Campus

_____ Door and window locks are secure.

_____ Halls and stairwells have adequate lighting.

_____ Dorm doors are not left unlocked or propped open.

_____ I do not give dorm or residence keys to others.

_____ I keep my door locked.

_____ I do not allow strangers into my room.

_____ I do not walk, jog, or exercise alone at night.

_____ I use campus escort services or walk with friends.

_____ I know the areas that security guards patrol and stay where they can see or hear me if possible.

Your answers here can help you identify behaviors that you should change. Consider planning a behavior change strategy to alter one or more of your risky behaviors.

CHAPTER 17
Environmental Health

Multiple Choice

1. Historically, the highest priority in environmental health was controlling:
   a. infectious diseases.
   b. air pollution.
   c. population growth.
   d. energy waste.

2. Approximately how many Americans become ill each year from contaminated drinking water?
   a. 1,000
   b. 10,000
   c. 100,000
   d. 1,000,000

3. Which of the following is a disadvantage of landfill?
   a. It becomes unstable when decomposition occurs.
   b. Buried chemicals leak into the soil.
   c. It is often a breeding ground for infectious diseases.
   d. All of the above.

4. The increase in the concentrations of greenhouse gases is primarily the result of:
   a. the release of CFCs.
   b. energy use in the developed world.
   c. heavy metal contamination.
   d. temperature inversions.

5. The ozone layer protects the earth from excessive:
   a. radon exposure.
   b. nuclear radiation.
   c. ultraviolet radiation.
   d. chlorofluorocarbons.

6. Which one of the following is a major source of acid precipitation pollutants?
   a. air conditioners
   b. lead-based paints
   c. synthetic building materials
   d. industrial combustion of coal

7. Lead poisoning is a serious problem among children who:
   a. live in older buildings.
   b. had low birth weights.
   c. have not been vaccinated.
   d. have poor diets.

8. All the following strategies can help reduce chemical pollution and its health effects EXCEPT:
    a. burning your trash.
    b. buying locally grown and/or organic produce.
    c. eating less meat.
    d. staying out of the house for a few days after fumigating.

9. A radioactive gas found in certain soils and rocks is:
    a. lead.
    b. asbestos.
    c. ozone.
    d. radon.

10. Which of the following is NOT a possible effect of exposure to excessive noise?
    a. higher blood pressure
    b. higher blood cholesterol
    c. deafness
    d. tinnitus

True or False

T F 1. You can minimize your water consumption by taking baths instead of showers.

T F 2. The bulk of our food garbage ends up in the sewage system.

T F 3. Plastic waste is the largest component (by weight) of household trash.

T F 4. The world's population is currently growing by about 25 people per minute.

T F 5. Dust storms contribute to air pollution.

T F 6. Damage to the ozone layer should reverse itself as soon as CFC production declines.

T F 7. The population growth rate is higher in developed countries than in developing countries.

T F 8. Using compact fluorescent bulbs instead of incandescent bulbs reduces air pollution.

T F 9. Exposure to asbestos can cause lung cancer.

T F 10. Prolonged exposure to sounds above 80–85 decibels can cause permanent hearing loss.

ANSWERS: Multiple Choice: 1. a (p. 391); 2. d (p. 392); 3. b (p. 393); 4. b (p. 397); 5. c (397); 6. d (p. 398); 7. a (p. 400); 8. a (p. 401); 9. d (p. 402); 10. b (p. 403); True or False: 1. F (p. 392); 2. T (p. 393); 3. F (p. 393); 4. F (p. 395); 5. T (p. 395); 6. F (p. 397); 7. F (p. 398); 8. T (p. 399); 9. T (p. 400); 10. T (p. 403).

Name _____ Section _____ Date _____

WELLNESS WORKSHEET 17

Environmental Health Checklist

The following list of statements relates to your impact on the environment. Put a check next to the statements that are true for you.

Conserving Energy and Improving the Air

_____ I ride my bike, walk, use public transportation, or carpool in a fuel-efficient vehicle whenever possible.

_____ I keep my car tuned up and well maintained.

_____ My vehicle is fuel efficient (city: _____ MPG; highway: _____ MPG).

_____ My car tires are inflated at the proper pressure.

_____ I avoid quick starts and drive within the speed limit.

_____ I don't use my car's air conditioner when opening the window would suffice.

_____ My residence is well insulated.

_____ Where possible, I use compact fluorescent bulbs instead of incandescent bulbs.

_____ I turn off lights and appliances when they are not in use.

_____ I avoid turning on heat or air conditioning whenever possible.

_____ I run the washing machine, dryer, and dishwasher only when they have full loads.

_____ I dry my hair with a towel rather than a hair dryer.

Saving the Ozone Layer

_____ I keep my car's air conditioner in good working order and have it serviced by a service station that recycles, rather than releases, CFCs.

_____ I check labels on aerosol cans and avoid those that contain CFCs.

_____ I avoid products containing methyl chloroform (1,1,1-trichloroethane).

_____ I don't have a halon fire extinguisher.

_____ I have an energy-efficient refrigerator, which I keep in good working order.

Reducing Garbage

_____ When shopping, I choose products with the least amount of packaging.

_____ I choose recycled and recyclable products and those sold in bulk.

_____ I avoid products packaged in plastic and unrecycled aluminum.

_____ I store food in glass jars and reusable plastic containers rather than using plastic wrap.

_____ I take my own bag along when I go shopping.

_____ Whenever possible, I use long-lasting or reusable products (such as refillable pens and rechargeable batteries).

_____ I use a ceramic mug and metal spoon for coffee and tea rather than disposable cups and stirrers.

_____ I recycle newpapers, glass, cans, paper, and other materials.

_____ I have a compost pile or bin for my organic garbage, or I take my organic garbage to a community composting center.

(over)

Insel/Roth, *Core Concepts in Health,* Brief Ninth Edition. © 2002 The McGraw-Hill Companies, Inc.

STUDY GUIDE

Reducing Chemical Pollution and Toxic Wastes

_____ When shopping, I read labels and try to buy the least toxic products available.

_____ I don't pour toxic materials (bleach, motor oil, etc.) down the sink.

_____ If I am unsure of the proper way to dispose of something, I contact my local health department or environmental health office.

_____ Whenever possible, I buy organic produce or produce that is in season and has been grown locally.

Saving Water

_____ I take showers instead of baths.

_____ I take short showers and switch off the water when I'm not actively using it.

_____ I do not run the water while brushing my teeth, shaving, or hand-washing clothes or dishes.

_____ My sinks have aerators installed in them.

_____ My shower has a low-flow showerhead.

_____ I have a water-saving toilet, or I have a water-displacement device in my toilet.

_____ I fix any faucets that leak.

Preserving Wildlife and the Natural Environment

_____ I snip or rip plastic six-pack rings before discarding them.

_____ I don't buy products made from endangered species.

_____ When hiking or camping, I never leave anything behind.

Statements that you have not checked can help you identify behaviors that you can change to improve environmental health. Consider planning a behavior change activity to alter one or more of your behaviors. To change some of the items listed, you may need the cooperation of your family and/or roommate(s). If there are environmental issues that are important to you, you can go beyond individual action by informing others, joining and volunteering your time to organizations working on environmental problems, and contacting your elected representatives.